WORLD HEALTH ORGANIZATION
INTERNATIONAL AGENCY FOR RESEARCH ON CANCER

IARC Monographs on the Evaluation of Carcinogenic Risks to Humans

VOLUME 91

Combined Estrogen–Progestogen Contraceptives and Combined Estrogen–Progestogen Menopausal Therapy

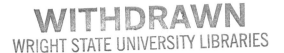

This publication represents the views and expert opinions
of an IARC Working Group on the
Evaluation of Carcinogenic Risks to Humans,
which met in Lyon,

7–14 June 2005

2007

QZ
202
I11
v.91
2007

IARC MONOGRAPHS

In 1969, the International Agency for Research on Cancer (IARC) initiated a programme on the evaluation of the carcinogenic risk of chemicals to humans involving the production of critically evaluated monographs on individual chemicals. The programme was subsequently expanded to include evaluations of carcinogenic risks associated with exposures to complex mixtures, life-style factors and biological and physical agents, as well as those in specific occupations.

The objective of the programme is to elaborate and publish in the form of monographs critical reviews of data on carcinogenicity for agents to which humans are known to be exposed and on specific exposure situations; to evaluate these data in terms of human risk with the help of international working groups of experts in chemical carcinogenesis and related fields; and to indicate where additional research efforts are needed.

The lists of IARC evaluations are regularly updated and are available on Internet: http://monographs. iarc.fr/

This programme has been supported by Cooperative Agreement 5 UO1 CA33193 awarded since 1982 by the United States National Cancer Institute, Department of Health and Human Services. Additional support has been provided since 1986 by the European Commission, Directorate-General EMPL (Employment, and Social Affairs), Health, Safety and Hygiene at Work Unit, and since 1992 by the United States National Institute of Environmental Health Sciences.

Published by the International Agency for Research on Cancer,
150 cours Albert Thomas, 69372 Lyon Cedex 08, France
©International Agency for Research on Cancer, 2007

Distributed by WHO Press, World Health Organization, 20 Avenue Appia, 1211 Geneva 27, Switzerland
(tel.: +41 22 791 3264; fax: +41 22 791 4857; e-mail: bookorders@who.int).

Publications of the World Health Organization enjoy copyright protection in accordance with the provisions of Protocol 2 of the Universal Copyright Convention. All rights reserved.

The International Agency for Research on Cancer welcomes requests for permission to reproduce or translate its publications, in part or in full. Requests for permission to reproduce or translate IARC publications – whether for sale or for noncommercial distribution – should be addressed to WHO Press, at the above address (fax: +41 22 791 4806; email: permissions@who.int).

The designations employed and the presentation of the material in this publication do not imply the expression of any opinion whatsoever on the part of the Secretariat of the World Health Organization concerning the legal status of any country, territory, city, or area or of its authorities, or concerning the delimitation of its frontiers or boundaries.

The mention of specific companies or of certain manufacturers' products does not imply that they are endorsed or recommended by the World Health Organization in preference to others of a similar nature that are not mentioned. Errors and omissions excepted, the names of proprietary products are distinguished by initial capital letters.

The IARC Monographs Working Group alone is responsible for the views expressed in this publication.

IARC Library Cataloguing in Publication Data

Combined Estrogen–Progestogen Contraceptives and
Combined Estrogen–Progestogen Menopausal Therapy/
IARC Working Group on the Evaluation of Carcinogenic Risks to Humans (2005 : Lyon, France)

(IARC monographs on the evaluation of carcinogenic risks to humans ; v. 91)

1. Contraceptives, Oral, Hormonal – adverse effects   2. Estrogens – adverse effects
3. Estrogens – therapeutic use   4. Hormone Replacement Therapy – adverse effects
5. Neoplasms – chemically induced 6. Neoplasms – prevention & control
7. Progestins – adverse effects 8. Progestins – therapeutic use
I. IARC Working Group on the Evaluation of Carcinogenic Risks to Humans   II. Series

ISBN 978 92 832 1291 1   (NLM Classification: W1)
ISSN 1017-1606

PRINTED IN FRANCE

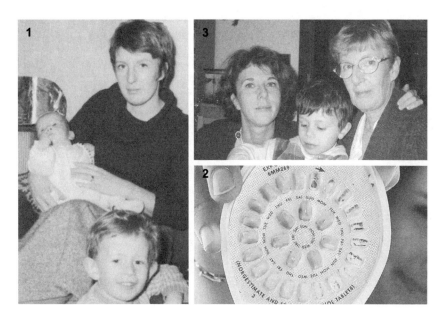

1 Oral contraceptives for family planning worldwide have revolutionized the reproductive lives of millions of women since their introduction in the 1960s.

2 Later on, a variety of side-effects including cardiovascular diseases was recognized. In response to these concerns, new generations of combined oral contraceptives were developed that featured lower doses of estrogen and newer, more potent progestogens.

3 The effectiveness and ease of use of combined hormonal contra-ceptives suggest that they will continue to be used to a significant extent in the future.

Cover design: Georges Mollon, IARC

CONTENTS

NOTE TO THE READER

The term 'carcinogenic risk' in the *IARC Monographs* series is taken to mean that an agent is capable of causing cancer under some circumstances. The *Monographs* evaluate cancer hazards, despite the historical presence of the word 'risks' in the title.

Inclusion of an agent in the *Monographs* does not imply that it is a carcinogen, only that the published data have been examined. Equally, the fact that an agent has not yet been evaluated in a monograph does not mean that it is not carcinogenic.

The evaluations of carcinogenic risk are made by international working groups of independent scientists and are qualitative in nature. No recommendation is given for regulation or legislation.

Anyone who is aware of published data that may alter the evaluation of the carcinogenic risk of an agent to humans is encouraged to make this information available to the Carcinogen Identification and Evaluation Group, International Agency for Research on Cancer, 150 cours Albert Thomas, 69372 Lyon Cedex 08, France, in order that the agent may be considered for re-evaluation by a future Working Group.

Although every effort is made to prepare the monographs as accurately as possible, mistakes may occur. Readers are requested to communicate any errors to the Carcinogen Identification and Evaluation Group, so that corrections can be reported in future volumes.

IARC MONOGRAPHS ON THE EVALUATION OF CARCINOGENIC RISKS TO HUMANS: COMBINED ESTROGEN–PROGESTOGEN CONTRACEPTIVES AND COMBINED ESTROGEN–PROGESTOGEN MENOPAUSAL THERAPY

Lyon, 7–14 June 2005

LIST OF PARTICIPANTS

Working Group Members[1]

Garnet L. Anderson, Women's Health Initiative, Clinical Coordinating Center, Fred Hutchinson Cancer Research Center, 1100 Fairview Avenue N, M3-A410, PO Box 19024, Seattle, WA 98109, USA

Philippe Autier, Unit of Epidemiology, Prevention and Screening, Jules Bordet Institute, Boulevard de Waterloo 125, Brussels 1000, Belgium

Valerie Beral, Cancer Epidemiology Unit, University of Oxford, Richard Doll Building, Roosevelt Drive, Headington, Oxford OX3 7LF, United Kingdom (*Subgroup Chair, Cancer in Humans*)

Maarten C. Bosland, Department of Environmental Medicine, New York University School of Medicine, 57 Old Forge Road, Tuxedo, NY 10987, USA (*Subgroup Chair, Other Relevant Data*)

Esteve Fernández, Cancer Prevention & Control Unit, Catalan Institute of Oncology, Avenue Gran Via s/n Km. 2.7, 08907 L'Hospitalet (Barcelona), Spain

Sandra Z. Haslam, Breast Cancer & the Environment Research Center, Department of Physiology, Michigan State University, 2201 Biomedical and Physical Sciences Building, East Lansing, MI 48824, USA

David G. Kaufman[2], Department Pathology & Laboratory Medicine, University of North Carolina at Chapel Hill, 620 Brinkhous-Bullitt Building, CB 7525, Chapel Hill, NC 27599-7525, USA

---

[1] Working Group Members and Invited Specialists serve in their individual capacities as scientists and not as representatives of their government or any organization with which they are affiliated. Affiliations are provided for identification purposes only.

[2] Received past research support from Organon (a unit of Akzo-Nobel). There are no discussions or expectations of future research support.

Carlo La Vecchia, Laboratory of General Epidemiology, Mario Negri Institute, via Eritrea 62, 20157 Milan, Italy (*Overall Chair*)

Alfredo A. Molinolo, Oral & Pharyngeal Cancer Branch, National Institute of Dental & Craniofacial Research, Building 30, Room 213, 30 Convent Drive, Bethesda, MD 20892-4340, USA (*Subgroup Chair, Cancer in Experimental Animals*)

Polly A. Newcomb (*not present for evaluations*), Fred Hutchinson Cancer Research Center, 1100 Fairview Avenue N, Seattle WA 98109, USA (*Subgroup Chair, Exposure Data*)

Fritz F. Parl, Department of Pathology, The Vanderbilt Clinic TVC 4918, Vanderbilt University Medical Center, 23rd Avenue South at Pierce Street, Nashville, TN 37232-5310, USA

Julian Peto, Department of Epidemiology & Population Health, London School of Hygiene & Tropical Medicine, Keppel Street, London WC1E 7HT, United Kingdom

Giuseppe Rosano[3] (*not present for evaluations*), Cardiovascular Research Unit, Department of Medical Sciences, San Raffaele-Tosinvest Sanita, Via Suvereto 10, 00139 Roma (RM) – Lazio, Italy

Deodutta Roy, Department of Environmental & Occupational Health, Robert Stempel School of Public Health, Florida International University, Building HLS 2, Room 591, 11200 SW 8th Street, Miami, FL 33199, USA

Frank Z. Stanczyk (*unable to attend*), Reproductive Endocrine Research Laboratory, Women's & Children's Hospital, Keck School of Medicine, University of Southern California, 1240 N. Mission Road, Room 1M2, Los Angeles, CA 90033, USA

David B. Thomas, Program in Epidemiology, Fred Hutchinson Cancer Research Center, 1100 Fairview Avenue North, Seattle, WA 98109-1024, USA

Lars Vatten, Department of Community Medicine & General Practice, Norwegian University of Science & Technology, Eirik Jarls Gate 10, 6th floor, 7489 Trondheim, Norway

Invited Specialists

Ted Junghans, Technical Resources International Inc, 6500 Rock Spring Drive, Suite 650, Bethesda, MD 20817-1197, USA

Steve Olin, ILSI Risk Science Institute, One Thomas Circle, NW, 9th Floor, Washington, DC 20005-5802, USA

Samuel Shapiro[4], Department of Public Health, University of Cape Town Medical School, Anzio Road, Observatory, South Africa

Randall S. Stafford[5], School of Population Health, University of Auckland, Private Bag 92019, Auckland 1020, New Zealand

---

[3] Receives a minor amount of travel support for talks sponsored by Solvay S.A. and Pfizer Inc.

[4] Serves as a scientific consultant to Schering AG. Also received a minor amount of travel support to talk at a meeting sponsored by Organon (a unit of Akzo Nobel).

[5] Received research support from Glaxo Smith Kline and is in discussions with them about future research support.

Representative

Charles William Jameson, Report on Carcinogens, National Institute of Environmental Health Sciences, PO Box 12233, 79, Alexander Drive, Research Triangle Park, NC 27709, USA

Observer

Observer for the European Federation of Pharmaceutical Industries and Associations (EFPIA)

Jens U. Meyer[6], Global Medical Development, Gynecology & Andrology, Central Medical Affairs, Schering AG, Müllerstrasse 178, 13342 Berlin, Germany

IARC Secretariat

Robert Baan, *IARC Monographs* programme (*Rapporteur, Subgroup on Other Relevant Data*)

Julien Berthiller, Gene–Environment Epidemiology

Vincent James Cogliano, *IARC Monographs* programme (*Head of Programme*)

Carolyn Dresler, Tobacco and Cancer

Fatiha El Ghissassi, *IARC Monographs* programme (*Co-Rapporteur, Subgroup on Other Relevant Data*)

Silvia Franceschi, Infections and Cancer Epidemiology

Maria-Alice G. Gonçalves, Gene–Environment Epidemiology

Yann Grosse, *IARC Monographs* programme (*Responsible Officer; Rapporteur, Subgroup on Cancer in Experimental Animals*)

Neela Guha, Gene–Environment Epidemiology

Manuela Marron, Gene–Environment Epidemiology

Jane Mitchell, *IARC Monographs* programme (*Editor*)

Nikolai Napalkov, *IARC Monographs* programme

Béatrice Secretan, *IARC Monographs* programme (*Rapporteur, Subgroup on Exposure Data*)

Kurt Straif, *IARC Monographs* programme (*Rapporteur, Subgroup on Cancer in Humans*)

Andreas Ullrich, Programme in Cancer Control, Department of Chronic Diseases and Health Promotion (CHP), World Health Organization, 20, Avenue Appia, 1211 Geneva 27, Switzerland

Administrative assistance

Sandrine Egraz

Brigitte Kajo

Martine Lézère

Helene Lorenzen-Augros

---

[6] Employed by Schering AG

PREAMBLE

IARC MONOGRAPHS PROGRAMME ON THE EVALUATION OF CARCINOGENIC RISKS TO HUMANS

PREAMBLE

1. BACKGROUND

In 1969, the International Agency for Research on Cancer (IARC) initiated a programme to evaluate the carcinogenic risk of chemicals to humans and to produce monographs on individual chemicals. The *Monographs* programme has since been expanded to include consideration of exposures to complex mixtures of chemicals (which occur, for example, in some occupations and as a result of human habits) and of exposures to other agents, such as radiation and viruses. With Supplement 6 (IARC, 1987a), the title of the series was modified from *IARC Monographs on the Evaluation of the Carcinogenic Risk of Chemicals to Humans* to *IARC Monographs on the Evaluation of Carcinogenic Risks to Humans*, in order to reflect the widened scope of the programme.

The criteria established in 1971 to evaluate carcinogenic risk to humans were adopted by the working groups whose deliberations resulted in the first 16 volumes of the *IARC Monographs series*. Those criteria were subsequently updated by further ad-hoc working groups (IARC, 1977, 1978, 1979, 1982, 1983, 1987b, 1988, 1991a; Vainio *et al.*, 1992).

2. OBJECTIVE AND SCOPE

The objective of the programme is to prepare, with the help of international working groups of experts, and to publish in the form of monographs, critical reviews and evaluations of evidence on the carcinogenicity of a wide range of human exposures. The *Monographs* may also indicate where additional research efforts are needed.

The *Monographs* represent the first step in carcinogenic risk assessment, which involves examination of all relevant information in order to assess the strength of the available evidence that certain exposures could alter the incidence of cancer in humans. The second step is quantitative risk estimation. Detailed, quantitative evaluations of epidemiological data may be made in the *Monographs*, but without extrapolation beyond the range of the data available. Quantitative extrapolation from experimental data to the human situation is not undertaken.

The term 'carcinogen' is used in these monographs to denote an exposure that is capable of increasing the incidence of malignant neoplasms; the induction of benign neoplasms may in some circumstances (see p. 19) contribute to the judgement that the exposure is carcinogenic. The terms 'neoplasm' and 'tumour' are used interchangeably.

Some epidemiological and experimental studies indicate that different agents may act at different stages in the carcinogenic process, and several mechanisms may be involved. The aim of the *Monographs* has been, from their inception, to evaluate evidence of carcinogenicity at any stage in the carcinogenesis process, independently of the underlying mechanisms. Information on mechanisms may, however, be used in making the overall evaluation (IARC, 1991a; Vainio *et al.*, 1992; see also pp. 25–27).

The *Monographs* may assist national and international authorities in making risk assessments and in formulating decisions concerning any necessary preventive measures. The evaluations of IARC working groups are scientific, qualitative judgements about the evidence for or against carcinogenicity provided by the available data. These evaluations represent only one part of the body of information on which regulatory measures may be based. Other components of regulatory decisions vary from one situation to another and from country to country, responding to different socioeconomic and national priorities. **Therefore, no recommendation is given with regard to regulation or legislation, which are the responsibility of individual governments and/or other international organizations.**

The *IARC Monographs* are recognized as an authoritative source of information on the carcinogenicity of a wide range of human exposures. A survey of users in 1988 indicated that the *Monographs* are consulted by various agencies in 57 countries. About 2500 copies of each volume are printed, for distribution to governments, regulatory bodies and interested scientists. The Monographs are also available from IARC*Press* in Lyon and via the Marketing and Dissemination (MDI) of the World Health Organization in Geneva.

3.   SELECTION OF TOPICS FOR MONOGRAPHS

Topics are selected on the basis of two main criteria: (a) there is evidence of human exposure, and (b) there is some evidence or suspicion of carcinogenicity. The term 'agent' is used to include individual chemical compounds, groups of related chemical compounds, physical agents (such as radiation) and biological factors (such as viruses). Exposures to mixtures of agents may occur in occupational exposures and as a result of personal and cultural habits (like smoking and dietary practices). Chemical analogues and compounds with biological or physical characteristics similar to those of suspected carcinogens may also be considered, even in the absence of data on a possible carcinogenic effect in humans or experimental animals.

The scientific literature is surveyed for published data relevant to an assessment of carcinogenicity. The IARC information bulletins on agents being tested for carcinogenicity (IARC, 1973–1996) and directories of on-going research in cancer epidemiology (IARC, 1976–1996) often indicate exposures that may be scheduled for future meetings. Ad-hoc working groups convened by IARC in 1984, 1989, 1991, 1993 and

1998 gave recommendations as to which agents should be evaluated in the IARC Monographs series (IARC, 1984, 1989, 1991b, 1993, 1998a,b).

As significant new data on subjects on which monographs have already been prepared become available, re-evaluations are made at subsequent meetings, and revised monographs are published.

4.   DATA FOR MONOGRAPHS

The *Monographs* do not necessarily cite all the literature concerning the subject of an evaluation. Only those data considered by the Working Group to be relevant to making the evaluation are included.

With regard to biological and epidemiological data, only reports that have been published or accepted for publication in the openly available scientific literature are reviewed by the working groups. In certain instances, government agency reports that have undergone peer review and are widely available are considered. Exceptions may be made on an ad-hoc basis to include unpublished reports that are in their final form and publicly available, if their inclusion is considered pertinent to making a final evaluation (see pp. 25–27). In the sections on chemical and physical properties, on analysis, on production and use and on occurrence, unpublished sources of information may be used.

5.   THE WORKING GROUP

Reviews and evaluations are formulated by a working group of experts. The tasks of the group are: (i) to ascertain that all appropriate data have been collected; (ii) to select the data relevant for the evaluation on the basis of scientific merit; (iii) to prepare accurate summaries of the data to enable the reader to follow the reasoning of the Working Group; (iv) to evaluate the results of epidemiological and experimental studies on cancer; (v) to evaluate data relevant to the understanding of mechanism of action; and (vi) to make an overall evaluation of the carcinogenicity of the exposure to humans.

Working Group participants who contributed to the considerations and evaluations within a particular volume are listed, with their addresses, at the beginning of each publication. Each participant who is a member of a working group serves as an individual scientist and not as a representative of any organization, government or industry. In addition, nominees of national and international agencies and industrial associations may be invited as observers.

6.   WORKING PROCEDURES

Approximately one year in advance of a meeting of a working group, the topics of the monographs are announced and participants are selected by IARC staff in consultation with other experts. Subsequently, relevant biological and epidemiological data are collected by the Carcinogen Identification and Evaluation Unit of IARC from recognized sources of information on carcinogenesis, including data storage and retrieval systems such as MEDLINE and TOXLINE.

For chemicals and some complex mixtures, the major collection of data and the preparation of first drafts of the sections on chemical and physical properties, on analysis, on production and use and on occurrence are carried out under a separate contract funded by the United States National Cancer Institute. Representatives from industrial associations may assist in the preparation of sections on production and use. Information on production and trade is obtained from governmental and trade publications and, in some cases, by direct contact with industries. Separate production data on some agents may not be available because their publication could disclose confidential information. Information on uses may be obtained from published sources but is often complemented by direct contact with manufacturers. Efforts are made to supplement this information with data from other national and international sources.

Six months before the meeting, the material obtained is sent to meeting participants, or is used by IARC staff, to prepare sections for the first drafts of monographs. The first drafts are compiled by IARC staff and sent before the meeting to all participants of the Working Group for review.

The Working Group meets in Lyon for seven to eight days to discuss and finalize the texts of the monographs and to formulate the evaluations. After the meeting, the master copy of each monograph is verified by consulting the original literature, edited and prepared for publication. The aim is to publish monographs within six months of the Working Group meeting.

The available studies are summarized by the Working Group, with particular regard to the qualitative aspects discussed below. In general, numerical findings are indicated as they appear in the original report; units are converted when necessary for easier comparison. The Working Group may conduct additional analyses of the published data and use them in their assessment of the evidence; the results of such supplementary analyses are given in square brackets. When an important aspect of a study, directly impinging on its interpretation, should be brought to the attention of the reader, a comment is given in square brackets.

7.   EXPOSURE DATA

Sections that indicate the extent of past and present human exposure, the sources of exposure, the people most likely to be exposed and the factors that contribute to the exposure are included at the beginning of each monograph.

Most monographs on individual chemicals, groups of chemicals or complex mixtures include sections on chemical and physical data, on analysis, on production and use and on occurrence. In monographs on, for example, physical agents, occupational exposures and cultural habits, other sections may be included, such as: historical perspectives, description of an industry or habit, chemistry of the complex mixture or taxonomy. Monographs on biological agents have sections on structure and biology, methods of detection, epidemiology of infection and clinical disease other than cancer.

For chemical exposures, the Chemical Abstracts Services Registry Number, the latest Chemical Abstracts primary name and the IUPAC systematic name are recorded; other synonyms are given, but the list is not necessarily comprehensive. For biological agents, taxonomy and structure are described, and the degree of variability is given, when applicable.

Information on chemical and physical properties and, in particular, data relevant to identification, occurrence and biological activity are included. For biological agents, mode of replication, life cycle, target cells, persistence and latency and host response are given. A description of technical products of chemicals includes trade names, relevant specifications and available information on composition and impurities. Some of the trade names given may be those of mixtures in which the agent being evaluated is only one of the ingredients.

The purpose of the section on analysis or detection is to give the reader an overview of current methods, with emphasis on those widely used for regulatory purposes. Methods for monitoring human exposure are also given, when available. No critical evaluation or recommendation of any of the methods is meant or implied. The IARC published a series of volumes, *Environmental Carcinogens: Methods of Analysis and Exposure Measurement* (IARC, 1978–93), that describe validated methods for analysing a wide variety of chemicals and mixtures. For biological agents, methods of detection and exposure assessment are described, including their sensitivity, specificity and reproducibility.

The dates of first synthesis and of first commercial production of a chemical or mixture are provided; for agents which do not occur naturally, this information may allow a reasonable estimate to be made of the date before which no human exposure to the agent could have occurred. The dates of first reported occurrence of an exposure are also provided. In addition, methods of synthesis used in past and present commercial production and different methods of production which may give rise to different impurities are described.

Data on production, international trade and uses are obtained for representative regions, which usually include Europe, Japan and the United States of America. It should not, however, be inferred that those areas or nations are necessarily the sole or major sources or users of the agent. Some identified uses may not be current or major applications, and the coverage is not necessarily comprehensive. In the case of drugs, mention of their therapeutic uses does not necessarily represent current practice, nor does it imply judgement as to their therapeutic efficacy.

Information on the occurrence of an agent or mixture in the environment is obtained from data derived from the monitoring and surveillance of levels in occupational environments, air, water, soil, foods and animal and human tissues. When available, data on the generation, persistence and bioaccumulation of the agent are also included. In the case of mixtures, industries, occupations or processes, information is given about all agents present. For processes, industries and occupations, a historical description is also given, noting variations in chemical composition, physical properties and levels of occupational exposure with time and place. For biological agents, the epidemiology of infection is described.

Statements concerning regulations and guidelines (e.g., pesticide registrations, maximal levels permitted in foods, occupational exposure limits) are included for some countries as indications of potential exposures, but they may not reflect the most recent situation, since such limits are continuously reviewed and modified. The absence of information on regulatory status for a country should not be taken to imply that that country does not have regulations with regard to the exposure. For biological agents, legislation and control, including vaccines and therapy, are described.

8.   STUDIES OF CANCER IN HUMANS

(a)   Types of studies considered

Three types of epidemiological studies of cancer contribute to the assessment of carcinogenicity in humans — cohort studies, case–control studies and correlation (or ecological) studies. Rarely, results from randomized trials may be available. Case series and case reports of cancer in humans may also be reviewed.

Cohort and case–control studies relate the exposures under study to the occurrence of cancer in individuals and provide an estimate of relative risk (ratio of incidence or mortality in those exposed to incidence or mortality in those not exposed) as the main measure of association.

In correlation studies, the units of investigation are usually whole populations (e.g. in particular geographical areas or at particular times), and cancer frequency is related to a summary measure of the exposure of the population to the agent, mixture or exposure circumstance under study. Because individual exposure is not documented, however, a causal relationship is less easy to infer from correlation studies than from cohort and case–control studies. Case reports generally arise from a suspicion, based on clinical experience, that the concurrence of two events — that is, a particular exposure and occurrence of a cancer — has happened rather more frequently than would be expected by chance. Case reports usually lack complete ascertainment of cases in any population, definition or enumeration of the population at risk and estimation of the expected number of cases in the absence of exposure. The uncertainties surrounding interpretation of case reports and correlation studies make them inadequate, except in rare instances, to form the sole basis for inferring a causal relationship. When taken together with case–control and cohort studies, however, relevant case reports or correlation studies may add materially to the judgement that a causal relationship is present.

Epidemiological studies of benign neoplasms, presumed preneoplastic lesions and other end-points thought to be relevant to cancer are also reviewed by working groups. They may, in some instances, strengthen inferences drawn from studies of cancer itself.

(b)   Quality of studies considered

The Monographs are not intended to summarize all published studies. Those that are judged to be inadequate or irrelevant to the evaluation are generally omitted. They may be mentioned briefly, particularly when the information is considered to be a useful supplement to that in other reports or when they provide the only data available. Their inclusion does not imply acceptance of the adequacy of the study design or of the analysis and interpretation of the results, and limitations are clearly outlined in square brackets at the end of the study description.

It is necessary to take into account the possible roles of bias, confounding and chance in the interpretation of epidemiological studies. By 'bias' is meant the operation of factors in study design or execution that lead erroneously to a stronger or weaker association than in fact exists between disease and an agent, mixture or exposure circumstance. By 'confounding' is meant a situation in which the relationship with disease is made to appear stronger or weaker than it truly is as a result of an association between the apparent causal factor and another factor that is associated with either an increase or decrease in the incidence of the disease. In evaluating the extent to which these factors have been minimized in an individual study, working groups consider a number of aspects of design and analysis as described in the report of the study. Most of these considerations apply equally to case–control, cohort and correlation studies. Lack of clarity of any of these aspects in the reporting of a study can decrease its credibility and the weight given to it in the final evaluation of the exposure.

Firstly, the study population, disease (or diseases) and exposure should have been well defined by the authors. Cases of disease in the study population should have been identified in a way that was independent of the exposure of interest, and exposure should have been assessed in a way that was not related to disease status.

Secondly, the authors should have taken account in the study design and analysis of other variables that can influence the risk of disease and may have been related to the exposure of interest. Potential confounding by such variables should have been dealt with either in the design of the study, such as by matching, or in the analysis, by statistical adjustment. In cohort studies, comparisons with local rates of disease may be more appropriate than those with national rates. Internal comparisons of disease frequency among individuals at different levels of exposure should also have been made in the study.

Thirdly, the authors should have reported the basic data on which the conclusions are founded, even if sophisticated statistical analyses were employed. At the very least, they should have given the numbers of exposed and unexposed cases and controls in a case–control study and the numbers of cases observed and expected in a cohort study. Further tabulations by time since exposure began and other temporal factors are also important. In a cohort study, data on all cancer sites and all causes of death should have been given, to reveal the possibility of reporting bias. In a case–control study, the effects of investigated factors other than the exposure of interest should have been reported.

Finally, the statistical methods used to obtain estimates of relative risk, absolute rates of cancer, confidence intervals and significance tests, and to adjust for confounding should have been clearly stated by the authors. The methods used should preferably have been the generally accepted techniques that have been refined since the mid-1970s. These methods have been reviewed for case–control studies (Breslow & Day, 1980) and for cohort studies (Breslow & Day, 1987).

(c)   Inferences about mechanism of action

Detailed analyses of both relative and absolute risks in relation to temporal variables, such as age at first exposure, time since first exposure, duration of exposure, cumulative exposure and time since exposure ceased, are reviewed and summarized when available. The analysis of temporal relationships can be useful in formulating models of carcino-genesis. In particular, such analyses may suggest whether a carcinogen acts early or late in the process of carcinogenesis, although at best they allow only indirect inferences about the mechanism of action. Special attention is given to measurements of biological markers of carcinogen exposure or action, such as DNA or protein adducts, as well as markers of early steps in the carcinogenic process, such as proto-oncogene mutation, when these are incorporated into epidemiological studies focused on cancer incidence or mortality. Such measurements may allow inferences to be made about putative mecha-nisms of action (IARC, 1991a; Vainio et al., 1992).

(d)   Criteria for causality

After the individual epidemiological studies of cancer have been summarized and the quality assessed, a judgement is made concerning the strength of evidence that the agent, mixture or exposure circumstance in question is carcinogenic for humans. In making its judgement, the Working Group considers several criteria for causality. A strong asso-ciation (a large relative risk) is more likely to indicate causality than a weak association, although it is recognized that relative risks of small magnitude do not imply lack of causality and may be important if the disease is common. Associations that are replicated in several studies of the same design or using different epidemiological approaches or under different circumstances of exposure are more likely to represent a causal relation-ship than isolated observations from single studies. If there are inconsistent results among investigations, possible reasons are sought (such as differences in amount of exposure), and results of studies judged to be of high quality are given more weight than those of studies judged to be methodologically less sound. When suspicion of carcino-genicity arises largely from a single study, these data are not combined with those from later studies in any subsequent reassessment of the strength of the evidence.

If the risk of the disease in question increases with the amount of exposure, this is considered to be a strong indication of causality, although absence of a graded response is not necessarily evidence against a causal relationship. Demonstration of a decline in risk after cessation of or reduction in exposure in individuals or in whole populations also supports a causal interpretation of the findings.

Although a carcinogen may act upon more than one target, the specificity of an association (an increased occurrence of cancer at one anatomical site or of one morphological type) adds plausibility to a causal relationship, particularly when excess cancer occurrence is limited to one morphological type within the same organ.

Although rarely available, results from randomized trials showing different rates among exposed and unexposed individuals provide particularly strong evidence for causality.

When several epidemiological studies show little or no indication of an association between an exposure and cancer, the judgement may be made that, in the aggregate, they show evidence of lack of carcinogenicity. Such a judgement requires first of all that the studies giving rise to it meet, to a sufficient degree, the standards of design and analysis described above. Specifically, the possibility that bias, confounding or misclassification of exposure or outcome could explain the observed results should be considered and excluded with reasonable certainty. In addition, all studies that are judged to be methodologically sound should be consistent with a relative risk of unity for any observed level of exposure and, when considered together, should provide a pooled estimate of relative risk which is at or near unity and has a narrow confidence interval, due to sufficient population size. Moreover, no individual study nor the pooled results of all the studies should show any consistent tendency for the relative risk of cancer to increase with increasing level of exposure. It is important to note that evidence of lack of carcinogenicity obtained in this way from several epidemiological studies can apply only to the type(s) of cancer studied and to dose levels and intervals between first exposure and observation of disease that are the same as or less than those observed in all the studies. Experience with human cancer indicates that, in some cases, the period from first exposure to the development of clinical cancer is seldom less than 20 years; studies with latent periods substantially shorter than 30 years cannot provide evidence for lack of carcinogenicity.

9.   STUDIES OF CANCER IN EXPERIMENTAL ANIMALS

All known human carcinogens that have been studied adequately in experimental animals have produced positive results in one or more animal species (Wilbourn et al., 1986; Tomatis et al., 1989). For several agents (aflatoxins, 4-aminobiphenyl, azathioprine, betel quid with tobacco, bischloromethyl ether and chloromethyl methyl ether (technical grade), chlorambucil, chlornaphazine, ciclosporin, coal-tar pitches, coal-tars, combined oral contraceptives, cyclophosphamide, diethylstilboestrol, melphalan, 8-methoxypsoralen plus ultraviolet A radiation, mustard gas, myleran, 2-naphthylamine, nonsteroidal estrogens, estrogen replacement therapy/steroidal estrogens, solar radiation, thiotepa and vinyl chloride), carcinogenicity in experimental animals was established or highly suspected before epidemiological studies confirmed their carcinogenicity in humans (Vainio et al., 1995). Although this association cannot establish that all agents and mixtures that cause cancer in experimental animals also cause cancer in humans, nevertheless, **in the absence of adequate data on humans, it is biologically plausible and prudent to regard agents and mixtures for which there is** *sufficient evidence* **(see p. 24) of carcinogenicity in experimental animals as if they presented a carcinogenic risk to humans**. The possibility that a given agent may cause cancer through a species-specific mechanism which does not operate in humans (see p. 27) should also be taken into consideration.

The nature and extent of impurities or contaminants present in the chemical or mixture being evaluated are given when available. Animal strain, sex, numbers per group, age at start of treatment and survival are reported.

Other types of studies summarized include: experiments in which the agent or mixture was administered in conjunction with known carcinogens or factors that modify carcinogenic effects; studies in which the end-point was not cancer but a defined precancerous lesion; and experiments on the carcinogenicity of known metabolites and derivatives.

For experimental studies of mixtures, consideration is given to the possibility of changes in the physicochemical properties of the test substance during collection, storage, extraction, concentration and delivery. Chemical and toxicological interactions of the components of mixtures may result in nonlinear dose–response relationships.

An assessment is made as to the relevance to human exposure of samples tested in experimental animals, which may involve consideration of: (i) physical and chemical characteristics, (ii) constituent substances that indicate the presence of a class of substances, (iii) the results of tests for genetic and related effects, including studies on DNA adduct formation, proto-oncogene mutation and expression and suppressor gene inactivation. The relevance of results obtained, for example, with animal viruses analogous to the virus being evaluated in the monograph must also be considered. They may provide biological and mechanistic information relevant to the understanding of the process of carcinogenesis in humans and may strengthen the plausibility of a conclusion that the biological agent under evaluation is carcinogenic in humans.

(a)   Qualitative aspects

An assessment of carcinogenicity involves several considerations of qualitative importance, including (i) the experimental conditions under which the test was performed, including route and schedule of exposure, species, strain, sex, age, duration of follow-up; (ii) the consistency of the results, for example, across species and target organ(s); (iii) the spectrum of neoplastic response, from preneoplastic lesions and benign tumours to malignant neoplasms; and (iv) the possible role of modifying factors.

As mentioned earlier (p. 11), the *Monographs* are not intended to summarize all published studies. Those studies in experimental animals that are inadequate (e.g., too short a duration, too few animals, poor survival; see below) or are judged irrelevant to the evaluation are generally omitted. Guidelines for conducting adequate long-term carcinogenicity experiments have been outlined (e.g. Montesano *et al.*, 1986).

Considerations of importance to the Working Group in the interpretation and evaluation of a particular study include: (i) how clearly the agent was defined and, in the case of mixtures, how adequately the sample characterization was reported; (ii) whether the dose was adequately monitored, particularly in inhalation experiments; (iii) whether the doses and duration of treatment were appropriate and whether the survival of treated animals was similar to that of controls; (iv) whether there were adequate numbers of animals per group; (v) whether animals of each sex were used; (vi) whether animals were allocated randomly to groups; (vii) whether the duration of observation was adequate; and (viii) whether the data were adequately reported. If available, recent data on the incidence of specific tumours in historical controls, as well as in concurrent controls, should be taken into account in the evaluation of tumour response.

When benign tumours occur together with and originate from the same cell type in an organ or tissue as malignant tumours in a particular study and appear to represent a stage in the progression to malignancy, it may be valid to combine them in assessing tumour incidence (Huff *et al.*, 1989). The occurrence of lesions presumed to be preneoplastic may in certain instances aid in assessing the biological plausibility of any neoplastic response observed. If an agent or mixture induces only benign neoplasms that appear to be end-points that do not readily progress to malignancy, it should nevertheless be suspected of being a carcinogen and requires further investigation.

(b)   Quantitative aspects

The probability that tumours will occur may depend on the species, sex, strain and age of the animal, the dose of the carcinogen and the route and length of exposure. Evidence of an increased incidence of neoplasms with increased level of exposure strengthens the inference of a causal association between the exposure and the development of neoplasms.

The form of the dose–response relationship can vary widely, depending on the particular agent under study and the target organ. Both DNA damage and increased cell division are important aspects of carcinogenesis, and cell proliferation is a strong determinant of dose–response relationships for some carcinogens (Cohen & Ellwein, 1990). Since many chemicals require metabolic activation before being converted into their reactive intermediates, both metabolic and pharmacokinetic aspects are important in determining the dose–response pattern. Saturation of steps such as absorption, activation, inactivation and elimination may produce nonlinearity in the dose–response relationship, as could saturation of processes such as DNA repair (Hoel *et al.*, 1983; Gart *et al.*, 1986).

(c)   Statistical analysis of long-term experiments in animals

Factors considered by the Working Group include the adequacy of the information given for each treatment group: (i) the number of animals studied and the number examined histologically, (ii) the number of animals with a given tumour type and (iii) length of survival. The statistical methods used should be clearly stated and should be the generally accepted techniques refined for this purpose (Peto *et al.*, 1980; Gart *et al.*, 1986). When there is no difference in survival between control and treatment groups, the Working Group usually compares the proportions of animals developing each tumour type in each of the groups. Otherwise, consideration is given as to whether or not appropriate adjustments have been made for differences in survival. These adjustments can include: comparisons of the proportions of tumour-bearing animals among the effective number of animals (alive at the time the first tumour is discovered), in the case where most differences in survival occur before tumours appear; life-table methods, when tumours are visible or when they may be considered 'fatal' because mortality rapidly follows tumour development; and the Mantel-Haenszel test or logistic regression, when occult tumours do not affect the animals' risk of dying but are 'incidental' findings at autopsy.

In practice, classifying tumours as fatal or incidental may be difficult. Several survival-adjusted methods have been developed that do not require this distinction (Gart *et al.*, 1986), although they have not been fully evaluated.

10.   OTHER DATA RELEVANT TO AN EVALUATION OF CARCINOGENICITY AND ITS MECHANISMS

In coming to an overall evaluation of carcinogenicity in humans (see pp. 25–27), the Working Group also considers related data. The nature of the information selected for the summary depends on the agent being considered.

For chemicals and complex mixtures of chemicals such as those in some occupational situations or involving cultural habits (e.g. tobacco smoking), the other data considered to be relevant are divided into those on absorption, distribution, metabolism and excretion; toxic effects; reproductive and developmental effects; and genetic and related effects.

Concise information is given on absorption, distribution (including placental transfer) and excretion in both humans and experimental animals. Kinetic factors that may affect the dose–response relationship, such as saturation of uptake, protein binding, metabolic activation, detoxification and DNA repair processes, are mentioned. Studies that indicate the metabolic fate of the agent in humans and in experimental animals are summarized briefly, and comparisons of data on humans and on animals are made when possible. Comparative information on the relationship between exposure and the dose that reaches the target site may be of particular importance for extrapolation between species. Data are given on acute and chronic toxic effects (other than cancer), such as organ toxicity, increased cell proliferation, immunotoxicity and endocrine effects. The presence and toxicological significance of cellular receptors is described. Effects on reproduction, teratogenicity, fetotoxicity and embryotoxicity are also summarized briefly.

Tests of genetic and related effects are described in view of the relevance of gene mutation and chromosomal damage to carcinogenesis (Vainio *et al.*, 1992; McGregor *et al.*, 1999). The adequacy of the reporting of sample characterization is considered and, where necessary, commented upon; with regard to complex mixtures, such comments are similar to those described for animal carcinogenicity tests on p. 18. The available data are interpreted critically by phylogenetic group according to the end-points detected, which may include DNA damage, gene mutation, sister chromatid exchange, micro-nucleus formation, chromosomal aberrations, aneuploidy and cell transformation. The concentrations employed are given, and mention is made of whether use of an exogenous metabolic system *in vitro* affected the test result. These data are given as listings of test systems, data and references. The data on genetic and related effects presented in the *Monographs* are also available in the form of genetic activity profiles (GAP) prepared in collaboration with the United States Environmental Protection Agency (EPA) (see also Waters *et al.*, 1987) using software for personal computers that are Microsoft Windows® compatible. The EPA/IARC GAP software and database may be downloaded free of charge from *www.epa.gov/gapdb*.

Positive results in tests using prokaryotes, lower eukaryotes, plants, insects and cultured mammalian cells suggest that genetic and related effects could occur in mammals. Results from such tests may also give information about the types of genetic effect produced and about the involvement of metabolic activation. Some end-points described are clearly genetic in nature (e.g., gene mutations and chromosomal aberrations), while others are to a greater or lesser degree associated with genetic effects (e.g. unscheduled DNA synthesis). In-vitro tests for tumour-promoting activity and for cell transformation may be sensitive to changes that are not necessarily the result of genetic alterations but that may have specific relevance to the process of carcinogenesis. A critical appraisal of these tests has been published (Montesano *et al.*, 1986).

Genetic or other activity detected in experimental mammals and humans is regarded as being of greater relevance than that in other organisms. The demonstration that an agent or mixture can induce gene and chromosomal mutations in whole mammals indicates that it may have carcinogenic activity, although this activity may not be detectably expressed in any or all species. Relative potency in tests for mutagenicity and related effects is not a reliable indicator of carcinogenic potency. Negative results in tests for mutagenicity in selected tissues from animals treated *in vivo* provide less weight, partly because they do not exclude the possibility of an effect in tissues other than those examined. Moreover, negative results in short-term tests with genetic end-points cannot be considered to provide evidence to rule out carcinogenicity of agents or mixtures that act through other mechanisms (e.g. receptor-mediated effects, cellular toxicity with regenerative proliferation, peroxisome proliferation) (Vainio *et al.*, 1992). Factors that may lead to misleading results in short-term tests have been discussed in detail elsewhere (Montesano *et al.*, 1986).

When available, data relevant to mechanisms of carcinogenesis that do not involve structural changes at the level of the gene are also described.

The adequacy of epidemiological studies of reproductive outcome and genetic and related effects in humans is evaluated by the same criteria as are applied to epidemiological studies of cancer.

Structure–activity relationships that may be relevant to an evaluation of the carcinogenicity of an agent are also described.

For biological agents — viruses, bacteria and parasites — other data relevant to carcinogenicity include descriptions of the pathology of infection, molecular biology (integration and expression of viruses, and any genetic alterations seen in human tumours) and other observations, which might include cellular and tissue responses to infection, immune response and the presence of tumour markers.

11. SUMMARY OF DATA REPORTED

In this section, the relevant epidemiological and experimental data are summarized. Only reports, other than in abstract form, that meet the criteria outlined on p. 11 are considered for evaluating carcinogenicity. Inadequate studies are generally not summarized: such studies are usually identified by a square-bracketed comment in the preceding text.

(*a*) *Exposure*

Human exposure to chemicals and complex mixtures is summarized on the basis of elements such as production, use, occurrence in the environment and determinations in human tissues and body fluids. Quantitative data are given when available. Exposure to biological agents is described in terms of transmission and prevalence of infection.

(*b*) *Carcinogenicity in humans*

Results of epidemiological studies that are considered to be pertinent to an assessment of human carcinogenicity are summarized. When relevant, case reports and correlation studies are also summarized.

(*c*) *Carcinogenicity in experimental animals*

Data relevant to an evaluation of carcinogenicity in animals are summarized. For each animal species and route of administration, it is stated whether an increased incidence of neoplasms or preneoplastic lesions was observed, and the tumour sites are indicated. If the agent or mixture produced tumours after prenatal exposure or in single-dose experiments, this is also indicated. Negative findings are also summarized. Dose–response and other quantitative data may be given when available.

(*d*)   *Other data relevant to an evaluation of carcinogenicity and its mechanisms*

Data on biological effects in humans that are of particular relevance are summarized. These may include toxicological, kinetic and metabolic considerations and evidence of DNA binding, persistence of DNA lesions or genetic damage in exposed humans. Toxicological information, such as that on cytotoxicity and regeneration, receptor binding and hormonal and immunological effects, and data on kinetics and metabolism in experimental animals are given when considered relevant to the possible mechanism of the carcinogenic action of the agent. The results of tests for genetic and related effects are summarized for whole mammals, cultured mammalian cells and nonmammalian systems.

When available, comparisons of such data for humans and for animals, and particularly animals that have developed cancer, are described.

Structure–activity relationships are mentioned when relevant.

For the agent, mixture or exposure circumstance being evaluated, the available data on end-points or other phenomena relevant to mechanisms of carcinogenesis from studies in humans, experimental animals and tissue and cell test systems are summarized within one or more of the following descriptive dimensions:

(i) Evidence of genotoxicity (structural changes at the level of the gene): for example, structure–activity considerations, adduct formation, mutagenicity (effect on specific genes), chromosomal mutation/aneuploidy

(ii) Evidence of effects on the expression of relevant genes (functional changes at the intracellular level): for example, alterations to the structure or quantity of the product of a proto-oncogene or tumour-suppressor gene, alterations to metabolic activation/inactivation/DNA repair

(iii) Evidence of relevant effects on cell behaviour (morphological or behavioural changes at the cellular or tissue level): for example, induction of mitogenesis, compensatory cell proliferation, preoplasia and hyperplasia, survival of premalignant or malignant cells (immortalization, immunosuppression), effects on metastatic potential

(iv) Evidence from dose and time relationships of carcinogenic effects and interactions between agents: for example, early/late stage, as inferred from epidemiological studies; initiation/promotion/progression/malignant conversion, as defined in animal carcinogenicity experiments; toxicokinetics

These dimensions are not mutually exclusive, and an agent may fall within more than one of them. Thus, for example, the action of an agent on the expression of relevant genes could be summarized under both the first and second dimensions, even if it were known with reasonable certainty that those effects resulted from genotoxicity.

12.   EVALUATION

Evaluations of the strength of the evidence for carcinogenicity arising from human and experimental animal data are made, using standard terms.

It is recognized that the criteria for these evaluations, described below, cannot encompass all of the factors that may be relevant to an evaluation of carcinogenicity. In considering all of the relevant scientific data, the Working Group may assign the agent, mixture or exposure circumstance to a higher or lower category than a strict inter-pretation of these criteria would indicate.

(*a*)   *Degrees of evidence for carcinogenicity in humans and in experimental animals and supporting evidence*

These categories refer only to the strength of the evidence that an exposure is carcino-genic and not to the extent of its carcinogenic activity (potency) nor to the mechanisms involved. A classification may change as new information becomes available.

An evaluation of degree of evidence, whether for a single agent or a mixture, is limited to the materials tested, as defined physically, chemically or biologically. When the agents evaluated are considered by the Working Group to be sufficiently closely related, they may be grouped together for the purpose of a single evaluation of degree of evidence.

(i)   *Carcinogenicity in humans*

The applicability of an evaluation of the carcinogenicity of a mixture, process, occu-pation or industry on the basis of evidence from epidemiological studies depends on the variability over time and place of the mixtures, processes, occupations and industries. The Working Group seeks to identify the specific exposure, process or activity which is considered most likely to be responsible for any excess risk. The evaluation is focused as narrowly as the available data on exposure and other aspects permit.

The evidence relevant to carcinogenicity from studies in humans is classified into one of the following categories:

Sufficient evidence of carcinogenicity: The Working Group considers that a causal relationship has been established between exposure to the agent, mixture or exposure circumstance and human cancer. That is, a positive relationship has been observed between the exposure and cancer in studies in which chance, bias and confounding could be ruled out with reasonable confidence.

Limited evidence of carcinogenicity: A positive association has been observed between exposure to the agent, mixture or exposure circumstance and cancer for which a causal interpretation is considered by the Working Group to be credible, but chance, bias or confounding could not be ruled out with reasonable confidence.

Inadequate evidence of carcinogenicity: The available studies are of insufficient quality, consistency or statistical power to permit a conclusion regarding the presence or absence of a causal association between exposure and cancer, or no data on cancer in humans are available.

Evidence suggesting lack of carcinogenicity: There are several adequate studies covering the full range of levels of exposure that human beings are known to encounter, which are mutually consistent in not showing a positive association between exposure to the agent, mixture or exposure circumstance and any studied cancer at any observed level of exposure. A conclusion of 'evidence suggesting lack of carcinogenicity' is inevitably limited to the cancer sites, conditions and levels of exposure and length of observation covered by the available studies. In addition, the possibility of a very small risk at the levels of exposure studied can never be excluded.

In some instances, the above categories may be used to classify the degree of evidence related to carcinogenicity in specific organs or tissues.

(ii)   *Carcinogenicity in experimental animals*

The evidence relevant to carcinogenicity in experimental animals is classified into one of the following categories:

Sufficient evidence of carcinogenicity: The Working Group considers that a causal relationship has been established between the agent or mixture and an increased incidence of malignant neoplasms or of an appropriate combination of benign and malignant neoplasms in (a) two or more species of animals or (b) in two or more independent studies in one species carried out at different times or in different laboratories or under different protocols.

Exceptionally, a single study in one species might be considered to provide sufficient evidence of carcinogenicity when malignant neoplasms occur to an unusual degree with regard to incidence, site, type of tumour or age at onset.

Limited evidence of carcinogenicity: The data suggest a carcinogenic effect but are limited for making a definitive evaluation because, e.g. (a) the evidence of carcinogenicity is restricted to a single experiment; or (b) there are unresolved questions regarding the adequacy of the design, conduct or interpretation of the study; or (c) the agent or mixture increases the incidence only of benign neoplasms or lesions of uncertain neoplastic potential, or of certain neoplasms which may occur spontaneously in high incidences in certain strains.

Inadequate evidence of carcinogenicity: The studies cannot be interpreted as showing either the presence or absence of a carcinogenic effect because of major qualitative or quantitative limitations, or no data on cancer in experimental animals are available.

Evidence suggesting lack of carcinogenicity: Adequate studies involving at least two species are available which show that, within the limits of the tests used, the agent or mixture is not carcinogenic. A conclusion of evidence suggesting lack of carcinogenicity is inevitably limited to the species, tumour sites and levels of exposure studied.

(b)   *Other data relevant to the evaluation of carcinogenicity and its mechanisms*

Other evidence judged to be relevant to an evaluation of carcinogenicity and of sufficient importance to affect the overall evaluation is then described. This may include data on preneoplastic lesions, tumour pathology, genetic and related effects, structure–activity relationships, metabolism and pharmacokinetics, physicochemical parameters and analogous biological agents.

Data relevant to mechanisms of the carcinogenic action are also evaluated. The strength of the evidence that any carcinogenic effect observed is due to a particular mechanism is assessed, using terms such as weak, moderate or strong. Then, the Working Group assesses if that particular mechanism is likely to be operative in humans. The strongest indications that a particular mechanism operates in humans come from data on humans or biological specimens obtained from exposed humans. The data may be considered to be especially relevant if they show that the agent in question has caused changes in exposed humans that are on the causal pathway to carcinogenesis. Such data may, however, never become available, because it is at least conceivable that certain compounds may be kept from human use solely on the basis of evidence of their toxicity and/or carcinogenicity in experimental systems.

For complex exposures, including occupational and industrial exposures, the chemical composition and the potential contribution of carcinogens known to be present are considered by the Working Group in its overall evaluation of human carcinogenicity. The Working Group also determines the extent to which the materials tested in experimental systems are related to those to which humans are exposed.

(c)   Overall evaluation

Finally, the body of evidence is considered as a whole, in order to reach an overall evaluation of the carcinogenicity to humans of an agent, mixture or circumstance of exposure.

An evaluation may be made for a group of chemical compounds that have been evaluated by the Working Group. In addition, when supporting data indicate that other, related compounds for which there is no direct evidence of capacity to induce cancer in humans or in animals may also be carcinogenic, a statement describing the rationale for this conclusion is added to the evaluation narrative; an additional evaluation may be made for this broader group of compounds if the strength of the evidence warrants it.

The agent, mixture or exposure circumstance is described according to the wording of one of the following categories, and the designated group is given. The categorization of an agent, mixture or exposure circumstance is a matter of scientific judgement, reflecting the strength of the evidence derived from studies in humans and in experimental animals and from other relevant data.

Group 1 — The agent (mixture) is carcinogenic to humans.
The exposure circumstance entails exposures that are carcinogenic to humans.

This category is used when there is *sufficient evidence* of carcinogenicity in humans. Exceptionally, an agent (mixture) may be placed in this category when evidence of carcinogenicity in humans is less than sufficient but there is *sufficient evidence* of carcinogenicity in experimental animals and strong evidence in exposed humans that the agent (mixture) acts through a relevant mechanism of carcinogenicity.

Group 2

This category includes agents, mixtures and exposure circumstances for which, at one extreme, the degree of evidence of carcinogenicity in humans is almost sufficient, as well as those for which, at the other extreme, there are no human data but for which there is evidence of carcinogenicity in experimental animals. Agents, mixtures and exposure circumstances are assigned to either group 2A (probably carcinogenic to humans) or group 2B (possibly carcinogenic to humans) on the basis of epidemiological and experimental evidence of carcinogenicity and other relevant data.

Group 2A — The agent (mixture) is probably carcinogenic to humans.
The exposure circumstance entails exposures that are probably carcinogenic to humans.

This category is used when there is *limited evidence* of carcinogenicity in humans and *sufficient evidence* of carcinogenicity in experimental animals. In some cases, an agent (mixture) may be classified in this category when there is *inadequate evidence* of carcinogenicity in humans, *sufficient evidence* of carcinogenicity in experimental animals and strong evidence that the carcinogenesis is mediated by a mechanism that also operates in humans. Exceptionally, an agent, mixture or exposure circumstance may be classified in this category solely on the basis of *limited evidence* of carcinogenicity in humans.

Group 2B — The agent (mixture) is possibly carcinogenic to humans.
The exposure circumstance entails exposures that are possibly carcinogenic to humans.

This category is used for agents, mixtures and exposure circumstances for which there is *limited evidence* of carcinogenicity in humans and less than *sufficient evidence* of carcinogenicity in experimental animals. It may also be used when there is *inadequate evidence* of carcinogenicity in humans but there is *sufficient evidence* of carcinogenicity in experimental animals. In some instances, an agent, mixture or exposure circumstance for which there is *inadequate evidence* of carcinogenicity in humans but *limited evidence* of carcinogenicity in experimental animals together with supporting evidence from other relevant data may be placed in this group.

Group 3 — The agent (mixture or exposure circumstance) is not classifiable as to its carcinogenicity to humans.

This category is used most commonly for agents, mixtures and exposure circumstances for which the *evidence of carcinogenicity* is *inadequate* in humans and *inadequate* or *limited* in experimental animals.

Exceptionally, agents (mixtures) for which the *evidence of carcinogenicity* is *inadequate* in humans but *sufficient* in experimental animals may be placed in this category when there is strong evidence that the mechanism of carcinogenicity in experimental animals does not operate in humans.

Agents, mixtures and exposure circumstances that do not fall into any other group are also placed in this category.

Group 4 — The agent (mixture) is probably not carcinogenic to humans.

This category is used for agents or mixtures for which there is *evidence suggesting lack of carcinogenicity* in humans and in experimental animals. In some instances, agents or mixtures for which there is *inadequate evidence* of carcinogenicity in humans but *evidence suggesting lack of carcinogenicity* in experimental animals, consistently and strongly supported by a broad range of other relevant data, may be classified in this group.

13.   REFERENCES

Breslow, N.E. & Day, N.E. (1980) *Statistical Methods in Cancer Research*, Vol. 1, *The Analysis of Case–Control Studies* (IARC Scientific Publications No. 32), Lyon, IARC*Press*

Breslow, N.E. & Day, N.E. (1987) *Statistical Methods in Cancer Research*, Vol. 2, *The Design and Analysis of Cohort Studies* (IARC Scientific Publications No. 82), Lyon, IARC*Press*

Cohen, S.M. & Ellwein, L.B. (1990) Cell proliferation in carcinogenesis. *Science*, **249**, 1007–1011

Gart, J.J., Krewski, D., Lee, P.N., Tarone, R.E. & Wahrendorf, J. (1986) *Statistical Methods in Cancer Research*, Vol. 3, *The Design and Analysis of Long-term Animal Experiments* (IARC Scientific Publications No. 79), Lyon, IARC*Press*

Hoel, D.G., Kaplan, N.L. & Anderson, M.W. (1983) Implication of nonlinear kinetics on risk estimation in carcinogenesis. *Science*, **219**, 1032–1037

Huff, J.E., Eustis, S.L. & Haseman, J.K. (1989) Occurrence and relevance of chemically induced benign neoplasms in long-term carcinogenicity studies. *Cancer Metastasis Rev.*, **8**, 1–21

IARC (1973–1996) *Information Bulletin on the Survey of Chemicals Being Tested for Carcinogenicity/Directory of Agents Being Tested for Carcinogenicity*, Numbers 1–17, Lyon, IARC*Press*

IARC (1976–1996), Lyon, IARC*Press*

Directory of On-going Research in Cancer Epidemiology 1976. Edited by C.S. Muir & G. Wagner

Directory of On-going Research in Cancer Epidemiology 1977 (IARC Scientific Publications No. 17). Edited by C.S. Muir & G. Wagner

Directory of On-going Research in Cancer Epidemiology 1978 (IARC Scientific Publications No. 26). Edited by C.S. Muir & G. Wagner

Directory of On-going Research in Cancer Epidemiology 1979 (IARC Scientific Publications No. 28). Edited by C.S. Muir & G. Wagner

Directory of On-going Research in Cancer Epidemiology 1980 (IARC Scientific Publications No. 35). Edited by C.S. Muir & G. Wagner

Directory of On-going Research in Cancer Epidemiology 1981 (IARC Scientific Publications No. 38). Edited by C.S. Muir & G. Wagner

Directory of On-going Research in Cancer Epidemiology 1982 (IARC Scientific Publications No. 46). Edited by C.S. Muir & G. Wagner

Directory of On-going Research in Cancer Epidemiology 1983 (IARC Scientific Publications No. 50). Edited by C.S. Muir & G. Wagner

Directory of On-going Research in Cancer Epidemiology 1984 (IARC Scientific Publications No. 62). Edited by C.S. Muir & G. Wagner

Directory of On-going Research in Cancer Epidemiology 1985 (IARC Scientific Publications No. 69). Edited by C.S. Muir & G. Wagner

Directory of On-going Research in Cancer Epidemiology 1986 (IARC Scientific Publications No. 80). Edited by C.S. Muir & G. Wagner

Directory of On-going Research in Cancer Epidemiology 1987 (IARC Scientific Publications No. 86). Edited by D.M. Parkin & J. Wahrendorf

Directory of On-going Research in Cancer Epidemiology 1988 (IARC Scientific Publications No. 93). Edited by M. Coleman & J. Wahrendorf

Directory of On-going Research in Cancer Epidemiology 1989/90 (IARC Scientific Publications No. 101). Edited by M. Coleman & J. Wahrendorf

Directory of On-going Research in Cancer Epidemiology 1991 (IARC Scientific Publications No.110). Edited by M. Coleman & J. Wahrendorf

Directory of On-going Research in Cancer Epidemiology 1992 (IARC Scientific Publications No. 117). Edited by M. Coleman, J. Wahrendorf & E. Démaret

Directory of On-going Research in Cancer Epidemiology 1994 (IARC Scientific Publications No. 130). Edited by R. Sankaranarayanan, J. Wahrendorf & E. Démaret

Directory of On-going Research in Cancer Epidemiology 1996 (IARC Scientific Publications No. 137). Edited by R. Sankaranarayanan, J. Wahrendorf & E. Démaret

IARC (1977) *IARC Monographs Programme on the Evaluation of the Carcinogenic Risk of Chemicals to Humans*. Preamble (IARC intern. tech. Rep. No. 77/002)

IARC (1978) *Chemicals with* Sufficient Evidence *of Carcinogenicity in Experimental Animals —* IARC Monographs *Volumes 1–17* (IARC intern. tech. Rep. No. 78/003)

IARC (1978–1993) *Environmental Carcinogens. Methods of Analysis and Exposure Measurement*, Lyon, IARC*Press*

Vol. 1. Analysis of Volatile Nitrosamines in Food (IARC Scientific Publications No. 18). Edited by R. Preussmann, M. Castegnaro, E.A. Walker & A.E. Wasserman (1978)

Vol. 2. Methods for the Measurement of Vinyl Chloride in Poly(vinyl chloride), Air, Water and Foodstuffs (IARC Scientific Publications No. 22). Edited by D.C.M. Squirrell & W. Thain (1978)

Vol. 3. Analysis of Polycyclic Aromatic Hydrocarbons in Environmental Samples (IARC Scientific Publications No. 29). Edited by M. Castegnaro, P. Bogovski, H. Kunte & E.A. Walker (1979)

Vol. 4. Some Aromatic Amines and Azo Dyes in the General and Industrial Environment (IARC Scientific Publications No. 40). Edited by L. Fishbein, M. Castegnaro, I.K. O'Neill & H. Bartsch (1981)

Vol. 5. Some Mycotoxins (IARC Scientific Publications No. 44). Edited by L. Stoloff, M. Castegnaro, P. Scott, I.K. O'Neill & H. Bartsch (1983)

Vol. 6. N-Nitroso Compounds (IARC Scientific Publications No. 45). Edited by R. Preussmann, I.K. O'Neill, G. Eisenbrand, B. Spiegelhalder & H. Bartsch (1983)

Vol. 7. Some Volatile Halogenated Hydrocarbons (IARC Scientific Publications No. 68). Edited by L. Fishbein & I.K. O'Neill (1985)

Vol. 8. Some Metals: As, Be, Cd, Cr, Ni, Pb, Se, Zn (IARC Scientific Publications No. 71). Edited by I.K. O'Neill, P. Schuller & L. Fishbein (1986)

Vol. 9. Passive Smoking (IARC Scientific Publications No. 81). Edited by I.K. O'Neill, K.D. Brunnemann, B. Dodet & D. Hoffmann (1987)

*Vol. 10. Benzene and Alkylated Benzenes (*IARC Scientific Publications No. 85). Edited by L. Fishbein & I.K. O'Neill (1988)

Vol. 11. Polychlorinated Dioxins and Dibenzofurans (IARC Scientific Publications No. 108). Edited by C. Rappe, H.R. Buser, B. Dodet & I.K. O'Neill (1991)

Vol. 12. Indoor Air (IARC Scientific Publications No. 109). Edited by B. Seifert, H. van de Wiel, B. Dodet & I.K. O'Neill (1993)

IARC (1979) *Criteria to Select Chemicals for* IARC Monographs (IARC intern. tech. Rep. No. 79/003)

IARC (1982) *IARC Monographs on the Evaluation of the Carcinogenic Risk of Chemicals to Humans*, Supplement 4, *Chemicals, Industrial Processes and Industries Associated with Cancer in Humans* (IARC Monographs, Volumes 1 to 29), Lyon, IARC*Press*

IARC (1983) *Approaches to Classifying Chemical Carcinogens According to Mechanism of Action* (IARC intern. tech. Rep. No. 83/001)

IARC (1984) *Chemicals and Exposures to Complex Mixtures Recommended for Evaluation in IARC Monographs and Chemicals and Complex Mixtures Recommended for Long-term Carcinogenicity Testing* (IARC intern. tech. Rep. No. 84/002)

IARC (1987a) *IARC Monographs on the Evaluation of Carcinogenic Risks to Humans*, Supplement 6, *Genetic and Related Effects: An Updating of Selected* IARC Monographs *from Volumes 1 to 42*, Lyon, IARC*Press*

IARC (1987b) *IARC Monographs on the Evaluation of Carcinogenic Risks to Humans*, Supplement 7, *Overall Evaluations of Carcinogenicity: An Updating of* IARC Monographs *Volumes 1 to 42*, Lyon, IARC*Press*

IARC (1988) *Report of an IARC Working Group to Review the Approaches and Processes Used to Evaluate the Carcinogenicity of Mixtures and Groups of Chemicals* (IARC intern. tech. Rep. No. 88/002)

IARC (1989) *Chemicals, Groups of Chemicals, Mixtures and Exposure Circumstances to be Evaluated in Future IARC Monographs, Report of an ad hoc Working Group* (IARC intern. tech. Rep. No. 89/004)

IARC (1991a) *A Consensus Report of an IARC Monographs Working Group on the Use of Mechanisms of Carcinogenesis in Risk Identification* (IARC intern. tech. Rep. No. 91/002)

IARC (1991b) *Report of an ad-hoc* IARC Monographs *Advisory Group on Viruses and Other Biological Agents Such as Parasites* (IARC intern. tech. Rep. No. 91/001)

IARC (1993) *Chemicals, Groups of Chemicals, Complex Mixtures, Physical and Biological Agents and Exposure Circumstances to be Evaluated in Future* IARC Monographs, *Report of an ad-hoc Working Group* (IARC intern. Rep. No. 93/005)

IARC (1998a) *Report of an ad-hoc* IARC Monographs *Advisory Group on Physical Agents* (IARC Internal Report No. 98/002)

IARC (1998b) *Report of an ad-hoc* IARC Monographs *Advisory Group on Priorities for Future Evaluations* (IARC Internal Report No. 98/004)

McGregor, D.B., Rice, J.M. & Venitt, S., eds (1999) *The Use of Short and Medium-term Tests for Carcinogens and Data on Genetic Effects in Carcinogenic Hazard Evaluation* (IARC Scientific Publications No. 146), Lyon, IARC*Press*

Montesano, R., Bartsch, H., Vainio, H., Wilbourn, J. & Yamasaki, H., eds (1986) *Long-term and Short-term Assays for Carcinogenesis — A Critical Appraisal* (IARC Scientific Publications No. 83), Lyon, IARC*Press*

Peto, R., Pike, M.C., Day, N.E., Gray, R.G., Lee, P.N., Parish, S., Peto, J., Richards, S. & Wahrendorf, J. (1980) Guidelines for simple, sensitive significance tests for carcinogenic effects in long-term animal experiments. In: *IARC Monographs on the Evaluation of the Carcinogenic Risk of Chemicals to Humans*, Supplement 2, *Long-term and Short-term Screening Assays for Carcinogens: A Critical Appraisal*, Lyon, IARC*Press*, pp. 311–426

Tomatis, L., Aitio, A., Wilbourn, J. & Shuker, L. (1989) Human carcinogens so far identified. *Jpn. J. Cancer Res.*, **80**, 795–807

Vainio, H., Magee, P.N., McGregor, D.B. & McMichael, A.J., eds (1992) *Mechanisms of Carcinogenesis in Risk Identification* (IARC Scientific Publications No. 116), Lyon, IARC*Press*

Vainio, H., Wilbourn, J.D., Sasco, A.J., Partensky, C., Gaudin, N., Heseltine, E. & Eragne, I. (1995) Identification of human carcinogenic risk in IARC Monographs. *Bull. Cancer*, **82**, 339–348 (in French)

Waters, M.D., Stack, H.F., Brady, A.L., Lohman, P.H.M., Haroun, L. & Vainio, H. (1987) Appendix 1. Activity profiles for genetic and related tests. In: *IARC Monographs on the Evaluation of Carcinogenic Risks to Humans*, Suppl. 6, *Genetic and Related Effects: An Updating of Selected IARC Monographs from Volumes 1 to 42*, Lyon, IARC*Press*, pp. 687–696

Wilbourn, J., Haroun, L., Heseltine, E., Kaldor, J., Partensky, C. & Vainio, H. (1986) Response of experimental animals to human carcinogens: an analysis based upon the IARC Monographs Programme. *Carcinogenesis*, **7**, 1853–1863

GENERAL REMARKS

This ninety-first volume of *IARC Monographs* contains evaluations of the carcinogenic hazard to humans of combined estrogen–progestogen contraceptives and combined estrogen–progestogen menopausal therapy. These hormonal drugs were evaluated previously in Supplement 7 (IARC, 1987) and Volume 72 (IARC, 1999). A recent *IARC Monographs* Advisory Group (IARC, 2003) recommended that they be re-evaluated with high priority, and cited on-going epidemiological studies at that time that might suggest possible associations with additional cancer sites.

The hormonal drugs reviewed in this volume involve co-administration of an estrogen and a progestogen. Studies that did not provide information on the use of combined estrogen–progestogen agents are not reviewed. This volume does not review studies of estrogen-only agents; because of the interactions between estrogens and progestogens, estrogen-only agents are less relevant to an evaluation of combined estrogen and progestogen agents and adequate information is available on such agents themselves. It should be noted that this volume reviews only studies that are publicly available and therefore does not include pharmaceutical test results that are not in the public domain.

Worldwide, 61% of all women of reproductive age (aged 15–49 years) who are married or in a consensual union use contraception. Nine in 10 women who use contraception rely on modern methods, including female sterilization (21%), intrauterine devices (14%) and oral pills (7%). Based on a compilation of sources, it appears that oral contraception is the most widely used method of contraception among married women in developed countries as well as in two-thirds of the developing countries. In 2000, approximately 100 million women worldwide were current users of combined hormonal contraceptives (Blackburn *et al.*, 2000; United Nations, 2004).

Hormonal menopausal therapy was developed during the first half of the twentieth century to control menopausal symptoms and mitigate ageing, and originally comprised estrogen only. Its use increased steadily in the 1960s and 1970s, almost exclusively in North America and western Europe, until 1975 when an increased risk for endometrial cancer was observed. Addition of progestogen to the treatment was found to alleviate the risk, and the use of hormonal menopausal therapy increased again, in a combined estrogen–progestogen form, to peak at about 50 million prescriptions per year in the USA in 2000. In 2002, the Women's Health Initiative identified the treatment as a risk factor for stroke and other heart disorders, and the use decreased dramatically as a consequence.

Comparison of risks and benefits

The conclusion that combined estrogen–progestogen contraceptives increase the risk for some forms of cancer and decrease the risk for others highlights the need for a rigorous quantitative assessment of risks and benefits. This would require quantitative risk estimates for each form of cancer that is increased or decreased, and calculation of absolute risks rather than the relative risks used in this volume to assess causality. A comprehensive assessment would also consider the availability and efficacy of screening for these cancers, the efficacy and side-effects of cancer treatments and the extent to which this information is known or uncertain. The efficacy of cancer screening and treatment varies between different parts of the world; accordingly, the preferred methods of contraception may be specific to a particular country and population. Cervical cancer screening and treatment, for example, vary widely between countries, and cervical cancer is more common in many countries of Africa, Asia and South America. A comprehensive assessment should also go beyond cancer to compare hormonal and non-hormonal methods of contraception, their effectiveness and cost, and adverse and beneficial health effects other than cancer. The evaluations developed in this volume identify specific forms of cancer for which the risk is increased or decreased by combined estrogen–progestogen contraceptives and provide information that will help address the health concerns and well-being of hundreds of millions of women worldwide. Such comprehensive assessments are outside the scope of the *IARC Monographs* but will have important implications for public health.

Uncertainties for women who use both contraceptives and menopausal therapy

This volume considers combined estrogen–progestogen contraceptives and combined estrogen–progestogen menopausal therapy because these two classes of pharmaceuticals have many similarities. Combined contraceptives and combined menopausal therapy both involve co-administration of an estrogen and a progestogen. There is also some concordance in the tumour sites at which the risks for cancer are increased by combined contraceptives and by combined menopausal therapy.

Consequently, there is a possibility that women who use both combined estrogen–progestogen contraceptives and menopausal therapy during their lifetime may experience effects that are greater than those experienced by women who use either contraceptives or menopausal therapy but not both. For example, the conclusion that the increased risk for breast cancer returns to background levels 10 years after cessation of use of combined contraceptives may or may not apply to women who have begun to use combined menopausal therapy. Epidemiological studies of women who have used both combined contraceptives and menopausal therapy will be important to elucidate their joint effects.

Implications for cervical cancer screening

This volume contains a conclusion that combined estrogen–progestogen contraceptives can increase the risk for cervical cancer in women who have a human papillomavirus infection. This suggests that women who use this form of hormonal contraception over a long period of time should be encouraged to participate in cervical cancer screening programmes.

Recent trends in breast cancer incidence

After the Working Group met to develop this volume of *IARC Monographs*, it has been reported that breast cancer incidence in the USA has been declining since 2003 (Jemal *et al.*, 2007; Colditz, 2007). Careful analysis is warranted to determine to what extent this decline may be attributed to the concurrent decline in the use of combined estrogen–progestogen menopausal therapy and whether similar trends are occurring in other countries.

References

Blackburn, R.D., Cunkelman, J.A. & Zlidar, V.M. (2000) *Oral Contraceptives — An Update* (Population Reports, Series A, No. 9), Baltimore, MD, Johns Hopkins University School of Public Health, Population Information Program

Colditz, G.A. (2007) Decline in breast cancer incidence due to removal of promoter: Combination estrogen plus progestin. *Breast Cancer Res.*, **9**, 401

IARC (1987) *IARC Monographs on the Evaluation of Carcinogenic Risks to Humans*, Suppl. 7, *Overall Evaluation of Carcinogenicity: An Updating of* IARC Monographs *Volumes 1 to 42*, Lyon, pp. 272–310

IARC (1999) *IARC Monographs on the Evaluation of Carcinogenic Risks to Humans*, Vol. 72, *Hormonal Contraception and Post-Menopausal Hormonal Therapy*, Lyon

IARC (2003) *Report of an ad-hoc* IARC Monographs *Advisory Group on Priorities for Future Evaluations* (IARC Internal Report No. 03/001), Lyon

Jemal, A., Ward, E. & Thun, M.J. (2007) Recent trends in breast cancer incidence rates by age and tumor characteristics among U.S. women. *Breast Cancer Res.*, **9**, R28

United Nations (2004) *World Population Monitoring 2002, Reproductive Rights and Reproductive Health* (ST/ESA/SER.A/215), New York, Department of Economic and Social Affairs, Population Division

THE MONOGRAPHS

COMBINED ESTROGEN–PROGESTOGEN CONTRACEPTIVES

COMBINED ESTROGEN–PROGESTOGEN CONTRACEPTIVES

These substances were considered by a previous Working Group, in June 1998 (IARC, 1999), under the title 'Oral contraceptives, combined'. Since that time, new data have become available, and these have been incorporated into the monograph and taken into consideration in the present evaluation.

1. Exposure Data

1.1 Introduction

Combined hormonal contraceptives consist of an estrogen and a progestogen, and act primarily by preventing ovulation through the inhibition of follicle-stimulating hormone and luteinizing hormone. The progestogen component also renders the cervical mucus relatively impenetrable to sperm and reduces the receptivity of the endometrium to implantation. These mechanisms render combined hormonal contraceptives very effective in the prevention of pregnancy. Annual failure rates vary between 0.02% (two per 10 000 women/year) when full adherence to instructions for use is assumed (Ketting, 1988) and 5% for typical use (Fu *et al.*, 1999).

A variety of innovations have been developed since combined hormonal contraceptives were first made available in the late 1950s, but not all of these have proved valuable in practice. Changes in drug components, doses used and the temporal sequencing of exposure to drugs have incorporated new technologies and responded to suggested risks. While regional variations in use are abundant, the dominant trends have been towards less androgenic progestogens, lower doses of estrogen and progestogen, the near abandonment of hormonal contraceptives with an estrogen-only phase, a proliferation of different product formulations and the continuing development of novel delivery systems.

In combined hormonal contraception, ethinylestradiol is the most common estrogen, although other are used occasionally. A variety of progestogens is available and these differ in their properties with regard to progestogenic and androgenic characteristics. The estrogen and progestogen contained in combined hormonal contraceptives are usually given in a monthly cycle, and a variety of regimens ensure that the doses of the two constituents produce menstrual cycling. In general, estrogen and progestogen are taken in combination for 21 days followed by 7 drug-free days (often placebo tablets) during which time withdrawal bleeding usually occurs. Other cyclic schedules may be used to reduce or eliminate menses. A constant combination of estrogen and progestogen doses may be used (monophasic) or the doses of progestogen and (less often) estrogen may vary in two (biphasic) or three (triphasic) phases. While oral administration predominates, combined hormonal contraceptives can also be administered by injection, a transdermal patch or a transvaginal device.

Although the primary indication of these medications is to prevent pregnancy through regular use, they are also used to regulate menstrual disorders, to treat acne vulgaris or for emergency contraception. Worldwide, more than 100 million women use combined hormonal contraceptives. While their use is more common in developed countries, substantial consumption also occurs in the developing world. Recent trends suggest that overall use has continued to increase slowly in some regions, while it has remained constant in others. The demographic and social characteristics of combined hormonal contraception users are known to differ from those of non-users of these drugs.

1.2   Historical overview

Researchers in the late nineteenth century noted that follicular development and ovulation were suppressed during pregnancy and that extracts of the corpus luteum inhibited ovulation in laboratory animals. In 1921, Ludwig Haberlandt proposed that similar extracts might act as a contraceptive (IARC, 1999; Fraser, 2000).

Three estrogens were identified in the late 1920s and 1930s — estrone, estriol and estradiol. Progesterone was identified in 1929 and was crystallized in 1934. An oral equivalent of progesterone was not available until 1941, when diosgenin was synthesized from extracts of the Mexican yam. Further experimentation yielded the synthesis of norethisterone (known as norethindrone in the USA) in 1951 and norethynodrel in 1952. These compounds were named progestogens (or progestins) due to their progesterone-like properties (IARC, 1999; Fraser, 2000; Junod & Marks, 2002).

In the early 1950s, the combination of estrogen and progestogen was tested as a treatment for infertility, and it was noted that women who took this combined formulation did not ovulate. In 1956, during clinical trials of oral norethynodrel (a progestogen) as a contraceptive, it was found that preparations that contained mestranol (an estrogen) as a contaminant were more effective in suppressing ovulation than those that contained pure norethynodrel. In 1957, the combination of mestranol and norethynodrel was approved for use in the USA for the regulation of menstruation. Even before this combination was approved as a contraceptive in the USA in 1960, it was already being used for such purposes by 0.5 million women. In the same year, it became available in the United Kingdom. Diffusion of this and a second combined hormonal contraceptive formulation (mestranol and norethisterone) to continental Europe and Latin America occurred somewhat later in 1964–68. By the early 1970s, over 25% of women of child-bearing age in many developed countries were using combined hormonal contraceptives (IARC, 1999; Fraser, 2000; Junod & Marks, 2002; Shampo & Kyle, 2004).

The doses of combined hormonal contraceptives during this early period were 150 µg mestranol and 9.35 mg norethynodrel (Enovid in 1957), but quickly declined to 100 µg mestranol and 2 mg norethisterone (Ortho-Novum in 1964). Doses were further reduced to 50 µg estrogen as confirmation was received that low-dose formulations remained effective with a consequent reduction in adverse effects that had tended to limit continued use. The ease of use, efficacy and reversibility of hormonal contraceptives, as well as changing sexual behaviours and new expectations regarding the regulation of fertility, contributed to the rapid increase in combined hormonal contraceptive use in the 1960s (IARC, 1999; Junod & Marks, 2002).

The upward trend in the use of combined hormonal contraceptives came to a temporary halt in the early 1970s when adverse events associated with their use were highlighted, particularly in women who smoked cigarettes (WHO, 1995). While a variety of side-effects and a risk for thromboembolic events had been recognized earlier, new reports also focused on the risk for cardiovascular disease (Fraser, 2000). As a result, use of combined hormonal contraceptives declined substantially in most developed nations throughout the 1970s. Partly in response to these concerns, a new generation of combined hormonal contraceptives was developed that featured lower doses of estrogen (30 and 35 µg) and newer, more potent progestogens.

Increased use of combined hormonal contraceptives resumed in 1979–81 in many countries, particularly in the light of studies that suggested their relative safety and potential benefits on some outcomes, including reductions in rates of ovarian and endometrial cancer rates (Burkman et al., 2004). At this time, use of combined hormonal contraceptives also increased in many countries in Asia, Africa and the Middle East, facilitated by international aid programmes that were aimed at alleviating the economic consequences of high rates of fertility (IARC, 1999).

At the same time, dose schedules were also modified and refined. With the introduction of biphasic (1982) and triphasic (1984) combined hormonal contraceptives, doses of progestogen were modulated in a manner thought to mimic physiological patterns, although the objective benefits are subject to debate (Van Vliet et al., 2006a,b,c). The previous practice of sequential exposure to estrogen only, followed by combined exposure to estrogen and progestogen, was abandoned after it was found to be associated with an increased risk for endometrial cancer (IARC, 1999).

Further modifications have been made more recently through the continued development of other progestogens, the use of even lower doses of estrogen and the use of alternative dose schedules. Newer progestogens, such as spironolactone-derived drospirenone and more potent and less androgenic gonanes (desogestrel, gestodene), became more common. These formulations were partly aimed at reducing androgenic side-effects such as hirsutism and weight gain. Estrogen doses were reduced to 20 µg and then 15 µg. These low doses may be unsatisfactory for many women because of breakthrough bleeding and they require stricter adherence to instructions for use in order to be effective (Gallo et al.,

2004). Other recent innovations in combined hormonal contraception include devices for transvaginal and transdermal administration, variations in length of schedule (both shorter and longer cycles) and combined injectable formulations.

The increase in the use of combined hormonal contraceptives appeared to diminish in the mid-1990s (IMS Health, 2005), possibly due to renewed concerns regarding adverse effects and the growth of alternative contraceptive technologies (e.g. progestogen-only contraception) in developed countries. Similar declining increases in developing countries may reflect a shift towards greater use of other longer-term contraception, including sterilization, injections of progestogen and intrauterine devices (United Nations, 2004a).

In the 1990s, concerns about potential risks of combined hormonal contraceptives for cardiovascular disease (Hannaford *et al.*, 1994) and thromboembolic events persisted. In addition, the risk for breast cancer, which had been a concern since the introduction of hormonal contraceptives, was also re-emphasized (Collaborative Group on Hormonal Factors in Breast Cancer, 1996a,b). Specific concerns were also raised about the increased incidence of thromboembolism associated with progestogens such as gestodene and desogestrel (Jick *et al.*, 1995; WHO, 1995). In spite of these qualms, the effectiveness, ease of use and the risk profile of combined hormonal contraceptives suggest that they will continue to be used to a significant extent in the future. As in the past, the nature of the exposure associated with the components of combined hormonal contraception will probably continue to evolve.

1.3   Preparations of combined hormonal contraceptives

A plethora of products is available for use in combined hormonal contraceptives. Products that are currently available differ in a number of important aspects, including the estrogen compound used and its dose, the progestogen used, the schedule of exposure to the drugs and the route of administration. In addition, identical formulations may carry different brand names in different countries or even within the same country. These products and their ingredients are presented in Annexes 1–3.

The most common estrogen in combined hormonal contraceptives is ethinylestradiol. Over time, other estrogens have been used, including initially mestranol (a pro-drug of ethinylestradiol) and, more recently, estradiol. In the early development of combined hormonal contraceptives, doses of estrogen in the range of 100–150 µg were commonly used. Contemporary combined hormonal contraceptives may be classified by estrogen dose into 'high-dose' (≥ 50 µg), 'moderate-dose' (30–35 µg) and 'low-dose' (15–20 µg).

A variety of progestogens is used in combined hormonal contraceptives. Currently, they are often distinguished as 'first-generation' estranes (such as norethynodrel or norethisterone), 'second-generation' gonanes (such as levonorgestrel or norgestimate), 'third-generation' gonanes (gestodene and desogestrel) and 'fourth-generation' drospirenone. An additional class of progestogens, the pregnanes (e.g. cyproterone and chlormadinone), may also be used. Estranes are highly androgenic, while pregnanes and drospirenone have anti-androgenic activity. The later gonanes are less androgenic than the earlier compounds in that series. Lower androgenic activity minimizes androgenic side-effects such as acne, hirsutism, nausea and lipid changes. The affinity of individual progestogens for progesterone receptors varies considerably and determines the daily doses required to produce endometrial differentiation. Drospirenone has the lowest affinity (typical daily dose, 3 mg), while the later gonanes have the greatest affinity (0.05–0.15 mg daily dose) (Hammond *et al.*, 2001).

The schedule by which exposure to the drugs occurs may also vary. Most commonly, a constant combination of estrogen and progestogen is used for 3 weeks of a 4-week cycle (monophasic). The doses of progestogen and (less often) estrogen may vary in two (biphasic) or three (triphasic) phases followed by a drug-free phase. While multiphasic schedules seek to mimic physiological variations in exposure to hormones, they may not produce objective benefits over monophasic schedules (Van Vliet *et al.*, 2006a,b). Sequential exposure regimens that used prolonged exposure to estrogen alone are no longer used (IARC, 1999), but a short, 5-day, estrogen-only sequence has been re-introduced. Cycle lengths shorter and longer than 4 weeks may be used with the aim of limiting the duration of menses or eliminating menses altogether (Sulak, 2004). One-day-only use of hormones may be used for emergency contraception.

While oral administration predominates in combined hormonal contraception, the drugs also can be provided by injection, transdermal patch or transvaginal device. Injection of an estrogen and progestogen was used early in the development of hormonal contraception and is still available. Innovations in drug delivery have generated transdermal patches and a vaginal device.

The vast array of products available allows combined hormonal contraception to be tailored to the specific needs and preferences of individual women. While some of the newer products may offer advantages over the older ones, differences in adverse effects and effectiveness are not clear. [In addition, the proliferation of products also represents market differentiation in a large and profitable, but competitive market.]

It is important to recognize that many products are relatively new to the market, particularly those that provide newer progestogens. These, together with products that are currently under development, create a challenge for the evaluation of long-term risk from this class of pharmaceuticals.

1.4   Patterns of use

This section includes the indications of combined hormonal contraceptives, their current prevalence of use globally and trends in the use of these preparations. The characteristics of women who use combined hormonal contraception are also described. Most information on patterns of use of combined hormonal contraceptives is limited to oral forms, and does not include other routes of exposure except for progestogen-only formulations. However, these non-oral forms are generally much less common and information on oral use provides a reasonable proxy for all combined hormonal contraceptive use.

1.4.1   *Prevalence of use*

Based on a compilation of data sources, Blackburn *et al.* (2000) concluded that approximately 100 million women were current users of combined hormonal contraceptives worldwide and, outside of India and China, which have a very low prevalence of use, that 32% of married women in the developing world had ever used them. While variations in their use were enormous, they were the most widely used method of contraception among married women in two-thirds (44/68) of developing countries.

The United Nations (2004b) has compiled data from multiple sources on worldwide patterns of combined hormonal contraceptive use (Table 1). It was estimated that, among women in marital or consensual unions, 7.3% currently use combined hormonal contraception orally and 2.9% currently use hormonal injections or implants. Together, these methods account for 17% of all women who use contraception. Current oral use of combined hormonal contraception is greater in developed nations (15.7%) than in less developed nations (5.8%) (see Table 1), while the converse is true of injectable preparations and implants (0.7% versus 3.3%).

Reported use in the late 1990s varied considerably by region, with a relatively high prevalence of use among women in northern Africa, South-East Asia, South America, North America, New Zealand/Australia and Europe (except eastern Europe) (United Nations, 2004b). On a national level, particularly high prevalences of use were noted in Algeria (44%), Bangladesh (23%), Brazil (21%), Hungary (38%), Iran (21%), Kuwait (29%), Morocco (32%), Thailand (23%) and Zimbabwe (36%). In addition, all countries in western Europe had a prevalence above 30%. In many cases, countries adjacent to those with high prevalence of use had low prevalence: China (2%), India (2%), Peru (7%), Poland (2%), Rwanda (1%), Sudan (5%) and Yemen (4%). A range of factors contribute to these striking differences, including level of economic development, patterns of foreign aid and national family planning programmes (United Nations, 2004c).

Lundberg *et al.* (2004) presented additional information on worldwide variations in use. Current use among women aged 25–44 years varied from < 1 to 58%. In general, the variations within countries were relatively small compared with those between countries. In accordance with other studies, particularly high oral use of combined hormonal contraceptives was noted in western Europe and Australia/New Zealand.

Ross *et al.* (2002) suggested that a hierarchy of preferences for contraceptive methods exists in developing countries and depends on availability of contraception. At the highest level of access, sterilization is generally the method of choice, followed by oral contraceptives, intrauterine devices and condoms in decreasing order of preference. On the contrary, oral contraceptives are the most prevalent method in those countries that have the lowest mean availability of contraception.

Ali and Cleland (2005) also noted substantial variations in oral use of combined hormonal contraceptives within South and Central America where it was fairly prevalent in Brazil and Nicaragua, but low in Peru and Bolivia.

Table 1. Prevalence of oral use of combined hormonal contraceptives worldwide

	No. of women included[a]	Prevalence of oral contraceptive use[b]		Proportion of oral contraceptive use among all forms of contraception (%)[c]	Year of survey
		Mean (%)	Range (%)		
World	1 043 265	7.3		12.1	1998
More developed[d]	170 043	15.7		22.9	1996
Less developed[e]	873 223	5.8		9.8	1998
Africa	117 120	7.3		27.2	1999
Eastern		5.9	1.4–35.5		
Middle		1.6	1.0–16.7		
Northern		17.7	5.1–44.3		
Southern		10.4	5.4–14.7		
Western		2.7	1.8–18.2		
Asia	293 294	4.5		7.1	1997
China		1.7			
India		2.1			
South Central Asia		4.8	0.6–23.0		
South-East Asia		12.8	6.2–23.1		
Western Asia		6.4	1.0–28.8		
Europe	109 277	17.4		26.0	1995
Eastern		6.9	2.3–37.7		
Northern		19.2	3.9–26.0		
Southern		11.8	4.5–21.7		
Western		48.2	30.8–58.6		
Latin America and Caribbean	81 810	13.8		19.5	1997
Caribbean		7.6	2.3–31.5		
Central America		7.5	5.0–18.0		
South America		17.1	3.8–24.5		
USA/Canada	42 029	15.5		20.3	1995
Australia/New Zealand	2 989	23.3		30.7	1998
Oceania (except Australia/ New Zealand)	1 303	4.7	4.4–22.6	17.6	1996

From United Nations (2004b)

[a] Women aged 15–49 in a marital or consensual union (in thousands)

[b] Includes all formulations of oral contraceptives.

[c] Includes oral contraceptives, male and female sterilization, injectable implants, intrauterine devices, condoms, vaginal barriers, other modern methods, rhythm, withdrawal and other traditional methods.

[d] More developed: Europe, USA/Canada, Australia/New Zealand, Japan

[e] Less developed: Latin America and the Caribbean, Africa, Asia (except Japan), Oceania (except Australia and New Zealand)

Yuzpe (2002) reported that 17% of women of reproductive age in the USA were current users of oral contraceptives in 1995. In 2000, it was estimated that there were more than 10 million users in the USA, and that use was more common among younger women. In the USA, 80% of women born after 1945 have used oral contraceptives at some time (Blackburn *et al.*, 2000).

1.4.2   Trends in prevalence

Information on trends over time also indicates substantial heterogeneity between countries. Different investigators have reached contradictory conclusions on whether world-wide use is increasing or remains constant. Bongaarts and Johansson (2000) tracked changes in combined oral contraceptive use in the developing world and projected that it would double between 1993 (11% of women) and 2015 (22%). This trend is attributed to improved access, changes in the characteristics of users with better education, a desire for smaller families and new and improved technology. In contrast, Zlidar *et al.* (2003) suggested that use among married women had been more or less constant in 38 developing countries since 1990. However, Blackburn *et al.* (2000) noted very large increases in oral contraceptive use in Bangladesh (from 3 to 21%), Kenya (from 3 to 9%) and Morocco (from 13 to 32%) between 1978 and 1998, while rates declined or remained similar in Colombia, India and Egypt during the same period. A United Nations analysis of data on trend suggested little net change over time. Substantial variations were noted, however, with sizeable increases or decreases in selected countries (United Nations, 2004a).

Data on sales of combined hormonal contraceptives (IMS Health, 2005) confirmed many of the data on prevalence observed in the United Nations data compilation, but indi-cated increasing use worldwide (Table 2). A worldwide increase of 19% between 1994 and 1999 and a subsequent 21% increase from 1999 to 2004 were noted. The largest relative increases occurred in eastern Europe, the eastern Mediterranean, South-East Asia and the western Pacific. Only modest increases were observed in Africa and South America. It should be noted that these data may not include large quantities of hormonal contraceptives that are provided by national and international family planning programmes. Several other trends are indicated from the sales data: (i) the use of higher estrogen doses (≥ 50 µg) has continued to decline; (ii) growth in the use of products that contain later progestogens (gestodene, desogestrel) has slowed down and in some countries there has been a shift back to earlier progestogens (norethynodrel, norethis-terone); and (iii) monophasic hormonal formulations have continued to predominate with some shift away from multiphasic forms (IMS Health, 2005).

On the basis of case–control data from several large cities in the USA, the most frequent duration of use among controls was 1–5 years, although some women reported use for more than 15 years (Marchbanks *et al.*, 2002).

While most use of combined hormonal contraception is for on-going contraception, additional common indications include emergency contraception, regulation of menstrual disorders and treatment of acne. In a study of use in Dutch adolescents (14–17 years old),

Table 2. Trends in sales of combined hormonal contraceptives for selected years (millions of standard units[a])

Regions[b]	1994	1999	2004
Africa	9.5	10.4	10.2
South Africa	8.9	9.7	9.5
West Africa	0.6	0.6	0.7
Eastern Mediterranean	14.8	16.7	20.7
Europe	259.3	293.4	338.1
Eastern Europe	14.3	31.9	46.0
Western Europe	245.0	261.5	292.2
North America	103.3	122.4	161.0
South America	91.1	103.6	110.9
South-East Asia	17.0	45.0	70.1
Bangladesh	6.4	4.2	6.9
India	0	22.1	15.4
Republic of Korea	2.7	2.3	2.9
Rest of South-East Asia	7.9	16.4	44.9
Western Pacific	21.7	24.7	34.6
Australia/New Zealand	16.5	16.6	15.9
China/Hong Kong	0.2	0.7	0.9
Japan	0	0.6	3.0
Taiwan, China	1.4	1.3	1.4
Rest of Western Pacific	3.6	5.4	13.5
Total	516.9	616.4	745.8

From IMS Health (2005)

[a] Standard units, sales in terms of standard dose units; the standard dose unit for oral products is one tablet or capsule.

[b] The countries were grouped according to the WHO classification:

West Africa includes: Benin, Burkina, Cameroon, Congo, Gabon, Guinea, Ivory Coast, Mali, Senegal, Togo;

Eastern Mediterranean includes: Egypt, Jordan, Kuwait, Lebanon, Morocco, Saudi Arabia, Tunisia, United Arab Emirates;

Eastern Europe includes: Belarus, Bulgaria, Czech Republic, Estonia, Hungary, Latvia, Lithuania, Poland, Russian Federation, Slovakia, Slovenia, Ukraine;

Western Europe includes: Austria, Belgium, Denmark, Finland, France, Germany, Greece, Ireland, Israel, Italy, Luxembourg, Netherlands, Norway, Portugal, Spain, Sweden, Switzerland, Turkey, United Kingdom;

North America includes: Canada, Central America (Costa Rica, El Salvador, Guatemala, Honduras, Nicaragua, Panama), Mexico, Puerto Rico, USA;

Rest of South-East Asia includes: Indonesia, Pakistan, Thailand;

South America includes: Argentina, Brazil, Chile, Colombia, Dominican Republic, Ecuador, Peru, Uruguay, Venezuela;

Rest of Western Pacific includes: Malaysia, Philippines, Singapore.

current use for indications other than contraception (34%) included use for irregular cycles (18%), dysmenorrhoea (25%) and acne (11%) (van Hooff *et al.*, 1998).

The characteristics of women who use combined contraceptives differ from those who do not. Use appears to be more frequent among women who are younger and more highly educated, and increases with access to modern contraceptives (Piccinino & Mosher, 1998; Ross *et al.*, 2002).

Characteristics of users depend on regional differences and have evolved over time. Women have gradually begun to use oral contraceptives at younger ages, and initiation of use at 15–19 years of age is now frequent, while in the past it tended to start at 20–24 years of age. One study in the Netherlands reported a large increase in use among 15–17-year-old girls (Van Hooff *et al.*, 1998). In contrast, Piccinino and Mosher (1998) observed a decline in use among teenagers between 1988 and 1995 in the USA.

2. Studies of Cancer in Humans

2.1   Breast cancer

2.1.1   *Background*

In the previous evaluation of exogenous hormones and risk for cancer in women (IARC, 1999), the overall assessment of the use of combined oral contraceptives and the risk for breast cancer relied heavily on the work of the Collaborative Group on Hormonal Factors in Breast Cancer (1996a,b) (Figure 1). More than 50 case–control and cohort studies that included over 53 000 women with breast cancer had assessed the relation between use of combined oral contraceptives and risk for breast cancer. The weight of the evidence suggested a small increase in the relative risk among current and recent users of combined oral contraceptives. The small increase in risk was not related to duration of use, type of use or dose of the preparation used. By 10 years after cessation of use, the risk for breast cancer in women who had used combined oral contraceptives was similar to that of women who had never used this type of contraception (Figure 2). It was concluded that, if the reported association was causal, the excess risk for breast cancer associated with typical patterns of current use of combined oral contraceptives was very small.

2.1.2   *Use of combined oral contraceptives and detection of breast cancer*

The increase in risk for breast cancer associated with the use of combined oral contraceptives in younger women could be due to more frequent contacts with doctors, which leads to earlier detection of breast cancer through mammography, breast examination or echography. An effect of early detection would normally lead to an increase in the number of women diagnosed with in-situ or early stage breast cancer (i.e. tumour node metastasis stage I or cancer < 2 cm in size).

Figure 1. Relative risk for breast cancer in ever-users compared with never-users of combined oral contraceptives

Median year of diagnosis	Study	Combined oral contraceptive use		Statistics		Relative risk of breast cancer in ever-users versus never-users	
		Ever Cases/Controls	Never Cases/Controls	(O-E)	var(O-E)	RR* & 99% CI	RR*±SD
	PROSPECTIVE STUDIES						
1980	RCGP[15]	198/728	128/576	13·0	55·6		1·26±0·151
1982	Oxford/FPA[26]	96/437	101/342	-9·7	26·6		0·69±0·162
1985	NursesHealth[22]	1105/4243	1645/6703	35·6	431·0		1·09±0·050
1985	CanadianNBSS[37]	741/2905	594/2418	11·5	209·2		1·06±0·071
1987	AmerCancSoc[42]	264/1091	907/3671	1·5	93·4		1·02±0·104
1988	Netherlands Cohort[46]	105/408	348/1248	2·9	46·1		1·06±0·152
	Other[5,11,14,19]	138/431	436/1576	2·5	25·4		1·10±0·208
	All prospective studies	2647/10243	4159/16534	57·3	887·3		1·07±0·035
	CASE-CONTROL STUDIES, WITH POPULATION CONTROLS						
1976	Brinton[24]	714/781	2503/2764	14·0	193·7		1·07±0·075
1980	Bernstein/Pike[3,27]	373/369	66/70	0·3	21·3		1·01±0·218
1981	Hislop[8]	370/414	579/535	-5·0	51·5		0·91±0·133
1981	CASH[34]	2815/2872	1879/1784	-27·9	394·7		0·93±0·049
1983	UKNational[25]	684/673	71/82	5·9	31·2		1·20±0·197
1983	Bain/Siskind[23]	197/424	343/671	-3·9	31·6		0·88±0·167
1983	Ewertz[35]	479/458	1066/941	-4·0	80·8		0·95±0·109
1984	Meirik/Lund[9]	289/338	133/189	8·7	42·0		1·23±0·171
1984	Long Island[33]	266/230	914/950	13·8	57·2		1·27±0·149
1984	Clarke[38]	257/543	350/669	-4·0	47·8		0·92±0·139
1985	Yu/Yuan/Wang[18,40]	184/180	650/654	6·7	44·0		1·16±0·163
1985	Paul/Skegg[28]	674/1521	217/343	4·5	69·2		1·07±0·124
1987	Daling[50]	685/875	62/86	-0·0	26·5		1·00±0·194
1988	4StateStudy[47]	2427/3726	4443/5793	8·9	416·6		1·02±0·050
1988	Rookus/van Leeuven[49]	781/782	137/136	2·5	40·0		1·07±0·163
1989	Yang/Gallagher[41]	407/441	609/584	-15·3	55·1		0·76±0·118
1989	Primic-Zakelj[48]	296/297	323/322	3·0	58·1		1·05±0·135
1991	WISH[53]	1532/1597	334/412	20·5	119·8		1·19±0·100
	Other[2,10,12,17,21,39,52]	1563/2029	1417/2141	16·3	168·5		1·10±0·081
	All case-control studies, with population controls	14993/18550	16096/19126	44·8	1949·6		1·02±0·023
	CASE-CONTROL STUDIES, WITH HOSPITAL CONTROLS						
1980	Vessey[4,13]	963/972	1420/1419	8·5	193·4		1·04±0·074
1981	Ravnihar[16]	161/460	370/1479	26·6	59·2		1·57±0·163
1983	WHO(developing)[30]	525/5117	1180/9936	27·6	177·1		1·17±0·081
	WHO (developed)[30]	667/1933	922/2116	10·9	157·6		1·07±0·082
1986	Clavel[31]	247/424	248/472	8·6	44·1		1·21±0·166
1987	LaVecchia[45]	366/238	2897/2490	30·2	94·1		1·38±0·121
1992	Franceschi[51]	382/314	2187/2274	25·3	104·7		1·27±0·111
	Other[6,7,20,29,32,36,43,44]	616/1378	1879/3543	10·1	102·5		1·10±0·104
	All case-control studies, with hospital controls	3927/10836	11103/23729	147·8	932·7		1·17±0·035
	ALL STUDIES·	21567/39629	31358/59389	249·8	3769·6		1·07±0·017

0.0 0.5 1.0 1.5 2.0

Test for heterogeneity between study designs: X^2 (2 df)=11·6; p=0·003
Test for heterogeneity between studies: X^2 (33 df)=51·8; p=0·02

From Collaborative Group on Hormonal Factors in Breast Cancer (1996a)
Separate results are given for individual studies. Each relative risk and its 99% confidence interval (CI) is plotted as a black square and a line. The area of the square is proportional to the amount of statistical information (i.e. to the inverse of the variance of the logarithm of the relative risk). Diamonds indicate 99% CIs for totals. The solid vertical line represents a relative risk of 1.0 and the broken vertical line indicates the overall relative risk estimate for all studies combined.
*Relative risk (given with 99% CI) relative to never-users, stratified by study, age at diagnosis, parity and, where appropriate, the age of a woman when her first child was born and her age when her risk for conception ceased.
The numbers next to the references refer to the citations in the original article.

Figure 2. Relative risk for breast cancer by time since last use of combined oral contraceptives

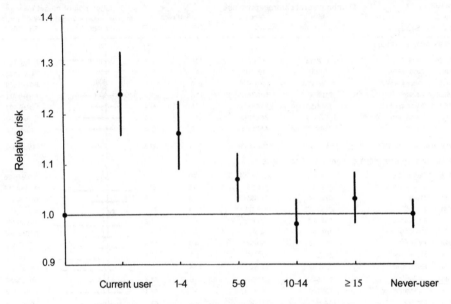

From Collaborative Group on Hormonal Factors in Breast Cancer (1996a,b)
Relative risk (given with 95% confidence interval [CI]) relative to no use, stratified by study, age at diagnosis, parity, age at first birth and age at which risk for conception ceased.

An analysis of the methods of detection of breast cancer in the Cancer and Steroid Hormone Study (CASH, 1986) found that, among women 20–44 years of age, 86% of breast cancers in oral contraceptive users and 84% of breast cancers in non-users were detected by the women themselves (Schlesselman *et al.*, 1992). In both groups, 2% or fewer of cancers were detected by mammography. Proportions of in-situ carcinomas were 4% and 5% in non-users and users, respectively. On average, the tumour diameter was 0.3 cm smaller in women who had used oral contraceptives ($p < 0.001$). Similar results were found in women aged 45–54 years. In clinical terms, however, that difference in size is small, and the authors concluded that the net effect of any diagnostic bias on advancing the date of diagnosis of cancer was less than 8 weeks. This corresponds to a spurious increase in the risk of early occurring breast cancer in oral contraceptive users of at most 2.4% (relative risk, 1.024).

Two large-scale studies of breast cancer and oral contraceptive use in the USA found significantly increased risks in women under 35 years of age who had used oral contraceptives for 5 years or more (Brinton *et al.*, 1995) or for 10 years or more (White *et al.*, 1994). Both studies examined breast screening and methods of diagnosis in case and control women, and concluded that the increased risks could not be explained by differences in screening or in biopsy rates between oral contraceptive users and non-users.

In the Women's CARE (Contraceptive and Reproductive Experience) study (Marchbanks *et al.*, 2002), the risk for invasive breast cancer with current low-estrogen oral contraceptive use was 1.5 (95% confidence interval [CI], 0.9–2.6) in women aged 45–64 years. In order to exclude a screening effect, the authors analysed the data after exclusion of women with stage I tumours. They did not report the data but stated that the relative risk did not decrease.

In the study conducted in Los Angeles, USA, cases of breast cancer included in-situ and invasive tumours (Ursin *et al.*, 1998). To examine the probability of early detection bias, the authors limited the analysis to invasive cancers and, although results were not reported, they stated that the findings remained unchanged.

2.1.3   *Cohort studies* (Table 3)

Grabrick *et al.* (2000) studied 426 families of women who were diagnosed with breast cancer at a tumour clinic in Minnesota, USA. Among a total of 6150 women who were studied, 239 cases of breast cancer were diagnosed. The aim of the study was to assess whether family history of breast cancer might modify the association between use of combined oral contraceptives and the risk for breast cancer. Among the entire cohort, ever use of oral contraceptives was associated with a relative risk of 1.4 (95% CI, 1.0–2.0) for breast cancer. The risk for 4 or more years of use was 1.3 (95% CI, 0.9–1.9). The relative risk for breast cancer associated with ever use of combined oral contraceptives was 3.3 (95% CI, 1.6–6.7) among sisters and daughters of the probands, 1.2 (95% CI, 0.8–2.0) among granddaughters and nieces of the probands and 1.2 (95% CI, 0.8–1.9) among women who had married into the families. The positive association with breast cancer among relatives of the probands was mainly confined to the use of oral contraceptives before 1975.

The long-term effects of oral contraceptives have been examined in a nested case–control study from the Netherlands. Van Hoften *et al.* (2000) studied the effect of past use of combined oral contraceptives and the long-term risk for developing breast cancer. Within a cohort of more than 12 000 women, 309 cases of breast cancer had developed during 7 years of follow-up, and these were compared with 610 controls. The risk for ever use of combined oral contraceptives was 1.31 (95% CI, 0.96–1.79). Duration of use was not associated with risk for breast cancer (relative risk, 1.43; 95% CI, 0.92–2.22) but, in a sub-analysis of women over 55 years of age who had used oral contraceptives for more than 10 years, the relative risk was 2.1 (95% CI, 1.1–4.0; based on 22 exposed cases) compared with never users.

The Women's Lifestyle and Health cohort combined data from Norway and Sweden, and included more than 103 000 women who were aged 30–49 years at entry into the study in the early 1990s (Kumle *et al.*, 2002). The population was followed up for breast cancer incidence by linkage to the Norwegian and the Swedish Cancer Registries; during 10 years of follow-up, 1008 women were diagnosed with invasive breast cancer. The relative risk was 1.3 (95% CI, 1.1–1.5) for ever use of combined oral contraceptives, 1.6 (95% CI, 1.2–2.1) for current use of any type of oral contraceptives at the beginning of follow-up and

Table 3. Cohort studies on the use of oral contraceptives and the risk for breast cancer

Reference	Country	Age at recruitment (years)	Size of cohort	Period of cohort	Histological diagnosis	No. of cases	Any use (%)	Relative risk (95% CI), any versus none	Relative risk (95% CI), longest duration	Relative risk (95% CI), current, recent use
Grabrick et al. (2000)[a]	USA	21–88	6 150	1991–96	NS	239	51	1.4 (1.0–2.0)	1.3 (0.9–1.9)	No difference between strata (data not shown)
Van Hoften et al. (2000)[b]	Netherlands	42–63	12 184	1982–96	NS	309	62.1	1.31 (0.96–1.79)	1.43 (0.92–2.22)	NS
Kumle et al. (2002)	Norway and Sweden	30–49	103 027	1991–99	Invasive	1008	74.11	1.3 (1.1–1.5)	1.3 (1.0–1.8)	1.6 (1.2–2.3)
Dumeaux et al. (2003)[c]	Norway	30–70	96 362	1991–97	Invasive	851	61.29	1.25 (1.07–1.46)	1.40 (1.09–1.79)	1.06 (0.39–2.87)
Dumeaux et al. (2004)[c,d]	Norway	30–70	86 948	1991–97	Invasive	1130	NS	NS	1.29 (1.05–1.60)	NS

CI, confidence interval; NS, not specified
[a] Cases included high-risk population
[b] Nested case–control study
[c] 63 patients were excluded from the multivariate analysis. Norwegian component of the study by Kumle et al. (2002)
[d] Update of Dumeaux et al. (2003), with adjustment for alcoholic beverage consumption. Included only women with complete information on alcoholic beverage consumption and duration of oral contraceptive use.

1.2 (95% CI, 1.1–1.4) for past use (before recruitment to the study). The results showed no increase in risk with longest duration of use. In relation to time since last use, the risk appeared to be higher in women who had used oral contraceptives within the last 2 years (relative risk, 1.6; 95% CI, 1.2–2.3) compared with women who had stopped using oral contraceptives 10–14 years previously (relative risk, 1.2; 95% CI, 1.0–1.6). Slightly stronger associations were related to early use (before the age of 20 years) and to relatively long-term use before first birth, but these were of borderline statistical significance.

In the Norwegian component of the previous study (Dumeaux *et al.*, 2003), the investigators studied whether specific types of estrogens and progestogens contained in oral contraceptives exert different effects on the risk for breast cancer. Among more than 96 000 women, 851 cases of invasive breast cancer were diagnosed during follow-up. The relative risk for ever use of combined oral contraceptives was 1.25 (95% CI, 1.07–1.46). An increased risk was related to use for 10 years or more (relative risk, 1.40; 95% CI, 1.09–1.79), but no trend in risk related to recency of use ($p = 0.42$) or to time since last use. In this study, the investigators examined the dose of estrogen contained in the respective brands of oral contraceptives, and reported a relative risk of 1.5 (95% CI, 1.1–2.0) associated with a cumulative dose of 100 mg or more. Within the same cohort, Dumeaux *et al.* (2004) studied whether the association with use of combined oral contraceptives may be modified by the use of alcoholic beverages. More than 86 000 women were followed up and included in the analysis, and 1130 cases of invasive breast cancer were diagnosed. The results suggested that combined oral contraceptives had an increasing effect on risk only among low consumers of alcoholic beverages (i.e. < 5 g per day) and not among women who reported regular use of alcoholic beverages ($p \leq 0.0001$).

2.1.4 *Case–control studies* (Table 4)

A case–control study in the USA assessed whether the combined use of oral contraceptives at a young age may increase the risk for breast cancer (Brinton *et al.*, 1998). The participants were under 55 years of age and included 1031 cases of breast cancer and 919 population controls. The study reported that the relative risk associated with ever use was 1.14 (95% CI, 0.9–1.4).

In Taiwan, China, where the incidence of breast cancer is generally low, Chie *et al.* (1998) studied the association between the use of combined oral contraceptives and subsequent risk for breast cancer in a case–control study of 174 cases and 453 hospital-based controls. The odds ratio for ever versus never use of oral contraceptives was 1.7 (95% CI, 0.9–3.2), and appeared to be somewhat higher among women who had started using oral contraceptives before the age of 25 years (odds ratio, 3.5; 95% CI, 1.2–9.7) and women who had used them for 5 years or more (odds ratio, 2.1; 95% CI, 0.8–5.6).

In a case–control study from California, Ursin *et al.* (1998) examined the use of combined oral contraceptives and the risk for breast cancer in young women. The aim of the study was to assess aspects of oral contraceptive use that may be important for the increased risk related to current or recent use in young women. The study included more

Table 4. Case–control studies of the use of oral contraceptives and the risk for breast cancer

Reference, location	Years of case diagnosis	Age (years)	Histology	Use	Ever versus never				Longest duration of use					Current/recent use				Time since last use
					Cases	Controls	Odds ratio	95% CI	Cases	Controls	Odds ratio	95% CI	Use (years)	Cases	Controls	Odds ratio	95% CI	
Brinton et al. (1998), USA	1990–92	<55	In-situ or invasive	Never	283	278	Ref.		283	278	Ref.							
				Ever	748	641	1.14	0.9–1.4	173	127	1.27	0.9–1.7	≥10					
Chie et al. (1998), Taiwan, China	1993–94	NS	NS	Never	149	406	Ref.		149	406	Ref.							
				Ever	25	47	1.7	0.9–3.2	9	15	2.1	0.8–5.6	≥5					
Ursin et al. (1998), USA	1983–88	≤40	In-situ and invasive	Never	124	116	Ref.		124	116	Ref.			124	116	Ref.		
				Ever	618	626	0.83	0.62–1.12	52	30	1.4	0.81–2.40	>12	111	84	1.14	0.75–1.72	<1 year
Magnusson et al. (1999), Sweden	1993–95	50–74	Invasive	Never	1733	1938	Ref.		1733	1938	Ref.			1733	1938	Ref.		
				Ever	898	889	0.98	0.86–1.12	357	353	0.98	0.82–1.18	≥5	73	59	1.0	0.69–1.44	<10 years
Ursin et al. (1999), USA	1983–87	20–55	NS	Never	383	594	Ref.		383	594	Ref.			383	594	Ref.		
				Ever	207	351	0.91	0.72–1.15	45	87	0.71	0.47–1.07	>5	29	63	0.68	0.41–1.14	<5 years
Shapiro et al. (2000), South Africa	1994–97	20–54	Invasive	Never	264	992	Ref.		264	992	Ref.			264	992	Ref.		
				Ever	220	633	1.2	1.0–1.5	16	39	1.2	0.7–2.3	>10	16	53	1.2	0.7–2.0	<5 years
Tessaro et al. (2001), Brazil	1995–98	20–60	NS	Never	45[a]	141[a]	Ref.		45[a]	141[a]	Ref.							
					42[b]	112[b]	Ref.		41[b]	111[b]	Ref.							
				Ever	127[a]	375[a]	1.1	0.7–1.6	38[a]	92[a]	1.2	0.7–2.0	>12					
					126[b]	392[b]	0.9	0.6–1.6	35[b]	123[b]	1.0	0.5–1.8						
Heimdal et al. (2002), Norway	1999	40–60	NS	Never	NR	NR	Ref.							NR	NR			
				Ever	NR	NR	0.9	0.68–1.18						NR	NR	1.99	0.80–4.98	0–4 years
Marchbanks et al. (2002), USA	1994–98	35–64	Invasive	Never	1032	980	Ref.		1032	980	Ref.			1032	980	Ref.		
				Ever	3497	3658	0.9	0.8–1.0	234	202	1.0	0.8–1.3	>15	200	172	1.0	0.8–1.3	<7 months

Table 4 (contd)

Reference, location	Years of case diagnosis	Age (years)	Histology	Use	Ever versus never				Longest duration of use					Current/recent use				Time since last use
					Cases	Controls	Odds ratio	95% CI	Cases	Controls	Odds ratio	95% CI	Use (years)	Cases	Controls	Odds ratio	95% CI	
Narod et al. (2002)[c], 11 countries	1977–2001	47.3 ± 10	Invasive	Never	NR	NR	Ref.							NR	NR	Ref.		
				Ever	NR	NR	1.2	1.02–1.52						NR	NR	0.83	0.66–1.04	< 1 year
Althuis et al. (2003), USA	1990–92	20–44	In-situ and invasive	Never	371	406	Ref.											
				Ever	1269	1086	1.24	1.0–1.5						309	258	1.47	1.2–1.9	≤ 5 years
Claus et al. (2003), USA	1994–98	20–79	Ductal carcinoma in situ	Never	425	465	Ref.		425	465	Ref.			425	465	Ref.		
				Ever	404	522	1.0	0.8–1.2	47	61	0.9	0.6–1.5	≥ 10	17	38	0.6	0.3–1.3	< 1 year
Newcomer et al. (2003), USA	NS	< 75	Lobular and ductal	Never	Lobular 334	5864	Ref.											
				Ever	159	3447	1.2	0.9–1.6						Lobular 6	141	2.6	1.0–7.1	
				Never	Ductal 3391	5864	Ref.											
				Ever	1676	3447	1.0	0.9–1.1						Ductal 47	141	1.2	0.8–1.9	

CI, confidence interval; NR, not reported; NS not specified; Ref., reference

[a] Hospital cases/controls

[b] Neighbourhood cases/controls

[c] Results only for *BRCA1* mutation carriers

than 700 women under 40 years of age who had invasive breast cancer or ductal carcinoma *in situ* and 744 population controls matched to the cases. The relative risk for ever versus never use was 0.83 (95% CI, 0.62–1.12) and that for use of oral contraceptives for 12 years or more was 1.4 (95% CI, 0.8–2.4). These results were adjusted for age, age at menarche, age at first birth, parity, duration of breast feeding and physical activity.

In another report restricted to Asian immigrants to California, Ursin *et al.* (1999) studied the relation between combined oral contraceptive use and risk for breast cancer. The study included nearly 600 cases of breast cancer and 1000 population controls. The results showed that the use of oral contraceptives increased with increasing time since migration, but there was no indication that use of oral contraceptives increased the risk for breast cancer. The relative risk for ever versus never use was 0.91 (95% CI, 0.72–1.15). The investigators conducted several subgroup analyses, according to age when the women started using oral contraceptives, duration of use and time since last use, but found no consistent association related to the use of oral contraceptives and the risk for breast cancer in any of these analyses.

In a large case–control study from Sweden, Magnusson *et al.* (1999) studied reproductive factors and the risk for breast cancer among women 50–74 years of age. As part of the study, the investigators also collected information on past use of combined oral contraceptives and were thus able to evaluate whether use in the past influenced the risk for breast cancer after the menopause. The study included 3016 women with invasive breast cancer and 3263 population controls without breast cancer, but information on oral contraceptives was available only for a subset of the population. The results showed no clear association with ever use of oral contraceptives (relative risk, 0.98; 95% CI, 0.86–1.12) and no association related to duration of use (*p* for trend = 0.88). The odds ratio for last use < 10 years previously was 1.00 (95% CI, 0.69–1.44) compared with never users. These results were adjusted for age, age at menarche, parity, age at first birth, menopausal status, age at menopause, height, body mass index and use of combined hormonal menopausal therapy.

The use of oral contraceptives in relation to the risk for breast cancer has been assessed in a case–control study in South Africa (Shapiro *et al.*, 2000). The primary aim of the study was to examine the effects of injectable contraceptives, but information was also collected on the use of oral contraceptives. Shapiro *et al.* (2000) included women aged 20–54 years who came from a defined area close to Cape Town, and were of either black or mixed racial descent. The odds ratio associated with ever use of oral contraceptives was 1.2 (95% CI, 1.0–1.5), that for use of 10 or more years was 1.2 (95% CI, 0.7–2.3) and that associated with use within the last 5 years was 1.2 (95% CI, 0.7–2.0). In analyses within age groups, the relative risk for ever use was 1.7 (95% CI, 1.0–3.0; based on 36 exposed cases) in women under 35 years of age, 1.2 (95% CI, 0.8–1.6; based on 91 exposed cases) in women aged 35–44 years and 1.1 (95% CI, 0.8–1.6; based on 93 exposed cases) in women aged 45–54 years.

A case–control study from Brazil (Tessaro *et al*., 2001) reported the use of combined oral contraceptives and the risk for breast cancer using different groups of controls, but the results showed no association with ever use or with duration of use.

In a case–control study of high-risk families, Heimdal *et al*. (2002) studied the use of combined oral contraceptives in carriers of the *BRCA1* mutation in relation to risk for breast cancer. The hazard ratio for ever use of oral contraceptives was 0.90 (95% CI, 0.68–1.18) in the total data set and 3.00 (95% CI, 0.36–10.2) in *BRCA1* carriers.

A large case–control study in the USA also aimed at studying whether the use of combined oral contraceptives at a relatively young age is associated with risk for breast cancer later in life (Marchbanks *et al*., 2002). The study included more than 4500 women with breast cancer and a similar number of controls from the same area as the cases, identified by random-digit dialling, aged 35–64 years. There was no association with ever use of oral contraceptives (odds ratio, 0.9; 95% CI, 0.8–1.0); the odds ratio was 1.0 (95% CI, 0.8–1.3) for current use and 0.9 (95% CI, 0.8–1.0) for use in the past. There was no increase in risk related to duration of use, age at first use or time since last use, and no increase in risk for breast cancer associated with any use of oral contraceptives that contained a relatively high dose of estrogen (relative risk, 0.8; 95% CI, 0.7–0.9; based on 1082 exposed cases). The relative risk associated with first use between 15 and 19 years was 1.0 (95% CI, 0.8–1.1; based on 1239 exposed cases). The results did not differ for black and white women, and there was no increase in risk associated with oral contraceptive use of women who had a family history of breast cancer. These results were adjusted for age, age at menarche, age at first birth, parity, body mass index, menopausal status and use of combined hormonal therapy.

Women who are carriers of *BRCA1* and *BRCA2* mutations have an inherited increase in risk for breast cancer. Narod *et al*. (2002) investigated whether women with these characteristics who have used combined oral contraceptives are at particularly high risk in a matched case–control study of 1311 pairs of women with known *BRCA1* or *BRCA2* mutations. Use of oral contraceptives was not associated with an increase in risk for those who were carriers of *BRCA2* mutations. However, the results suggested that *BRCA1* carriers may be at slightly elevated risk if they had used oral contraceptives before 1975, if they had used them before the age of 30 years and if the use had lasted for at least 5 years.

Althuis *et al*. (2003) studied risk for breast cancer related to current or recent use of combined oral contraceptives in a case–control study of women aged 20–44 years. The study involved more than 1600 women with invasive breast cancer and a comparable number of community controls. The odds ratio for ever use of oral contraceptives was 1.24 (95% CI, 1.0–1.5). Women who had used oral contraceptives within the last 5 years had a relative risk of 1.47 (95% CI, 1.2–1.9) and the odds ratio in women who had stopped taking oral contraceptives at least 10 years previously was 1.13 (95% CI, 0.9–1.4). Compared with never users, women who had used oral contraceptives that contained more than 35 µg ethinylestradiol were at higher risk (relative risk, 1.99; 95% CI, 1.2–3.2; based on 54 exposed cases) than women who used lower-dose preparations (relative risk, 1.27; 95% CI,

0.9–1.7; based on 161 exposed cases). In the subgroup of women under 35 years of age, the relative risk associated with ever use was 2.05 (95% CI, 1.3–3.2; based on 209 exposed cases), that for use within the last 5 years was 2.22 (95% CI, 1.4–3.5; based on 135 exposed cases) and that for cessation of use 10 or more years previously was 1.52 (95% CI, 0.8–3.0; based on 31 exposed cases). In this subgroup, dose of estrogen was also associated with an increased risk for breast cancer: the odds ratio associated with using oral contraceptives that contained high-dose estrogen was 3.62 (95% CI, 1.7–7.9; based on 27 exposed cases) and that for use of low-dose estrogen contraceptives was 1.91 (95% CI, 1.1–3.2; based on 81 exposed cases), compared with the risk in never users.

In a case–control study in the USA, Claus *et al.* (2003) assessed whether the use of combined oral contraceptives was associated with the development of ductal breast carcinoma *in situ* by comparing more than 800 cases with this condition and approximately 1000 control women aged 20–79 years. The results showed no association between any use of oral contraceptives and the risk for breast cancer *in situ* (odds ratio, 1.0; 95% CI, 0.8–1.2).

The association between oral contraceptive use and the risk for breast cancer was investigated in a population-based case–control study in the USA (Norman *et al.*, 2003) that included 1847 postmenopausal women with invasive breast cancer and 1932 controls (not shown in Table 4). The aim of the study was to assess the combined effect of use of oral contraceptives at a young age and use of hormonal therapy after the menopause. The report did not present detailed results related to the use of oral contraceptives alone, but stated that the use of oral contraceptives, independent of the use of hormonal therapy, was not associated with a risk for breast cancer.

Whether the use of combined oral contraceptives has different effects on various histological subtypes of breast cancer was investigated by Newcomer *et al.* (2003) in a case–control study of women under 75 years of age (mean age, 57.5 years). The study involved 493 women with lobular breast cancer, 5510 women with ductal carcinoma and 9311 randomly selected controls. The odds ratio for ever versus never use of oral contraceptives was 1.2 (95% CI, 0.9–1.6) for lobular breast carcinoma and 1.0 (95% CI, 0.9–1.1) for ductal carcinoma. The odds ratio associated with current use was 2.6 (95% CI, 1.0–7.1; based on six exposed cases) for lobular carcinoma, and there was a significant trend ($p = 0.02$) of increased risk with more recent use. Current use of oral contraceptives was not clearly associated with risk for ductal carcinoma (odds ratio, 1.2; 95% CI, 0.8–1.9). Among women who had started using oral contraceptives before the age of 20 years, the odds ratio was 1.0 (95% CI, 0.5–1.9; based on 17 exposed cases) for lobular carcinoma and 1.0 (95% CI, 0.8–1.2; based on 217 exposed cases) for ductal carcinoma.

2.2   Endometrial cancer

When the association between endometrial cancer and use of combined oral contraceptives was last reviewed, relevant data were available from three cohort studies and 16 case–control studies (IARC, 1999). The results from these studies consistently showed that the risk for endometrial cancer was reduced in women who had used oral contraceptives, and the reduction in risk was greater with longer duration of use. The evidence for combined oral contraceptives (including studies that were reviewed in 1999) is summarized here, together with new studies.

The cohort and case–control studies in which use of combined oral contraceptives and the risk for endometrial cancer has been investigated are summarized below and, when available, the risk associated with duration and recency of use is given. Risk estimates for women of different weight and parity (or gravidity) or who are users of hormonal meno-pausal therapy are given when available.

2.2.1   *Descriptive studies*

Several analyses have suggested that increased use of combined oral contraceptives can partially explain the decreasing rates of mortality from cancer of the uterine corpus (i.e. excluding those from cervical cancer) seen between 1960 and the 1980s (Beral *et al.*, 1988; Persson *et al.*, 1990; dos Santos Silva & Swerdlow, 1995). The decrease is particularly evident among women aged 55 years or younger, who most probably used combined oral contraceptives. Interpretation of these trends is complicated by improvements in cancer treatment over time and by a lack of correction for the proportion of women who had their uterus removed and were no longer at risk for developing (or dying from) endometrial cancer. Furthermore, the rates of death from cancer of the uterine corpus have generally decreased since the early 1950s, a decade before oral contraceptives were available. Thus, while it is plausible that increased use of combined oral contraceptives could have preceded and then paralleled the decrease in mortality from endometrial cancer, the magni-tude of any decrease in the rate of death from cancer of the uterine corpus that is related to increased use of oral contraceptives remains unclear.

2.2.2   *Cohort studies*

A questionnaire to obtain information on oral contraceptive use was sent to approxi-mately 97 300 married women aged 25–57 years in eastern Massachusetts, USA, in 1970, who were identified from the 1969 Massachusetts residence lists (Trapido, 1983). The age-standardized rate ratio for women who had ever used oral contraceptives relative to non-users was 1.4 (95% CI, 0.9–2.4); there was no consistent pattern of a risk with longer or more recent use (Table 5). Among nulliparous women, the age-adjusted rate ratio for oral contraceptive users relative to non-users was 2.4 (95% CI, 0.6–9.2), whereas the analogous rate ratio for parous women was 1.4 (95% CI, 0.8–2.4). Among women who also reported any use of menopausal estrogen therapy, the age-adjusted rate ratio for oral contraceptive users relative to non-users was 2.0 (95% CI, 0.9–4.3). No distinction was made between sequential and combined oral contraceptive use, and both preparations were available to the cohort before and during the study follow-up.

Beral *et al.* (1988) followed up approximately 23 000 oral contraceptive users and a similar number of non-users identified in 1968 and 1969 by the Royal College of General

Table 5. Cohort studies of the use of oral contraceptive pills[a] and the risk for endometrial cancer

Reference, location	Age (range/median)	Source population	Follow-up	Type/measure of therapy	No. of cases	No. of person-years	Relative risk (95% CI)
Trapido (1983), USA	25–57 years	97 300 residents of Boston and 14 contiguous towns	1970–76	No use	75	296 501	1.0
				Any use	18	124 851	1.4 (0.9–2.4)
				Duration (months)			
				1–11	6	33 997	1.7 (NR)
				12–23	4	21 978	1.9 (NR)
				24–35	3	21 437	1.6 (NR)
				36–59	2	28 705	0.6 (NR)
				≥ 60	3	18 734	1.5 (NR)
Beral et al. (1988), United Kingdom	49 years	46 000 British women identified by general practitioners	1968–87 (incidence) Dec. 1993 (mortality)	No use	16	182 866	1.0
				Any use	2	257 028	0.2 (0.0–0.7)
				No use	6	335 998	1.0
				Any use	2	517 519	0.3 (0.1–1.4)
Vessey & Painter (1995), United Kingdom	25–39 years	17 032 patients at 17 family planning clinics	1968–93	No use	14	NR	1.0
				Any use	1	NR	0.1 (0.0–0.7)
Kumle et al. (2003), Norway	30–70 years	102 443 Norwegian women	1991–99	No use			1.0
				Ever use			0.59 (0.38–0.92)
				Duration (years)			
				< 5	23	28 115	0.66 (0.39–1.10)
				5–9	8	12 159	0.65 (0.31–1.39)
				> 10	5	8 840	0.41 (0.15–1.13)
				No information	38	53 328	

CI, confidence interval; NR, not reported
[a] May be use of either combined or sequential oral contraceptive pills, but the majority of women used combined

Practitioners. Use of oral contraceptives (not otherwise specified) and the occurrence of uterine cancer were both determined from physicians' reports. Endometrial cancer was diagnosed in two of the oral contraceptive users and 16 of the non-users, which resulted in a rate ratio of 0.2 (95% CI, 0.0–0.7) after adjustment for age, parity, tobacco smoking, social class, number of previously normal Papanicolaou (Pap) smears and history of sexually transmitted disease. In a 25-year follow-up of deaths in the cohort (Beral *et al.*, 1999), eight deaths from endometrial cancer occurred, two among women who had ever used oral contraceptives and six among women who had never used them (rate ratio, 0.3; 95% CI, 0.1–1.4).

The Oxford Family Planning Association Study included 17 032 white married women identified at 17 family planning clinics in England and Scotland (Vessey & Painter, 1995) who had used oral contraceptives (not otherwise specified), a diaphragm or an intrauterine device for at least 5 months. Information on contraceptive history and any hospital referrals was obtained from physicians or from the women themselves (for those who stopped attending the clinics) during the study follow-up. A total of 15 292 women remained under observation until the age of 45 years; only those who had never used oral contraceptives (5881) or had used them for 8 years or more (3520) were followed from that time onwards. Endometrial cancer was diagnosed in 15 women, only one of whom had used oral contraceptives (age-adjusted rate ratio, 0.1; 95% CI, 0.0–0.7). In a previous analysis of mortality in this cohort (Vessey *et al.*, 1989), none of the oral contraceptive users but two of those who used a diaphragm or an intrauterine device (the comparison group) had died from endometrial cancer.

Kumle *et al.* (2003) followed 102 443 Norwegian women aged 30–70 years who were recruited into a cohort study in 1991–97. Endometrial cancers were identified by linkage to the Cancer Registry of Norway. Follow-up was through to December 1999, during which time 110 endometrial cancers were diagnosed. The relative risk associated with use of combined oral contraceptives was 0.59 (95% CI, 0.38–0.92). For use of less than 5 years, 5–9 years and more than 10 years, the relative risks were 0.66 (95% CI, 0.39–1.10), 0.65 (95% CI, 0.31–1.39) and 0.41 (95% CI, 0.15–1.13), respectively. Among the users of oral contraceptives, there was a significant trend of decreasing risk for endometrial cancer with increasing duration of use of oral contraceptives ($p = 0.03$).

2.2.3 *Case–control studies* (Table 6)

Among 152 women who had endometrial cancer and 516 controls in a hospital-based study in the USA and Canada (Kaufman *et al.*, 1980), a 60% reduction in risk was seen among women who used combined oral contraceptives relative to non-users. The risk for endometrial cancer declined with increasing duration of use, and a sustained reduction in risk was suggested among women who had stopped using oral contraceptives during the previous 5 years or more.

Weiss and Sayvetz (1980), in a population-based case–control study from western Washington State (USA), found that women who had used combined oral contraceptives for

Table 6. Case–control studies of use of combined oral contraceptives and the risk for endometrial cancer (by duration and recency of use when available)

Reference, location	Age	Source of controls	Ascertainment of use	Participation (%) Cases	Participation (%) Controls	Type/measure of use	No. of subjects Cases	No. of subjects Controls	Odds ratio (95% CI)
Kaufman et al. (1980), Canada and USA	< 60 years	Hospital patients	Personal interviews	96[a]	96[a]	No use	136	411	1.0
						Any use	16	105	[0.4 (0.2–0.8)[b]]
						Duration (years)			
						< 1	5	14	0.8 (NR)
						1–2	6	32	0.5 (NR)
						≥ 3	5	53	0.3 (NR)
						Unknown	0	6	
						Recency of use			
						≥ 5 years	12	60	0.6 (0.3–1.2)
						Use ≥ 1 year	8	52	0.5 (0.2–1.0)
Weiss & Sayvetz (1980), Washington State, USA	36–55 years	General population	Personal interviews	83	96	No use or < 1 year of use	93	173	1.0
						≥ 1 year of use	17	76	0.5 (0.1–1.0)
Hulka et al. (1982), North Carolina, USA	< 60 years	General population	Personal interviews and medical record reviews	90[a]	90[a]	No use or < 6 months' use	74	172	1.0
						≥ 6 months' use	5	31	0.4 (NR)
						Duration (years)			
						< 5	3	14	0.6 (NR)
						≥ 5	2	17	0.3 (NR)
						Recency (years)			
						< 1	0	13	–
						≥ 1	5	14	0.9 (NR)
Kelsey et al. (1982), Connecticut, USA	45–74 years	Hospital patients	Personal interviews	67	72	No use	NR	NR	1.0
						Each 5 years of use	NR	NR	0.6 (0.3–1.5)
						Age 45–55 years			
						No use	31	256	1.0
						Duration (years)			
						≤ 2.5	4	42	0.9 (NR)
						> 2.5	2	44	0.5 (NR)

Table 6 (contd)

Reference, location	Age	Source of controls	Ascertainment of use	Participation (%) Cases	Participation (%) Controls	Type/measure of use	No. of subjects Cases	No. of subjects Controls	Odds ratio (95% CI)
Henderson et al. (1983a), Los Angeles county, USA	≤ 45 years	Residents in neighbourhood of cases	Telephone interviews	81	NR	No use	67	50	1.0
						Duration (years)			
						< 2	23	22	0.8 (NR)
						2–3	12	11	0.8 (NR)
						4–5	4	9	0.3 (NR)
						≥ 6	4	18	0.1 (NR)
La Vecchia et al. (1986), greater Milan, Italy	< 60 years	Hospital patients	Personal interviews	98[c]	98[c]	Non-user	163	1104	1.0
						Any use	7	178	0.50 (0.23–1.12)
Pettersson et al. (1986), Uppsala, Sweden	≤ 60 years	General population	Personal interviews	93	80	No use	96	91	1.0
						Any use	12	22	0.5 (0.2–1.1)
						Duration (years)			
						< 1	5	6	0.8 (0.2–2.7)
						≥ 1	7	16	0.4 (0.2–1.0)
CASH (1987a), eight US areas	20–54 years	General population	Personal interviews	73	84	No use	250	1147	1.0
						Ever use	NR	NR	0.5 (0.4–0.6)
						Duration (months)			
						3–6	24	186	0.9 (0.5–1.5)
						7–11	13	80	1.3 (0.6–2.6)
						12–23	20	266	0.7 (0.4–1.2)
						24–71	26	576	0.4 (0.3–0.7)
						72–119	12	317	0.4 (0.2–0.8)
						≥ 120	15	241	0.4 (0.2–0.8)
						Recency (years)			
						< 5	12	471	0.3 (0.1–0.5)
						5–9	22	417	0.4 (0.2–0.6)
						10–14	30	368	0.5 (0.3–0.8)
						≥ 15	9	144	0.3 (0.2–0.6)

Table 6 (contd)

Reference, location	Age	Source of controls	Ascertainment of use	Participation (%)		Type/measure of use	No. of subjects		Odds ratio (95% CI)
				Cases	Controls		Cases	Controls	
WHO Collaborative Study (1988); Rosenblatt et al. (1991), nine centers in seven countries: Australia, Chile, China, Israel, Mexico, the Philippines, Thailand	< 60 years	Hospital patients	Personal interviews	87	93	No use	182	1072	1.0
						Progestogen content			
						High			
						Ever use	3	156	0.1 (0.1–0.4)
						Duration (months)			
						1–24	1	85	0.1 (0.0–0.7)
						≥25	2	69	0.2 (0.0–0.8)
						Recency (months)			
						1–120	1	61	0.1 (0.0–0.8)
						≥121	2	93	0.2 (0.0–0.7)
						Low			
						Ever use	9	132	0.6 (0.3–1.2)
						Duration (months)			
						1–24	8	69	1.0 (0.5–2.4)
						≥25	1	56	0.1 (0.0–1.1)
						Recency (months)			
						1–120	2	72	0.3 (0.0–1.1)
						≥121	7	54	1.1 (0.5–2.8)
Koumantaki et al. (1989), Athens, Greece	40–79 years	Hospital patients	Personal interviews	80	95	No use or ≤ 6 months' use	80	151	1.0
						> 6 months' use	3	13	0.6 (0.2–2.0)[d]
Levi et al. (1991), Canton of Vaud, Switzerland	32–75 years	Hospital patients	Personal interviews	85[a]	85[a]	No use	105	227	1.0
						Any use	17	82	0.5 (0.3–0.8)
						Duration (years)			
						< 2	9	19	1.0 (0.5–2.3)
						2–5	3	18	0.5 (0.1–1.2)
						> 5	5	45	0.3 (0.1–0.7)
						Recency (years)			
						< 10	4	30	0.3 (0.1–0.9)
						10–19	7	37	0.4 (0.2–1.0)
						> 19	5	15	0.8 (0.3–2.2)

Table 6 (contd)

Reference, location	Age	Source of controls	Ascertainment of use	Participation (%)		Type/measure of use	No. of subjects		Odds ratio (95% CI)
				Cases	Controls		Cases	Controls	
Shu et al. (1991), Shanghai, China	18–74 years	General population	Personal interviews	91	96	No use of any birth control	84	72	1.0
						Any use of oral contraceptives	32	46	0.8 (0.4–1.8)
						Duration (years)			
						≤ 2	NR	NR	1.4 (0.6–3.0)
						> 2	NR	NR	0.4 (0.1–1.2)
Jick et al. (1993), Washington State, USA	50–64 years	Members of health maintenance organization	Mailed form and pharmacy database	83	79	No use	110	737	1.0
						Any use	26	270	0.5 (0.3–0.9)
						Duration (years)			
						1	7	65	0.4 (0.1–1.4)
						2–5	11	90	0.8 (0.3–1.7)
						≥ 6	8	115	0.3 (0.1–0.9)
						Recency (years)			
						1–10	5	67	0.4 (0.1–1.1)
						11–15	6	82	0.4 (0.1–1.2)
						16–20	4	57	0.5 (0.1–1.8)
						≥ 21	9	54	0.6 (0.2–2.1)
Stanford et al. (1993), five US areas	20–74 years	General population	Personal interviews	87	66	No use	321	187	1.0
						Any use	81	107	0.4 (0.3–0.7)
						Duration (years)			
						< 1	27	21	0.7 (0.3–1.4)
						1–2	16	33	0.3 (0.1–0.6)
						3–4	12	16	0.3 (0.1–0.8)
						5–9	14	15	0.7 (0.3–1.6)
						≥ 10	7	19	0.2 (0.1–0.5)
						Recency (years)			
						< 10	6	18	0.1 (0.0–0.3)
						10–14	15	27	0.3 (0.1–0.7)
						15–19	24	32	0.4 (0.2–0.8)
						≥ 20	33	27	0.7 (0.4–1.3)

Table 6 (contd)

Reference, location	Age	Source of controls	Ascertainment of use	Participation (%) Cases	Participation (%) Controls	Type/measure of use	No. of subjects Cases	No. of subjects Controls	Odds ratio (95% CI)
Voigt et al. (1994)[e], Washington State, USA	40–59 years	General population	Personal interviews	83	95 and 73[f]	No use or < 1 year of use	117	284	1.0
						Recency of use			
						> 10 years			
						Duration (years)			
						1–5	14	30	0.9 (0.4–1.9)
						> 5	4	16	0.4 (0.1–1.2)
						≤ 10 years			
						Duration (years)			
						1–5	7	28	1.0 (0.4–2.4)
						> 5	7	74	0.3 (0.1–0.6)
						Progestogen content			
						Low			
						Duration (years)			
						1–5	10	22	1.1 (0.5–2.6)
						> 5	3	32	0.2 (0.1–0.8)
						High			
						Duration (years)			
						1–5	3	14	0.8 (0.2–3.1)
						> 5	3	28	0.3 (0.1–0.9)
Kalandidi et al. (1996), Athens, Greece	< 59–≥ 70 years	Hospital patients	Personal interviews	83	88	No use	143	293	1.0
						Any use	2	5	1.3 (0.2–7.7)
Salazar-Martinez et al. (1999), Mexico City, Mexico	37.1 (mean) years	Hospital patients	Personal interviews	100	93	No use	71	473	1.0
						Duration (years)			
						< 1	6	78	0.56 (0.22–1.30)
						> 1	7	117	0.36 (0.15–0.83)
Weiderpass et al. (1999), Sweden	50–74 years	General population	Self-completed questionnaire	75	80	No use	551	2252	1.0
						Duration (years)			
						< 3	91	421	1.0 (0.7–1.3)
						> 3	45	518	0.5 (0.3–0.7)

Table 6 (contd)

Reference, location	Age	Source of controls	Ascertainment of use	Participation (%)		Type/measure of use	No. of subjects		Odds ratio (95% CI)
				Cases	Controls		Cases	Controls	
Jain et al. (2000), Ontario, Canada	30–79 years	Population	Personal interview	70	59	No use Any use	317 195	265 248	1.0 0.66 (0.51–0.84)
Parslov et al. (2000), Denmark	> 50 years	Population	Self-completed questionnaire	93	91	No use *Duration (years)* < 1 1–5 > 5	90 52 50 45	75 95 210 158	1.0 0.4 (0.3–0.7) 0.2 (0.1–0.3) 0.2 (0.1–0.4)
Newcomb & Trentham-Deitz (2003), Wisconsin, USA	40–79 years	Population	45-min telephone interview	87	85.2	No use *Duration (years)* < 3 > 3	460 74 54	1494 260 275	1.0 1.04 (0.74–1.40) 0.73 (0.52–1.02)

CI, confidence interval; NR, not reported

[a] Responses reported for case and control women combined
[b] Crude odds ratio and 95% CI calculated from data provided in the published paper by exact methods
[c] Methods state that less than 2% of eligible case and control women refused an interview.
[d] 90% confidence interval
[e] Includes women from the study of Weiss & Sayvetz (1980).
[f] Response for controls identified in 1985–87

1 year or more had half the risk for endometrial cancer of women who were either non-users or had used combined oral contraceptives for less than 1 year (odds ratio, 0.5; 95% CI, 0.1–1.0). The risk estimates were adjusted for age and use of menopausal estrogen therapy. No further difference in duration of use was seen between cases and controls. In stratified analyses, the reduced risk was present only for women who had never used menopausal estrogen therapy (odds ratio, 0.4; 95% CI, 0.1–1.1) or who had used it for 2 years or less (odds ratio, 0.1; 95% CI, 0.01–1.1); no risk reduction was noted among women who had used it for 3 years or more (odds ratio, 1.3; 95% CI, 0.3–6.6).

Among 79 women treated at a hospital in North Carolina, USA, for endometrial cancer, 6.3% had used combined oral contraceptives for 6 months or longer compared with 15.3% of the 203 controls from 52 counties in the State (the main referral area for the hospital) (Hulka *et al.*, 1982).

Kelsey *et al.* (1982) studied women who were admitted to seven hospitals in Connecticut, USA. A total of 167 newly diagnosed cases of endometrial cancer were compared with 903 control women admitted for non-gynaecological surgery. Among the study participants aged 45–55 years — women who had had the opportunity to use oral contraceptives — those who had used oral contraceptives for 2.5 years or more had a 50% decrease in risk for endometrial cancer.

Henderson *et al.* (1983a) identified women with endometrial cancer from the population-based cancer registry for Los Angeles County and matched them to control women of similar age who lived in the same neighbourhood as the case. The risk for endometrial cancer decreased with increasing duration of use of combined oral contraceptives, and this pattern remained after further adjustment for parity, current weight, infertility and amenorrhoea. Neither the recency of use of oral contraceptives nor their relative estrogen and progestogen content had a clear impact on the risk, beyond that explained by duration of use (data not shown). When the analysis was stratified by body weight, a reduction in risk with longer duration of use was seen among women who weighed less than 170 lbs [77 kg] but not among women who weighed more.

In a hospital-based study in the area of greater Milan, Italy, La Vecchia *et al.* (1986) compared the use of combined oral contraceptives by women admitted for endometrial cancer and by women admitted for traumatic, orthopaedic, surgical and other conditions. Seven (4%) of the 170 case women and 178 (14%) of the 1282 control women reported use of combined oral contraceptives, which resulted in an odds ratio of 0.50 (95% CI, 0.23–1.12) after adjustment for age, marital status, education, parity, age at menarche, age at first birth, age at menopause, body mass index, cigarette smoking and use of non-contraceptive female hormones.

Pettersson *et al.* (1986) studied 254 women who resided in the health care region of Uppsala (Sweden) and who were referred to the Department of Gynaecologic Oncology with a newly diagnosed endometrial malignancy; each case was matched by age and county of residence to one control woman who was identified from a population registry. Use of combined oral contraceptives was analysed for women aged 60 years or under, and 108 cases and 113 controls were analysed. Women who had ever used contraceptives and users for 1 year or more had a lower risk than non-users (odds ratios, 0.5; 95% CI, 0.2–1.1; and 0.4; 95% CI, 0.2–1.0, respectively). [The Working Group noted that it is unclear whether the estimates were adjusted for potentially confounding factors.]

In a population-based study conducted by the Centers for Disease Control and the National Institute of Child Health and Human Development in the USA, women 20–54 years of age with newly diagnosed endometrial cancer were identified from eight cancer registries (Atlanta, Detroit, San Francisco, Seattle, Connecticut, Iowa, New Mexico and four urban counties in Utah) in the US Surveillance, Epidemiology and End Results (SEER) Program; 3191 controls were selected from the general population (CASH, 1987a). Women who had used only combined oral contraceptives had half the risk for endometrial cancer of non-users (age-adjusted odds ratio, 0.5; 95% CI, 0.4–0.6). The risk generally decreased with increasing duration of oral contraceptive use, and the greatest reduction in risk was seen among women who had used combined oral contraceptives for 2 years or more. The strength of the association was similar after adjustment for age alone and after multivariate adjustment for age, parity, education, body mass, menopausal status, geographical region, exogenous estrogen use and infertility. The risk for endometrial cancer did not vary with recency of use of combined oral contraceptives or with time since first use; women who had ceased use of oral contraceptives 15 years or more before the study interview and women who had first used oral contraceptives more than 20 years before the interview had a lower risk than non-users (age-adjusted odds ratios, 0.3 [95% CI, 0.2–0.6] and 0.4 [95% CI, 0.2–0.7], respectively). When the analysis was stratified by formulation of the oral contraceptive, all formulations that had been used for at least 6 months or more were associated with a decreased risk for endometrial cancer.

In a worldwide multicentre hospital-based study (nine centres in seven countries), the use of combined oral contraceptives was compared in 132 women who had endometrial cancer and 836 control women who were admitted to units other than obstetrics and gynaecology in each centre between 1979 and 1986 (WHO Collaborative Study of Neoplasia and Steroid Contraceptives, 1988). Women who had used combined oral contraceptives only had a lower risk for endometrial cancer than non-users (odds ratio, 0.5; 95% CI, 0.3–1.0), after adjustment for socioeconomic status, source of referal, use of injectable contraceptives, menopausal status, age of menopause, total number of pregnancies and years until becoming pregnant after infertility. The numbers of cases (total, 220) and control women (total, 1537) in this study continued to accrue through to 1988 and these were then further evaluated by Rosenblatt et al. (1991). Oral contraceptives were classified as being low-estrogen dose if they contained less than 50 µg ethinylestradiol or less than 100 µg mestranol and as being high-estrogen dose if they contained larger amounts of these estrogens. Based on their ability to induce subnuclear vacuolization in the endometrium, progestogens in oral contraceptives were classified as being high and low potency. The level of reduction in risk for endometrial cancer was related to both the estrogen dose and progestogen potency of the preparation: odds ratios for ever use were 1.1 (95% CI, 0.1–9.1) for high estrogen–low progestogen, 0.6 (95% CI, 0.3–1.3) for low estrogen–low progestogen,

0.2 (95% CI, 0.05–0.5) for high estrogen–high progestogen and 0.0 (95% CI, 0.0–1.1) for low estrogen–high progestogen preparations.

Koumantaki *et al.* (1989) studied women who had endometrial cancer and were admitted to two hospitals in Athens, Greece, and control women who were admitted to the Athens Hospital for Orthopaedic Disorders. Only three (4%) of the 83 case women and 13 (8%) of the 164 controls had used combined oral contraceptives for 6 months or longer (odds ratio, 0.6; 90% CI, 0.2–2.0, adjusted for age, parity, age at menarche, age at meno-pause, menopausal estrogen use, years of smoking, height and weight).

Among 122 women who were treated at a major referral hospital in the Canton of Vaud (Switzerland) for endometrial cancer, 14% had used combined oral contraceptives, as had 27% of the 309 control women admitted to the same hospital for non-neoplastic, non-gynaecological conditions (Levi *et al.*, 1991). The risk decreased from 1.0 (95% CI, 0.5–2.3) for use of less than 2 years to 0.5 (95% CI, 0.1–1.2) for use of 2–5 years and 0.3 (95% CI, 0.1–0.7) for use of more than 5 years. Oral contraceptive use within the previous 10 years (odds ratio, 0.3; 95% CI, 0.1–0.9) or within the previous 10–19 years (odds ratio, 0.4; 95% CI, 0.2–1.0) and first use before the age of 30 years (odds ratio, 0.3; 95% CI, 0.1–0.7) were all associated with a reduction in the risk for endometrial cancer. Women who had used oral contraceptives for 5 years or longer had a reduction in risk even when use had occurred 20 or more years previously. The risk estimates were adjusted for age, area of residence, marital status, education, parity, body mass, cigarette smoking and use of menopausal estrogen therapy. Little variation in risk was seen by categories of body mass (odds ratios, 0.6 for < 25 kg/m² and 0.2 for ≥ 25 kg/m²) or cigarette smoking (odds ratios, 0.5 for ever smokers and 0.6 for never smokers). Stratification by use of menopausal estrogen therapy was also presented (odds ratios, 0.4 for ever use and 0.5 for never use). There was no significant difference in the relative risk between nulliparous women (six cases and 14 controls) who used oral contraceptives (age-adjusted odds ratio, 0.8; 95% CI, 0.2–2.9) and the parous oral contraceptive users (11 cases and 68 controls; age-adjusted odds ratio, 0.3; 95% CI, 0.1–0.7).

Shu *et al.* (1991) studied 116 Chinese women who had endometrial cancer identified from the population-based Shanghai Cancer Registry and 118 control women identified from the Shanghai Residents' Registry. The odds ratio for use of oral contraceptives (not otherwise specified) compared with never use of this type of contraception, after adjustment for age, gravidity and weight, was 0.8 (95% CI, 0.4–1.8). When the duration of use was evaluated, there was a suggestion that oral contraceptive use for more than 2 years was associated with a greater reduction in the risk for endometrial cancer (odds ratio, 0.4; 95% CI, 0.1–1.2).

Jick *et al.* (1993) studied women who were members of a large health maintenance organization in western Washington State, USA. Women in whom endometrial cancer had been diagnosed were identified from the organization's tumour registry; the controls were also members of the organization. Both groups included only women who used the phar-macies of the organization and who had previously completed a questionnaire sent to all female members for a mammography study. Use of oral contraceptives (not otherwise specified), determined from the questionnaire, was reported by 18% of cases and 26% of controls which gave an odds ratio of 0.5 (95% CI, 0.3–0.9), adjusted for age, date of enrolment in the organization, body mass, age at menopause, parity and current use of menopausal estrogen therapy. In comparison with non-users, the reduced risk for endometrial cancer was most pronounced for women who had used oral contraceptives for 6 years or more (odds ratio, 0.3; 95% CI, 0.1–0.9) or within the last 10 years (odds ratio, 0.4; 95% CI, 0.1–1.1).

In the USA, 402 women who had endometrial cancer diagnosed at seven hospitals (in Chicago, IL; Hershey, PN; Irvine and Long Beach, CA; Minneapolis, MN; and Winston-Salem, NC) and 294 age-, race- and residence-matched control women from the general population agreed to be interviewed (Stanford et al., 1993). Use of combined oral contraceptives was reported by 20% of the cases and 36% of the controls (odds ratio, 0.4; 95% CI, 0.3–0.7, after adjustment for age, education, parity, weight and use of menopausal estrogen therapy). There was no clear pattern of decreasing risk with increasing duration of use. Relative to non-users, a strong reduction in risk was noted for women who had used these preparations within the last 10 years (odds ratio, 0.1; 95% CI, 0.0–0.3) and for those who had first used them less than 15 years previously (odds ratio, 0.1; 95% CI, 0.0–0.4); both of these effects waned with more distant oral contraceptive use. The risk estimates varied little by age at first use (< 25, 25–29, 30–34, ≥ 35 years). When duration and recency were evaluated jointly, use within the previous 20 years was more strongly predictive of a reduction in risk than longer duration of use (≥ 3 years). In a joint evaluation with other possible modifying factors, 3 or more years of use of combined oral contraceptive was associated with a reduced risk for endometrial cancer among women of high parity (odds ratio for women with five or more births, 0.2; 95% CI, 0.0–0.6), women who weighed less than 150 lbs [68 kg] (odds ratio, 0.4; 95% CI, 0.2–0.9) and women who had never (odds ratio, 0.2; 95% CI, 0.1–0.6) or briefly (< 3 years) (odds ratio, 0.8; 95% CI, 0.2–3.2) used menopausal estrogen therapy.

Voigt et al. (1994) combined the study population described in the study of Weiss and Sayvetz (1980) with a similar study population identified between 1985 and 1987 in western Washington State, USA. A reduction in risk for endometrial cancer associated with combined oral contraceptive use was present only among users of 5 or more years of duration, and even then only in women who were not long-term users of unopposed postmenopausal estrogens. Among these women, the risk did not substantially vary according to progestogen potency of the combined oral contraceptive used. When duration and recency of use of combined oral contraceptives were evaluated jointly, longer use (> 5 years) was associated with a reduced risk for endometrial cancer irrespective of recency (last use, ≤ 10 years ago versus > 10 years ago). When duration and the relative potency of the progestogens in the formulation were evaluated jointly, a longer duration of use (> 5 years), and not progestogen dose, was most predictive of a reduced risk.

Kalandidi et al. (1996) studied 145 women who had endometrial cancer and were admitted to two hospitals in Athens, Greece, and 298 control women who were admitted to the major accident hospital in Athens with bone fractures or other orthopaedic disorders.

Only two (1%) of the cases and five (1.7%) of the controls had ever used oral contraceptives (not otherwise specified). The multivariate-adjusted risk estimate was 1.3 (95% CI, 0.2–7.7).

Salazar-Martinez *et al.* (1999) conducted a hospital-based case–control study in Mexico City that involved 84 women who had endometrial cancer diagnosed in 1995–97 and 668 controls from 63 hospitals. The odds ratio for use of oral contraceptives for less than 1 year was 0.56 (95% CI, 0.22–1.30) and that for use for more than 1 year was 0.36 (95% CI, 0.15–0.83).

Weiderpass *et al.* (1999) conducted a population-based case–control study in Sweden that involved 687 women aged 50–74 years who had had endometrial cancer diagnosed in 1994–95 and 3191 controls. The odds ratio for use of oral contraceptives of less than 3 years was 1.0 (95% CI, 0.7–1.3) and that for use of 3 or more years was 0.5 (95% CI, 0.3–0.7; based on 45 exposed cases and 518 exposed controls). All analyses were adjusted for age, age at menopause, parity and age at last birth, body mass index and duration of previous use of various types of menopausal hormonal therapy.

Jain *et al.* (2000) conducted a case–control study in Ontario, Canada, that involved 512 women who had had endometrial cancer diagnosed in 1994–98 and 513 controls. The odds ratio for ever use of oral contraceptives was 0.66 (95% CI, 0.51–0.84). The estimate of relative risk was adjusted for age, education, parity, weight, age at menarche, tobacco smoking, education, calorie intake and expenditure. No results were given according to duration or recency of use of oral contraceptives.

Parslov *et al.* (2000) conducted a population-based case–control study in Denmark that involved 237 women aged under 50 years who had had endometrial cancer diagnosed in 1987–94 and 538 controls. The odds ratio was 0.4 (95% CI, 0.3–0.7) for use of oral contraceptives of less than 1 year, 0.2 (95% CI, 0.1–0.3) for use of 1–5 years and 0.2 (95% CI, 0.1–0.4) for use of more than 5 years.

Newcomb and Trentham-Deitz (2003) conducted a population-based case–control study in Wisconsin, USA, that involved 591 women aged 40–79 years who had had endometrial cancer diagnosed in 1991–94 and 2045 controls. The relative risk for endometrial cancer was 1.04 (95% CI, 0.74–1.40) for use of oral contraceptives of less than 3 years and 0.73 (95% CI, 0.52–1.02) for use of more than 3 years.

2.3   Cervical cancer

2.3.1   *Introduction*

Five cohort and 16 case–control studies of oral contraceptive use and cervical cancer were evaluated previously (IARC, 1999). On aggregate, the studies showed a small increase in relative risk associated with long-term use. This was observed in four studies in which some analyses were restricted to cases and controls who tested positive for human papillomavirus (HPV) infection. However, the Working Group concluded that biases related to sexual behaviour, screening and other factors could not be ruled out as possible explanations for the observed associations.

Studies to determine whether the use of hormonal oral contraceptives increases the risk for HPV infection have been reviewed previously (IARC, 1999); it was concluded that oral contraceptives probably do not enhance susceptibility to HPV infection (although in some cultures the sexual behaviours of oral contraceptive users may be more conducive to the acquisition of HPV infection than that of non-users).

It is now generally accepted that persistent infection by one of several carcinogenic strains of sexually transmitted HPV is prerequisite for the development of most cervical carcinomas. However, most infected women do not develop cervical cancer, which indicates that additional co-factors may play an etiological role. The uterine cervical epithelium at the squamocolumnar junction is the tissue from which cervical carcinomas arise and is responsive to estrogens and progestogens. It is therefore reasonable to question whether combined oral contraceptives that contain these two types of hormone act as co-factors to alter the risk for cervical cancer.

Invasive cervical cancer is the final result of a presumed series of events: initial HPV infection, establishment of a persistent infection, resultant development of cervical intraepithelial neoplasia (CIN) of increasing severity (from dysplasia or low-grade CIN to carcinoma in situ or CIN3) and finally invasive carcinoma. In-situ and invasive carcinomas are classified histologically as squamous-cell carcinoma, adenocarcinoma or adenosquamous carcinoma if they have both squamous and adenomatous elements. Combined hormonal contraceptives could theoretically increase the risks for cervical cancer by increasing susceptibility to an HPV infection, increasing the probability of persistence in infected women, enhancing the development of mild intraepithelial lesions in women with persistent infection, increasing progression from mild intraepithelial lesions to carcinoma in situ or promoting in-situ lesions to invade surrounding tissues (development of invasive carcinomas). Studies of different design are thus needed to address different hypotheses regarding the possible role of hormonal contraceptives in the development of cervical cancer.

It was long acknowledged that cervical cancer was probably caused by one or more sexually transmitted agent (IARC, 2007). A major difficulty in studying the possible role of oral use of combined hormonal contraceptives in the development of cervical cancer was to account adequately for the potential confounding influence of sexual behaviour on the results. After the establishment of the role of HPV in the genesis of cervical carcinoma, studies of oral use of hormonal contraceptives as a possible co-factor were conducted in which HPV infection was assessed using serological tests for HPV antibodies or tests for HPV DNA in cervical scrapings. Cases and controls were classified as HPV-positive or HPV-negative, and estimates of the relative risk for cervical cancer in relation to various features of oral contraceptive use were either calculated separately for HPV-positive women or controlled for HPV status. However, this has been of limited value in assessing the role of oral use of hormonal contraceptives in cervical carcinogenesis because of the lack of sensitivity of the serological tests, and the difficulty in interpreting both negative and positive HPV DNA assays in controls. Another problem in assessing observed associations of cervical cancer with the oral use of hormonal contraceptives has been the difficulty to rule out the possible effect of selective screening of users (IARC, 2007).

2.3.2   Meta-analysis

Since the previous evaluation (IARC, 1999), Smith *et al.* (2003) performed a meta-analysis of data from 28 studies or groups of studies that had been reported up to July 2002; results of the meta-analysis are summarized in Table 7 by duration of use. Risk for cervical cancer was found to increase significantly with duration of oral contraceptive use in most, but not all, case–control and cohort studies, and there was a statistically significant divergence of results in some of the analyses. The combined relative risks from all studies for in-situ and invasive cancers combined in women who used oral contraceptives for < 5, 5–9 and ≥ 10 years were 1.1 (95% CI, 1.1–1.2), 1.6 (95% CI, 1.4–1.7) and 2.2 (95% CI, 1.9–2.4), respectively. The association was stronger in the cohort studies, and risks were higher for in-situ than invasive carcinomas and for adenocarcinomas than squamous-cell carcinomas. An increase in risk with duration of use was apparent in most studies and in all studies combined, but the risk tended to decline with time since cessation of oral contraceptive use regardless of duration of use (Table 8). Invasive and in-situ carcinomas were not separated in these analyses. The association was stronger in women who tested positively for HPV DNA than in those who tested negatively, and the trend in risk with duration of use remained after adjustment for HPV status. The associations were not materially

Table 7. Summary of results of a meta-analysis of data from 28 studies on the risk for cervical cancer in relation to years of oral use of hormonal contraceptives

Type of study or carcinoma	Approximate duration of use (years)		
	< 5	5–9	≥ 10
All cervical cancer types			
Cohort	1.8 (1.4–2.4)	2.2 (1.7–2.9)	3.3 (2.4–4.5)
Case–control	1.1 (1.0–1.2)	1.5 (1.4–1.7)	2.0 (1.8–2.3)
All studies	1.1 (1.1–1.2)	1.6 (1.4–1.7)	2.2 (1.9–2.4)
HPV positive subjects	0.9 (0.7–1.2)	1.3 (1.0–1.9)	2.5 (1.6–3.9)
HPV negative subjects	0.9 (0.6–1.4)	0.9 (0.5–1.4)	1.3 (0.9–1.9)
Adjusted for HPV status[a]	0.9 (0.7–1.1)	1.3 (1.0–1.7)	1.7 (1.3–2.3)
Invasive carcinoma	1.1 (1.0–1.2)	1.4 (1.2–1.6)	2.0 (1.8–2.4)
Carcinoma *in situ*	1.3 (1.2–1.4)	2.1 (1.4–2.4)	2.4 (1.9–2.9)
Squamous-cell carcinoma	1.1 (1.0–1.2)	1.5 (1.3–1.7)	2.0 (1.7–2.3)
Adenocarcinoma	1.5 (1.2–1.8)	1.7 (1.2–2.3)	2.8 (2.0–3.9)

From Smith *et al.* (2003)
[a] Nine studies measured HPV DNA using polymerase chain reaction (PCR)-based assays, one study used HPV antibodies.

Table 8. Summary of results of a meta-analysis of data from four studies[a] on the risk for cervical cancer in relation to years of use and time since last use of oral hormonal contraceptives

Years since last use	Approximate duration of use (years)	
	< 5	≥ 5
< 8	1.4 (1.2–1.5)	2.1 (1.8–2.4)
≥ 8	1.1 (1.0–1.2)	1.4 (1.1–1.9)

From Smith *et al.* (2003)
[a] Including two multicentre collaborative studies

altered after adjustment for numbers of sexual partners, cervical cancer screening, tobacco smoking and use of barrier contraceptives, and were observed in selected studies in both developed and developing countries.

2.3.3 *Methodological considerations*

In some of the analyses of Smith *et al.* (2003), cases of in-situ and invasive carcinoma were not distinguished. Since bias due to selective screening of users of oral contraceptives more probably affected results of studies of in-situ diseases, they were considered separately in this review. In addition, studies of carcinomas *in situ* in screened women were considered separately from studies in general populations.

Although Green *et al.* (2003) reviewed the prevalence of HPV DNA in cancer-free women in 19 case–control studies of cervical cancer and in surveys of HPV prevalence, such studies cannot distinguish between recent, transient HPV infections and persistent infections. Women who have long-term (persistent) infections are more likely to test positive at a single point in time than those who have short-term transient infections; therefore, women who tested positive in these studies may represent persistent infections. No consistent associations were found between prevalence of high- or low-risk types of HPV and any use, current use or long-term use of oral contraceptives. One prospective study of 1995 women in Bogota, Colombia (Molano *et al.*, 2003), reported that clearance of HPV infection was slightly more frequent among women who had ever used oral contraceptives than among non-users (hazard ratio adjusted for age, HPV type, multiplicity of HPV types and parity, 1.38; 95% CI, 1.07–1.77), whereas another prospective study of 621 female university students followed over 24 months (Richardson *et al.*, 2005) found that the use of oral contraceptives was unrelated to clearance of high-risk (age-adjusted hazard ratio, 0.8; 95% CI, 0.3–1.3) or low-risk (hazard ratio, 1.1; 95% CI, 0.6–1.9) HPV infection. It thus seems unlikely that oral contraceptives play a role in the persistence of HPV infections. These results provide evidence that associations of cervical cancer with oral contraceptive use are probably not a result of confounding by detection of HPV.

Infection by high-risk types of HPV has been assessed in two ways: serological tests for HPV antibodies and tests for HPV DNA in cervical tissue (usually using polymerase chain reaction (PCR)-based technology). A small proportion of DNA-based assays and approximately half of the serological tests in cases of cervical cancer give negative results, although nearly all cases are presumably a result of HPV infection, which indicates that these tests are not 100% sensitive (IARC, 2007). Therefore, in some case–control analyses, either all cases (on the assumption that they are all HPV-related) or HPV-positive cases have been compared with HPV-positive controls. In this review, studies based on HPV serology and those based on HPV DNA assays are considered separately, and studies in which cases are compared with HPV-positive controls are distinguished from those in which HPV status is controlled for in the statistical analyses (IARC, 2007).

2.3.4   *Studies of in-situ and invasive cervical cancer in which HPV antibodies were measured*

In two of the most recent studies that presumably used the most sensitive tests available, only 43 (19.5%) of 221 women who had invasive cervical cancer tested positive for antibodies to HPV 16-E7 in an enzyme-linked immunosorbant assay (ELISA) with synthetic peptides (Berrington *et al.*, 2002) and 156 (66.4%) of 235 women who had invasive squamous-cell cervical carcinoma tested positive for antibodies to types 16, 18, 31, 45 or 52 using a polymer-based viral-like particle ELISA (Shields *et al.*, 2004). Since these tests do not identify correctly all women who have been infected with a high-risk type of HPV, residual confounding can occur in studies in which relative risk estimates are stratified on or controlled for HPV status (IARC, 2007). It has been proposed that all cases (regardless of their HPV antibody status) be compared with HPV-positive controls, but if the proportion of controls that test positive for HPV antibodies varies by use of oral contraceptives, spurious associations with oral contraceptives can occur.

The results of three studies of cervical neoplasia and the use of oral contraceptives, in which HPV antibodies were measured, that have been published since the previous review (IARC, 1999) are summarized in Table 9.

Two studies provided estimates of relative risk for cervical carcinoma in relation to duration of oral contraceptive use after controlling for HPV antibody status. Madeleine *et al.* (2001) compared 150 cases of adenocarcinoma *in situ* in western Washington State, USA, with 651 controls selected from the same population. Berrington *et al.* (2002) compared 221 women aged 20–44 years who had invasive cervical cancer diagnosed in the United Kingdom between 1984 and 1988 with 393 control women selected from the same general practitioners' registers as the cases. In contrast to the study of Shields *et al.* (2004), the percentage of controls with HPV antibodies decreased with duration of oral contraceptive use in this study. [The trend in risk ratios for seropositivity was not statistically significant, but the variables that were controlled for in their calculation was not indicated.] In both of these studies, risk increased with duration of use before controlling for HPV antibody status. Berrington *et al.* (2002) found similar trends in women with and

Table 9. Relative risks for three types of cervical cancer in relation to duration of oral use of hormonal contraceptives controlled for the presence or absence of human papillomavirus (HPV) antibodies

Reference	Lesion	Years of use	No. of subjects		Relative risk adjusted for HPV serology	
			Cases	Controls	No	Yes
Madeleine	Adeno-	None	8	74	1.0	–
et al. (2001)	carcinoma	Ever	124	384	2.7 (1.2–5.8)	4.0 (1.7–9.4)
	in situ	1–5	64	250	2.1 (1.0–4.8)	–
		6–11	40	101	3.4 (1.5–8.0)	–
		≥ 12	20	33	5.5 (2.1–14.6)	–
					p for trend < 0.0001	
Berrington	Invasive	None	12	49	[1.0][a]	1.0 (0.5–2.1)
et al. (2002)	cervical	1–4	73	159	[1.9][a]	1.6 (1.2–2.2)
	cancer	5–9	76	117	[2.6][a]	1.9 (1.3–2.6)
		≥ 10	60	68	[3.6][a]	2.8 (1.9–4.2)
Shields et al.	Invasive	None	123	81		1.0[b]
(2004)	squamous	< 5	59	69	Data not given	0.6 (0.4–0.9)[b]
	- cell	5–10	33	30		0.7 (0.4–1.3)[b]
		> 10	20	26		0.5 (0.3–1.0)[b]

[a] Crude estimates calculated by the Working Group from the numbers of cases and controls shown in the table
[b] Results restricted to women with a positive test for HPV antibodies

without HPV antibodies (data not shown) but, after controlling for HPV antibodies, the trend was slightly attenuated; however, Madeleine et al. (2001) found that the risk estimate in women who ever had used oral contraceptives was increased after controlling for HPV antibodies.

A case–control study in the USA (Shields et al., 2004) compared 235 cases of invasive squamous-cell cancer (all reasonably presumed to have been exposed to HPV) with 206 (43.0%) of 486 population-based controls who tested positive for antibodies against HPV types 16, 18, 31, 45 or 52. In relation to duration of oral contraceptive use, there was no trend in risk for cervical cancer when cases were compared with all controls [data not presented in the published report], but the prevalence of HPV antibodies in the controls increased, which resulted in a decrease in risk in analyses that compared cases with sero-positive controls. [Although the results of the US study were controlled for time since last Pap smear, screening bias could have influenced the results if most cases were detected at screening and if oral contraceptive users were more likely to have been screened than non-users. The discrepant results in the relationship of HPV antibody prevalence in the controls with duration of oral contraceptive use in the studies of Berrington et al. (2002) and Shields et al. (2004) render the results of both investigations questionable.]

2.3.5   *Studies in which cervical tissue was assayed for HPV DNA*

(a)   *Cervical carcinoma* in situ

Among women with HPV infection at enrolment into a cohort in Manchester, United Kingdom (Deacon *et al.*, 2000), relative risks for subsequent development of CIN3 in current and former users of oral contraceptives were 1.3 (95% CI, 0.7–2.5) and 1.2 (95% CI, 0.6–2.1), respectively. Risk did not vary linearly with increasing duration of use or with time since last use, although the relative risk in women with more than 8 years of use was 1.5 (95% CI, 0.8–2.9).

Castle *et al.* (2002) followed 1812 women who had tested positive for high-risk HPV DNA when they enrolled in a 10-year prospective study of cervical neoplasia at Kaiser Permanente in Portland, OR, USA, for a period of 122 months. The risks for developing CIN3 in current users of oral contraceptives versus non-users was 0.84 (95% CI, 0.49–1.5).

It was shown in the studies below that women who tested positive for HPV DNA in their cervical tissue had an increasing risk for in-situ cervical cancer with increasing duration of oral contraceptive use (Table 10).

In a multicentre case–control study of squamous-cell carcinoma and adenocarcinoma of the cervix in the USA (Lacey *et al.*, 1999), cases were selected from hospital admissions and population controls were selected by random-digit dialling. Forty-eight cases of squamous-cell carcinoma *in situ* and 33 cases of adenocarcinoma *in situ* (regardless of their HPV DNA status) were compared with 48 controls who tested positive to one or more of 18 high-risk types of HPV. As shown in Table 10, the relative risk in current users was increased for in-situ adenocarcinoma but not significantly for in-situ squamous-cell carcinoma, and a trend in risk with duration of use was observed only for adenocarcinoma (*p* for trend = 0.03).

In a study nested in a cohort of screened women in Uppsala county, Sweden, Ylitalo *et al.* (1999) compared 178 cases of carcinoma *in situ* (most presumably squamous-cell) who had HPV type 16 or 18 in pre-diagnostic smears with 178 matched controls with the same HPV types. Risk was higher in current than in former users of oral contraceptives and increased with duration of use (*p*-value of test for trend = 0.12). A similar trend was observed for women who tested negative for HPV 16 or 18.

In a collaborative study in Colombia and Spain (Moreno *et al.*, 2002), 211 cases of squamous-cell carcinoma *in situ* (selected from hospitals, pathology laboratories and screening clinics) who tested positive for one of 14 high-risk types of HPV were compared with 28 controls with normal cervical cytology (selected from the same place of recruitment as the cases) but who had similar positive tests for a high-risk type of HPV. Risk increased with duration of use of oral contraceptives.

[The Working Group noted that the results of the studies of Lacey *et al.* (1999) and Moreno *et al.* (2002) were based on a very small number of controls who were HPV-positive. The relative risk estimates therefore had wide confidence intervals.]

In conclusion, the results from two case–control studies of screened women (Ylitalo *et al.*, 1999; Moreno *et al.*, 2002) showed a significant increase in risk for squamous-cell

Table 10. Relative risks for in-situ cervical neoplasia in relation to oral use of hormonal contraceptives in case–control studies in which cases were compared with controls with high-risk types of HPV DNA in their cervical tissue

Reference, country	Type of study	Reported diagnosis in the cases	Oral contra-ceptive use	No. of subjects		Relative risk (95% CI)
				Cases	Controls	
Lacey et al. (1999), USA	Population-based case–control	Squamous-cell carcinoma in situ	Never	7	11	1.0 (reference)
			Former	32	27	1.0 (0.4–2.8)
			Current	9	10	1.3 (0.5–3.6)
			Years of use			
			≤ 2	10	9	0.9 (0.3–3.0)
			3–6	15	12	0.9 (0.3–2.8)
			> 6	16	16	1.2 (0.3–3.9)
		Adeno-carcinoma in situ	Never	2	11	1.0 (reference)
			Former	13	27	2.0 (0.4–9.9)
			Current	18	10	12.6 (2.5–64.2)
			Years of use			
			≤ 2	7	9	3.2 (0.6–17.2)
			3–6	7	12	1.7 (0.3–9.5)
			> 6	17	16	6.0 (1.2–30.7)
Ylitalo et al. (1999), Sweden	Case–control nested in screening cohort	Carcinoma in situ	Never	48	84	1.0 (reference)
			Former	241	239	1.5 (0.8–3.1)
			Current	77	48	2.7 (1.1–6.7)
			Years of use			
			< 2			1.6 (0.7–3.7)
			2–9			2.2 (1.0–4.9)
			≥ 10			2.8 (1.1–6.9)
Moreno et al. (2002), Spain and Columbia	Screening-based case–control	Squamous-cell carcinoma in situ	Never	65	14	1.0 (reference)
			Ever	146	14	2.5 (1.0–6.8)
			> 5 years of use	92	9	2.9 (1.2–7.1)

CI, confidence interval; HPV, human papillomavirus

intraepithelial cervical lesions with duration of oral contraceptive use, but the population-based (but not screening-based) study did not show such an association (Lacey et al., 1999); two prospective studies showed no significant association of use of oral contraceptives with risk for CIN3 (Deacon et al., 2000; Castle et al., 2002). The studies of Lacey et al. (1999) and Madeleine et al. (2001) showed a strong increasing trend in risk for adenocarcinoma in situ with duration of oral contraceptive use, but in neither study were the controls selected from screening programmes. [Since most cases of adenocarcinoma in situ are detected at screening, these studies could have yielded spurious results if the probability of being screened is related to duration of oral contraceptive use.]

(b)   *Invasive cervical neoplasia*

In a study in Thailand (Thomas *et al*., 2001a), 126 women with in-situ or invasive cervical cancer that contained HPV 16 and 42 women with HPV 18-associated adenomatous cervical carcinoma were compared with 250 hospital control women who had no evidence of HPV infection in their cervical scrapings. Relative risks for HPV 16- and HPV 18-associated tumours in women who had ever used oral contraceptives were estimated to be 1.3 (95% CI, 0.8–2.0) and 1.4 (95% CI, 0.7–2.7), respectively. No trends in risk with duration of oral contraceptive use were found. [Thus, if oral contraceptives do enhance the risk for cervical cancer, they appear to do so equally for women who are infected with HPV types 16 and 18.]

Two case–control studies of invasive cervical cancer, in which PCR-based assays for HPV DNA were used and in which there was sufficient use of oral contraceptives for meaningful analysis, are summarized in Table 11 (Moreno *et al*., 2002; Shapiro *et al*., 2003).

Moreno *et al*. (2002) conducted a multinational pooled analysis with studies from Brazil, Columbia, Morocco, Paraguay, Peru, the Philippines, Spain and Thailand which included overall more than 1400 cases and 1900 controls. Cases were women who had been newly diagnosed with invasive squamous-cell cervical carcinoma and admitted to participating hospitals and controls were women with no cervical cancer who were selected from

Table 11. Relative risks for invasive cervical carcinoma in relation to oral use of hormonal contraceptives in two case–control studies in which cases were compared with controls with high-risk types of HPV DNA in their cervical tissue

Reference, country	Oral contraceptive use	No. of women		Relative risk (95% CI)
		Cases	Controls	
Moreno *et al*. (2002), eight countries	Never	1006	149	1.0
	Ever	459	78	1.3 (0.88–1.91)
	> 5 years of use	239	19	4.0 (2.0–8.0)
Shapiro *et al*. (2003), South Africa	Never	364	166	1.0
	Ever	160	88	0.9 (0.7–1.3)
	Years of use			
	< 1	63	41	0.8 (0.5–1.2)
	1–4	58	32	0.9 (0.6–1.6)
	≥ 5	32	13	1.3 (0.6–2.7)
	Years since last use			
	current/< 1	16	9	1.3 (0.7–2.4)
	1–4	17	8	1.9 (1.0–3.5)
	5–9	20	11	1.0 (0.6–1.6)
	10–14	25	19	0.8 (0.5–1.3)
	≥ 15	73	38	0.7 (0.5–0.9)

CI, confidence interval; HPV, human papillomavirus

the same hospitals as the cases. Cervical tissue from all cases and controls was tested for high-risk types of HPV DNA using PCR-based technology. In analyses in which HPV DNA-positive cases and controls were compared, the estimate of the relative risk in women who had ever used oral contraceptives was 1.3 (95% CI, 0.88–1.91), and the individual estimates among the participating countries were significantly heterogeneous (not shown). However, there was a clear increase in risk for more than 5 years of duration of use, and the estimates of relative risks in such users were not significantly heterogeneous among the study centres.

In a large study of invasive cervical cancer published after the meta-analysis by Smith *et al.* (2003), Shapiro *et al.* (2003) recruited 484 women who had invasive squamous-cell cervical cancer and 40 women who had invasive cervical adenocarcinoma from two tertiary care hospitals in South Africa. A total of 1541 control women were recruited from the same hospitals, or from local hospitals or community health centres from which the cases were referred. The overall results are consistent with those of the meta-analysis of Smith *et al.* (2003). No significant trend in risk was seen with duration of use, but a statistically non-significant increase in risk was observed for duration of use of ≥ 5 years. The relative risks for users of oral contraceptives for < 1, 1–4, ≥ 5 years were 0.8 (95% CI, 0.5–1.2), 0.9 (95% CI, 0.6–1.6) and 1.3 (95% CI, 0.6–2.7), respectively. As in the meta-analysis, the risk declined with time since last use: the relative risks for current users and for women who had last used oral contraceptives < 1, 1–4, 5–9, 10–14 and ≥ 15 years previously were 1.3 (95% CI, 0.7–2.4), 1.9 (95% CI, 1.0–3.5), 1.0 (95% CI, 0.6–1.6), 0.8 (95% CI, 0.5–1.3) and 0.7 (95% CI, 0.5–0.9), respectively. Cervical scrapings from all controls were tested for 13 high-risk types of HPV and 254 (16.5%) were positive. As shown in Table 11, when the cases (all reasonably presumed to be HPV-positive) were compared with the HPV-positive controls, risk was not significantly increased in women who had ever used oral contraceptives. Among the controls, the proportions that tested positive for HPV DNA in users and non-users of oral contraceptives were 14.6 and 17.7%, respectively. Although this proportion declined slightly with duration of oral contraceptive use (16.3, 14.7 and 10.7% in users of < 1, 1–4 and ≥ 5 years), it did not vary consistently by time since last use, and the relative risks did not differ appreciably from those based on the comparison of cases to all controls (not shown).

In a study in Latvia (Silins *et al.*, 2004), 223 women who had invasive cervical carcinoma were identified in the oncology centre, which treats about 90% of all cases in the country, and were compared with 239 healthy controls selected from the Latvian population registry. Serum from all women were tested for immunoglobulin G (IgG) antibodies to HPV types 6, 11, 16, 18 and 33, and cervical scrapings were tested for 18 high-risk and nine low-risk HPV types. The relative risk for cervical cancer in women who had ever used oral contraceptives was 0.4 before controlling for HPV, 0.4 (95% CI, 0.2–1.0) after controlling for HPV 16/18 antibodies and 0.4 (95% CI, 0.2–1.1) after controlling for HPV in cervical tissue.

In a hospital-based study of 198 cases of invasive cervical cancer and 202 controls conducted in Algeria (Hammouda *et al.*, 2005), relative risks for users of oral contraceptives for < 5, 5–9 and ≥ 10 years were 0.6 (95% CI, 0.3–1.2), 0.5 (95% CI, 0.3–1.1) and 0.8 (95% CI, 0.4–1.6), respectively. Although cases and controls were tested for HPV DNA, the results were presented separately or were adjusted for HPV DNA status.

On aggregate, there is inconsistent evidence that the oral use of hormonal contraceptives alters the risk for invasive cervical carcinoma, although studies in which all (Shapiro *et al.*, 2003) or most (Moreno *et al.*, 2002) cases were compared with HPV-positive controls should theoretically be the best design to attempt to determine such an alteration in women with an HPV infection.

2.3.6   *Studies conducted to determine whether oral contraceptives alter the risk for progression of cervical lesions*

In a prospective study in Brazil (Cavalcanti *et al.*, 2000), 280 women who were initially diagnosed with intraepithelial lesions were tested for HPV types by in-situ hybridization. The risk for progression to carcinoma *in situ* or invasive carcinoma was 1.4 (95% CI, 0.4–5.6) in users of oral contraceptives compared with non-users. [The methods used in this study could not be evaluated adequately from the published report.]

Two studies have been conducted in which cases of invasive cancer were directly compared with cases of carcinoma *in situ*. Relative risk estimates from such studies can be interpreted as risks for progression from in-situ to invasive disease.

Thomas *et al.* (2002) analysed data from five centres in Chile, Mexico and Thailand that participated in the WHO Collaborative Study of Neoplasia and Steroid Contraceptives. Based on data from more than 1300 women who had squamous-cell carcinoma *in situ* and more than 2000 women who had invasive squamous-cell carcinoma, those who had ever used oral contraceptives and those who had used them for 1–12, 13–60 and > 60 months had relative risks for invasive versus in-situ disease of 1.0 (95% CI, 0.8–1.2), 1.0 (95% CI, 0.8–1.3), 0.9 (95% CI, 0.7–1.1) and 1.0 (95% CI, 0.8–1.3), respectively, compared with non-users. [Although HPV assays were not performed in this study, since HPV is a necessary cause of cervical carcinoma, this would only be needed in the improbable event that oral contraceptive use was related differently to various types of high-risk HPVs with different potentials to cause progression to invasive disease.]

In a study in Thailand (Thomas *et al.*, 2001b), HPV assays were performed on 190 women who had invasive squamous-cell cervical carcinoma and 75 women who had carcinoma *in situ*. After controlling for HPV types, the relative risk in women who had ever used oral contraceptives was 1.3 (95% CI, 0.8–2.0) for HPV-16 and 1.4 (95% CI, 0.7–2.7) for HPV 18 positivity.

2.4   Ovarian cancer

This section reviews studies on the use of combined oral contraceptives and ovarian cancer that have been published or updated since the last evaluation (IARC, 1999). On the basis of four cohort studies and 21 case–control studies, the previous Working Group

(IARC, 1999) found a substantially reduced incidence of ovarian cancer among combined oral contraceptive users, with a consistent inverse duration–risk relationship.

2.4.1   Descriptive studies

Analyses of mortality trends in several areas of Europe (Adami et al., 1990; La Vecchia et al., 1998; Levi et al., 2004; Bray et al., 2005) and in the USA (Gnagy et al., 2000; Tarone & Chu, 2000) showed that women born after 1920 — i.e. the generations who had used oral contraceptives — experienced reduced rates of ovarian cancer. The downward trends were larger in countries where oral contraceptives had been used more widely (Bray et al., 2005).

2.4.2   Cohort studies

Two cohort studies have been updated (Beral et al., 1999; Vessey et al., 2003) and an additional study has been published (Kumle et al., 2004). The main findings from these are given in Table 12.

The Royal College of General Practitioners' study was based on 46 000 women recruited in 1968 from 1400 British general practices (Beral et al., 1988); 30 cases of ovarian cancer were observed up to 1987, which corresponded to multivariate relative risks of 0.6 (95% CI, 0.3–1.4) for women who had ever used oral contraceptives and of 0.3 for those who had used them for 10 years or longer. Adjustment was made for age, parity,

Table 12. Cohort studies of oral use of combined contraceptives and ovarian cancer, 1998–2004

Reference, country	No. of cases	Relative risk (95% CI)	
		Ever use	Longest use
Ramcharan et al. (1981), USA	16	0.4 (0.1–1.0)	–
Beral et al. (1988, 1999), United Kingdom	55	0.6 (0.3–1.0)	0.2 (0.1–1.3) (≥ 10 years)
Hankinson et al. (1995), USA	260	1.1 (0.8–1.4)	0.7 (0.4–1.1) (≥ 5 years)
Vessey & Painter (1995), Vessey et al. (2003), United Kingdom	61	0.4 (0.2–0.7)	0.2 (0.1–0.6) (> 8 years)
Kumle et al. (2004), Norway and Sweden	214[a]	0.6 (0.5–0.7)	0.1 (0.01–0.6) (> 15 years)

CI, confidence interval
[a] 135 invasive, 79 borderline

smoking and social class. At the 25-year follow-up for mortality (Beral *et al.*, 1999), 55 deaths from ovarian cancer were observed, which corresponded to relative risks of 0.6 (95% CI, 0.3–1.0) for women who had ever used oral contraceptives and 0.2 (95% CI, 0.1–1.3) for ≥ 10 years of use, based on one death. The protection persisted for ≥ 20 years since cessation of use (relative risk, 0.7; 95% CI, 0.4–1.4).

The Oxford Family Planning Association study was based on 17 032 women who were enrolled between 1968 and 1976 from various family planning clinics in the United Kingdom (Vessey & Painter, 1995). Adjustment was made for age and parity. At the 32-year follow-up of the same cohort at 31 December 2000, 61 deaths from ovarian cancer were observed. The relative risks for oral use of combined hormonal contraceptives were 0.4 (95% CI, 0.2–0.7) for ever use, 1.1 (95% CI, 0.6–2.0; 17 deaths) for a duration of ≤ 48 months, 0.2 (95% CI, 0.0–0.5; three deaths) for 49–96 months and 0.2 (95% CI, 0.1–0.6; five deaths) for ≥ 97 months (Vessey *et al.*, 2003).

The Norwegian-Swedish Women's Lifestyle and Health cohort included 103 551 women aged 30–49 years in 1991–92 (Kumle *et al.*, 2004). During the follow-up through to 2000, 214 incident cases of ovarian epithelial neoplasms were observed (135 invasive, 79 borderline). Relative risks were adjusted for country, age, parity, menopausal status and use of menopausal hormonal therapy. Compared with women who had never used oral contraceptives, the overall relative risk for those who ever had was 0.6 (95% CI, 0.5–0.7); the relative risk for progestogen-only preparations was 0.5 (95% CI, 0.2–1.2). Ever use was associated with relative risks of 0.6 (95% CI, 0.4–0.8) for invasive cancers and 0.7 (95% CI, 0.5–1.2) for borderline cases. For duration of use, the relative risks were 0.9 for < 1 year of use, 0.5 for 1–4 years, 0.6 for 5–9 years, 0.5 for 10–14 years and 0.1 for ≥ 15 years. The trend in risk with duration of use was significant, and the relative risk per year of use was 0.91 (95% CI, 0.85–0.96). Corresponding values per year of use were 0.89 (95% CI, 0.84–0.94) for invasive and 0.96 (95% CI, 0.91–1.0) for borderline tumours.

2.4.3 *Case–control studies*

Studies that include information on oral contraceptives and ovarian cancer that have been published or updated since the previous evaluation (IARC, 1999) are summarized in Table 13.

In a population-based study of 824 cases and 860 controls diagnosed between 1990 and 1993 in three Australian states (New South Wales, Victoria and Queensland), Purdie *et al.* (1995) found a relative risk of 0.5 (95% CI, 0.4–0.7) for any use of oral contra-ceptives and 0.3 (95% CI, 0.2–0.4) for ≥ 10 years of use. The response rate was 90% for cases and 73% for controls. Adjustment was made for sociodemographic factors, family history of cancer, use of talc, smoking and reproductive and hormonal factors. A sub-sequent analysis of the same dataset (Siskind *et al.*, 2000) indicated that the reduction in risk was 7% (95% CI, 4–9%) per year of use, that the protection was observed in various strata of age at first use and that there was little evidence that the effect waned with time since last use. When this dataset was analysed separately by histological type, the relative risk was 0.62 (95% CI, 0.37–1.04) for mucinous and 0.52 (95% CI, 0.39–0.68) for non-mucinous ovarian cancers (Purdie *et al.*, 2001).

Table 13. Case–control studies of oral use of combined contraceptives and ovarian cancer

Reference, country	Type of study	Relative risk (95% CI)[a]			
		No. of cases (age in years)	Ever use	Longest use	Duration (years)
Hildreth *et al.* (1981), USA	Hospital-based	62 (45–74)	0.5 (0.1–1.7)	NR	
Weiss *et al.* (1981a), USA	Population-based	112 (36–55)	0.6 (NR)	0.5 (0.2–1.3)	≥ 9
Willett *et al.* (1981), USA	Nested in a cohort	47 (< 60)	0.8 (0.4–1.5)	0.8 (0.3–2.1)	> 3
Cramer *et al.* (1982), USA	Population-based	144 (< 60)	0.4 (0.2–1.0)	0.6	> 5
Franceschi *et al.* (1982), Italy	Hospital-based	161 (19–69)	0.7 (0.4–1.1)	NR	
Rosenberg *et al.* (1982), USA	Hospital-based	136 (< 60)	0.6 (0.4–0.9)	0.3 (0.1–0.8)	≥ 5
Risch *et al.* (1983), USA	Population-based	284 (20–74)	[0.5] (NR)	NR	
Tzonou *et al.* (1984), Greece	Hospital-based	150 (NR)	0.4 (0.1–1.1)	NR	
CASH (1987b), USA	Population-based	492 (20–54)	0.6 (0.5–0.7)	0.2 (0.1–0.4)	≥ 10
Harlow *et al.* (1988), USA	Population-based	116 (20–79)	0.4 (0.2–0.9)	0.4 (0.2–1.0)	> 4
Wu *et al.* (1988), USA	Hospital- and population-based	299 (18–74)	0.7 (0.5–1.1)	0.4 (0.2–0.7)	> 3
Booth *et al.* (1989), United Kingdom	Hospital-based	235 (< 65)	0.5 (0.3–0.9)	0.1 (0.01–1.0)	> 10
Hartge *et al.* (1989), USA	Hospital-based	296 (20–79)	1.0 (0.7–1.7)	0.8 (0.4–1.5)	> 5
Shu *et al.* (1989), China	Population-based	229 (18–70)	1.8 (0.8–4.1)	1.9 (0.4–9.3)	> 5
WHO Collaborative Study (1989a), 7 countries	Hospital-based	368 (< 62)	0.8 (0.6–1.0)	0.5 (0.3–1.0)	> 5
Parazzini *et al.* (1991a), Italy	Hospital-based	505 (22–59)	0.7 (0.5–1.0)	0.5 (0.3–0.9)	≥ 2
Parazzini *et al.* (1991b), Italy	Hospital-based	91 (23–64)	0.3 (0.2–0.6)	0.2 (0.1–0.6)	≥ 2

Table 13 (contd)

Reference, country	Type of study	Relative risk (95% CI)[a]			
		No. of cases (age in years)	Ever use	Longest use	Duration (years)
Polychronopoulou et al. (1993), Greece	Hospital-based	189 (< 75)	0.8 (0.2–3.7)	NR	
Risch et al. (1994, 1996), Canada	Population-based	450 (35–79)	0.5 (0.4–0.7)	0.3 (0.2–0.6)	≥ 10
Rosenberg et al. (1994), USA	Hospital-based	441 (< 65)	0.8 (0.6–1.0)	0.5 (0.2–0.9)	≥ 10
Purdie et al. (1995), Australia	Population-based	824 (18–79)	0.5 (0.4–0.7)	0.3 (0.2–0.4)	≥ 1
Godard et al. (1998), Canada	Population-based	170 (20–84)	p = 0.038	0.33 (0.13–0.82)	> 10
Salazar-Martinez et al. (1999), Mexico	Hospital-based (outpatient controls)	84 (mean, 54.6)	0.4 (0.2–0.8)	0.4 (0.2–0.8)	> 1
Wittenberg et al. (1999), USA	Population-based	322 (20–79)	0.9 (0.4–2.1)[b] 0.8 (0.6–1.3)[c]	0.4 (0.1–1.4)[b] 0.6 (0.4–1.0)[c]	≥ 5
Beard et al. (2000), USA	Population-based	103 (15–85+)	1.1 (0.6–2.3)	0.8 (0.4–1.1)	≥ 0.5
Cramer et al. (2000), USA	Population-based	563 (mean, 51)	0.7 (0.5–0.8)	–	–
Greggi et al. (2000), Italy	Hospital-based	440 (≤ 80)	0.4 (0.3–0.6)	0.3 (0.2–0.5)	≥ 2
Ness et al. (2000), USA	Population-based	767 (< 70)	0.6 (0.3–0.8)	0.3 (0.1–0.5)	≥ 10
Chiaffarino et al. (2001), Italy	Hospital-based	1031 (< 80)	0.9 (0.7–1.2)	0.5 (0.3–0.9)	≥ 5
Riman et al. (2001), Sweden	Population-based	193 (50–74) borderline	1.2 (0.9–1.8)	1.2 (0.6–2.1)	≥ 10
Royar et al. (2001), Germany	Population-based	282 (< 75)	0.5 (0.3–0.7)	0.4 (0.3–0.6)	> 5
Riman et al. (2002), Sweden	Population-based	655 (50–74)	0.7 (0.6–0.9)	0.4 (0.2–0.6)	≥ 10
Schildkraut et al. (2002), USA	Population-based	390 (20–54)	1.0 referent[d] 0.0[e] 2.1 (1.2–3.7)[f] 1.6 (0.9–3.0)[g] 2.9 (1.8–4.5)[h]		

Table 13 (contd)

Reference, country	Type of study	Relative risk (95% CI)[a]			
		No. of cases (age in years)	Ever use	Longest use	Duration (years)
Tung et al. (2003), USA (Hawaii and California)	Population-based	558 (mean, borderline, 48; invasive, 58)	0.6 (0.4–0.8)	0.4 (0.3–0.6)	> 5
Mills et al. (2004), USA	Population-based	256 (mean, 56.6)		0.4 (0.2–0.7)	> 10
Pike et al. (2004), USA	Population-based	477 (18–74)		0.5 (0.2–0.8)	≥ 10
Pooled analyses					
Franceschi et al. (1991a), Greece, Italy, United Kingdom	Three hospital-based studies	971 (< 65)	0.6 (0.4–0.8)	0.4 (0.2–0.7)	≥ 5
Harris et al. (1992), USA	Pooled analysis of 12 US population- and hospital-based case–control studies	327 (NR)	0.8 (0.6–1.1)	0.6 (0.4–0.9)	> 5
Whittemore et al. (1992), USA	Same pooled analysis as Harris et al. (1992)	2197 (NR)	0.7 (0.6–0.8)	0.3 (0.2–0.4)	≥ 6
John et al. (1993), USA	Pooled analysis of 7 of the 12 studies in the pooled analysis of Whittemore et al. (1992)	110 (mean, invasive, 53.3; borderline, 37.1)	0.7 (0.4–1.2)	0.6 (0.2–1.6)	≥ 6
Bosetti et al. (2002), Greece, Italy, United Kingdom	Re-analysis of 6 studies	2768 (< 40–69)	0.7 (0.6–0.8)	0.4 (0.3–0.6)	≥ 5

CI, confidence interval; NR, not reported
[a] Whenever available
[b] Mucinous
[c] Non-mucinous
[d] Potency progestogen/estrogen high/high
[e] Potency progestogen/estrogen high/low
[f] Potency progestogen/estrogen low/high
[h] Non-users, potency progestogen/estrogen low/low

A case–control study was conducted in 1995–96 in Montréal, Canada, on 170 women aged 20–84 years with invasive or borderline ovarian cancer and 170 population controls (Godard *et al.*, 1998). Fifty-eight cases were familial (i.e. with a history of breast or ovarian cancer in first-degree relatives) and 111 were non-familial. Overall, 50% of cases versus 61.8% of controls reported ever having used oral contraceptives ($p = 0.038$). The multivariate model was based on 152 cases (101 sporadic, 51 familial) and 152 controls. Compared with women who had used oral contraceptives for < 1 year (66 cases, 88 controls), the relative risk was 0.77 (95% CI, 0.44–1.36) for use of 1–5 years, 0.49 (95% CI, 0.27–0.91) for use of 6–10 years and 0.33 (95% CI, 0.13–0.82) for use of 11–25 years.

A case–control study was conducted in Mexico city in 1995–97 on 84 cases of ovarian epithelial cancer and 668 outpatient controls (Salazar-Martinez *et al.*, 1999). The response rate was 100% for cases and 93% for controls. Overall, 13 (15.4%) cases versus 195 (29.2%) controls had ever used oral contraceptives (odds ratio, 0.36; 95% CI, 0.15–0.83). Compared with never users of oral contraceptives, the multivariate relative risks, adjusted for age, parity, breast-feeding, smoking, diabetes mellitus, physical activity, menopausal status and body mass index, were 0.56 (95% CI, 0.22–1.3) for ≤ 1 year of use and 0.36 (95% CI, 0.15–0.83) for > 1 year of use.

An extraction from a previously published case–control study from western Washington State, USA, included a separate analysis of 43 mucinous and 279 non-mucinous ovarian epithelial cancers compared with 426 population controls aged 20–79 years (Wittenberg *et al.*, 1999). The participation rate was approximately 64% for cases and 68% for controls. After adjustment for age and parity, the relative risk for ever use of oral contraceptives was 0.9 (95% CI, 0.4–2.1) for mucinous and 0.8 (95% CI, 0.6–1.3) for non-mucinous cancers. Corresponding values for duration of use of ≥ 5 years were 0.4 (95% CI, 0.1–1.4) and 0.6 (95% CI, 0.4–1.0) and for time since last use ≥ 15 years were 1.2 (95% CI, 0.5–3.0) and 1.0 (95% CI, 0.7–1.7), respectively.

In a population-based case–control study of 103 incident cases of ovarian cancer diagnosed between 1975 and 1991 and 103 controls from Olmsted County, MN, USA, the age-matched relative risk was 1.1 (95% CI, 0.6–2.3) for ever having used oral contraceptives and 0.8 (95% CI, 0.4–1.1) for ≥ 6 months of use (Beard *et al.*, 2000).

A population-based case–control study conducted between 1992 and 1997 in Massachusetts and New Hampshire, USA, included 563 incident cases and 523 controls (Cramer *et al.*, 2000). The overall participation rate was about 55% for both cases and controls. Ever (≥ 3 months) use of oral contraceptives was reported by 226 (40%) cases and 276 (53%) controls [which corresponded to a crude odds ratio of 0.66 (95% CI, 0.52–0.84)].

A hospital-based case–control study of ovarian cancer was conducted between 1992 and 1997 in the Rome area, Italy, and included 440 cases and 868 hospital controls, with a response rate over 97% for both cases and controls (Greggi *et al.*, 2000). The multivariate odds ratio (adjusted for age, education, parity and family history of ovarian cancer) for ever having used oral contraceptives was 0.4 (95% CI, 0.3–0.6) and that for long-term use (≥ 2 years) was 0.3.

A study was conducted in Delaware Valley, USA, which included contiguous counties in Pennsylvania, New Jersey and Delaware, between 1994 and 1998 (Ness *et al.*, 2000) on 767 cases and 1367 community controls under the age of 70 years; the response rate was 88% for incident cases and 72% for controls. A relative risk of 0.6 (95% CI, 0.3–0.8) for ever having used oral contraceptives and 0.3 (95% CI, 0.1–0.5) for ≥ 10 years of use was found after adjustment for age, parity and family history of ovarian cancer. The protection was similar for use of low-estrogen/low-progestogen and for high-estrogen (≥ 50 μg ethinylestradiol)/high-progestogen (≥ 0.5 mg norgestrel) formulations (relative risk ranged between 0.5 and 0.7 for women who had ever used various combinations). The reduced risk was similar across strata of gravidity and when hormonal preparations were used for contraceptive or non-contraceptive uses (e.g. endometriosis) (Ness *et al.*, 2001). Another report from the same dataset considered 616 invasive and 151 borderline tumours and various histotypes separately (Modugno *et al.*, 2001). The relative risk per year of oral contraceptive use was 0.94 (95% CI, 0.91–0.96) for all invasive cancers, 0.93 (95% CI, 0.90–0.97) for serous (218 cases), 0.93 (95% CI, 0.85–1.02) for mucinous (52 cases), 0.93 (95% CI, 0.88–0.97) for endometrioid (136 cases) and 0.98 for other invasive tumours (150 cases), 0.92 (95% CI, 0.88–0.98) for all borderline cancers, 0.91 (95% CI, 0.85–0.98) for serous (79 cases) and 0.94 (95% CI, 0.88–1.01) for mucinous (60 cases) ovarian borderline tumours. In this dataset, information on androgenicity of oral contraceptives was available for 568 cases and 1026 controls (Greer *et al.*, 2005). The relative risk was 0.52 (95% CI, 0.35–0.76) for use of androgenic oral contraceptives and 0.58 (95% CI, 0.45–0.78) for use of non-androgenic oral contraceptives. No difference in risk between androgenic and non-androgenic formulations was observed in relation to duration of use, age at first use or time since last use. Another report (Walker *et al.*, 2002) showed a protective effect in both women with and those without a family history of ovarian cancer, although the number of women with a family history was small (three cases, nine controls).

In a case–control study conducted in Italy between 1983 and 1991 on 971 incident cases under 75 years of age and 2758 hospital controls that was included in the previous evaluation (IARC, 1999), no appreciable difference in the relation between oral use of hormonal contraceptives and the risk for ovarian cancer was observed between women with and those without family history of ovarian and breast cancer (Tavani *et al.*, 2000). The response rate was over 95% for both cases and controls. The relative risk for women who had ever used oral contraceptives was 0.7 in those with and 0.8 in those without a family history. Adjustment was made for age and area of residence. When different histological types of ovarian cancer were considered in the same dataset, the relative risk for ever use of oral contraceptives was 0.7 (95% CI, 0.5–1.0) for serous, 1.4 (95% CI, 0.6–3.4) for mucinous and 0.8 (95% CI, 0.2–2.9) for endometrioid neoplasms (Parazzini *et al.*, 2004).

A multicentric study was conducted between in 1992 and 1997 in four areas of northern, central and southern Italy and included 1031 cases of ovarian cancer and 2441 hospital controls under the age of 80 years (Chiaffarino *et al.*, 2001). The response rate was over 95% for both cases and controls. Adjustment was made for age, centre, education, parity and family history of ovarian and breast cancer. The multivariate relative risk was

0.9 for ever having used hormonal contraceptives and 0.5 for ≥ 5 years of use. In the same dataset, the relative risk for ≥ 5 years of oral contraceptive use was 0.9 for women with a family history of breast or ovarian cancer in first-degree relatives and 0.5 for those without (Tavani *et al.*, 2004).

A case–control study was conducted between 1993 and 1996 in two regions of Germany and included 282 patients with ovarian cancer (invasive and borderline) aged 20–75 years and 533 population controls (Royar *et al.*, 2001). [The overall response rate was approximately 58% for cases and 53% for controls.] The multivariate relative risk for ever having used oral contraceptives was 0.5, after adjusting for parity, breast-feeding, family history of ovarian cancer, tubal ligation and hysterectomy; the decrease in risk was 7% per year of use (95% CI, 4–10%). The reduced risk was observed for oral contraceptives that contained < 35 µg (relative risk, 0.14; 95% CI, 0.06–0.36), 35–45 µg (relative risk, 0.33; 95% CI, 0.15–0.72) and ≥ 50 µg (relative risk, 0.57; 95% CI, 0.34–0.89) ethinylestradiol.

The potency of progestogen and estrogen in oral contraceptives in relation to the risk for ovarian cancer was also considered in a re-analysis of the CASH Study that was conducted between 1980 and 1982 in eight population-based cancer registries of the US SEER Program and included 390 cases and 2869 controls. This highest risk was found for non-users compared with users of high-potency oral contraceptives (odds ratio, 2.9; 95% CI, 1.8–4.5) (Schildkraut *et al.*, 2002). Compared with women who did not use oral contraceptives, the relative risk for long-term (≥ 5 years) use was 0.2 (95% CI, 0.1–0.5) for high-potency progestogen, 0.4 (95% CI, 0.2–0.6) for high-potency estrogen, 0.4 (95% CI, 0.2–0.6) for low-potency progestogen and 0.3 (95% CI, 0.1–0.6) for low-potency estrogen formulations.

In a population-based case–control study of 655 incident cases of ovarian cancer and 3899 controls aged 50–74 years conducted between 1993 and 1995 in Sweden (Riman *et al.*, 2002), the relative risk for ever having used oral contraceptives was 0.73 (95% CI, 0.59–0.90) and that for longest use (≥ 10 years) was 0.36 (95% CI, 0.22–0.59). The response rate was 76% for cases and 83% for controls. Adjustment was made for age, parity, body mass index and age at menopause. The inverse association with oral use of hormonal contraceptives tended to decrease with time since last use, although the risk remained below unity 25 years or more after last use. The inverse association was observed for serous (odds ratio, 0.56; 95% CI, 0.42–0.71 for ever use), endometrioid (odds ratio, 0.71; 95% CI, 0.49–1.03) and clear-cell (odds ratio, 0.66; 95% CI, 0.31–1.43) cancers but not for mucinous tumours (relative risk, 1.96; 95% CI, 1.04–3.67). The same group of 3899 controls was used in a case–control study of 193 cases of borderline ovarian tumours (including 110 serous and 81 mucinous) aged 50–74 years (Riman *et al.*, 2001). The refusal rate for cases was less than 25%. Oral use of hormonal contraceptives conferred no protection against borderline ovarian cancers. The multivariate risks for ever having used oral contraceptives, adjusted for age, parity, body mass index, age at menopause and use of various types of hormonal therapy, were 1.23 (95% CI, 0.9–1.8) overall, 1.40 (95% CI, 0.87–2.26) for serous borderline tumours and 1.04 (95% CI, 0.61–1.79) for mucinous borderline tumours. No relation was observed with duration of or time since last use of oral contraceptives; the relative risk for ≥ 10 years of use was 1.16 (95% CI, 0.61–2.10). [The apparent difference from other studies on borderline cancers may be related to the older age of these users.]

A multicentric case–control study conducted between 1993 and 1999 in Hawaii, HI, and Los Angeles, CA, USA, included 558 histologically confirmed ovarian epithelial cancers and 601 population controls (Tung et al., 2003). The participation rate was 62% for cases and 67% for controls. Adjustment was made for age, ethnicity, study site, education, pregnancy and tubal ligation. The relative risk for ever having used oral contraceptives was 0.6 (95% CI, 0.4–0.8) and that for > 5 years of use was 0.4 (95% CI, 0.3–0.6). The inverse relation was similar for mucinous (relative risk, 0.5; 95% CI, 0.3–0.9) and non-mucinous (relative risk, 0.6; 95% CI, 0.4–0.8) neoplasms, as well as for invasive (relative risk, 0.6; 95% CI, 0.4–0.8) and borderline ovarian tumours (relative risk, 0.6; 95% CI, 0.4–1.0). The protection appeared to level off with time since last use, and no protective effect was evident 10 years or more after last use.

A population-based case–control study was conducted in 2000–01 in 22 counties of central California and included 256 ovarian cancer cases (182 invasive, 74 borderline) and 1122 controls who were frequency-matched on age and ethnicity (Mills et al., 2004). Compared with women who had never used oral contraceptives, the relative risks adjusted for age, race or ethnicity and breast-feeding were 0.89 (95% CI, 0.59–1.36) for ≤ 1 year of use, 0.82 (95% CI, 0.55–1.21) for 2–5 years of use, 0.62 (95% CI, 0.38–1.00) for 6–10 years of use and 0.37 (95% CI, 0.20–0.68) for > 10 years of use. The results did not differ materially for invasive and borderline tumours, but the numbers were small.

A case–control study was conducted between 1992 and 1998 in Los Angeles County, CA, USA, on 477 cases of invasive ovarian epithelial cancer and 660 population controls aged 18–74 years (Pike et al., 2004). The participation rate was approximately 80% of cases and 70% of controls approached. Multivariate relative risks were adjusted for age, ethnicity, socioeconomic status, education, family history of ovarian cancer, tubal ligation, use of talc, nulliparity, age at last birth, menopausal status, age at menopause and type of hormonal therapy. Compared with women who had never used oral contraceptives, the relative risks were 1.00 (95% CI, 0.72–1.39) for < 5 years of use, 0.72 (95% CI, 0.46–1.13) for 5–9 years of use and 0.48 (95% CI, 0.23–0.78) for ≥ 10 years of use. The relative risk per year of use was 0.94 (95% CI, 0.91–0.97) overall and 0.88 (95% CI, 0.81–0.97) for high-estrogen/high-progestogen, 0.94 (95% CI, 0.88–1.00) for high-estrogen/low-progestogen, 0.66 (95% CI, 0.36–1.21) for low-estrogen/high-progestogen and 0.95 (95% CI, 0.92–0.99) for low-estrogen/low-progestogen preparations.

A collaborative re-analysis (Bosetti et al., 2002) of use of oral contraceptives and risk for ovarian cancer was based on 2768 cases and 6274 controls from six studies conducted in three European countries (Greece, Italy and the United Kingdom; Tzonou et al., 1984; Booth et al., 1989; Polychronopoulou et al., 1993; Parazzini et al., 1994; Greggi et al., 2000; Chiaffarino et al., 2001). Adjustment was made for age and other sociodemographic factors, calendar year of interview, menopausal status and parity. The multivariate relative risk was 0.7 (95% CI, 0.6–0.8) for ever use and 0.4 (95% CI, 0.3–0.6) for longest use

(≥ 5 years), which corresponded to a decrease in risk of approximately 5% per year of use. The protective effect appeared to persist for at least 20 years after last use of oral contraceptives in the absence of any significant trend of decreasing risk with time since cessation of use.

Oral hormonal contraceptives are commonly used in the treatment of endometriosis. Data from four population-based case–control studies conducted in the USA between 1993 and 2001 were pooled to analyse risk factors for ovarian cancer in women with no endometriosis (Modugno et al., 2004). These included 2759 cases of ovarian cancer with no endometriosis, 184 cases with endometriosis, 1972 controls with no endometriosis and 177 controls with endometriosis. Multivariate relative risks were computed with adjustment for study centre, age and family history of ovarian cancer. Compared with women who had never used oral contraceptives, the relative risk was 0.58 (95% CI, 0.33–1.03) for < 10 years and 0.21 (95% CI, 0.08–0.58) for ≥ 10 years of use among women with endometriosis and 0.70 (95% CI, 0.60–0.80) for < 10 years and 0.47 (95% CI, 0.37–0.61) for ≥ 10 years of use among women with no endometriosis.

2.4.4   Case–control studies among breast cancer gene (BRCA1/2) carriers (Table 14)

A study conducted in North America and Europe on 207 susceptible women with hereditary ovarian cancer (179 with BRCA1 and 28 with BRCA2 mutations) and 161 sister controls found a relative risk of 0.5 (95% CI, 0.3–0.8) for ever use of oral contraceptives; the risk decreased with increasing duration of use (relative risk, 0.4; 95% CI, 0.2–0.7 for > 6 years). Adjustment was made for geographical area of residence, year of birth, parity and age at first birth. The results were similar (relative risk, 0.4 for ever use and 0.3 for > 6 years of use) when the comparison was made with control carriers of BRCA1 or BRCA2 only (Narod et al., 1998).

In a population-based case–control study from Israel (Modan et al., 2001), 240 cases of ovarian cancer with BRCA1 or BRCA2 mutations and 592 cases with no mutations were compared with 2257 controls. Oral use of hormonal contraceptives and duration of use were inversely related to the risk for ovarian cancer in women with no mutations, but not in those with BRCA1 or BRCA2 mutations. The relative risk for ≥ 5 years of use was 1.07 (95% CI, 0.63–1.83) in mutation carriers and 0.53 (95% CI, 0.34–0.84) in non-carriers.

In a case–control study of 36 BRCA1-carrier cases of ovarian cancer, 381 non-carrier cases and 568 population controls conducted between 1997 and 2001 in the San Francisco Bay Area, CA, USA (McGuire et al., 2004), the relative risk for ever having used oral contraceptives was 0.54 (95% CI, 0.26–1.13) among BRCA1 mutation carriers and 0.55 (95% CI, 0.41–0.75) among non-carriers. The relative risk for use of ≥ 7 years was 0.22 (95% CI, 0.07–0.71) among BRCA1 carriers and 0.43 (95% CI, 0.30–0.63) among non-carriers. The response rate was 75% among cases and 72% among controls. Adjustment was made for age, ethnicity and parity.

Table 14. Case–control studies on combined oral contraceptives and ovarian cancer among *BRCA1/2* carrier cases

Reference, country	Type of study	Relative risk (95% CI)		
		No. of cases (age in years)	Ever use	Longest use (duration)
Narod *et al.* (1998), USA	Hereditary cancers	207 (< 75) with *BRCA1* (179) or *BRCA2* (28) mutations	0.5 (0.3–0.8)	0.4 (0.2–0.7) (> 6 years)
Modan *et al.* (2001), Israel	Population-based	240 with *BRCA1/2* mutations	1.1 (0.7–1.9) (0.1–1.9 years) 0.8 (0.4–1.4) (2.0–4.9 years)	1.1 (0.6–1.8) (≥ 5 years)
McGuire *et al.* (2004), USA	Population-based	36 *BRCA1* carriers 381 *BRCA1* non-carriers	0.5 (0.3–1.1) 0.6 (0.4–0.8)	0.2 (0.1–0.7) (≥ 7 years) 0.4 (0.3–0.6) (≥ 7 years)
Whittemore *et al.* (2004), Australia and United Kingdom	Registry-based *BRCA1/2* carriers	147 with *BRCA1* or *BRCA2* mutations	0.9 (0.5–1.4)	0.6 (0.4–1.1) (≥ 6 years)

CI, confidence interval

A study based on registers of women with *BRCA1* or *BRCA2* germline mutations from Australia and the United Kingdom included 147 cases of ovarian cancer and 304 controls. The multivariate relative risk for ever having used oral contraceptives was 0.85 (95% CI, 0.53–1.4) and that for ≥ 6 years of use was 0.62 (95% CI, 0.35–1.1). Adjustment was made for study centre, parity and age. The continuous relative risk per year of use among users was 0.95 (95% CI, 0.91–0.99) (Whittemore *et al.*, 2004).

2.5   Liver cancer

The majority of primary liver cancers are hepatocellular carcinomas. The major risk factor for these cancers in areas of high incidence is chronic infection with hepatitis B (HBV) virus, but the continuing increase seen in low-risk western populations is due at least in part to the increasing prevalence of hepatitis C virus, which also causes hepato-cellular carcinoma (IARC, 1994). Aflatoxin on mouldy food, liver cirrhosis, consumption of alcoholic beverages (IARC, 1988; Baan *et al.*, 2007) and tobacco smoking (IARC, 2004) are also important causes of this disease. Cholangiocarcinoma is less common than hepatocellular carcinoma, although it frequently occurs in parts of South-East Asia, and can be caused by infection with liver flukes (Parkin *et al.*, 1991).

2.5.1 Descriptive studies

Forman *et al.* (1983) analysed the rates of mortality from primary liver cancer among men and women in England and Wales between 1958 and 1981. The age-standardized death rate in women aged 20–39 years increased from 0.9 per million in 1970–75 to 1.8 per million in 1976–81 ($p < 0.005$), whereas changes in death rates between these periods among women aged 40–54 years and among men were small and were not statistically significant. The authors suggested that the change was consistent with the idea that combined oral contraceptives caused some cases of liver cancer, but noted that no such trend was apparent in Australia, western Germany, the Netherlands or the USA — other countries where the use of combined oral contraceptives had been similar to that in England and Wales. In an analysis of subsequent secular trends in mortality in England and Wales, Mant and Vessey (1995) concluded that the rate of mortality from liver cancer had remained constant in age groups of women who had had major exposure to oral contraceptives, and Waetjen and Grimes (1996) found no evidence for an effect of the oral use of hormonal contraceptives on secular trends in death rates from liver cancer in Sweden or the USA.

2.5.2 Cohort studies

In the Nurses' Health Study in the USA, Colditz *et al.* (1994) studied a cohort of 121 700 female registered nurses aged 30–55 years in 1976 who were followed up for deaths until 1988. Women who reported angina, myocardial infarct, stroke or cancer at baseline were excluded, which left 116 755 women for follow-up. Of these, 55% reported having used combined oral contraceptives and 5% reported current use. Incidence rates with person–months of follow-up were used as the denominator and oral contraceptive use at recruitment as the exposure. The risks associated with any use of oral contraceptives relative to no use, adjusted for age, tobacco smoking, body mass index and follow-up interval, was 0.9 (95% CI, 0.8–1.0) for death from any cancer. Ten deaths from primary liver or biliary-tract cancer occurred during the 12 years of follow-up, two of which were among women who had used oral contraceptives, with a relative risk of 0.4 (95% CI, 0.1–2.4). No information was provided on infection with hepatitis viruses.

Hannaford *et al.* (1997) described the relationships between use of oral contraceptives and liver disease in two British prospective studies conducted by the Royal College of General Practitioners and the Oxford Family Planning Association. In the first study, 46 000 women, half of whom were using combined oral contraceptives, were recruited in 1968–69 and followed up until they changed their general practitioner or until 1995. Five cases of liver cancer were observed, comprising one hepatocellular carcinoma in a woman who had never used oral contraceptives, three cholangiocarcinomas in women who had formerly used oral contraceptives and one cholangiocarcinoma in a woman who had never used oral contraceptives. The risk for cholangiocarcinoma associated with former use of oral contraceptives in relation to no use was 3.2 (95% CI, 0.3–31). In a study of mortality in the same cohort after 25 years of follow-up, five deaths from liver cancer occurred among women who had used combined oral contraceptives and one in a woman who had never used them, to give a relative risk of 5.0 (95% CI, 0.6–43) (Beral *et al.*, 1999). In the study of the Oxford Family Planning Association, 17 032 women were recruited between 1968 and 1974, and most were followed up until 1994. Three liver cancers were reported, comprising two hepatocellular carcinomas and one cholangiocarcinoma, all in women who had formerly used oral contraceptives. No information on infection with hepatitis viruses was provided.

2.5.3   Case–control studies

(a)   Benign neoplasms of the liver

Edmondson *et al.* (1976) interviewed by telephone 34 of 42 eligible women who had undergone surgery for hepatocellular adenoma in Los Angeles, CA, USA, between 1955 and 1976. One age-matched friend control was interviewed for each case. Twenty-eight of the 34 (82%) cases and 19 of 34 (56%) controls had used oral contraceptives for more than 12 months. The risks relative to use of combined oral contraceptives for less than 12 months were 1.3 for 13–36 months of use, 5.0 for 61–84 months of use, 7.5 for 85–108 months of use and 25 for 109 months of use and longer.

Rooks *et al.* (1979) interviewed 79 of 89 eligible women aged 16–50 years in whom hepatocellular adenoma had been diagnosed between 1960 and 1976 at the Armed Forces Institute of Pathology, Washington DC, USA. Three age-matched neighbourhood controls were sought for each case, and 220 were interviewed. Seventy-two of the 79 (91%) cases and 99 of 220 (45%) controls had used oral contraceptives for more than 12 months. The risks relative to use of oral contraceptives for less than 12 months were 0.9 for 13–36 months of use, 1.16 for 37–60 months of use, 1.29 for 61–84 months of use and 5.03 for 85 months of use and longer.

Gemer *et al.* (2004) conducted a case–control study of liver haemangioma in women that included 40 cases diagnosed between 1995 and 2002 at the Barzilai Medical Centre, Ashkelon, Israel, and 109 control women with normal liver scans. The odds ratio for liver lesions was 1.2 (95% CI, 0.5–2.6) for women who had ever used oral contraceptives and 0.7 (95% CI, 0.2–3.0) for use within the last 2 years.

(b)   Malignant tumours of the liver

The studies on malignant tumours of the liver described below are summarized in Table 15.

Henderson *et al.* (1983b) studied women in Los Angeles County, CA, USA, in whom liver cancer had been diagnosed and confirmed histologically during 1975–80 when they were 18–39 years of age. Two neighbourhood controls were sought for each case and matched on age and ethnic group. Twelve cases of liver cancer were identified, and interviews were obtained with 11 of the patients: eight with hepatocellular carcinoma, one with a giant-cell carcinoma, one with a sclerosing duct-forming carcinoma and one with a papillary carcinoma. Four of 22 identified controls refused to be interviewed and were replaced, to give a response rate among those first selected of 82%; the true response rate was probably lower because the census information used to identify controls could not be

Table 15. Case–control studies of use of combined oral contraceptives and liver cancer

Reference, study area	Age (years)	No. of cases	No. of controls	Odds ratio[a] (95% CI)	Comments
Henderson et al. (1983b), California, USA	18–39	11	22	[7.0 (0.7–71)]	
Forman et al. (1986), England and Wales	20–44	30	147	3.8 (1.0–14.6)	Adjusted for age, year of birth
Neuberger et al. (1986), United Kingdom	< 50	26	1333	1.0 (0.4–2.4)	Not adjusted for tobacco smoking or alcoholic beverage consumption. Three cases are also included in Forman et al. (1986).
Palmer et al. (1989), USA	19–54	12	60	[15 (1.7–126)]	No information on tobacco smoking
WHO Collaborative Study (1989b), Chile, China, Colombia, Israel, Kenya, Nigeria, Philippines, Thailand	15–56 (mean, 41.8)	122	802	0.7 (0.4–1.2)	Adjusted for alcoholic beverage consumption, number of live births, occupation
Kew et al. (1990), South Africa	15–54	46	92	1.9 (0.6–5.6)	No effect of alcoholic beverage or tobacco consumption on risk estimates
Vall Mayans et al. (1990), Catalonia region, Spain	No age limits	29	57	[4.7 (1.1–20)]	86.5 % of cases had liver cirrhosis. Tobacco and alcohol adjustment did not alter risk estimates.
Yu et al. (1991), California, USA	18–74	25	58	3.0 (1.0–9.0)	Adjustment for tobacco and alcohol did not alter risk estimates.
Hsing et al. (1992), USA	25–49	72	549	1.6 (0.6–2.6)	Adjusted for age, education, parity
Tavani et al. (1993), Italy	28–60	43	194	2.6 (1.0–7.0)	
Collaborative MILTS (1997), France, Germany, Greece, Italy, Spain, United Kingdom	< 65	293	1779	0.8 (0.5–1.0)	No association for duration of use, type of formulation; significantly increased risk for > 6 years of use in individuals with no hepatitis infection or liver cirrhosis
Yu et al. (2003), Taiwan (China)	≥ 35	218	729	0.75 (0.44–1.28)	No association for ≥ 2 years' duration of use

CI, confidence interval; MILTS, Multicentre International Liver Tumour Study
[a] Odds ratios are given for never versus ever use of oral contraceptives.

obtained for 4.3% of the houses surveyed. None of the patients or controls reported a prior history of hepatitis or jaundice; none of the four cases had HBV surface antigens (HBsAg); none of the patients reported exposure to any known hepatotoxin, and there was no difference in the frequency of alcoholic beverage consumption between cases and controls. Tobacco smoking histories were not reported. Ten of the 11 patients (including seven of the eight cases of hepatocellular carcinoma) had used oral contraceptives, and the 11th had received hormone injections of an undetermined type; 13 of the 22 controls had used oral contraceptives. The average duration of use of oral contraceptives was 64.7 months for the patients and 27.1 months for the controls (one-sided matched $p < 0.005$). [The relative risk for any use of oral contraceptives was 7.0 (95% CI, 0.7–71) for hepatocellular carcinoma and 6.9 (95% CI, 0.7–64) for all liver cancers (unmatched analyses).]

Forman *et al.* (1986) identified all women certified to have died from primary liver cancer at the age of 20–44 years in England and Wales between 1979 and 1982. Two controls were selected for each case from among women who had died from cancer of the kidney, cancer of the brain or acute myeloid leukaemia, and, for 1982 only, two further controls were selected for each case from among women who had died as a result of a road traffic accident. Information on exposure was obtained from a questionnaire sent to the general practitioners of cases for 46 of 85 (54.1%) potential cases and for 147 of 233 (63.1%) eligible controls. Eighteen of 30 (60%) cases had used oral contraceptives compared with 79 of 147 (54%) controls. Information on tobacco smoking and alcoholic beverage consumption was not available. The relative risks, adjusted for age and year of birth, were: for hepatocellular carcinoma, 3.8 for any use, 3.0 for < 4 years, 4.0 for 4–7 years and 20.1 for ≥ 8 years of use; for cholangiocarcinoma, 0.3 for any use, 0.1 for < 4 years and 0.9 for ≥ 4 years of use. [The published risks were adjusted for age and year of birth, but CIs were not given. The unadjusted relative risks and 95% CIs, calculated from the published data, were: hepatocellular carcinoma, any use, 3.2 (95% CI, 1.0–10); < 4 years, 2.4 (95% CI, 0.7–8.5); 4–7 years, 3.6 (95% CI, 0.8–16); and ≥ 8 years, 13 (95% CI, 2.1–78); cholangiocarcinoma, any use, 0.3 (95% CI, 0.1–1.3); < 4 years, 0.2 (95% CI, 0.0–1.3); and ≥ 4 years, 0.7 (95% CI, 0.2–3.7).] There was no information on infection with hepatitis viruses. Three cases in this study were also included in the study of Neuberger *et al.* (1986), described below.

Neuberger *et al.* (1986) studied 26 women in whom hepatocellular carcinoma had been diagnosed and confirmed histologically in a non-cirrhotic liver when they were under the age of 50 years. The cases were referred from all over the United Kingdom to the Liver Unit at King's College School of Medicine and Dentistry, London, between 1976 and 1985. The controls were 1333 women who had been hospital controls in a case–control study of breast cancer and had been interviewed during 1976–80. The results were not adjusted for tobacco smoking or alcoholic beverage use. Eighteen of the 26 (69%) cases had taken hormonal contraceptives orally. The controls were used to calculate the expected numbers of cases for each duration of oral contraceptive use, within age and calendar groups. The expected number of women who had ever used oral contraceptives was 18.7, which gave a relative risk of 1.0 (95% CI, 0.4–2.4). The relative risks by duration of use were 0.3 (95% CI, 0.1–1.1) for < 4 years, 0.9 (95% CI, 0.3–3.4) for 4–7 years and 4.4 (95% CI, 1.5–13) for ≥ 8 years. None of the cases had HBsAg, but one had antisurface antibodies and three had anticore antibodies. Exclusion of these four cases changed the relative risks associated with oral contraceptive use to 1.5 (95% CI, 0.5–4.4) for any use, 0.5 (95% CI, 0.1–1.9) for < 4 years, 1.5 (95% CI, 0.4–6.3) for 4–7 years and 7.2 (95% CI, 2.0–26) for ≥ 8 years. Three cases in this study were also included in the study of Forman *et al.* (1986), described above.

Palmer *et al.* (1989) conducted a hospital-based case–control study of women in whom liver cancer had been diagnosed when they were 19–54 years of age in five cities in the USA in 1977–85. They identified 12 cases of liver cancer, of which nine were hepatocellular carcinoma, two were cholangiocarcinoma and one was undetermined. None of the cases reported a history of hepatitis, nor was there mention in their hospital discharge summaries of HBV infection; liver cirrhosis was discovered at the time of surgery in one case of hepatocellular carcinoma. Five controls were selected for each case and matched on hospital, age and date of interview. Tobacco smoking status was not reported, but alcoholic beverage intake was similar in cases and controls. Eleven of the 12 cases (including eight of the nine cases of hepatocellular carcinoma) and 20 of the 60 controls had used oral contraceptives. The risk for hepatocellular carcinoma relative to women who had used oral contraceptives for < 2 years was 20 (95% CI, 2.0–190) for 2–4 years of use and 20 (95% CI, 1.6–250) for ≥ 5 years of use. [The unmatched relative risk for any use was 15 (95% CI, 1.7–126).]

The WHO Collaborative Study of Neoplasia and Steroid Contraceptives (1989) was a hospital-based case–control study conducted in eight countries between 1979 and 1986. A total of 168 eligible cases were identified; 122 (72.6%) of the diagnoses were confirmed, and these women were interviewed. Histological typing was available for 69 cases: 36 were hepatocellular carcinoma, 29 were cholangiocarcinoma, one was an adenocarcinoma and three were not specified. Controls were selected from among individuals admitted to the same hospitals as the cases with conditions not thought to be related to the use of oral contraceptives. The overall response rate of controls was 94.3%. Information on tobacco smoking was not collected; there was no statistically significant difference in alcoholic beverage consumption between cases and controls (17.2% of the cases and 26% of the controls had ever drunk alcoholic beverages). The finding that 25 of 122 cases (20.5%) and 216 of 802 controls (26.9%) had used oral contraceptives gave odds ratios, adjusted for number of live births and occupation, of 0.7 (95% CI, 0.4–1.2) for any use, 0.8 (95% CI, 0.4–1.5) for use of 1–12 months, 0.7 (95% CI, 0.3–1.7) for use of 13–36 months and 0.7 (95% CI, 0.3–1.7) for use of ≥ 37 months. The odds ratios for any use by histological subtype were 0.6 (95% CI, 0.2–1.6) for hepatocellular carcinoma, 1.2 (95% CI, 0.5–3.1) for cholangiocarcinoma and 0.5 (95% CI, 0.2–1.3) for a clinical diagnosis with no histological confirmation. Information on prior infection with hepatitis viruses was not collected, but all except one of the study centres were in countries with high rates of liver cancer where HBV infection is endemic.

Kew *et al.* (1990) conducted a hospital-based case–control study in Johannesburg, South Africa, among patients in whom histologically confirmed hepatocellular carcinoma had been diagnosed when they were aged 19–54 years. Two controls per case were selected and matched by age, race, tribe, rural or urban birth, hospital and ward. Patients with diseases in which contraceptive steroids might be causally implicated were not considered eligible as controls. Tobacco smoking and alcoholic beverage intake were associated with the risk for liver cancer, but inclusion of these variables in the analysis did not alter the results. Seven of 46 (15.2%) cases and eight of 92 (8.7%) controls had ever used oral contraceptives, to give an overall relative risk of 1.9 (95% CI, 0.6–5.6). The relative risks were 2.1 (95% CI, 0.4–11) for use of < 4 years, 2.0 (95% CI, 0.1–33.1) for use of 4–8 years and 1.5 (95% CI, 0.3–7.2) for use of > 8 years. Nineteen of 46 cases were HBsAg-positive, 25 had evidence of past infection with HBV and two had never been infected. The odds ratio for hepatocellular carcinoma in HBsAg-negative patients who used contraceptive steroids of any type was 0.4 (95% CI, 0.2–1.0).

Vall Mayans *et al.* (1990) conducted a hospital-based case–control study in the Catalonia region of northeastern Spain, where 96 patients admitted to the Liver Unit of the University Hospital in Barcelona between 1986 and 1988 were identified, 74 of whom had histologically or cytologically confirmed hepatocellular carcinoma. Liver cirrhosis was present in 83 (86.5%) cases. For the 29 female cases, two controls were selected per case and matched on sex, age, hospital and time of admission. Patients with diagnoses related to the use of oral contraceptives were considered ineligible as controls. One control was excluded from the analysis because of later confirmation of liver cirrhosis. Serum from all patients was tested for HBsAg, antibody to hepatitis B core antigen and antibody to hepatitis surface antigen. All patients were interviewed, but the response rates were not given. Tobacco smoking was not associated with risk, and adjustment for alcoholic beverage intake did not alter the results. Six of 29 female cases (20.7%) and three of 57 female controls (5.3%) had used oral contraceptives [unmatched relative risk, 4.7 (95% CI, 1.1–20)]. Overall, 9.4% of cases and 2.1% of controls were HBsAg-positive, and all of the users of oral contraceptives were HBsAg-negative.

Yu *et al.* (1991) used a population-based cancer registry to identify cases of histologically confirmed hepatocellular carcinoma diagnosed in black or white non-Asian women aged 18–74 years resident in Los Angeles County, CA, USA, between 1984 and 1990. Two neighbourhood controls were sought for each case and matched on sex, year of birth and race. Adjustment for tobacco smoking and alcoholic beverage consumption did not alter the results. Thirteen of 25 (52%) cases and 18 of 58 (31%) controls had used oral contraceptives. The odds ratios were 3.0 (95% CI, 1.0–9.0) for any use, 2.3 (95% CI, 0.5–11) for use of ≤ 12 months, 1.7 (95% CI, 0.3–9.1) for use of 13–60 months and 5.5 (95% CI, 1.2–25) for use of ≥ 61 months. For the 11 cases who had formerly used oral contraceptives, the mean time since last use was 14.5 years. Seven cases had antibodies to one or more markers of hepatitis viral infection; when these cases were excluded, the association between the use of oral contraceptives and the risk for hepatocellular carcinoma became stronger.

Hsing *et al.* (1992) studied deaths from primary liver cancer among women aged 25–49 years in the USA (except the State of Oregon) in 1985 and in the National Mortality Followback Survey in 1986. The study included 98 cases for analysis, of which 76 were primary liver cancer and 22 were cholangiocarcinoma. Controls were selected from among women in the National Mortality Followback Study who had died in 1986 from causes other than liver cancer and whose next of kin returned the questionnaire. Potential controls with evidence of chronic liver disease or whose causes of death were thought to be associated with oral contraceptive use were excluded, which left 629 controls for analysis. The odds ratios were adjusted for tobacco smoking and alcoholic beverage use. For all subjects with complete data, 39 of 72 (54.2%) cases and 243 of 549 (44.3%) controls had ever used oral contraceptives; the odds ratios were 1.6 (95% CI, 0.9–2.6) for any use, 1.2 (95% CI, 0.6–2.4) for use of < 5 years, 2.0 (95% CI, 1.0–4.4) for use of 5–9 years and 2.0 (95% CI, 0.8–4.8) for use of ≥ 10 years. For subjects whose spouse or parent responded, the relative risks were 2.7 (95% CI, 1.4–5.3) for any use, 2.1 (95% CI, 0.9–4.6) for use of < 5 years, 3.9 (95% CI, 1.6–9.6) for use of 5–9 years and 4.8 (95% CI, 1.7–14) for use of ≥ 10 years. When the four Asian cases and 10 controls from populations who were presumed to have a higher prevalence of HBV infection were excluded from the analysis, higher risk estimates were seen for any use (2.8; 95% CI, 1.4–5.5) and for long-term (≥ 10 years) use (5.2; 95% CI, 1.7–15). The relative risks for the 13 cases of cholangiocarcinoma were 0.8 (95% CI, 0.3–2.7) for any use, 0.5 (95% CI, 0.1–2.7) for < 5 years of use, 0.6 (95% CI, 0.1–5.4) for 5–9 years of use and 3.3 (95% CI, 0.7–16) for ≥ 10 years of use.

Tavani *et al.* (1993) conducted a hospital-based case–control study of women who had histologically or serologically confirmed hepatocellular carcinoma diagnosed at the age of 28–73 years in the greater Milan area, Italy, between 1984 and 1992. Controls were women admitted to hospital for acute non-neoplastic diseases (37% traumas, 13% other orthopaedic disorders, 40% acute surgical conditions, 10% other). Since none of the women aged 60 years or over had ever used oral contraceptives, the analysis was restricted to women under that age. Nine of 43 (20.9%) cases and 21 of 194 (10.8%) controls had ever used oral contraceptives. The odds ratios, adjusted for age, education and parity, were 2.6 (95% CI, 1.0–7.0) for any use, 1.5 (95% CI, 0.5–5.0) for use of ≤ 5 years and 3.9 (95% CI, 0.6–25) for use of > 5 years. In relation to time since oral contraceptives were last used, the odds ratios were 1.1 (95% CI, 0.3–4.6) for ≤ 10 years and 4.3 (95% CI, 1.0–18) for > 10 years. No information was available on infection with hepatitis viruses.

The Multicentre International Liver Tumour Study (Collaborative MILTS Project Team, 1997) included women who had hepatocellular carcinoma and were diagnosed before the age of 65 years between 1990 and 1996 in seven hospitals in Germany and one each in France, Greece, Italy, Spain and the United Kingdom. The diagnoses were based on histological examination or on imaging and increased α-fetoprotein concentration. An average of four controls was sought for each case: two general hospital controls without cancer, one hospital control with a diagnosis of an eligible tumour and one population control. The controls were frequency-matched for age, and living controls were obtained for cases who had died. Of the 368 eligible cases, 317 (86.1%) were included. Oral contraceptive use was reported for 148 of the 293 (50.5%) cases and 1086 of the 1779 (61.0%) controls. The odds ratio for any use of oral contraceptives was 0.8 (95% CI, 0.5–1.0); those by duration of use were 0.8 (95% CI, 0.5–1.3) for 1–2 years, 0.6 (95% CI, 0.3–1.1) for 3–5 years and 0.8 (95% CI, 0.5–1.1) for ≥ 6 years of use. For use of oral contraceptives that contained cyproterone acetate, the odds ratios were 0.9 (95% CI, 0.5–1.6) for any use, 0.9 (95% CI, 0.4–2.4) for use of 1–2 years, 0.9 (95% CI, 0.3–2.4) for use of 3–5 years and 0.9 (95% CI, 0.4–2.0) for use of ≥ 6 years. When the analysis was restricted to the 51 cases who had no liver cirrhosis or evidence of infection with hepatitis viruses, the odds ratios increased to 1.3 (95% CI, 0.4–4.0) for use of any oral contraceptives of 1–2 years, 1.8 (95% CI, 0.5–6.0) for use of 3–5 years and 2.8 (95% CI, 1.3–6.3) for use of ≥ 6 years.

Yu *et al.* (2003) conducted a multicentre case–control study on reproductive risk factors for hepatocellular carcinoma in women in Taiwan, China, where this disease is common. Cases were 218 women aged 35 years or over who had hepatocellular carcinoma and were recruited through four large hospitals; 729 controls were selected from first-degree or non-biological relatives. Twenty cases (9.2%) and 110 (15%) controls had used oral contraceptives, to give an adjusted odds ratio of 0.75 (95% CI, 0.44–1.28) for ever having used and 0.38 (95% CI, 0.13–1.09) for more than 2 years of use of oral contraceptives.

2.6   Colorectal cancer

Several studies have provided information on the use of combined oral contraceptives and the risk for colorectal cancer. The previous evaluation of exogenous hormones and risk for cancer reviewed four cohort and 10 case–control studies, none of which showed significantly elevated risks in women who used these preparations for any length of time (Tables 16 and 17). The relative risks were below unity for nine studies, and statistically significant in two (IARC, 1999).

Some aspects, however, remain undefined, including the risk related to duration and recency of use and more adequate allowance for confounding, which left the issue of a causal inference for the observed association open to discussion. This section reviews data on oral contraceptives and colorectal cancer that have been published since the last evaluation (IARC, 1999).

2.6.1   Cohort studies

In addition to the four cohort studies reviewed previously (IARC, 1999), four cohort studies have provided new data on the potential association between oral contraceptives and colorectal cancer (Table 16).

van Wayenburg *et al.* (2000) analysed the mortality from colorectal cancer according to several reproductive variables in the Diagnostisch Onderzoek Mammacarcinoom (DOM) cohort study, a population-based breast cancer screening programme in Utrecht, The Netherlands. Between 1974 and 1977, 14 697 women who lived in Utrecht were enrolled in the DOM study, and 12 239 women who attended the second screening visit

Table 16. Cohort studies of oral use of contraceptives and colorectal cancer

Reference	Country and study	Population (follow-up); no. of cases/ deaths	Relative risk (95% CI) (ever versus never users)			Comments
			Colorectal	Colon	Rectum	
Chute et al. (1991); Martinez et al. (1997)	USA Nurses' Health Study	89 448 (12 years); 501 cases	0.84 (0.69–1.02)	0.64 (0.40–1.02)	0.76 (0.49–1.18)	Adjusted for age, body mass index, exercise, family history of cancer, aspirin, alcohol, meat intake, menstrual factors; significant inverse trend with duration of use
Bostick et al. (1994)	Iowa State, USA	35 215 (4 years); 212 cases	–	1.0 (0.7–1.4)	–	Adjusted for age, height, parity, caloric intake, vitamin intake
Troisi et al. (1997)	USA BCDDP	57 528 (10 years); 95 cases	1.0 (0.7–1.4)	–	–	Adjusted for age only; adjustment for education, body mass index did not alter relative risk; no significant effect with duration of use.
Beral et al. (1999); Hannaford & Elliot (2005)[a]	United Kingdom RCGP OCS	46 000 (25 years); 146 cases, 438 controls	0.84 (0.56–1.24) < 5 years: 0.85 (0.52–1.38) 5–9 years: 0.75 (0.44–1.30) ≥ 10 years: 0.97 (0.52–1.80)			Adjusted for social class, smoking, parity, hormonal menopausal therapy (age and length of follow-up by matching)
van Wayenburg et al. (2000)	Netherlands DOM Study	10 671 (18 years); 95 deaths	0.68 (0.21–2.21)			Adjusted for age at entry, age at first birth, smoking, type of menopause, socioeconomic status, body mass index
Vessey et al. (2003)	United Kingdom OPFA Study	17 032 (30 years); 46 deaths	0.9 (0.4–2.1)			Relative risk of death for use < 24 months versus never use; no trend with duration of use; adjusted for age, parity, social class, smoking
Rosenblatt et al. (2004)	Shanghai, China	267 400 (10 years); 655 cases	–	1.09 (0.86–1.37)		No trend with duration of use; adjustment for age, parity

BCDDP, Breast Cancer Detection Demonstration Project; CI, confidence interval; DOM, Diagnostich Onderzoek Mammacarcinoom; OFPA, Oxford Family Planning Association; RCGP OCS, Royal College of General Practitioners Oral Contraceptive Study
[a] Nested case-control study within the RCGP OCS

were followed up over a median of 18 years. Few women in the cohort (5%) had ever used oral contraceptives and 95 women in the cohort died of colorectal cancer [number of deaths among exposed and unexposed not provided]. The relative risk for death from colorectal cancer was 0.68 (95% CI, 0.21–2.21), after adjustment for age at entry, age at first birth, tobacco smoking habits, natural or artificial menopause, socioeconomic status and body mass index (analysis according to duration of use not presented).

The Oxford Family Planning Association study was based on 17 032 women, aged 25–39 years at entry, who were recruited between 1968 and 1974 from various family planning clinics in the United Kingdom (Vessey & Painter, 1995) and followed up for mortality until the end of 2000. A total of 889 deaths were noted during 479 400 woman–years of observation. Only 8% of the woman–years related to women aged 60 years or more; 16% represented current or recent (within 1 year) users of oral contraceptive and 33% related to women who had not used such contraceptives in the preceding 96 months. From the total mortality observed, 46 women died from colorectal cancer, 18 of whom had never and 28 had ever used oral contraceptives. The multivariate relative risks for mortality from colorectal cancer were 0.9 (95% CI, 0.3–2.3) for < 4 years of oral contraceptive use, 1.1 (95% CI, 0.5–2.5) for 4–8 years of use and 0.8 (95% CI, 0.4–1.9) for > 8 years of use compared with no use. Adjustment was made for age, parity, social class and tobacco smoking (Vessey et al., 2003). [The relative risk for mortality from colorectal cancer was 0.90 (95% CI, 0.38–2.11) for ever versus never use, as computed by the Working Group.]

Rosenblatt et al. (2004) reported on a 10-year follow-up of 267 400 female textile workers at 519 factories in Shanghai, China, who were administered a questionnaire at enrolment into a randomized trial of breast self-examination between 1989 and 1991 and who were followed up until 2000. At the end of follow-up, 655 women had been diagnosed with incident colon cancer (563 who had never and 92 who had ever used oral contraceptives). The relative risk for colon cancer was 1.09 (95% CI, 0.86–1.37) for women who had ever used oral contraceptives (adjusted for age and parity), 0.97 (95% CI, 0.64–1.47) for < 6 months of oral contraceptive use, 0.96 (95% CI, 0.67–1.38) for 7–24 months of use, 1.13 (95% CI, 0.65–1.97) for 25–36 months of use and 1.56 (95% CI, 1.01–2.40) for > 36 months of use (p for trend = 0.16).

Hannaford and Elliot (2005) conducted a nested case–control study within the Royal College of General Practitioners' Oral Contraceptive Cohort Study. This cohort included 46 000 women who were recruited in 1968–69 by general practitioners throughout the United Kingdom and were followed up for 25 years. This nested case–control study updated data from a previous report (Beral et al., 1999). In this analysis, 146 cases of fatal and non-fatal colorectal cancer [separate number of colon and rectal cases not given] and 438 controls matched by age and length of follow-up (three controls for each case) were identified. Of these, 76 cases and 247 controls had used oral contraceptives. The odds ratio for colorectal cancer, adjusted for social class, tobacco smoking, parity and use of hormonal therapy, was 0.84 (95% CI, 0.56–1.24). The reduction in risk was greater but not significant among current users (odds ratio, 0.38; 95% CI, 0.11–1.32) than among former users (odds ratio, 0.89; 95% CI, 0.59–1.31). The trend in risk by duration of use was not significant and no clear trend with time since last or first use was observed.

2.6.2 Case–control studies

In addition to the 10 case–control studies reviewed in the last evaluation (IARC, 1999), three case–control studies on the use of oral contraceptives and colorectal cancer have been published (Table 17).

Kampman *et al.* (1994) conducted a population-based case–control study of 102 women who had incident colon cancer and 123 controls in the Netherlands. Of these, 46 cases and 58 controls had ever used oral contraceptives, which gave an odds ratio for colon cancer of 0.97 (95% CI, 0.46–2.03). Adjustment was made for age, urbanization grade, energy intake, energy-adjusted intake of fat, carbohydrate, dietary fibre and vitamin C, cholecystectomy, family history of colon cancer and socioeconomic level. [Estimates for duration of use and time since first and last use were not provided.]

Levi *et al.* (2003) conducted a hospital-based case–control study of 131 women who had incident colorectal cancer (71 colon cancers, 60 rectal cancers) and 373 control women in the Swiss Canton of Vaud. Of these, 14 cases and 65 controls had ever used oral contraceptives, to give an odds ratio of 0.8 (95% CI, 0.4–1.7) [separate odds ratios for colon and rectal cancers were not given]. Adjustment was made for age, education, family history of colorectal cancer, parity, fibre intake and physical activity. There was no consistent relation with duration of or time since first or last use (most odds ratios were non-significantly below unity).

Nichols *et al.* (2005) conducted a population-based case–control study in the State of Wisconsin, USA, of 1488 women aged 20–74 years who had incident colorectal (1122 colon, 366 rectal) cancer and were enrolled in either 1988–91 or 1997–2001. Of these women, 426 cases and 1968 controls had ever used combined oral contraceptives, which gave an odds ratio for colorectal cancer of 0.89 (95% CI, 0.75–1.06). The odds ratio was conditional on age and date of enrolment and was adjusted for family history of colorectal cancer, body mass index, education, screening, tobacco smoking, use of hormonal therapy and age at first birth. The odds ratio for colon cancer was 0.87 (95% CI, 0.72–1.06), conditional on age and date of enrolment, and adjusted for family history of colorectal cancer, body mass index, education, screening, tobacco smoking, use of hormonal therapy, age at first birth, alcoholic beverage consumption and menopausal status; that for rectal cancer was 0.87 (95% CI, 0.65–1.17), conditional on age and date of enrolment, and adjusted for family history of colorectal cancer, physical activity, education, screening, smoking and use of hormonal therapy. No pattern in risk was seen according to duration of use or age at starting use. Recency of use was not related to risk for colon cancer. Among women who had rectal cancer, a reduction in risk was seen (odds ratio, 0.53; 95% CI, 0.28–1.00) in the category of most recent (i.e. < 14 years) oral contraceptive use.

Table 17. Case–control studies of use of oral contraceptives and colorectal cancer

Reference	Country and study	Cases: controls	Relative risk (95% CI) (ever versus never users)			Comments
			Colorectal	Colon	Rectum	
Weiss et al. (1981b)	Washington State, USA	143:707	≤ 5 years: 1.3 (0.5–3.1) > 5 years: 2.0 (0.7–5.2)	1.0	2.6 ($p = 0.09$)	Adjusted for age; no significant trends with duration of use
Potter & McMichael (1983)	Adelaide, Australia	155:311		0.5 (0.3–1.2)	0.7 (0.3–1.8)	Adjusted for reproductive variables; inverse trend with duration of use
Furner et al. (1989)	Chicago, USA	90:208	0.6 (0.3–1.3)			Unadjusted
Kune et al. (1990)	Melbourne, Australia	190:200	–	1.2 (0.6–2.6)	2.04 (1.0–4.1)	Adjusted for age, parity, age at first child; no significant trend with duration of use
Peters et al. (1990)	Los Angeles, USA	327:327	–	< 5 years: 1.0 (0.6–1.8) ≥ 5 years: 1.1 (0.4–2.9)	–	Family history of cancer, parity, exercise, fat, alcohol, calcium intake; no effect of duration of use
Franceschi et al. (1991b)	Northeastern Italy	89:148	0.2 (0.0–2.0)			Unadjusted; only 1 case and 9 controls had ever used oral contraceptives.
Wu-Williams et al. (1991)	North America (NAm) and China (Ch)	395:1112	–	NAm: 1.2 ($p = 0.67$) Ch: 0.55 ($p = 0.27$)	NAm: 0.4 ($p = 0.04$) Ch: 0.7 ($p = 0.34$)	Unadjusted (but unaltered by exercise, saturated fat, duration of residence in NAm); no trend with duration of use
Jacobs et al. (1994)	Seattle, USA	193:194	–	1.2 (0.70–1.90)	–	Adjusted for age, age at birth of first birth, vitamin intake; no trend with duration of use

Table 17 (contd)

Reference	Country and study	Cases: controls	Relative risk (95% CI) (ever versus never users)			Comments
			Colorectal	Colon	Rectum	
Kampman et al. (1994)	The Netherlands	102:123	–	0.97 (0.46–2.03)	–	Adjusted for age, urbanization, cholecystectomy, socio-economic level, colon cancer, family history, dietary habits
Kampman et al. (1997)	USA, KPMCP	894:1120	–	0.86 (0.67–1.10)	–	Adjusted for age, cancer family history, aspirin, caloric intake, hormonal menopausal therapy, exercise
Fernandez et al. (1998)	Italy	1232:2793	0.6 (0.5–0.9)	0.7 (0.5–0.9)	0.7 (0.5–1.1)	Adjusted for age, education, family history of cancer, body mass index, estrogen replacement therapy, energy intake; no effect with duration of use; stronger protection in recent users
Levi et al. (2003)	Canton of Vaud, Switzerland	131:373		0.8 (0.4–1.7) ≤ 5 years: 0.7 (0.2–2.4) > 5 years: 0.9 (0.4–2.0)		Adjusted for age, education, family history of colorectal cancer, parity, fibre intake, physical activity; no trend with duration, time since first or last use
Nichols et al. (2005)	Wisconsin State, USA	1488:4297	0.89 (0.75–1.06)	0.87 (0.72–1.06)	0.87 (0.65–1.17)	Adjusted for age, study enrollment, family history of colorectal cancer, body mass index, education, screening, smoking, hormonal menopausal therapy, alcohol, age at first birth; no effect with duration of use; greater reduced risk in recent users (rectal)

CI, confidence interval; KPMCP, Kaiser Permanente Medical Care Program

2.7   Cutaneous malignant melanoma

The previous evaluation (IARC, 1999) omitted several studies and contained inaccuracies in the reporting of some results. The four cohort and 18 case–control studies of oral contraceptive use and cutaneous melanoma have therefore been re-assessed.

2.7.1   *Cohort studies* (Table 18)

Beral *et al.* (1977) and Ramcharan *et al.* (1981) first reported on a study of oral contraceptive use and cutaneous melanoma that comprised a cohort and a case–control component. Cohort data were derived from a prospective study on non-contraceptive effects of oral contraceptive use among 17 942 women aged 17–59 years at baseline, who were members of the Kaiser Permanente Health Plan, California, USA. Between 1968 and 1976, 22 cases of melanoma were found; eight had never used oral contraceptives, eight had used oral contraceptives for less than 4 years and six had used them for 4 years or more.

In the United Kingdom, 17 032 white married women aged 25–39 years were recruited between 1968 and 1974 at 17 family planning clinics within the framework of a study by the Oxford Family Planning Association (Adam *et al.*, 1981; Hannaford *et al.*, 1991). On entry, 56% of women were taking oral contraceptives, 25% were using a diaphragm and 19% were using an intrauterine device. Since each woman's oral contraceptive status could change during the course of the study, users of these preparations may have contributed periods of observation as either current or former users. After 266 866 woman–years of follow-up, 32 new cases of cutaneous malignant melanoma were recorded, 17 of which occurred among women who had ever used oral contraceptives (relative risk, 0.8; 95% CI, 0.4–1.8). None of the rates observed in any category of duration of use was materially different from that seen in women who had never used these preparations. The relative risks, adjusted for age, parity, social class and tobacco smoking, were 0.6 (95% CI, 0.2–1.6) for < 5 years of use, 1.0 (95% CI, 0.4–2.6) for 5–9 years of use and 1.0 (95% CI, 0.2–3.1) for ≥ 10 years of use. There was no relationship between time since cessation of use of oral contraceptives and the risk for cutaneous malignant melanoma, and none of the formulations resulted in a specific pattern of risk.

In the United Kingdom, 1400 general practitioners recruited 23 000 women who were using oral contraceptives and an equal number of age-matched women who had never used them between 1968 and 1969 within the framework of the study of the Royal College of General Practitioners (Kay, 1981; Hannaford *et al.*, 1991). After 482 083 woman–years of follow-up, 58 new cases of cutaneous malignant melanoma had been recorded, 31 of which occurred among women who had ever used combined oral contraceptives; the relative risk, adjusted for age, parity, social class and tobacco smoking, was 0.9 (95% CI, 0.6–1.5). No significant trend of increasing risk with duration of use was seen, with a relative risk for 10 years or more of use of 1.8 (95% CI, 0.8–3.9). Relative risks did not vary according to recency of use, estrogen or progestogen content of the contraceptives or the site of cutaneous malignant melanoma.

Table 18. Cohort studies of the use of combined oral contraceptives and the risk for cutaneous malignant melanoma

Reference, location	Population cohort	Age (years)	No. of cases	Type of exposure	No. of cases	Relative risk (95% CI)	Comments
Beral et al. (1977); Ramcharan et al. (1981), USA	17 942 white women	17–59	22	Never used Ever used for < 4 years Ever used for ≥ 4 years	8 8 6	NR NR NR	Walnut Creek Contraceptive Drug Study; hospital-based cases diagnosed in 1968–76; interviews based on postal, telephone and direct interviews; median follow-up, 6 years
Hannaford et al. (1991), United Kingdom	17 032 married white women	25–39	32	Never used Ever use *Duration of use* < 5 years 5–9 years ≥ 10 years	15 17 5 8 4	1.0 0.8 (0.4–1.8) 0.6 (0.2–1.6) 1.0 (0.4–2.6) 1.0 (0.2–3.1)	Oxford Family Planning Association (1968–74); interviews based on postal questionnaire, telephone and home visits; maximum follow-up, 21 years; adjusted for age, parity, social class, tobacco smoking
Hannaford et al. (1991), United Kingdom	46 000 women	NR	58	Never used Ever use *Duration of use* < 5 years 5–9 years ≥ 10 years	27 31 15 8 8	1.0 0.9 (0.6–1.5) 0.8 (0.4–1.5) 0.7 (0.3–1.5) 1.8 (0.8–3.9)	Royal College of General Practitioners; based on questionnaires provided by physicians; maximum follow-up, 21 years; adjusted for age, parity, social class, tobacco smoking
Feskanish et al. (1999), USA	183 693 pre-menopausal white women	25–55	252	Never used Ever use Current use < 10 years ≥ 10 years Past use < 5 years 5–9 years ≥ 10 years	64 374 23 9 14 165 98 47 18	1.0 1.4 (0.8–1.6) 2.0 (1.2–3.4) 1.0 (0.4–2.8) 3.4 (1.7–7.0) 1.1 (0.8–1.5) 1.0 (0.7–1.4) 1.2 (0.8–1.9) 1.4 (0.8–2.5)	Nurses' Health Study I and II; self-reported cases by nurses; adjusted for age, skin reaction to sun exposure; history of sunburn, mole counts, hair colour, family history of melanoma, parity, height, body mass index

CI, confidence interval; NR, not reported

The Nurses' Health study in the USA (Feskanich *et al.*, 1999) included two cohorts of 79 571 and 104 122 pre-menopausal white women. Response rates were 90% in both cohorts. Two hundred and fifty-two cases of melanoma were confirmed in both cohorts (146 in the first cohort from 1976 to 1994 and 106 in the second cohort from 1989 to 1995). All relative risks were adjusted for age, skin reaction to sun exposure, history of sunburn, mole counts, hair colour, family history of melanoma, parity, height and body mass index. The risk for cutaneous melanoma was 2.0 (95% CI, 1.2–3.4) among current users of oral contraceptives compared with women who had never used them. The increase in risk for melanoma was concentrated in the subgroup of current oral contraceptive users with 10 or more years of use, in whom 14 cutaneous melanomas occurred during the follow-up period (5.5% of all verified cases), which led to an adjusted relative risk of 3.4 (95% CI, 1.7–7.0). A higher estrogen dose did not appear to be associated with a higher risk for melanoma (assessed only in the second cohort). Risk did not appear to be elevated among past oral contraceptive users, even with longer duration of use. In women who had stopped taking oral contraceptives, no progressive decline in risk was observed with time since last use. No significant increase in risk was found in users who began taking oral contraceptives at 20 years of age or less.

2.7.2   *Case–control studies* (Table 19)

Beral *et al.* (1977) reported on oral contraceptive use and cutaneous melanoma in a study that was developed at a medical centre for the Kaiser Permanente Health Plan, California, USA. Thirty-seven cases aged 20–59 years at the time of diagnosis were registered at the medical centre. Two age-matched controls per case were recruited from administrative records of the plan. The crude risk for cutaneous melanoma for ever having used versus never having used oral contraceptives was 1.8 (95% CI, 0.7–4.6).

Adam *et al.* (1981) investigated 169 cases of cutaneous malignant melanoma in women aged 15–49 years who had been recorded at the cancer registries of southwestern England during 1971–76 and 342 age-matched control women drawn from the lists of the same general practitioners as the cases. Data were obtained from the general practitioners' records and from postal questionnaires for approximately 70% of the study women. The risk for cutaneous malignant melanoma was 1.1 (95% CI, 0.7–1.8) for ever having used combined oral contraceptives and [1.1 (95% CI, 0.4–2.8)] for current use. There was no increase in risk with duration of past or current use. Cases were moderately more sensitive to the sun and more likely to engage in outdoor tanning activities; 8% of cases had ever used sunlamps compared with 3% of controls ($p < 0.05$). No adjusted risks were presented, but the authors stated that adjustment did not affect the estimated risks.

In a case–control study of cutaneous melanoma in Seattle, USA (Holly *et al.*, 1983), use of combined oral contraceptives for 5 years or longer was more common among cases than controls, which gave a relative risk of 3.1 (95% CI, 1.3–7.3) for duration of use of 10 years or more, with a highly significant trend ($p = 0.004$) with duration of use. The risk for melanoma increased steeply in women who had taken oral contraceptives for 5 years or

Table 19. Case–control studies of the use of combined oral contraceptives and malignant melanoma

Reference, location	No. of cases	Age (years)	No. of controls	Exposure	No. of cases/no. of controls	Odds ratios (95% CI)	Adjustment/comments
Beral et al. (1977), USA	37 from hospital-based cancer register	20–59	74	Never used Ever used No information	22/33 13/36 2/5	1.0 1.8 [0.7–4.6] –	Walnut Creek Contraceptive Drug Study; review of medical records
Adam et al. (1981), United Kingdom	169	15–49	342	Never used Ever used *Current or past use* 1 month–4 years ≥ 5 years No information	66/214 44/126 22/72 17/35 5/19	1.0 [1.1 (0.7–1.8)] [1.0 (0.6–1.8)] 1.6 (0.8–3.1)]	Unadjusted; cases were moderately more sensitive to sun and more likely to engage in outdoor tanning activities; 8% of cases and 3% of controls had ever used sunlamps (*p* < 0.05); postal questionnaire
Holly et al. (1983), Seattle, USA	87	35–74	863	Never used *Current or past use* 1–4 years 5–9 years ≥ 10 years *For SSM only; use for ≥ 5 years, and* Current use 1–4 years since last use ≥ 5 years since last use	38/621 6/118 9/78 9/47 NR NR NR	1.0 [0.8 (0.3–2.2)] [1.9 (0.8–4.2)] [3.1 (1.3–7.3)] 0.9 (0.1–9.7) 2.5 (0.8–7.0) 5.1 (2.0–12.8)	Age; no data on exposure to sun
Lew et al. (1983), Massachusetts State, USA	111	23–81	107	–	–	–	No data reported but authors stated that there was no difference in combined oral contraceptive use between cases and controls.

Table 19 (contd)

Reference, location	No. of cases	Age (years)	No. of controls	Exposure	No. of cases/no. of controls	Odds ratios (95% CI)	Adjustment/comments
Beral et al. (1984), Sydney, Australia	287	15–24	574	Never used	79/159	1.0	No adjustment made, but authors stated that education, phenotype, history of sunburn and exposure to sun did not alter results; no difference by body location, thickness or histological type of melanoma
				Current or past use			
				1–4 years	124/274	[0.9 (0.6–1.3)]	
				5–9 years	56/103	[1.1 (0.7–1.7)]	
				≥ 10 years	28/36	[1.6 (0.9–2.9)]	
Helmrich et al. (1984), Canada and USA	160	20–59	640	Never used	97/370	1.0	Adjusted for age, area, religion, education, hormone-related variables
				Ever used	63/270	0.9 (0.6–1.3)	
				Use during year before study	8/52	0.5 (0.2–1.3)	
				Use for 5 years before study	4/18	0.9 (0.3–2.9)	
				Current or past use			
				< 1 year	15/82	0.7 (0.4–1.3)	
				1–4 years	23/106	0.8 (0.5–1.4)	
				5–9 years	11/49	0.8 (0.4–1.7)	
				≥ 10 years	5/21	1.0 (0.4–2.9)	
				Unknown	9/12		
				Use for ≥ 5 years, starting 10 years before study	12/46	1.0 (0.5–2.1)	
Holman et al. (1984), Western Australia	276	18–79	276	Never used	NR	1.0	Adjusted for sensitivity to sun, migration status, sun exposure; no difference in risk estimates for the different histological types; no association with time since last use; home interviews
				Ever used	NR	1.0 (0.6–1.6)	
				Current or past use			
				< 2 years	NR	0.8 (0.3–2.0)	
				2–4 years	NR	2.2 (0.7–6.8)	
				≥ 5 years	NR	1.6 (0.5–4.9)	

Table 19 (contd)

Reference, location	No. of cases	Age (years)	No. of controls	Exposure	No. of cases/no. of controls	Odds ratios (95% CI)	Adjustment/comments
Gallagher et al. (1985), Canada	361	20–79	361	Never used	NR	1.0	Adjusted for age, education, phenotype, freckling; no difference in risk estimates for the different histological types; home interviews
				Current or past use			
				< 1 year	NR	1.0 (NR)	
				1–4 years	NR	0.9 (NR)	
				≥ 5 years	NR	0.8 (NR)	
						Trend NS	
Green & Bain (1985), Queensland, Australia	91	15–81	91	Never used	48/42	1.0	Adjustment for phenotypic characteristics, solar exposure did not change results; no trend with time since last use and age at last use
				Ever used	43/49	0.7 (0.4–1.5)	
				Current and past use			
				1 month–4 years	31/30	[0.9 (0.5–1.8)]	
				> 4 years	12/19	0.4 (0.2–1.1)	
Østerlind et al. (1988), Denmark	280	20–79	536	Never used	167/299	1.0	Adjusted for age, sensitivity to sun, sunbathing; no difference according to type and potency of combined oral contraceptives
				Ever used	111/237	0.8 (0.5–1.2)	
				Current or past use			
				< 2 years	24/58	0.8 (0.4–1.4)	
				2–4 years	30/68	0.8 (0.4–1.3)	
				5–9 years	27/59	0.8 (0.4–1.4)	
				≥ 10 years	30/52	1.0 (0.6–1.7)	
Zanetti et al. (1990), Province of Turin, Italy	186	19–92	205	Never used	83/88	1.0	Analysed only in women aged 60 or younger; adjusted for age, education, phenotype, sunbathing; risk did not change according to type or location of melanoma, age or potency of combined oral contraceptive; hospital and home interviews.
				Ever used	NR	1.0 (0.5–1.9)	
				Current or past use			
				< 3 years	14/18	0.9 (0.4–1.8)	
				≥ 3 years	13/17	0.9 (0.3–2.0)	

Table 19 (contd)

Reference, location	No. of cases	Age (years)	No. of controls	Exposure	No. of cases/no. of controls	Odds ratios (95% CI)	Adjustment/comments
Lê et al. (1992), France	91	18–44	149	Never used	24/38	1.0	Adjusted for sensitivity, exposure to sun for a subgroup of cases and controls with no substantial changes in risk estimates for duration of use; no association with time since first use, age at first use or combined duration of use and time since first use
				Current or past use			
				1–9 years	54/97	1.1 (0.6–2.0)	
				≥ 10 years	13/14	2.1 (0.7–5.9)	
Palmer et al. (1992), New York and Philadelphia, USA	615	18–64	2107	Never used	313/800	1.0	Adjusted for age, education, body mass index, menopause, phenotype; elevated risk among non-severe cases of melanoma was attributed to surveillance bias; similar relative risk for different types
				Current or past use			
				< 3 years	201/447	[1.2 (0.9–1.4)]	
				≥ 3 years	73/193	[1.0 (0.7–1.3)]	
				Unknown	23/57		
				Severe cases with			
				5–9 years of use	12/80	1.0 (0.5–2.0)	
				≥ 10 years of use	29/187	1.1 (0.6–2.1)	
				Non-severe cases with			
				5–9 years of use	11/79	1.5 (0.8–2.6)	
				≥ 10 years of use	6/80	2.0 (0.9–4.3)	
Zaridze et al. (1992), Moscow, Russian Federation	54	NR	54	Never used	53/47	1.0	Adjusted for phenotype, naevi and sunbathing
				Ever used	1/7	0.04 (0.00–0.5)	

Table 19 (contd)

IARC MONOGRAPHS VOLUME 91

Reference, location	No. of cases	Age (years)	No. of controls	Exposure	No. of cases/no. of controls	Odds ratios (95% CI)	Adjustment/comments
Holly et al. (1995), San Francisco, USA	452	25–59	930	**CMM** Never used	NR	1.0	Adjusted for age; authors stated that risk estimates were unaltered by education, phenotype or exposure to sun.
				Ever used	NR	0.7 (0.5–1.0)	
				Current or past use			
				< 5 years	NR	0.6 (0.4–0.9)	
				5–9 years	NR	0.9 (0.6–1.4)	
				≥ 10 years	NR	1.0 (0.6–1.6)	
				SMM Ever used	NR	0.7 (0.5–0.9)	
				Current or past use			
				< 5 years	NR	0.6 (0.4–0.8)	
				5–9 years	NR	0.8 (0.6–1.1)	
				≥ 10 years	NR	0.8 (0.5–1.3)	
Westerdahl et al. (1996), Sweden	180	15–75	292	Never used	108/182	1.0	Adjusted for phenotype, naevi, sunburn; age at use and timing of use in relation to first child did not influence risk.
				Ever used	65/78	1.6 (0.9–2.8)	
				Current or past use			
				< 4 years	26/30	2.2 (0.9–4.6)	
				4–7 years	20/28	1.5 (0.7–3.5)	
				≥ 8 years	19/40	1.0 (0.5–2.0)	
Smith et al. (1998), Connecticut State, USA	308	≥ 18	233	Never used	170/131	1.0	Adjusted for age, marital status, hair colour, number of arm naevi, sun exposure index; no trend with duration of use and no association with age at first use
				Ever used	138/72	1.1 (0.6–1.7)	
				Current or past use			
				≤ 2 years	60/40	1.3 (0.7–2.3)	
				> 2–5 years	29/7	0.6 (0.3–1.2)	
				> 5 years	49/25	1.4 (0.7–2.8)	
Naldi et al. (2005), Italy	316	≥ 18	308	Never used	266/258	1.0	Adjusted for age, education, body mass index, number of melanocytic naevi, pigmentary traits, history of sunburn and reaction to sun exposure
				Ever used	50/60	1.1 (0.6–1.7)	

CI, confidence interval; CMM, cutaneous malignant melanoma; NR, not reported; NS, not significant; SMM, superficial spreading melanoma more and had stopped since 1–4 or 5 years or more. There was no increase in risk among current users. The highest risk was found for superficial spreading melanoma. No adjustment was made for sensitivity or exposure to the sun. [Category-specific risks were not presented in the publication and were calculated by the Working Group.]

In a study in Sydney, Australia (Beral et al., 1984), increasing duration of oral contraceptive use was not associated with increased risk for cutaneous malignant melanoma. An increased risk was found for a subgroup of women who had used these formulations for 5 years or longer and who had begun use at least 10 years before diagnosis of cutaneous malignant melanoma, with a relative risk of 1.5 (95% CI, 1.0–2.1). The increase in risk persisted after control for phenotypic characteristics, number of moles and measures of exposure to ultraviolet light. The risk did not vary according to the location, thickness or type of melanoma.

A case–control study carried out in several parts of the USA and Canada between 1976 and 1982 (Helmrich et al., 1984) included 160 women aged 20–59 years who had a recent histological diagnosis of cutaneous malignant melanoma and 640 control women aged 20–59 years who were admitted to hospital for trauma or orthopaedic and surgical conditions. The age-adjusted relative risk for women who had ever used combined oral contraceptives was 0.9 (95% CI, 0.6–1.3). There was no trend in risk with increasing duration of use, and the relative risk for ≥ 10 years of use was 1.0 (95% CI, 0.4–2.9). For the 40 cases and 140 controls who had first used combined oral contraceptives at least 10 years previously, the relative risk was 1.1 (95% CI, 0.7–1.8). For women with more advanced cutaneous malignant melanoma (i.e. Clark's level IV and V), the relative risk was 0.6 (95% CI, 0.2–2.3).

In Australia (Holman et al., 1984), a study was conducted in 276 women with melanoma and age-matched controls. The risk for melanoma for ever having used oral contraceptives was 1.0 (95% CI, 0.6–1.6). Extensive adjustement for sensitivity and exposure to the sun and migration status was made. For all melanoma and for the different types of melanoma, no association was observed with duration of use or with time since last use.

In a Canadian study (Gallagher et al., 1985), no association was found between the risk for cutaneous malignant melanoma and the use of combined oral contraceptives in 361 cases and an equal number of controls aged 20–69 years. The relative risks for < 1, 1–4 and ≥ 5 years of use, adjusted for age, phenotypic characteristics and freckling, were 1.0, 0.9 and 0.8, respectively. No association was seen between the histological type of superficial spreading melanoma and duration of use or years since last use; the relative risk for women who had used combined oral contraceptives for 10 or more years before diagnosis of cutaneous malignant melanoma was 1.0.

A study in Queensland, Australia, in 1979–80 (Green & Bain, 1985) included 91 women aged 15–81 years who had melanoma and 91 age-matched controls chosen at random from the population. No increased risk for cutaneous malignant melanoma was found in relation to ever having used combined oral contraceptives (age-adjusted odds ratio, 0.7; 95% CI, 0.4–1.5), and no trend in risk was found with increasing duration of use, age at last use or time since last use. Adjustment for sensitivity and exposure to the sun did not affect the risk estimates.

In a study from Denmark (Østerlind et al., 1988), all risk estimates were adjusted for age, phenotypic characteristics and sunbathing. The risk from ever having used oral contraceptives was 0.8 (95% CI, 0.5–1.2) for all melanoma and 0.9 (95% CI, 0.6–1.3) for superficial spreading melanoma. There was no evidence of an increased risk for cumulative exposure; the relative risk for ≥ 10 years of use was 1.0 (95% CI, 0.6–1.7). No specific pattern of risk was seen with the type of oral contraceptive, such as sequential progestogen-only or high-potency combined oral contraceptives, when these were assessed separately, but there were few women in each group.

Zanetti et al. (1990) carried out a case–control study in the Province of Turin, Italy, of 186 of 211 women aged 19–92 years who had histologically confirmed cutaneous malignant melanoma and were identified from the Turin Cancer Registry between 1984 and 1987 and 205 control women aged 17–92 years drawn from the National Health Service Registry. Use of combined oral contraceptives was analysed only in women aged 60 years or younger. Adjustment was made for age, education, phenotypic characteristics and sunbathing. The risk for cutaneous malignant melanoma of ever having used combined oral contraceptives was 1.0 (95% CI, 0.5–1.9) for all melanoma and 1.3 (95% CI, 0.4–4.5) for superficial spreading melanoma. No association was observed with duration of use. The longest duration of use (≥ 3 years) that began 10 or more years before the diagnosis of cutaneous malignant melanoma was not associated with an increased risk [risk estimates not reported]. The relative risks were identical for use of combined oral contraceptives that contained high estrogen doses (≥ 50 µg) and low estrogen doses.

Lê et al. (1992) assessed the effect of the use of combined oral contraceptives on the risk for cutaneous malignant melanoma in France between 1982 and 1987. The 91 cases from five hospitals were women under 45 years of age who had newly diagnosed histologically confirmed melanomas. Controls were 149 age-matched women who consulted in the same hospital for diagnosis or treatment of diseases that were unrelated to the use of combined oral contraceptives, including skin diseases. The risk for cutaneous malignant melanoma for ≥ 10 years of use of oral contraceptives was 2.1 (95% CI, 0.7–5.9). No association was found with time since first use (relative risk for 15–20 years since first use, 1.9; 95% CI, 0.8–4.5). No difference was found between superficial spreading melanoma and other types of cutaneous malignant melanoma. In the subgroup of 49 cases and 78 controls who were aged 30–40 years, a risk for melanoma of 4.4 (95% CI, 1.1–17) was found, based on 10 cases and eight controls who had used oral contraceptives for 10 years or more.

A case–control study of cutaneous malignant melanoma was carried out between 1979 and 1991 in Philadelphia and New York, USA (Palmer et al., 1992); the cases were 615 women under the age of 70 years (median age, 40 years) who had recently received a first diagnosis of cutaneous malignant melanoma. Patients with melanoma in situ were not included. Two control groups of white women (median age, 41 years) with other malignancies (610 patients) or non-malignant illnesses (1497 patients) that were judged to be unrelated to the use of combined oral contraceptives were selected. In order to address the possibility of selection bias due to differential surveillance of combined oral contraceptive users and non-users, the cases were subdivided by severity. For severe cases (thickness ≥ 0.75 mm, or Clark's level IV or V), the relative risks adjusted for age, education, menopause and phenotypic characteristics were 1.1 (95% CI, 0.8–1.5) for any use and 1.1 (95% CI, 0.6–2.1) for ≥ 10 years of use. For non-severe cases, duration of use was not associated with the risk.

Zaridze *et al.* (1992) evaluated risk factors in 96 cases of cutaneous malignant melanoma in Moscow, Russian Federation. Controls were recruited from among persons who were visiting cancer patients and matched by age. Use of combined oral contraceptives was analysed for 54 women with cutaneous malignant melanoma and 54 controls and showed a strong inverse association: the relative risk, adjusted for phenotypic characteristics, naevi and sunbathing, was 0.04 (95% CI, 0.0–0.5), based on one case and seven controls who had ever used combined oral contraceptives.

In the study of Holly *et al.* (1995), 72% of cases of cutaneous malignant melanoma and 79% of control subjects in San Francisco, USA, reported ever having used combined oral contraceptives. The age-adjusted relative risk was 0.7 (95% CI, 0.5–1.0) for all cutaneous malignant melanoma and 0.7 (95% CI, 0.5–0.9) for superficial spreading melanoma. Examination by latency and duration of use showed no significant trend. The relative risk for ≥ 10 years of use was 0.8 (95% CI, 0.5–1.3) for all cutaneous malignant melanoma and 1.0 (95% CI, 0.6–1.6) for superficial spreading melanoma. Use beginning ≥ 17 years before diagnosis was associated with relative risks of 0.6 (95% CI, 0.4–0.7) for all cutaneous malignant melanoma and 0.6 (95% CI, 0.4–0.8) for superficial spreading melanoma.

In the Swedish study of Westerdahl *et al.* (1996), use of combined oral contraceptives (40% of cases and 37% of controls) was associated with a non-significantly elevated risk of 1.6 (95% CI, 0.9–2.8) after adjustment for phenotypic characteristics, naevi and sunburn. No trend in risk was seen with duration of use (relative risk for > 8 years of use, 1.0; 95% CI, 0.5–2.0), age at first use or age at last use.

In Connecticut State, USA, Smith *et al.* (1998) investigated 308 women with melanoma aged ≥ 18 years and 233 control women in 1987–89. Cases were drawn from hospital-based records and controls were chosen from the general population by random-digit dialling. The risk for cutaneous melanoma among women who had ever used oral contraceptives was 1.1 (95% CI, 0.7–1.8) after adjustment for age, hair colour, marital status, number of arm naevi and sun exposure index. No association was found with duration of oral contraceptive use or with age at first use.

In Italy, Naldi *et al.* (2005) investigated 316 cases of melanoma in women of all ages and 308 control women in 1992–94. Cases were drawn from hospital-based records and controls were chosen from among non-dermatological and non-oncological patients who attended the same hospitals. The participation rate for cases and controls was 99%. The risk for cutaneous melanoma among women who had ever used oral contraceptives was 1.1 (95% CI, 0.6–1.7) after adjustment for age, education, body mass index, number of melanocytic naevi, pigmentary traits, history of sunburn and reaction to sun exposure.

2.7.3   *Meta- and pooled analyses*

A meta-analysis of 18 published case–control studies of cutaneous malignant melanoma and the use of combined oral contraceptives showed a pooled relative risk of 1.0 (95% CI, 0.9–1.0) (Gefeller *et al.*, 1998). The data for 3796 cases and 9442 controls showed no significant variation in the effect of combined oral contraceptives in the different studies, and analysis of various subgroups, defined by the design characteristics of the studies, did not materially alter this result.

In 2002, the investigators of case–control studies of cutaneous melanoma agreed to pool their original data in order to perform a new analysis of associations between melanoma and oral contraceptive use, using the same categories for exposure (Karagas *et al.*, 2002). The analyses were limited to studies that ascertained data on major risk factors for melanoma including pigmentary characteristics and exposure to sunlight. Analysis was further restricted to studies that involved a personal interview because questions designed for postal surveys may have been phrased differently or have been less complex. Studies that were limited to hospitalized cases were also excluded since these cases might have been biased by over-representation of advanced lesions. Finally, only studies that included at least 100 cases and 100 controls were retained, as smaller studies would have required a similar analytical effort, but would have contributed little to the overall analysis. Eleven case–control studies met the analytical criteria (Beral *et al.*, 1984; Holman *et al.*, 1984; Gallagher *et al.*, 1985; Green & Bain, 1985; Østerlind *et al.*, 1988; Swerdlow *et al.*, 1986; Elwood *et al.*, 1990; Zanetti *et al.*, 1990; Kirkpatrick *et al.*, 1994; Holly *et al.*, 1995; Langholz *et al.*, 2000) and data were available for all but one of these (Beral *et al.*, 1984). Two studies had never published their results on oral contraceptive use (Kirkpatrick *et al.*, 1994; Langholz *et al.*, 2000). The 10 pooled studies totalled 2110 women with melanoma and 3178 control women. Overall, no excess risk was associated with oral contraceptive use for 1 year or longer compared with never use or use for less than 1 year (pooled odds ratio, 0.86; 95% CI, 0.74–1.01) and there was no evidence of variation between studies. No relation was found between incidence of melanoma and duration of oral contraceptive use, age at starting use, year of use, years since first use or last use or specifically current oral contraceptive use.

2.8   Thyroid cancer

The results of 13 case–control studies of thyroid cancer and the use of oral contraceptives, 10 of which were reviewed in the previous evaluation (IARC, 1999), were pooled by La Vecchia *et al.* (1999) (see Table 20). The overall odds ratio was 1.5 (95% CI, 1.0–2.1) for current users, and declined to 1.1 over 10 years after cessation of oral contraceptive use.

Six subsequent studies are also summarized in Table 20. The largest (Sakoda & Horn-Ross, 2002), in which 544 cases and 558 population controls from the San Francisco Bay area, USA, were interviewed, yielded a slightly reduced risk for ever users (odds ratio, 0.7; 95% CI, 0.5–1.0). A hospital-based case–control study in Serbia of 204 matched case–control pairs reported ever use of oral contraceptives in 52 cases and 25 controls,

Table 20. Studies of the use of combined oral contraceptives and thyroid cancer

Reference, location	Age (years)	Cancer type	Oral contraceptive use	Cases	Controls	Odds ratio (95% CI)	Comments
Rossing et al. (1998), Washington State, USA	18–64	Papillary thyroid	*Age < 45 years* Never Ever *Age 45–64 years* Never Ever	48 247 34 81	40 341 62 131	1.0 0.6 (0.4–0.9) 1.0 1.2 (0.7–2.2)	
La Vecchia et al. (1999), North America, Europe and Asia	All ages	Thyroid	Never Ever Current	1324 808 91	2011 1290 118	1.0 1.2 (1.0–1.4) 1.5 (1.0–2.1)	Pooled data from 13 studies
Mack et al. (1999), Los Angeles County, USA	15–54	Thyroid	Never Ever	81 211	90 202	1.0 1.0 (0.6–1.6)	
Iribarren et al. (2001), San Francisco Bay area, USA	10–89	Thyroid	Use in last year	NR	NR	1.07 (0.69–1.67)	Kaiser Permanente cohort
Sakoda & Horn-Ross (2002), San Francisco Bay Area, USA	20–74	Papillary thyroid	Never Ever Current	204 337 79	177 380 83	1.0 0.7 (0.5–1.0) 0.7 (0.5–1.1)	
Haselkorn et al. (2003), San Francisco Bay Area, USA	20–74	Thyroid	*Age < 50 years* Never Ever *Age ≥ 50 years* Never Ever	121 246 79 69	97 239 62 87	1.0 0.8 (0.6–1.2) 1.0 0.5 (0.3–0.8)	No effect of duration; cases were Caucasian and Asian.
Zivaljevic et al. (2003), Serbia	14–87	Thyroid	Never Ever	152 52	179 25	1.0 2.5 (1.4–4.2)	

CI, confidence interval; NR, not reported

which gave a significant excess risk for ever users (odds ratio, 2.5; 95% CI, 1.4–4.2) (Zivaljevic et al., 2003). The remaining four studies gave odds ratio estimates for ever use of oral contraceptives of between 0.6 and 1.2 (Rossing et al., 1998; Mack et al., 1999; Iribarren et al., 2001; Haselkorn et al., 2003).

2.9   Other cancers

Twenty-one studies of cancers at other sites (lung, gallbladder, pancreas, lymphomas, gestational trophoblastic diseases, neuroblastoma, oesophagus and kidney) are summarized in Table 21. Marginally significant reductions in risk among ever users of oral contraceptives were reported in two studies of lung cancer and in single studies for cancer of the pancreas, B-cell non-Hodgkin lymphoma and oesophageal cancer. All overall confidence intervals for other studies included unity.

3.   Studies of Cancer in Experimental Animals

In this section, only relevant studies on estrogens and progestogens alone and in combination that were published subsequent to or were not included in the previous evaluation (IARC, 1999) are reviewed in detail. Studies that were reviewed previously are summarized briefly.

3.1   Estrogen–progestogen combinations

The results of studies reviewed previously (IARC, 1979, 1999) on the carcinogenicity of combinations of estrogens and progestogens that are used in combined oral contraceptives are summarized below (see Tables 22 and 23).

The incidence of pituitary adenomas in female and male mice was increased by administration of mestranol plus chlormadinone acetate, mestranol plus ethynodiol diacetate, ethinylestradiol plus ethynodiol diacetate, mestranol plus norethisterone, ethinylestradiol plus norethisterone (females only) and mestranol plus norethynodrel. The latter combination also increased the incidence of pituitary adenomas in female rats.

The incidence of benign mammary tumours was increased in intact and castrated male mice by ethinylestradiol plus chlormadinone acetate and in castrated male mice by mestranol plus norethynodrel. In male rats, the incidence of benign mammary tumours was increased by administration of ethinylestradiol plus norethisterone acetate. This combination did not cause tumour formation in any tissue in one study in female monkeys.

The incidence of malignant mammary tumours was increased in female and male mice by ethinylestradiol plus megestrol acetate, in female and male rats by ethinylestradiol plus ethynodiol diacetate, and in female rats by mestranol plus norethisterone and mestranol plus norethynodrel.

Table 21. Association between oral contraceptive use and the risk for other cancers

Reference, location	Age (years)	Cancer type	Oral contraceptive use	Cases	Controls	Odds ratio (95% CI)	Comments
Nelson et al. (2001), Los Angeles, USA	18–75	Intermediate or high-grade B-cell non-Hodgkin lymphoma	Never Ever < 5 years ≥ 5 years	111 66 43 21	93 84 53 29	1.00 0.47 (0.26–0.86) 0.50 (0.26–0.95) 0.35 (0.15–0.82)	Matched, fitting education, place of birth
Glaser et al. (2003), San Francisco Bay Area, USA	19–79	Hodgkin lymphoma	Never ≤ 2.2 years 2.3–5.3 years > 5.3 years	87 91 72 62	91 79 73 82	1.0 1.2 (0.8–1.9) 0.9 (0.6–1.5) 0.8 (0.5–1.3)	Multivariate parsimonious model that includes variables significant at $p < 0.10$ (reproductive history, socio-economic status)
Vessey et al. (2003), England and Scotland	25–39	Lymphoma/ haemopoietic cancer	Never < 4 years 4–8 years > 8 years	16 6 8 11	– – – –	1.0 0.9 (0.3–2.5) 1.0 (0.4–2.5) 1.2 (0.5–2.7)	OFPA cohort of 17 032 Caucasian women; adjusted for parity, social class, smoking
Schiff et al. (1998), Rochester, MN, USA	≥ 20	Central nervous system lymphoma	Never Ever	35 3	52 19	1.0 0.3	
Gago-Dominguez et al. (1999), Los Angeles, USA	25–74	Renal-cell cancer	Never Ever	258 164	255 167	1.0 1.0 (0.7–1.4)	Adjusted for age, education, hysterectomy
Olshan et al. (1999), Canada and USA	< 20	Neuroblastoma	Maternal use during first trimester No Yes	442 17	444 15	1.0 1.0 (0.5–2.1)	Odds ratios also unity for oral contraceptive use in previous year or ever

Table 21 (contd)

IARC MONOGRAPHS VOLUME 91

Reference, location	Age (years)	Cancer type	Oral contraceptive use	Cases	Controls	Odds ratio (95% CI)	Comments
Schüz et al. (2001), Germany	≤7	Neuroblastoma	*Maternal use during pregnancy*				
			No	159	1671	1.0	
			Yes	4	26	5.7 (1.5–23)	
			Unspecified	16	70	NR	
Palmer et al. (1999), USA	≥18	GTD	Never	36	98	1.0	Matched analysis; $p = 0.03$ for trend with duration
			Ever	199	315	1.8 (1.2–2.8)	
Parazzini et al. (2002), Greater Milan area, Italy	13–56	GTD	Never	164	306	1.0	Risk increased with duration
			Ever	104	130	1.5 (1.1–2.1)	
Taioli & Wynder (1994), USA	20–89	Lung adeno-carcinoma	Never	134	229	1.0	
			Ever	46	74	0.8 (0.5–1.5)	
Beral et al. (1999), United Kingdom	16–79	Lung	Never	40	–	1.0	RCGP cohort of 46 000 women
			Ever	75	–	1.2 (0.8–1.8)	
Kreuzer et al. (2003), Germany	≤75	Lung	Never	528	557	1.00	Adjusted for age, region, education, smoking variables
			Ever	279	354	0.69 (0.51–0.92)	
			< 5 years	86	105	0.69 (0.46–1.03)	
			5–11 years	87	130	0.65 (0.44–0.95)	
			≥ 12 years	102	115	0.69 (0.47–1.02)	
			Nonsmokers				Adjusted for age, region, education, time since stopped smoking
			Never	–	–	1.00	
			Ever	–	–	1.18 (0.78–1.79)	
			Smokers				
			Never	–	–	1.00	
			Ever	–	–	0.50 (0.34–0.74)	

Table 21 (contd)

Reference, location	Age (years)	Cancer type	Oral contraceptive use	Cases	Controls	Odds ratio (95% CI)	Comments
Vessey et al. (2003), England and Scotland	25–39	Lung	Never	15	—	1.0	OFPA cohort of 17 032 Caucasian women; adjusted for parity, social class, smoking
			< 4 years	9	—	1.4 (0.6–3.5)	
			4–8 years	12	—	1.2 (0.5–2.6)	
			> 8 years	18	—	1.3 (0.6–2.8)	
Kreiger et al. (2001), Ontario, Canada	20–74	Pancreas	< 6 months	41	160	1.00	Multivariate, fitting age, oral contraceptives, hormonal menopausal therapy, obstetric history, body mass index, diet, smoking
			≥ 6 months	9	64	0.36 (0.13–0.96)	
Skinner et al. (2003), USA	30–55	Pancreas	Never	159	—	1.00	Nurses Health Study; multivariate, fitting age, period, smoking, diabetes, body mass index, parity; age at baseline, 30–55 and followed up to 1998
			Ever	83	—	1.21 (0.91–1.61)	
			< 1 year	26	—	1.45 (0.94–2.21)	
			1–2.9 years	13	—	0.78 (0.44–1.39)	
			3–7.9 years	27	—	1.38 (0.85–1.99)	
			≥ 8 years	17	—	1.26 (0.76–2.10)	
Duell & Holly (2005), San Francisco Bay Area, USA	21–85	Pancreas	Never	135	402	1.00	Adjusted for age, education, smoking
			Ever	102	394	0.95 (0.65–1.4)	
			< 1 year	18	70	0.85 (0.47–1.5)	
			1–2 years	25	140	0.67 (0.39–1.2)	
			3–7 years	18	73	0.92 (0.50–1.7)	
			≥ 8 years	41	103	1.4 (0.89–2.3)	
Yen et al. (1987), Rhode Island State, USA	< 60	Gallbladder	Never	6	70	1.0	
			Ever	4	6	7.8 (2.0–30)	

Table 21 (contd)

Reference, location	Age (years)	Cancer type	Oral contraceptive use	Cases	Controls	Odds ratio (95% CI)	Comments
WHO Collaborative Study (1989c), Chile, China, Columbia, Israel, Kenya, Mexico	NR	Gallbladder	Never Ever Current	49 9 1	269 86 8	1.0 0.6 (0.3–1.3) 0.9 (0.1–7.4)	
Moerman et al. (1994), Netherlands	35–79	Gallbladder and biliary tract	Never Ever	61 14	203 49	1.0 1.1 (0.5–2.4)	
Zatonski et al. (1997), Australia, Canada, Netherlands, Poland	64.9 (mean)	Gallbladder	Never Ever	132 20	558 142	1.0 1.0 (0.5–2.0)	
Gallus et al. (2001), Italy and Switzerland	<79	Squamous-cell oesophageal cancer	Never Ever	110 4	392 33	1.0 0.24 (0.06–0.96)	Three hospital-based case–control studies pooled; adjusted for age, education, body mass index, energy intake, tobacco, alcoholic beverages

CI, confidence interval; GTD, gestational trophoblastic diseases; OFPA, Oxford Family Planning Association; RCGP, Royal College of General Practitioners

Table 22. Effects of combinations of various progestogens and estrogens on tumour incidence in mice

Combination	Pituitary adenomas		Mammary tumours			Uterine tumours	Cervical/ vaginal tumours
	Male	Female	Benign (males)	Malignant			
				Male	Female		
Chlormadinone acetate + mestranol	+	+					
Chlormadinone acetate + ethinylestradiol			+/c				
Ethynodiol diacetate + mestranol	+	+					
Ethynodiol diacetate + ethinylestradiol	+	+				+	
Lynestrenol + mestranol					+/−		
Lynestrenol + ethinylestradiol + 3-methylcholanthrene							+[a]
Megestrol acetate + ethinylestradiol				+	+		
Norethisterone acetate + ethinylestradiol	+/?	+/?					
Norethisterone + ethinylestradiol		+					
Norethisterone + mestranol	+	+					
Norethynodrel + mestranol	+	+	c		+/?	+	+
Norethynodrel + mestranol + 3-methylcholanthrene							−
Norgestrel + ethinylestradiol + 3-methylcholanthrene							+[a]

From IARC (1979, 1999)

+, increased tumour incidence; +/−, slighly increased tumour incidence; +/c, increased tumour incidence; c, increased tumour incidence in castrated animals; +/?, increased tumour incidence, but not greater than that with the estrogen or progestogen alone

[a] Protection at doses 1/2000th and 1/200th that of a contraceptive pill for women; enhancement at a dose of 1/20th that of a contraceptive pill for women

Table 23. Effects of combinations of various progestogens and estrogens on tumour incidence in rats

Combination	Pituitary adenomas		Mammary tumours			Liver				Foci (females)
			Benign (males)	Malignant		Adenoma		Carcinoma		
	Male	Female		Male	Female	Male	Female	Male	Female	
Ethynodiol diacetate + ethinylestradiol				+	+					
Ethynodiol diacetate + mestranol				?	?					
Megestrol acetate + ethinylestradiol			+/−	+/−	+/−	+/?	+/?			
Norethisterone acetate + ethinylestradiol			+		+	+			+	
Norethisterone + mestranol						+	−	−		
Norethynodrel + mestranol	+/?	+	+/?	+/?	+	+/?	−	−	−	+
Norethynodrel + mestranol + N-nitroso-diethylamine							−	−	−	+
Norgestrel + ethinylestradiol			+/−							

From IARC (1979, 1999)

+, increased tumour incidence; +/−, slightly increased tumour incidence; +/?, increased tumour incidence; +/?, increased tumour incidence, but not greater than that with the estrogen or progestogen alone; ? conflicting result; −, no effect

In female mice, the incidence of malignant non-epithelial uterine tumours was increased by ethinylestradiol plus ethynodiol diacetate and that of vaginal or cervical tumours by norethynodrel plus mestranol. In mice treated with 3-methylcholanthrene to induce genital tumours, ethinylestradiol plus lynestrenol, ethinylestradiol plus norgestrel and mestranol plus norethynodrel increased the incidence of uterine tumours; however, this occurred only at the highest doses of ethinylestradiol plus lynestrenol and ethinylestradiol plus norgestrel that were tested. Lower doses inhibited the tumorigenesis induced by 3-methylcholanthrene alone.

In male rats, the incidence of liver adenomas was increased by mestranol plus norethisterone and by ethinylestradiol plus norethisterone acetate; the latter combination also increased the incidence of hepatocellular carcinomas in female rats. Liver foci, which are putative preneoplastic lesions, were induced in female rats by mestranol plus norethynodrel. In rats initiated for hepatocarcinogenesis with N-nitrosodiethylamine, mestranol plus norethynodrel increased the formation of altered hepatic foci.

Subcutaneous implantation and oral administration in rabbits

Virgin female New Zealand white rabbits, about 6 months of age and weighing 3.2–4.7 kg, were randomized into groups of five. Steroids (estradiol plus levonorgestrel or ethinylestradiol plus levonorgestrel) were delivered by subdermal implants in the neck or, in one case, by oral administration. The estimated dose of levonorgestrel was based on its loss from implants of the same type in women. Estimates of the doses of estradiol or ethinylestradiol delivered were based on measurements of in-vitro release from the implants used. Because of the high release and early exhaustion of steroid supply, the progestogen implants were replaced at 20-day intervals. The steroids administered orally were the commercially available combination pill Lo Femenal®; each tablet contained 30 µg ethinylestradiol and 300 µg norgestrel. Norgestrel contained equal amounts of levonogestrel and its inactive isomer. The pills were dispersed in 2 mL water and were administered intragastrically, but evaluation of the effects was confounded by the very low bioavailability of ethinylestradiol in this species when given orally. Hence, a new experiment was conducted in which levonorgestrel was delivered by oral pill and 30 µg of ethinylestradiol per day was delivered by implant for 8 weeks. At necropsy, lesions were noted and the weights of the uterus, liver and spleen were determined. Samples for tissue block preparation were taken from all lesions identified in organs or tissues, and samples were routinely taken from the uterus, spleen, lung, liver and bone marrow. Tissues were stained with haematoxylin and eosin and were studied microscopically. The animals were killed after 2 or 4.5 months. The incidences of tumours among the groups treated subcutaneously with a combination of estradiol and levonorgestrel are shown in Table 24. Estradiol alone resulted in decidualization, but did not induce deciduosarcoma, nor did tumours develop when estradiol was supplemented with lower doses of levonorgestrel, with the exception of an early atypical deciduosarcoma in one group. All animals in the groups treated with 66 or 233 µg/day levonorgestrel for 2 or 4.5 months had multiple deciduosarcomas. Neoplastic decidual cells were found in the uterine blood vessels of many animals of these groups. In the other experiments by subcutaneous administration, ethinylestradiol was substituted for estradiol. The implants were in place for 6 months before the animals were killed. The experimental design and histological findings are summarized in Table 25. Ethinylestradiol alone induced deciduosarcomas in the spleen and ovary of one animal. In combination with a high dose of levonorgestrel (150 μg/day), even 10 μg/day ethinylestradiol produced many

Table 24. Incidence of malignant tumours in female New Zealand white rabbits treated subcutaneously with estradiol (E$_2$) and levonorgestrel (LNG)

Treatment time	E$_2$ (μg/day)	LNG (μg/day)	% of animals with deciduosarcomas ($n = 4$–5)				
			Uterus	Spleen	Liver	Ovary	Lung
2 months	0	0	0	0	0	0	0
	60	0	0	0	0	0	0
	60	8	0	25[a]	0	0	0
	60	25	0	0	0	0	0
	60	66	80	100	60	40	40[b]
	60	233	100	100	40	20	0
4.5 months	0	0	0	0	0	0	0
	6	233	20	0	0	0	0
	20	233	100	40	20	0	0
	60	233	100	75	25	0	25
	200	233	100	100	40	40	20

From Jänne *et al.* (2001)
[a] Atypical deciduosarcoma
[b] Metastasis

Table 25. Incidence of malignant tumours in female New Zeland white rabbits treated subcutaneously with ethinylestradiol (EE) and levonorgestrel (LNG)

Treatment time	EE (μg/day)	LNG (μg/day)	Proliferation of hepatic bile ductules (%)	% of animals with deciduosarcomas ($n = 5$)				
				Uterus	Spleen	Liver	Ovary	Lung
6 months	0	0	0	0	0	0	0	0
	30	0	80	0	20	0	20	0
	10	150	20	100	100	20	0	0
	30	150	20	100	100	100	20	20[a]

From Jänne *et al.* (2001)
[a] Metastasis

deciduosarcomas. As in the experiments cited earlier, hyperplasia of splenic mesenchymal cells was seen in most animals in all groups that received estrogen. Proliferation of hepatic bile ductules was observed in 40% of rabbits that received ethinylestradiol. This lesion was not seen in any other test or control rabbits. In the experiment in which levonorgestrel was delivered by an oral pill and 30 μg/day ethinylestradiol were delivered by implant, one of five animals developed a spleen deciduosarcoma (Jänne *et al.*, 2001). [This study clearly shows the carcinogenic effects of combinations of levonorgestrel with ethinylestradiol as well as with estradiol. It is interesting to note that, although the study is well designed, there is no human counterpart for deciduosarcomas. Hepatic bile duct proliferation is a more relevant lesion in this context.]

3.2   Estrogens used in combined oral contraceptives

The results of studies reviewed previously (IARC, 1979, 1999) on the carcinogenicity of estrogens used in combined oral contraceptives are summarized below (see Tables 26 and 27).

The incidence of pituitary adenomas was increased by ethinylestradiol and mestranol in female and male mice and by ethinylestradiol in female rats.

The incidence of malignant mammary tumours was increased by ethinylestradiol and mestranol in female and male mice and female rats; however, mestranol did not increase the incidence of mammary tumours in female dogs in a single study.

Ethinylestradiol increased the incidence of cervical tumours in female mice.

In female and male mice, ethinylestradiol increased the incidence of hepatocellular adenomas. In female rats, ethinylestradiol and mestranol increased the numbers of altered hepatic foci. In rats, ethinylestradiol increased the incidence of hepatocellular adenomas in females and males and of hepatocellular carcinomas in females, whereas mestranol increased the incidence of hepatic nodules and carcinomas combined in females.

The incidence of microscopic malignant kidney tumours was increased in male hamsters exposed to ethinylestradiol.

In female mice initiated for liver carcinogenesis and exposed to unleaded gasoline, ethinylestradiol increased the number of altered hepatic foci; however, when given alone after the liver carcinogen, it reduced the number of altered hepatic foci.

In female rats initiated for liver carcinogenesis, ethinylestradiol and mestranol increased the number of altered hepatic foci and the incidence of adenomas and carcinomas. Ethinylestradiol also increased the incidence of kidney adenomas, renal-cell carcinomas and liver carcinomas in male rats initiated with *N*-nitrosoethyl-*N*-hydroxyethylamine. In female hamsters initiated with *N*-nitrosobis(2-oxopropyl)amine, ethinylestradiol increased the incidence of renal tumours and the multiplicity of dysplasias.

Table 26. Effects of ethinylestradiol and mestranol alone and with known carcinogens on tumour incidence in mice

Estrogen	Pituitary adenoma		Malignant mammary tumours		Uterine tumours	Vaginal/ cervical tumours	Liver		
							Adenoma		Foci (females)
	Male	Female	Male	Female			Male	Female	
Ethinylestradiol	+	+	+	+	+	+	+	+	
Mestranol	+	+	+	+			−	−	
Ethinylestradiol + *N*-nitrosodiethylamine									
Ethinylestradiol + *N*-nitrosodiethylamine + unleaded gasoline									Protective +

From IARC (1979, 1999)

+, increased tumour incidence; −, no effect

Table 27. Effects of ethinylestradiol and mestranol alone and with known carcinogens on tumour incidence in rats

Estrogen	Pituitary adenoma (females)	Malignant mammary tumours (females)	Liver Adenoma Male	Adenoma Female	Carcinoma Male	Carcinoma Female	Foci (females)	Kidney Adenoma (males)	Carcinoma (females)
Ethinylestradiol	+	+	+	+		+	+		
Mestranol		+				+/−	+		
Ethinylestradiol + N-nitrosoethyl-N-hydroxyethylamine					+			+	+
Ethinylestradiol + N-nitroso-diethylamine			+	+	+	+	+[a]		
Mestranol + N-nitrosodiethylamine			+	+	+	+	+		

From IARC (1979, 1999)

+, increased tumour incidence; −, no effect; +/−, slightly increased tumour incidence
[a] In one of three studies, ethinylestradiol initiated hepatocarcinogenesis.

3.2.1   *Subcutaneous implantation*

(*a*)   *Mouse*

A total of 272 female CD-1 (ICR) mice, 9 weeks of age, were divided equally into 17 groups and received subcutaneous implants into the back of cholesterol pellets (31.84 mg) that contained 0 or 0.16 mg estrone, estradiol, estriol, 2-hydroxyestrone, 2-hydroxyestradiol, 2-hydroxyestriol, 2-methoxyestrone, 2-methoxyestradiol, 2-methoxyestriol, 4-hydroxy-estrone, 4-hydroxyestradiol, 16β-hydroxyestrone diacetate, 16-epiestriol, 16,17-epiestriol, 16α-hydroxyestrone or 17-epiestriol. The pellets were renewed every 7 weeks throughout the experiment. At 10 weeks of age, each mouse received a single injection of 12.5 mg/kg bw *N*-ethyl-*N'*-nitro-*N*-nitrosoguanidine (ENNG) dissolved at a concentration of 1.5% (w/v) in polyethylene glycol into one of the uterine cavities via the vagina. The experiment was terminated at 30 weeks of age, when all surviving animals were autopsied to obtain repro-ductive organs, and the uterus and ovaries were weighed and processed for histological exa-mination. Endometrial proliferative lesions were classified histologically into two categories — hyperplasia and adenocarcinoma — and the incidence is given in Table 28. The results indicated that estrogens and their metabolites affect endometrial carcinogenesis in mice ini-tiated with ENNG in a manner that is dependent on their metabolic attributes. Estrogens (estrone, estradiol and estriol) and their metabolites that belong to the 16α-hydroxylation pathway (16α-hydroxyestrone and 17-epiestriol) and the upstream of the 16β-hydroxylation pathway (16β-hydroxyestrone diacetate) exerted both promoting and additive co-carcino-genic effects on endometrial carcinogenesis in ENNG-initiated mice as shown by the deve-lopment of invasive adenocarcinomas. Estrogen metabolites that belong to the downstream of the 16β-hydroxylation pathway exerted mainly promoting effects in this experimental model, as shown by the enhanced development of endometrial hyperplasia (16-epiestrol), or exerted no effect (16,17-epiestriol) (Takahashi *et al.*, 2004).

(*b*)   *Hamster*

Groups of 10 male Syrian hamsters, 4–6 weeks of age, were implanted subcutaneously with 25-mg pellets of estradiol, 17α-estradiol, ethinylestradiol, menadione, a combination of 17α-estradiol and ethinylestradiol or a combination of ethinylestradiol and menadione [no effective dose provided]. The hamsters received a second identical pellet 3 months after the initial treatment. A control group of 10 animals was sham-operated and left untreated. The animals were killed after 7 months and inspected macroscopically for tumour nodules on the surface of each kidney (see Table 29). No tumour nodules were detected in untreated hamsters or in groups of hamsters that were treated with 17α-estradiol, ethinylestradiol, menadione or a combination of 17α-estradiol and ethinylestradiol for 7 months. In contrast, hamsters treated with either estradiol or a combination of ethinylestradiol and menadione for 7 months developed renal tumours. The tumour incidence was 90% in the group treated with estradiol (versus 0% in untreated controls; $p < 0.05$, Fisher's exact test) and 30% in the group treated with a combination of ethinylestradiol and menadione. The mean number of tumour nodules per hamster was higher in the group treated with estradiol compared

Table 28. Incidence of endometrial proliferative lesions in female CD-1 mice treated with a single dose of ENNG and various estrogens

Treatment	Effective no. of animals	Endometrial hyperplasias[a,b]				Adeno-carcinomas[b]	Total[b]
		+	++	+++	Total		
Control	16	2 (13)	6 (38)	1 (6)	9 (56)	0	9 (56)
Estrone	16	1 (6)	1 (6)	2 (13)	4 (25)	12 (75)*	16 (100)*
Estradiol	16	0	2 (13)	1 (6)	3 (19)	13 (81)*	16 (100)*
Estriol	16	1 (6)	7 (44)	2 (13)	10 (63)	6 (38)*	16 (100)*
2-Hydroxyestrone	16	5 (31)	6 (38)	2 (13)	13 (81)	0	13 (81)
2-Hydroxyestradiol	16	7 (44)	4 (25)	1 (6)	12 (75)	0	12 (75)
2-Hydroxyestriol	16	6 (38)	8 (50)	1 (6)	15 (93)*	0	15 (93)*
2-Methoxyestrone	16	7 (44)	3 (19)	0	10 (62)	0	10 (62)
2-Methoxyestradiol	16	7 (44)	7 (44)	1 (6)	15 (93)*	0	15 (93)*
2-Methoxyestriol	16	8 (50)	8 (50)	0	16 (100)*	0	16 (100)*
4-Hydroxyestrone	15	4 (27)	5 (33)	1 (7)	10 (67)	0	10 (67)
4-Hydroxyestradiol	16	6 (38)	4 (25)	2 (13)	12 (75)	0	12 (75)
16β-Hydroxyestrone diacetate	15	2 (13)	7 (47)	2 (13)	11 (73)	4 (27)*	15 (100)*
16-Epiestriol	16	9 (56)*	5 (31)	2 (13)	16 (100)*	0	16 (100)*
16,17-Epiestriol	16	5 (31)	6 (38)	1 (6)	12 (75)	0	12 (75)
16α-Hydroxyestrone	15	1 (7)	6 (40)	4 (27)	11 (73)	4 (27)*	15 (100)*
17-Epiestriol	15	1 (7)	2 (13)	1 (7)	4 (27)	11 (73)*	15 (100)*

From Takahashi et al. (2004)

ENNG, N-ethyl-N-nitro-N-nitrosoguanidine

[a] Hyperplasias are classified based on the degree of cellular atypism into three subcategories: +, slight; ++, moderate; +++, severe

[b] Numbers of animals (percentage incidence)

* Significantly different from control value ($p < 0.05$, Fisher's exact test)

Table 29. Influence of different estrogens and menadione on renal carcinogenesis in male Syrian hamsters

Treatment	No. of animals with tumours/ no. of animals	Mean no. of tumour nodules per hamster
Estradiol	9/10[a]	7.0 ± 3.16[b]
17α-Estradiol	0/10	0
Ethinylestradiol	0/10	0
17α-Estradiol + ethinylestradiol	0/10	0
Menadione	0/10	0
Menadione + ethinylestradiol	3/10[c]	1.6 ± 2.67
Untreated	0/10	0

From Bhat *et al.* (2003)
[a] $p < 0.05$ compared with untreated controls and the menadione + ethinylestradiol-treated group by Fisher's exact test
[b] $p < 0.05$ compared with untreated controls by the χ^2 test; $p < 0.05$ compared with the menadione + ethinylestradiol-treated group by using the unpaired t test
[c] $p < 0.10$ compared with untreated controls by Fisher's exact test

with the group treated with a combination of ethinylestradiol and menadione or the untreated control group (Bhat *et al.*, 2003).

3.2.2   *Subcutaneous injection*

Mouse

Groups of outbred female CD-1 mice [initial number of animals per group not specified] were given daily subcutaneous injections of 2 µg estrogen (2- or 4-hydroxyestradiol, estradiol or ethinylestradiol) dissolved in corn oil or corn oil alone (as a control) on days 1–5 of life. Mice were killed at 12 or 18 months of age. Tissue sections were stained and evaluated by light microscopy. The number of mice with reproductive tract tumours was determined. The incidence of uterine adenocarcinomas was compared by Fisher's exact tests (see Table 30). Both of the catechol estrogens examined (2- and 4-hydroxyestradiol) induced tumours in CD-1 mice. 2-Hydroxyestradiol was more carcinogenic than estradiol: 14 and 11% of the rodents developed uterine adenocarcinomas at 12 and 18 months, respectively, after neonatal administration of catechol estrogen. In contrast, 4-hydroxyestradiol was considerably more carcinogenic than 2-hydroxyestradiol and produced a 74% (12 months) and 56% (18 months) tumour incidence after treatment during the neonatal period. Ethinylestradiol also induced more tumours (38% at 12 months and 50% at 18 months) than estradiol. This study, which was designed to demonstrate the carcinogenic properties of catechol estrogens, also included a group that was treated with ethinylestradiol in which uterine adenocarcinomas were induced at a high incidence (Newbold & Liehr, 2000). [It should be

Table 30. Uterine adenocarcinomas in groups of female CD-1 mice injected subcutaneously with various estrogens during the neonatal period

Compound	Incidence of uterine adenocarcinoma No. of animals with tumour/total no. of animals (%)		
	12 months	18 months	Total
Control (corn oil)	0/12 (0)	0/22 (0)	0/34 (0)
2-Hydroxyestradiol	3/21 (14)	2/19 (11)	5/40 (12)*
4-Hydroxyestradiol	14/19 (74)	9/16 (56)	23/35 (66)**
Estradiol	0/5[a]	1/10 (10)	1/15 (7)
Ethinylestradiol	9/24 (38)	9/18 (50)	18/42 (43)**

From Newbold & Liehr (2000)
* $p < 0.05$ versus corn oil controls (Fisher's exact test)
** $p < 0.01$ versus corn oil controls (Fisher's exact test)
[a] These data were published previously (Newbold *et al.*, 1990).

noted that studies in neonatal mice could have additional limitations for the extrapolation of the effects of hormones in adult women who take oral contraceptives.]

3.2.3 *Oral administration to transgenic mice*

Sixty female *p53* (+/–) mice (heterozygous female *p53*-deficient CBA mice, in which exon 2 of the lateral *p53* allele was inactivated, were the F_1 offspring of heterozygous *p53*-deficient male C57 BL/6J mice that had been back-crossed with female CBA mice (Tsukada *et al.*, 1993)) and 60 female wild-type *p53* (+/+) litter mates, 6 weeks of age, were each divided into four groups of 15 animals. [The Working Group noted the small number of animals.] All mice received an intraperitoneal injection of 120 mg/kg bw *N*-ethyl-*N*-nitrosourea (ENU) in physiological saline, followed by no further treatment (Group 1) or were fed *ad libitum* diets that contained 1 ppm ethinylestradiol (Group 2), 2.5 ppm ethinylestradiol (5 ppm for the first 4 weeks reduced to 2.5 ppm thereafter because of marked body weight depression; Group 3) or 2000 ppm methoxychlor [a weakly estrogenic pesticide] (Group 4) for 26 weeks. Individual body weights in each group were measured every week. One of the 15 *p53* (+/–) mice in Group 2 died during the early period of the experiment. After the end of the 26-week experiment, surviving animals were killed and autopsied. The uterine tissues were sectioned and stained for microscopic examination. The differences in the incidence of uterine proliferative lesions were assessed by the Fisher's exact test. Multiple nodules (5–20 mm in diameter) of the uterine horn suggestive of uterine tumours were observed in seven, nine, 12 and seven *p53* (+/–) mice in Groups 1, 2, 3 and 4, respectively. The absolute uterine weights and uterine weight/body weight ratios of *p53* (+/–) and *p53* (+/+) mice in Groups 2, 3 and 4 were significantly higher than those in the Group 1 mice. The uterine weights of *p53* (+/–) mice, especially in Group 3, were considerably increased because of marked growth of uterine tumours. Uterine proliferative lesions were classified into endometrial stromal polyps, endometrial stromal sarcomas, adenocarcinomas, atypical hyperplasias and endometrial glandular hyperplasias. Atypical hyperplasias were classified into two cell types — clear and basophilic — characterized by small proliferative foci of endometrial glandular epithelia with atypia. Non-atypical endometrial glandular hyperplasias were composed of increased numbers of endometrial glands with occasional cysts. The incidence of uterine stromal tumours in *p53* (+/–) mice was 87% (47% stromal sarcomas, 40% polyps), 85% (64% stromal sarcomas, 21% polyps), 87% (stromal sarcomas) and 53% (stromal sarcomas) in Groups 1, 2, 3 and 4, respectively; there was a significant difference in the incidence of stromal sarcomas between Groups 1 and 3 (see Table 31). In *p53* (+/+) mice, only stromal polyps were seen at an incidence of 20, 13, 0 and 0% in Groups 1, 2, 3 and 4, respectively; these values displayed a clear decrease compared with the incidence of stromal tumours in the groups of *p53* (+/–) mice. The incidence of clear-cell type atypical hyperplasias in *p53* (+/–) mice was 0, 14, 60 and 0% in Groups 1, 2, 3 and 4, respectively; that in *p53* (+/+) mice was 0, 7, 53, and 0%; the difference between Groups 1 and 3 was significant in both cases ($p < 0.05$, Fisher's exact test). For atypical hyperplasias of the basophilic cell type, there were no significant differences among the groups [incidence not specified]. One *p53* (+/–) mouse in Group 3 developed a clear-cell adenocarcinoma. The incidence of glandular hyperplasias in *p53* (+/–) mice was 60, 79, 60 and 27% in Groups 1, 2, 3 and 4, respectively, whereas that in *p53* (+/+) mice was 60, 80, 100 and 100%; the incidence in Group 3 and Group 4 *p53* (+/+) mice showed significant differences from values in Group 1 (Mitsumori *et al.*, 2000). [This study suggests that ethinylestradiol possibly exerts tumour-promoting (co-carcinogenic) effects on stromal and epithelial proliferative lesions of the uterus in *p53*-deficient mice initiated with ENU.]

3.3   Progestogens used in combined oral contraceptives

The results of studies that were reviewed previously (IARC, 1979, 1999) on the carcinogenicity of progestogens used in combined oral contraceptives are summarized below (see Tables 32, 33 and 34).

The incidence of pituitary adenomas was increased by norethisterone in female mice and by norethynodrel in female and male mice and male rats.

The incidence of malignant mammary tumours was increased in female mice by lynestrenol, megestrol acetate and norethynodrel. In female rats, lynestrenol and norethisterone slightly increased the incidence of malignant mammary tumours. In male rats, norethisterone also slightly increased the incidence of malignant mammary tumours, while norethynodrel increased the incidence of both benign and malignant mammary tumours. In female dogs, chlormadinone acetate, lynestrenol and megestrol acetate increased the incidence of benign and malignant mammary tumours; however, lynestrenol had a protective effect at a low dose but enhanced tumour incidence at two higher doses. Levonorgestrel did not increase the incidence of mammary tumours in one study in dogs.

Table 31. Incidence of lesions (percentage) in female *p53* (+/+) and (+/–) CBA mice injected intraperitoneally with ENU and given EE or MXC in the diet

Treatment	*p53* (+/–) Mice (n = 15)[a]					*p53* (+/+) Mice (n = 15)				
	Uterine stromal tumours		Atypical hyperplasias		Glandular hyperplasias	Uterine stromal tumours		Atypical hyperplasias		Glandular hyperplasias
	Polyps	Stromal sarcomas	Clear-cell type	Basophilic cell type[b]		Polyps	Stromal sarcomas	Clear-cell type	Basophilic cell type[b]	
ENU	40	47	0	NR	60	20	0	0	NR	60
ENU + 1 ppm EE	21	64*	14	NR	79	13	0	7	NR	80
ENU + 2.5 ppm EE	0	87*	60*c	NR	60	0	0	53*	NR	100*
ENU + MXC	0	53	0	NR	27	0	0	0	NR	100*

From Mitsumori *et al.* (2000)

ENU, *N*-ethyl-*N*-nitrosourea; EE, ethinylestradiol; MXC, methoxychlor; NR, not reported

* Significantly different from the ENU group (*p* < 0.05, Fisher's exact test)

[a] ENU + 1 ppm EE group (n = 14)

[b] Crude number not specified in the paper, but the authors state that there were no significant differences among treatment groups.

[c] One animal in this group developed a clear-cell adenocarcinoma.

Table 32. Effects of various progestogens alone or with a known carcinogen on tumour incidence in mice

Progestogen	Pituitary adenoma		Mammary tumours		Uterine tumours	Vaginal/cervical tumours	Liver			
							Adenoma		Carcinoma	
	Male	Female	Benign (males)	Malignant (females)			Male	Female	Male	Female
Chlormadinone acetate							+/−			
Cyproterone acetate							+[a]	+/−[a]	+[a]	+[a]
Ethynodiol diacetate			c				+/−			
Lynestrenol				+			+			
Megestrol acetate				+				+		
Norethisterone acetate		+					+/−			
Norethisterone	+	+					+/−	+/−		
Norethynodrel			c	+						
Norethynodrel + 3-methyl-cholanthrene					+	−				

From IARC (1979, 1999)

+, increased tumour incidence; +/−, slightly increased tumour incidence; −, no effect; c, increased incidence in castrated males

[a] Dose exceeded the maximum tolerated daily dose

Table 33. Effects of various progestogens alone or with a known carcinogen on tumour incidence in rats

Progestogen	Pituitary adenoma (males)	Mammary tumours			Liver				
		Benign (males)	Malignant		Adenoma		Carcinoma (males)	Foci	
			Male	Female	Male	Female		Male	Female
Cyproterone acetate					+[a]	+[a]			+[b]
Ethynodiol diacetate		+							
Lynestrenol				+/−					
Norethisterone acetate					+	+		+	+ or −[c]
Norethisterone		+/−	+/−	+/−	+	+			
Norethynodrel		+	+		+	+			−[c]
Norethynodrel + N-nitrosodiethylamine	+						+		+

From IARC (1979, 1999)

+, increased tumour incidence; +/−, slightly increased tumour incidence; −, no effect

[a] Liver adenomas detected only at high doses

[b] Tested for initiating activity; the results were positive in one study in which it was administered for 5 days and negative when it was administered as a single dose.

[c] Tested as a single dose for initiating activity

Table 34. Effects of various progestogens on mammary tumour incidence in female dogs

Progestogen	Benign	Malignant
Chlormadinone acetate	+	+
Lynestrenol	+[a]	+[a]
Megestrol acetate	+	+

From IARC (1979, 1989)
+, increased tumour incidence
[a] In this study, lynestrenol had a biphasic effect, with protection at the low dose (10 times the human contraceptive dose) and enhancement at 50 and 125 times the human contraceptive dose.

In female mice treated with 3-methylcholanthrene to induce uterine tumours, norethynodrel further increased the tumour incidence.

In male mice treated with chlormadinone acetate, ethynodiol diacetate, lynestrenol, norethisterone or norethisterone acetate, the incidence of liver adenomas was increased. Megestrol acetate increased the incidence of adenomas in female mice. Cyproterone acetate increased the incidence of liver adenomas and that of hepatocellular carcinomas in male and female mice, but at levels that exceeded the maximum tolerated dose. In rats, the incidence of liver adenomas was increased by norethisterone acetate (males and females), norethisterone (males), norethynodrel and cyproterone acetate (males and females). The numbers of altered hepatic foci in female rats were also increased by norethisterone acetate and cyproterone acetate. In female rats treated with N-nitrosodiethylamine to initiate hepatocarcinogenesis, norethynodrel increased the number of altered hepatic foci. Norethynodrel alone was shown to increase the incidence of hepatocarcinomas in male rats.

Levonorgestrel in combination with N-nitrosobis(2-oxopropyl)amine did not increase the incidence of renal dysplastic lesions or tumours in female hamsters.

Oral administration to dogs

Groups of three female beagle dogs, 9–10 months old, were treated orally for 91 days with 0.03, 0.3 or 3 mg/kg bw per day dienogest. Three control animals were given the vehicle (0.5% carboxymethylcellulose) alone. On the day after the last treatment, the animals were killed and their mammary glands and pituitary glands were removed. The mammary glands from dogs treated with dienogest for 91 days showed dose-dependent proliferation. Dogs given 3 mg/kg bw per day showed severe alveoli hyperplasia and a large number of vacuoles in the alveolar cells. The pituitary glands from dienogest-treated dogs showed slight hypertrophy compared with those from control dogs (Ishikawa et al., 2000). [Dienogest has progestational activity and caused proliferation of mammary gland epithelial cells in dogs, although no conclusive evidence of a carcinogenic effect was provided. As part of this same study, and with a similar design, dienogest showed no effects in female rats or monkeys.]

4. Other Data Relevant to an Evaluation of Carcinogenicity and its Mechanisms

4.1 Absorption, distribution, metabolism and excretion in humans

The metabolism and disposition of various formulations of oral contraceptives used in humans differ. After entering the small intestine, estrogenic and progestogenic compounds in combined oral contraceptives undergo metabolism by bacterial enzymes and enzymes in the intestinal mucosa to varying extents. The mixture of metabolized and unmetabolized compounds then undergoes intestinal absorption, and thus enters the portal vein blood, which perfuses the liver. In the liver, the compounds can be metabolized extensively, which leads to variations in the amount of active drug. A fraction of the absorbed dose of ethinyl-estradiol and some progestogens is also excreted in the bile during its first transit through the liver. Although some of these compounds are partially reabsorbed via the enterohepatic circulation, a fraction may also be excreted in this 'first pass', which reduces overall bio-availability.

Since steroids penetrate normal skin easily, various systems have also been developed that deliver estrogens and progestogens parenterally, e.g. transdermal patches, nasal sprays, subcutaneous implants, vaginal rings and intrauterine devices (Fanchin et al., 1997; Dezarnaulds & Fraser, 2002; Meirik et al., 2003; Sarkar, 2003; Wildemeersch et al., 2003; Sturdee et al., 2004). These different modes of administration have been described previously (IARC, 1999). In general, all parenteral routes avoid loss of the drug by hepatic first-pass metabolism and minimally affect hepatic protein metabolism.

The absorption rates of orally administered estrogens and progestogens are usually rapid; peak serum values are observed between 0.5 and 4 h after intake. Serum concentrations rise faster with multiple treatments than with single doses and achieve higher steady-state levels, which are still punctuated by rises after each daily dose. The rise in steady-state levels with multiple doses may reflect the inhibitory effect of both estrogens and progestogens on cytochrome P450 (CYP) metabolic enzyme activities. Alternatively, estrogens may induce the production of sex hormone-binding globulin (SHBG), which may increase the capacity of the blood to carry progestogens. The metabolism of progestogens and ethinylestradiol typically involves reduction, hydroxylation and conjugation. In some cases, metabolism converts an inactive pro-drug into a hormonally active compound. Hydroxylated metabolites are typically conjugated as glucuronides or sulfates and most are eliminated rapidly, with half-lives of 8–24 h (IARC, 1999).

Little is known about the effect of hormonal therapy on aromatase (CYP 19), which is responsible for the synthesis of estrogens. Aromatase is expressed in both normal and malignant breast tissues and its activity in the breast varies widely. However, the mechanisms and extent of regulation of aromatase in breast tissues have not been fully established and, to investigate the potential role of estrogen in this regulation, studies were carried out in an in-vitro model (Yue *et al.*, 2001) in which MCF-7 cells were cultured in long-term estrogen-deprived medium (LTED cells). It was found that long-term estrogen deprivation enhanced aromatase activity by three- to fourfold compared with that in wild-type MCF-7 cells. Re-exposure of LTED cells to estrogen reduced aromatase activity to the levels of wild-type MCF-7 cells. The authors also measured aromatase activity in 101 frozen breast carcinoma specimens and compared tumour aromatase activities in premenopausal patients with those in postmenopausal patients and in postmenopausal patients who did or did not take hormonal therapy. Although not statistically significant, a trend was observed that paralleled that in the in-vitro studies. Aromatase activity was higher in breast cancer tissues from patients who had lower levels of circulating estrogen. These data suggest that estrogen may be involved in the regulation of aromatase activity in breast tissues.

Two epidemiological studies examined the association of a common aromatase poly-morphism (intron 4 TTTA repeat) and osteoporosis in postmenopausal women who did or did not take hormonal menopausal therapy. The Danish Osteoporosis Prevention Study showed an increase in bone mineral density in women who had long TTTA repeats and who received therapy (Tofteng *et al.*, 2004). In untreated women, no association was observed between bone mass or bone loss and the TTTA polymorphism. In contrast, a Finnish study found that the TTTA polymorphism did not influence bone mineral density, which is a risk for fracture, or circulating levels of estradiol in treated or untreated women (Salmen *et al.*, 2003).

4.1.1   *Ethinylestradiol and mestranol*

Structural modification of the estradiol molecule by insertion of an ethinyl group at carbon 17 yields ethinylestradiol, which is considerably more potent than estradiol and has high activity following oral administration. This compound is used frequently as the estrogenic component of oral contraceptives.

Modification of ethinylestradiol by formation of a methyl ether at carbon 3 gives rise to mestranol, which was widely used in the early years of oral contraception, but is now rarely employed. Mestranol binds poorly to the estrogen receptor and its estrogenic effect is due to its rapid demethylation in the liver to form ethinylestradiol; however, demethy-lation is not complete and more mestranol must be administered than ethinylestradiol to achieve similar effects.

Goldzieher and Brody (1990) studied the pharmacokinetics of doses of 35 µg ethinyl-estradiol (24 women) and 50 µg mestranol (27 women) in combination with 1 mg nore-thisterone. Serum concentrations of ethinylestradiol were measured after treatment with either estrogen, each of which produced an average serum concentration of approximately 175 pg/mL ethinylestradiol, with wide inter-individual variation. The maximal serum con-centrations were achieved within about 1–2 h, and the half-life for elimination ranged from 13 to 27 h. The oral bioavailability of ethinylestradiol was 38–48%, and a 50-µg dose of mestranol was shown to be bioequivalent to a 35-µg dose of ethinylestradiol.

Hümpel *et al.* (1990) obtained serum samples from one group of 30 women who were taking a cycle of a combined oral contraceptive that contained ethinylestradiol and desogestrel and from another group of 39 women who were taking ethinylestradiol and gestodene. The serum concentrations of ethinylestradiol reached mean maximal levels of 106–129 pg/mL 1.6–1.8 h after intake. The mean serum concentrations of SHBG were 186–226 nmol/L, those of cortisol-binding globulin were 89–93 mg/L and those of cortisol were 280–281 μg/L.

Kuhnz *et al.* (1990a) compared the pharmacokinetics of ethinylestradiol administered as a single dose in combination with either gestodene or desogestrel to 18 women. In contrast to previous reports (Goldzieher & Brody, 1990; Hümpel *et al.*, 1990), which showed that the bioavailability of ethinylestradiol differed according to the associated progestogen, this study showed no significant difference.

The major pathway of ethinylestradiol metabolism in the liver of humans and animals is 2-hydroxylation, which is presumably catalysed by CYP 3A4 (Guengerich, 1988; see Section 4.1 of the monograph on Combined estrogen–progestogen menopausal therapy).

4.1.2   *Norethisterone*

Most of the data that pertain to the pharmacokinetics of norethisterone derive from a study (Back *et al.*, 1978) in which 1 mg norethisterone acetate and 0.05 mg ethinylestradiol were administered orally and intraveneously as a single dose or at 4-weekly intervals to a group of six premenopausal women. The results show that the absolute bioavailability of norethisterone after administration ranged from 47 to 73% (mean, 64%) compared with intravenous administration. The half-life [of the β phase of a two-component model] of elimination ranged from 4.8 to 12.8 h (mean, 7.6 h) with no significant differences between oral and intravenous administration.

Data from two different studies (Odlind *et al.*, 1979; Stanczyk *et al.*, 1983; Stanczyk, 2003) showed a dose–response in circulating levels of norethisterone following oral administration to premenopausal women of 5 mg, 1 mg (combined with 0.12 mg ethinylestradiol), 0.5 mg and 0.3 mg norethisterone. Mean peak plasma levels were approximately 23, 16, 6 and 4 ng/mL, respectively, within 1–2 h after treatment.

Norethisterone undergoes extensive ring A reduction to form dihydro- and tetrahydronorethisterone metabolites that undergo conjugation; it can also be aromatized. Low serum levels of ethinylestradiol have been measured in postmenopausal women following oral administration of relatively large doses of norethisterone acetate or norethisterone (Kuhnz *et al.*, 1997). On the basis of the area-under-the-curve (AUC) values that were determined for ethinylestradiol and norethisterone, it was shown that the mean conversion ratio of norethisterone to ethinylestradiol was 0.7 and 1.0% at doses of 5 and 10 mg, respectively. The authors calculated that this corresponds to an oral dose equivalent of about 6 μg ethinylestradiol/mg of norethisterone acetate. Similarly, it was shown that a dose of 5 mg norethisterone administered orally was equivalent to about 4 μg ethinylestradiol/mg norethisterone. On the basis of these calculations, it was estimated that lower doses of norethisterone or its acetate (e.g. 0.5–1.0 mg) in combination with ethinylestradiol would add between 0.002 and 0.01 mg ethinylestradiol to that already present. [The estimations for these lower doses were extrapolated from high doses of these compounds, which were not combined with ethinylestradiol. Nevertheless, it appears that significant amounts of ethinylestradiol are formed from norethisterone, and that the amount formed appears to be highly variable.]

No information on the pharmacokinetics of ethinylestradiol or mestranol via the dermal route (patch) was available to the Working Group.

4.1.3   *Norethisterone acetate, ethynodiol diacetate, norethynodrel and lynestrenol*

It is generally considered that progestogens that are structurally related to norethisterone are pro-drugs and that their progestational activity is due to their conversion to norethisterone. After oral administration, norethisterone acetate and ethynodiol diacetate are rapidly converted to norethisterone by esterases during hepatic first-pass metabolism. Although less is known about the transformation of lynestrenol and norethynodrel (Stanczyk & Roy, 1990), it appears that lynestrenol first undergoes hydroxylation at carbon 3 and then oxidation of the hydroxyl group to form norethisterone. Although there is no convincing evidence for the in-vivo transformation of norethynodrel to norethisterone, data from receptor-binding tests and bioassays suggest that norethynodrel is also a pro-drug.

4.1.4   *Levonorgestrel*

Stanczyk and Roy (1990) reviewed the metabolism of levonorgestrel in women treated orally with the radioactively labelled compound. Levonorgestrel was found mostly un-transformed in serum within 1–2 h after administration, but the concentrations of conjugated metabolites increased progressively between 4 and 24 h after ingestion. Most of the conjugates were sulfates and glucuronides. In addition to the remaining unconjugated levonorgestrel, considerable amounts of unconjugated and sulfate-conjugated forms of 3α,5β-tetrahydrolevonorgestrel were found; smaller quantities of conjugated and unconjugated 3α,5α-tetrahydrolevonorgestrel and 16β-hydroxylevonorgestrel were also identified (Sisenwine *et al.*, 1975a). Approximately 45% of radioactively labelled levonorgestrel was excreted via the urine and about 32% via the faeces. The major urinary metabolites were glucuronides (the most abundant was 3α,5β-tetrahydrolevonorgestrel glucuronide) and smaller quantities of sulfates were found (Sisenwine *et al.*, 1975b).

A dose–response has been demonstrated for circulating levels of levonorgestrel (Stanczyk, 2003) following administration of single oral doses of 0.25, 0.15 and 0.075 mg levonorgestrel to six, 24 and 24 women, respectively (Humpel *et al.*, 1977; Goebelsmann *et al.*, 1986; Stanczyk *et al.*, 1990). When the three doses were combined with 30–50 µg ethinylestradiol, mean peak levonorgestrel levels of 6.0, 3.5 and 2.5 ng/mL were attained at 1–3 h with the decreasing order of doses. At 24 h, the mean levonorgestrel level was 1.2 ng/mL with the highest dose and less than 0.5 ng/mL with the other two doses.

The bioavailability of levonorgestrel is generally accepted to be 100%. This generalization is based on two studies that used only a small number of women (Humpel *et al.*, 1978; Back *et al.*, 1981). In one of the studies (Back *et al.*, 1981), absolute bioavailabilities were determined for doses of 0.25 and 0.15 mg levonorgestrel, each of which was administered to five women in combination with ethinylestradiol (0.05 mg). The results show that the bioavailability for the 0.15-mg dose of levonorgestrel ranged from 72 to 125% (mean, 99%); that for the 0.15-mg dose ranged from 63 to 108% (mean, 89%). When the individual bioavailabilities for the 0.25-mg dose were examined, it was noted that 60% of the subjects had bioavailabilities greater than 100%. [This demonstrates that, for each of these subjects, the AUC for levonorgestrel obtained by the oral route was greater than that obtained intravenously, and implies that there was a methodological problem in the study.] In the same study, the mean half-life of elimination was found to be 13.2 h and 9.9 h for the 0.15-mg and 0.25-mg doses of levonorgestrel, respectively, when administered intravenously. These values were similar after oral dosing.

Carol *et al.* (1992) evaluated the pharmacokinetics of levonorgestrel in groups of 11–20 women who were given single or multiple treatments with combined oral contraceptive preparations that contained 0.125 mg levonorgestrel plus 0.03 or 0.05 mg ethinylestradiol. The serum concentrations of levonorgestrel reached a maximum of about 4 ng/mL at 1–2 h after a single treatment with either preparation. After 21 days of treatment, the peak and sustained concentrations of levonorgestrel were about twice as high as those after a single treatment. The serum concentration of SHBG increased after treatment with both contraceptives (but to a greater extent with the contraceptive containing 0.05 mg ethinylestradiol), which indicates the important role of estrogen in the induction of this protein.

Kuhnz *et al.* (1992) treated a group of nine women with a single dose of a combined oral contraceptive that contained 0.15 mg levonorgestrel plus 0.03 mg ethinylestradiol; eight of these women received the same regimen for 3 months after an abstention period of 3 months. The peak concentrations of levonorgestrel were found 1 h after single or multiple treatments. The peak serum concentrations of levonorgestrel were 3.1 and 5.9 ng/mL, respectively. The AUC concentration for total and free levonorgestrel increased by two- to fourfold after a single dose compared with multiple treatments. The distribution of free, albumin-bound and SHBG-bound levonorgestrel was similar in women who had received one or multiple treatments, but the serum concentration of the globulin increased significantly after multiple treatments.

Kuhnz *et al.* (1994a) treated 14 women with a combined oral contraceptive that contained 0.125 mg levonorgestrel plus 0.03 mg ethinylestradiol as a single dose and for 3 months as a triphasic regimen (Triquilar®) after an abstention period of 1 week. The serum concentration of free levonorgestrel reached a peak of 0.06–0.08 ng/mL about 1 h after treatment with a single dose or on day 1 of the first or third cycle. In contrast, the calculated values of the AUC more than doubled, from 0.32 (single dose) to 0.75 (multiple treatment, first cycle)–0.77 (multiple treatment, third cycle) ng × h/mL. The serum concentrations of cortisol-binding globulin and SHBG more than doubled after multiple treatments with the contraceptive. After a single dose, 1.4% of the levonorgestrel in serum was free, 43% was bound to albumin and 55% was bound to SHBG. After multiple treatments, only 0.9–1.0% levonorgestrel in serum was free and 25–30% was bound to albumin and the amount that was bound to SHBG increased to 69–74%. The concentrations of free and total testosterone decreased from 3 and 460 pg/mL, respectively, before treatment to 1 and 270 pg/mL, respectively, at the end of one treatment cycle and increased again to 2 and 420 pg/mL, respectively, by the 1st day of the third cycle. Thus, the treatment-free interval of 1 week was sufficient to restore pretreatment values for testosterone.

4.1.5   Desogestrel

Desogestrel is a pro-drug and its progestational activity is mediated by one of its metabolites, 3-ketodesogestrel. In a study in which 10 women ingested single doses of 0.15 mg desogestrel combined with 0.03 mg ethinylestradiol and another group of women ingested single doses of 0.15 mg 3-ketodesogestrel combined with 0.03 mg ethinylestradiol (Hasenack et al., 1986), serum 3-ketodesogestrel levels were essentially the same in both groups of women, whereas desogestrel was not found in significant amounts.

Following administration of a single oral dose of 0.15 mg desogestrel combined with 0.03 mg ethinylestradiol to a group of 25 women, the mean maximum concentration of 3-ketodesogestrel was 3.69 ng/mL, which was reached at a mean time of 1.6 ± 1.0 h (Bergink et al., 1990). The mean bioavailability of 3-ketodesogestrel in two cross-over studies, in which women received either a single oral or intravenous dose of 0.15 mg desogestrel combined with 0.03 mg ethinylestradiol, was reported to be 76 and 62%, respectively (Back et al., 1987; Orme et al., 1991). The mean half-life of elimination for 3-ketodesogestrel, calculated from two studies (Back et al., 1987; Bergink et al., 1990) in which women were given a single oral dose of 0.15 mg desogestrel combined with 0.03 mg ethinylestradiol, was not consistent (23.8 h versus 11.9 h); the longer half-life was calculated from serum 3-ketodesogestrel levels that were obtained up to 72 h (Bergink et al., 1990) whereas frequent blood sampling was carried out only up to 24 h in the other study. [The lack of data beyond 24 h is a deficiency of most studies of progestogen pharmacokinetics in which the half-life of elimination is calculated.]

A multiple dosing study (Kuhl et al., 1988a) was carried out in 11 women who ingested 0.15 mg desogestrel in combination with 0.03 mg ethinylestradiol daily for 12 continuous treatment cycles and whose blood was sampled at frequent intervals on days 1, 10 and 21 of cycles 1, 3, 6 and 12. The results showed that 3-ketodesogestrel levels were relatively low on day 1 but rose progressively and were higher on day 21 of the treatment cycles. This increase was attributed to the elevated serum levels of SHBG induced by the estrogenic component of the pill.

A group of 19 women were given three cycles of a triphasic oral contraceptive that contained combinations of desogestrel and ethinylestradiol at doses of 0.15, 0.05 and 0.035 mg for the first 7 days, 0.10 and 0.03 mg for days 8–14 and 0.15 and 0.03 mg for days 15–21, respectively, followed by 7 days without hormone. Multiple blood samples were taken from the women throughout this interval, and serum concentrations of 3-ketodesogestrel, ethinylestradiol and SHBG were determined, together with the elimination half-life and dose proportionality. The concentration of 3-ketodesogestrel reached steady-state levels at each desogestrel dose, and the pharmacokinetics was proportional to the dose. The concentration of ethinylestradiol also reached a steady state, and the pharmacokinetics was constant thereafter. The concentration of SHBG was significantly increased between days 1 and 7 of the cycle but not between days 7, 14 and 21 (Archer *et al.*, 1994).

4.1.6   *Gestodene*

Gestodene is metabolized primarily in the liver by CYP 3A4 and is a strong inducer of this enzyme. Although ethinylestradiol is also metabolized by CYP 3A4, gestodene does not appear to inhibit its metabolism. Known metabolites of gestodene include di-hydrogestodene, 3,5-tetrahydrogestodene and hydroxygestodene.

Gestodene is not a pro-drug. Following administration of a single oral dose of 0.025, 0.075 or 0.125 mg gestodene in combination with or without 0.03 mg ethinylestradiol to six women, a dose–response was observed. The half-life of elimination of gestodene was shown to range from 12 to 14 h for the three doses studied (Tauber *et al.*, 1989). Mean maximum concentration values of 1.0, 3.6 and 7.0 ng/mL gestodene were attained between 1.4 and 1.9 h, respectively. The mean absolute bioavailability was calculated to be 99% (range, 86–112%) for the commonly prescribed dose of 0.075 mg gestodene. In another similar study (Orme *et al.*, 1991), the mean absolute bioavailability was reported to be 87% (range, 64–126%).

The same experimental design that was used for the multiple dosing studies with desogestrel (Kuhl *et al.*, 1988a) was also used for gestodene (Kuhl *et al.*, 1988b). The results showed a dramatic rise in mean gestodene levels between day 1 and day 10, and a further rise between day 10 and day 21 in all study cycles. These findings were attributed to increased levels of SHBG and were similar to those obtained when multiple dosing was performed with desogestrel.

Following oral administration of 0.075 mg gestodene combined with 0.03 mg ethinyl-estradiol, either as a single dose or as multiple doses, the circulating levels of gestodene were relatively high compared with similar treatments with other progestogens in combination with ethinylestradiol (Fotherby, 1990). [This finding was surprising because the 0.075-mg dose of gestodene is the lowest dose of any progestogen used in a combined oral contraceptive pill. The major factor responsible for the elevated levels of gestodene appears to be the high affinity of SHBG for gestodene, which results in a lower metabolic clearance and consequently a higher concentration of this progestogen in the blood. It has been reported that approximately 75% of gestodene is bound to SHBG after oral treatment with gestodene/ethinylestradiol, which is considerably higher than that observed with other progestogens combined with ethinylestradiol.]

Kuhnz *et al.* (1990b) studied the binding of gestodene to serum proteins in 37 women who had taken a combined oral contraceptive that contained gestodene plus ethinylestradiol for at least 3 months: 0.6% was free, 24% was bound to albumin and 75% was bound to SHBG.

Kuhnz *et al.* (1991) examined the effects of a single administration followed by multiple administrations over one cycle (after an abstention period of 1 week) of a tri-phasic combined oral contraceptive that contained gestodene and ethinylestradiol on the concentrations of ethinylestradiol and testosterone in 10 women. After a single oral dose of 0.10 mg gestodene plus 0.03 mg ethinylestradiol, the serum ethinylestradiol concentration reached 100 pg/mL in about 1.9 h; thereafter, the concentration declined, with a half-life of 11 h. On day 21 of the treatment cycle, the maximum concentrations reached 140 pg/mL 1.6 h after intake. In comparison with day 21 after the single dose treatment, the levels of total and free testosterone were reduced by about 60% on day 21 of the treatment cycle.

Kuhnz *et al.* (1993) treated 14 women with a combined oral contraceptive that contained 0.10 mg gestodene plus 0.03 mg ethinylestradiol as a single dose and for 3 months as a triphasic regimen after an abstention of 1 week. The maximum serum concentrations of gestodene 30 min after dosing were 4.3 ng/mL after a single dose, 15 ng/mL at the end of the first cycle and 14.4 ng/mL at the end of three cycles. A half-life for clearance of 18 h was observed after a single treatment, with a volume of distribution of 84 L. Multiple treatments increased the clearance half-life to 20–22 h and reduced the distribution volume to about 19 L. The serum concentration of SHBG increased with multiple treatments, presumably as an effect of ethinylestradiol, which is thought to account for the observed change in the distribution of gestodene (from 1.3% free, 69% bound to SHBG and 29% bound to albumin after a single treatment to 0.6% free, 81% bound to SHBG and 18% bound to albumin after multiple treatments).

Heuner *et al.* (1995) treated 14 women with a combined oral contraceptive that contained 0.075 mg gestodene plus 0.02 mg ethinylestradiol by a single administration or for 3 months as a triphasic regimen. The serum concentrations of gestodene, ethinylestradiol, cortisol-binding globulin, SHBG and testosterone were followed after the single treatment and through cycles 1 and 3. The concentration of gestodene reached a maximum of 3.5 ng/mL within 0.9 h after a single dose and 8.7 ng/mL within 0.7 h after multiple doses. The clearance half-time for a single dose of gestodene also increased from 12.6 h to nearly 20 h after multiple treatments. There was a large increase in the concentration of SHBG with time after multiple treatments. After a single dose, 1.3% of gestodene in serum was free, 30% was bound to albumin and 68% was bound to SHBG.

4.1.7   *Norgestimate*

Very little is known about the pharmacokinetics of orally administered norgestimate except that it is a relatively complex pro-drug. After its oral administration, the acetate group at carbon 17 is rapidly removed during hepatic first-pass metabolism. The product formed — levonorgestrel-3-oxime — has progestational activity. It has also been referred to as deacetylated norgestimate and, more recently, has been assigned the common name norelgestromin. Rapid formation of norelgestromin from norgestimate was demonstrated by McGuire *et al.* (1990); serum levels of norelgestromin were measured after administration of single and multiple oral doses of 0.36 mg norgestimate combined with 0.07 mg ethinylestradiol to 10 women. Mean peak serum levels of 17-deacetylnorgestimate (norelgestromin) were approximately 4 ng/mL and were attained after about 1.4 h; the levels remained elevated up to 36 h after treatment. In contrast, peak levels of norgestimate were only ~100 pg/mL 1 h after treatment; the concentration declined rapidly thereafter and none was detectable 5 h after treatment.

Norgestimate is converted to levonorgestrel. In a randomized, comparative pharmacokinetic study by Kuhnz *et al.* (1994b), 12 women received single oral doses of 0.25 mg norgestimate combined with 0.035 mg ethinylestradiol and 0.25 mg levonorgestrel combined with 0.05 mg ethinylestradiol. The levonorgestrel AUC ratios were determined after administration of both formulations and were used to calculate the bioavailability of norgestimate-derived levonorgestrel: on average, about 22% of the administered dose of norgestimate became systemically available as levonorgestrel.

In addition to norelgestromin and levonorgestrel, a third progestationally active metabolite of orally administered norgestimate is formed, which is probably levonorgestrel-17-acetate (Kuhnz *et al.*, 1994b).

4.1.8 *Newly developed progestogens*

In recent years, new progestogens have been synthesized that may improve the performance of combined hormones. Two of these that are currently in use (Sitruk-Ware, 2004a) are discussed below. Other members of this group, e.g. nesterone, nomegestrol acetate and trimegestone, are used much less frequently, although their pharmacological profile is similar with respect to receptor binding (see Tables 17 and 18 in Section 4.2 of the monograph on Combined estrogen–progestogen menopausal therapy) (Kuhl, 1996; Couthino *et al.*, 1999; Kumar *et al.*, 2000; Tuba *et al.*, 2000; Lepescheux *et al.*, 2001; Shields-Botella *et al.*, 2003).

(*a*) *Dienogest*

Dienogest (17α-cyanomethyl-17β-hydroxyestra-4,9-dien-3-one) is a derivative of 19-nortestosterone. It has progestational activity but no androgenic, estrogenic, anti-estrogenic or corticoid activity. It strongly suppresses endometrial proliferation and does not antagonize the beneficial effects of estrogens. Dienogest binds highly selectively to the progesterone receptor, but does not bind to SHBG. As a result, it does not compete with testosterone for binding, and thereby helps to minimize the free serum levels of the androgen. Relatively high levels of the compound (approximately 9%) are free in the serum. After oral intake, a maximum serum concentration of dienogest is reached after about 1 h and does not accumulate after repeated dosing. The compound has an elimination half-life of 9.1 h. Studies of receptor binding have shown that the anti-androgenic activity of dienogest is similar to that of cyproterone acetate and progesterone (Teichmann, 2003).

Studies on the pharmacokinetics of dienogest have been carried out following oral and intravenous administration of different doses (Oettel *et al.*, 1995). A dose–response in serum dienogest levels was observed in 12 women after oral administration of four single doses (1, 2, 4 and 8 mg) in randomized order during four consecutive menstrual cycles. Following administration of the 1-mg dose, the mean maximum concentration was 23.4 ng/mL and the time to reach this level was 2.2 ± 1.1 h; half-life of elimination was 6.5 h. The absolute bioavailability of dienogest was determined in 16 healthy male volunteers who ingested a single dose of two tablets, each of which contained 2 mg dienogest and 0.03 mg ethinylestradiol; the average bioavailability value was 96.2%. In the same study, the average terminal half-life was reported to be 10.8 and 11.6 h after oral and intravenous doses, respectively.

From the two studies described above and other related studies by Oettel *et al.* (1995), it can be concluded that circulating levels of dienogest are relatively high compared with those found with similar doses of other progestogens. The clearance of dienogest appears to be lower than that of other progestogens, although most of it is weakly bound to albumin in the blood (Oettel *et al.*, 1995). No significant accumulation of dienogest was observed in serum during its daily intake (Oettel *et al.*, 1995).

(b)   Drospirenone

The pharmacokinetic characteristics of drospirenone (3 mg) combined with ethinylestradiol (0.03 mg) were assessed in 13 women during 13 continuous cycles, each of which consisted of 21 continuous days of treatment followed by a 7-day treatment-free interval (Blode *et al.*, 2000). Frequent blood sampling was carried out on day 21 of treatment cycles 1, 6, 9 and 13. After administration of the first tablet, the mean maximum concentration of drospirenone was 36.9 ng/mL, which rose to 87.5 ng/mL on day 21 of the first cycle and ranged from 78.7 to 84.2 ng/mL on day 21 of the next three sampling cycles. The corresponding time to reach peak levels ranged from 1.6 to 1.8 h, and the half-life of elimination values were 31.1–32.5 h.

Other pharmacokinetic characteristics of drospirenone, based on data obtained by the manufacturer of an oral contraceptive that contained 3 mg drospirenone combined with 0.03 mg ethinylestradiol, have been reviewed (Krattenmacher, 2000). It was reported that a steady-state in circulating drospirenone levels is achieved after 1 week of treatment, and a dose–response in circulating drospirenone levels is obtained following oral administration of doses ranging from 1 to 10 mg. In addition, the absolute bioavailability was reported to be on average 76%.

4.1.9   Interactions of other drugs with oral contraceptives

Kopera (1985) reviewed the drug interactions associated with the administration of progestogens to patients who received other medications. Progestogens adversely affect the metabolism of certain drugs and, in turn, the metabolism of progestogens is affected by other drugs. These effects presumably occur as a consequence of the induction of metabolic enzymes, or competition for metabolic pathways or for binding to serum carrier proteins (Shenfield *et al.*, 1993).

Data on the effects of some oral contraceptive estrogens and progestrogens in animals were reviewed previously (IARC, 1999) (see also Section 4.2 of this monograph and Sections 4.1 and 4.2 of the monograph on Combined estrogen–progestogen menopausal therapy in this volume).

4.2   Receptor-mediated effects

There is evidence that not all the effects of estrogens and progestogens that are used in combined hormonal (oral) contraceptives are mediated through nuclear or other receptors. In addition, the effects of these steroids probably involve several molecular pathways and cross-talk between receptor- and/or non-receptor-mediated pathways. During the past decade, research on the mechanisms of hormonal action and on hormones and cancer has grown immensely. Two different subtypes of the progesterone receptor, subtypes A and B (Kazmi *et al.*, 1993; Vegeto *et al.*, 1993), and several estrogen receptors that have different functions — the nuclear estrogen receptors-α and -β and their subtypes — have been identified (Kuiper *et al.*, 1996; Mosselman *et al.*, 1996; Kuiper *et al.*, 1997). In addition, estrogen receptors-α and other estrogen-binding proteins that are located in the plasma membrane appear to be responsible for rapid non-genomic estrogen responses (Pietras *et al.*, 2001; Song *et al.*, 2002; Razandi *et al.*, 2003) and may activate signal transduction pathways by estrogens (Razandi *et al.*, 2003; Song *et al.*, 2004). There is also some evidence to suggest that a non-genomically acting progesterone receptor is responsible for rapid progestogen responses (Castoria *et al.*, 1999; Sutter-Dub, 2002; Sager *et al.*, 2003). However, the literature on specific interactions of constituents of combined oral contraceptive preparations with these receptor subtypes is still limited.

Increased attention to the various components of combined oral contraceptives in recent years has resulted in the availability of more information on the progestogens used with respect to their hormonal activities and binding to various receptors and other binding proteins. This information is summarized in Tables 35 and 36.

4.2.1   *Combined oral contraceptives*

(*a*)   *Humans*

(i)   *Breast epithelial cell proliferation*

It was concluded previously that exposure to combined oral contraceptives increases breast epithelial cell proliferation and that, when ethinylestradiol is the estrogen component, this effect is dose-dependent (IARC, 1999). Increased breast epithelial cell proliferation may be associated with an increased risk for breast cancer (Russo & Russo, 1996; Pihan *et al.*, 1998). Isaksson *et al.* (2001) confirmed and extended these conclusions which are consistent with an increase in risk for breast cancer: all 53 women who had taken combined

Table 35. Overview of the spectrum of hormonal activities of progestogens used in combined oral contraceptives[a]

Progestogen	Progesto-genic	Anti-estrogenic	Estrogenic	Androgenic	Anti-androgenic	Gluco-corticoid	Antimineralo-corticoid
Chlormadinone acetate	−	+	−	−	+	+	−
Cyproterone acetate	−	+	−	−	+, +	+	−
Desogestrel	−	+	−	+	−	±, −	−
Dienogest	−	+, ±	−, ±	−	+	−	−
Drospirenone	−, +	+	−	−	+	?, −	+
Gestodene	−	+	−	+	−	±, +	+
Levonorgestrel	−	+	−	+	−	−	−
Norethisterone acetate	−, +	+	+	+	−	−	−

Adapted from Wiegratz & Kuhl (2004); second value for progestogenic activity only from Sitruk-Ware (2002); second value, except for progestogenic activity from Schindler et al. (2003)

+, effective; ±, weakly effective; −, ineffective; ?, unknown

[a] Data are based mainly on animal experiments. The clinical effects of progestogens are dependent on their tissue concentrations.

No comparable data were available for ethynodiol diacetate or lynestrenol.

Note: This information should be viewed as only an indication of the hormonal activity (and its order of magnitude) of the various progestogens.

Table 36. Relative binding affinities of progestogens used in combined oral contraceptives to steroid receptors and serum binding globulins[a]

Progestogen	PR	AR	ER	GR	MR	SHBG	CBG
Chlormadinone acetate	134	5	0	8	0	0	0
Cyproterone acetate	180	6	0	6	8	0	0
Desogestrel (as 3-ketodesogestrel)	300	20	0	14	0	15	0
Dienogest	10	10	0	1	0	0	0
Drospirenone	70, 19	65, 2	0, < 0.5	6, 3	230, 500	0	0
Gestodene	180, 864	85, 71	0, < 0.02	27, 38	290, 97	40	0
Levonorgestrel	300, 323	45, 58	0	1, 7.5	75, 17	50	0
Norethisterone acetate	150, 134	15, 55	0.015	0, 1.4	0, 2.7	16	0
Reference compounds (100%)	Progesterone	Metribolone R1881	Estradiol-17β	Dexamethasone (or cortisol)	Aldosterone	5α-dihydro-testosterone	Cortisol

Adapted from Wiegrazt & Kuhl (2004); second value from Sitruk-Ware (2004)

AR, androgen receptor; CBG, corticoid-binding globulin; ER, estrogen receptor; GR, glucocorticoid receptor; MR, mineralocorticoid receptor; PR, progesterone receptor; SHBG, sex hormone-binding globulin

[a] Values were compiled by these authors by cross-comparison of the literature. Because the results of the various in-vitro experiments depend largely on the incubation conditions and biological materials used, the published values are inconsistent. These values do not reflect the biological effectiveness, but should be viewed as only an indication of the order of magnitude of the binding affinities of the various progestogens. No comparable data were available for ethinodiol acetate or lynestrenol.

oral contraceptives had used preparations that contained ethinylestradiol combined with levonorgestrel, desogestrel, lynestrenol or norethisterone; however, the actual dose levels were not provided. Data from these women were compared with those from 54 women who had not used hormonal contraception. Fine needle aspirates were obtained between days 16 and 21 on the first cycle of treatment or, for control women, during the second half of the menstrual cycle. The mean percentage of breast epithelial cells that stained for Ki-67 (using the MIB-1 antibody that reacts with a human nuclear antigen present in proliferating cells) was 4.8% (median, 3.0%; range, 0–50%) in women exposed to combined oral contraceptives and 2.2% (median, 1.5%; range, 0–8%) in control women, a difference that was statistically significant. In 37 women who had taken ethinylestradiol plus levonorgestrel, the correlation between serum levonorgestrel levels and breast epithelial cell proliferation was found to be statistically significant in a positive direction (Spearman $r = 0.43$; $p = 0.02$). For 16 women who had taken ethinylestradiol plus levonorgestrel, fine needle aspirates were obtained both before the start of the oral contraceptive treatment and 2 months afterwards. The mean percentage of breast epithelial cells that stained for Ki-67 was 1.4% (median, 0.5%; range, 0–5%) before treatment and 5.8% (median, 0.8%; range, 0–50%) after 2 months of treatment; this change was of borderline significance ($p = 0.055$).

(ii)   Effects on the endometrium

Four independent studies have investigated the effects of combined oral contraceptives on the endometrium. Moyer and Felix (1998) obtained endometrial biopsies from two groups of nine women who were exposed for an unreported duration to a regimen that consisted of oral treatment with either 0.06 mg mestranol plus 5 or 10 mg norethisterone acetate or 0.075 mg mestranol plus 5 mg norethynodrel for 21 days, followed by 7 days with no treatment. Biopsies were taken during the 7 days with no treatment. For comparison, biopsies were also taken from 10 untreated premenopausal women between days 5 and 14 of the menstrual cycle. Mitotic counts were significantly reduced from 12.3/1000 glandular cells in untreated women to 1.6 and 0.01/1000 cells in women exposed to mestranol plus norethynodrel and norethisterone acetate, respectively. [The Working Group noted that the timing of biopsy in the treated and untreated women probably does not permit an adequate comparison.]

Archer (1999) studied 11 women who took a triphasic oral regimen of 0.02 mg ethinylestradiol plus 0.05 mg desogestrel for 21 days, placebo for 2 days and 0.01 g ethinylestradiol for the last 5 days of each 28-day cycle. Endometrial biopsies were taken after 13–14 cycles. A progestational effect on endometrial histology was observed with secretory changes in samples obtained between days 11 and 21 of the treatment cycle. However, this was benign and no endometrial hyperplasia or metaplasia was observed.

Oosterbaan (1999) reported a study of women who took an oral preparation that consisted of 0.05 mg ethinylestradiol plus 0.06 mg gestodene for 24 days followed by 4 days with no treatment. Endometrial biopsies were taken during the late luteal phase before treatment (baseline biopsies) and between days 15 and 24 of the treatment cycle during cycle 3 or 6. Histological evidence of endometrial atrophy was observed in three of nine subjects during cycle 3 and in four of nine subjects during cycle 6, whereas 11 of 13 baseline biopsies showed a secretory endometrium.

A regimen that consisted of 21 days of 0.03 mg ethinylestradiol plus 3 mg drospirenone followed by 7 days of no treatment was studied by Lüdicke et al. (2001). Endometrial biopsies were taken at baseline (26 women) and after 3 (11 women), 6 (10 women) and 13 cycles (26 women); endometrial thickness was also assessed by ultrasound at these four time-points ($n = 26$). Morphometry and ultrasound showed endometrial atrophy following the treatment: after 3, 6 and 13 cycles, 41, 44 and 63% of subjects, respectively, had an atrophic endometrium. Glandular mitotic activity (normally 0.3/1000 cells) was also absent at these three time-points.

Collectively, these four studies indicate atrophic and anti-proliferative endometrial effects of progestogen-containing combined oral contraceptives, apparently regardless of the regimen and the actual progestogen used. This anti-proliferative effect may be associated with a reduction in the risk for endometrial cancer.

(iii)   *Effects on the colon*

In addition to a range of growth factor receptors, the human colon has both estrogen and progesterone nuclear receptors and expresses known estrogen-inducible genes (*pS2* and *ERD5*) (Di Leo et al., 1992; Hendrickse et al., 1993; Singh et al., 1998). However, some studies did not confirm these findings; in addition, there are conflicting results on the expression of these receptors in stromal versus epithelial cells which are perhaps related to differences in the methodology used between studies (Waliszewski et al., 1997; Slattery et al., 2000). Nevertheless, these observations suggest that there may be a link between exposures to hormones in combined oral contraceptives and menopausal therapy and colon cancer, but they do not predict the nature of such a relationship.

(iv)   *Effects on hormonal systems*

Several new studies have investigated the relationship between combined oral contraceptives and hormonal parameters. In four of these, serum levels of SHBG and free testosterone were measured. Levels of SHBG were increased by two- to fourfold and free testosterone levels were reduced by 40–80%, regardless of the combined oral contraceptive regimen used (Piérard-Franchimont et al., 2000; Boyd et al., 2001; Isaksson et al., 2001; Wiegratz et al., 2003). Wiegratz et al. (2003) studied women who were taking four different contraceptive regimens for 21 days followed by 7 days with no treatment: 0.03 mg ethinylestradiol plus 2 mg dienogest, 0.02 mg ethinylestradiol plus 2 mg dienogest, 0.01 mg ethinylestradiol plus 2 mg estradiol valerate plus 2 mg dienogest or 0.02 mg ethinylestradiol plus 0.10 mg levonorgestrel. In addition to reducing free testosterone and increasing the levels of SHBG, all treatments reduced levels of dehydroepiandrosterone sulfate and increased those of corticoid-binding globulin by approximately twofold and of thyroxin-binding globulin by approximately 50%, while prolactin was not affected. All four regimens had comparable effects, except that ethinylestradiol plus levonorgestrel increased levels of SHBG by only 50–100% and ethinylestradiol plus estradiol valerate plus dienogest increased levels of prolactin by up to 40%. In the study by Isaksson *et al.* (2001), levels of androstenedione and total testosterone were also reduced as well as that of serum progesterone by 10-fold; levels of insulin-like growth factor-1 in the serum were not affected. Chatterton *et al.* (2005) found an even stronger reduction in nipple aspirate fluid progesterone from the breast (98%) and in serum progesterone (96.5%) in women who took a variety of triphasic contraceptives, but observed no effect on dehydroepiandrosterone or its sulfate or androstenedione, which are the potential precursors of 17β-estradiol. Levels of 17β-estradiol and estrone sulfate were also substantially reduced. These data suggest the possible involvement of reduced androgenic and estrogenic stimulation of responsive tissue, e.g. the breast. However, all combined oral contraceptives contain estrogens and several of the progestogens used, such as levonorgestrel and norethisterone, have androgenic activity. These studies highlight the possibility of complex interactions with other hormonal systems.

(b)   Experimental systems

Rodriguez *et al.* (1998, 2002) examined the effects of a triphasic oral contraceptive regimen on the ovary of cynomolgus macaque monkeys. The treatment was equivalent to human doses of 0.03 mg ethinylestradiol plus 0.05 mg levonorgestrel per day for 6 days, followed by 0.04 mg ethinylestradiol plus 0.075 mg levonorgestrel for 5 days, followed by 0.03 mg ethinylestradiol plus 0.125 mg levonorgestrel for 10 days, followed by 7 days with no treatment. Parallel groups received ethinylestradiol only, levonorgestrel only or no treatment (control). This cyclic regimen was repeated every 28 days continuously for 35 months. The percentage of ovarian epithelial (surface) cells that stained positively for a reaction indicative of apoptosis was reduced by ethinylestradiol alone to a mean value of 1.8% compared with the mean control value of 3.9%. In contrast, apoptosis was increased more than sixfold by levonorgestrel alone and almost fourfold by the contraceptive combination of ethinylestradiol and levonorgestrel (Rodriguez *et al.*, 1998). The treatments also affected the protein (immunohistochemical) expression of isoforms of transforming growth factor-β (TGF-β) that are known to be associated with apoptosis. TGF-β1 expression was reduced in epithelial cells, whereas expression of TGF-β2/3 was increased (Rodriguez *et al.*, 2002). These findings may be consistent with a protective effect of combined oral contraceptives against the risk for ovarian cancer.

In cell culture, 0.01 nM, 1 nM and 100 nM gestodene, levonorgestrel and the active metabolite of gestodene, 3-ketodesogestrel, given together either for 7 days or for the last 4 days of a 7-day estrogen treatment, all inhibited the cell proliferation induced by 10^{-10}M 17β-estradiol in estrogen receptor-positive MCF-7 breast cancer cells (Seeger *et al.*, 2003). The inhibition was dose-dependent for the combined 7-day treatment, but was similar regardless of dose when given on the last 4 days of estrogen treatment. A concentration of 10 µM had a lesser (continuous progestogen) or no (sequential progestogen) inhibitory effect. This study suggests that the progestogen components of combined oral contraceptives may reduce the stimulation of breast cell proliferation by the estrogen component, but no human studies are available.

4.2.2   *Oral contraception and HPV*

(*a*)   *Humans*

Both estrogen and progesterone receptors are expressed in normal human uterine cervix epithelium; in many cases, estrogen receptors, but not progesterone receptors, are lost during the development of cervical carcinoma *in situ* and invasive cancer (Nonogaki *et al.*, 1990; Monsonego *et al.*, 1991). Expression of progesterone receptors is increased in carcinoma *in situ* and greatly diminished in invasive cancer (Monsonego *et al.*, 1991). Infection with HPV is an essential causative component of human cervical cancer in more than 90% of cases (see IARC, 2007). HPV has more than 100 genotypes, some of which are associated with high risk for cancer and others with lower risk (see IARC, 2007). The loss of estrogen receptors may be associated with infection with specific types of HPV (Nonogaki *et al.*, 1990). These observations suggest that estrogen and progesterone may be involved in cervical carcinogenesis (de Villiers, 2003).

(*b*)   *Experimental systems*

Transcription of HPV is regulated by the long control region of the viral genome (see IARC, 2007). Expression of the E6 and E7 genes of HPV is affected by progesterone (and glucocorticoids for which there are also receptors in cervical epithelium) through hormone response elements on the long control region (Chan *et al.*, 1989). This appears to occur in both high-risk (HPV 16 and 18) and low-risk HPV (HPV 11) types. There is also evidence that E6 and E7 expression is regulated by estrogen but there are no known estrogen-response elements on the long control region. Plasmids for the expression of chloramphenicol acetyl transferase (CAT) in the HPV 16 and 18 long control regions that were transfected into HeLa cells that contain progesterone but no estrogen receptors responded differentially to different estrogen and progestogens, but combinations of these were not tested (Chen *et al.*, 1996). 17β-Estradiol and estriol, but not estrone, induced HPV 16 CAT expression (2.3- and 2.7-fold, respectively) and, to a lesser extent, HPV 18 CAT expression (1.3- and 1.5-fold, respectively) at concentrations of 100 nM. HPV 18 CAT expression was only minimally increased by some progestogens (cyproterone acetate, norethynodrel and ethynodiol diacetate), hardly increased by progesterone itself and not increased by norethisterone acetate or norgestrel (all tested at concentrations of 100 nM). In contrast, HPV 16 CAT expression was increased by all of these progestogens (except norgestrel); progesterone and norethisterone acetate were the least active (1.7- and 1.8-fold increase, respectively) and ethynodiol diacetate, cyproterone acetate and northynodrel were the most active (2.3-, 2.5- and 2.5-fold increase, respectively).

In cervical epithelial cells transfected with and immortalized by HPV 16, 17β-estradiol was metabolized to a greater extent to 16α-hydroxy metabolites than to 2-hydroxy metabolites; 4-hydroxy metabolites were not detected (Auborn *et al.*, 1991). 17β-Estradiol and 16α-hydroxyestrone stimulated cell proliferation and caused increased growth in soft agar of cervical epithelial cells transfected with and immortalized by HPV 16 (Newfield *et al.*, 1998). In both studies, human foreskin epithelial cells (which do not express estrogen receptors) transfected with and immortalized by HPV 16 did not metabolize or respond to estrogen. Fifty women who had moderate or high-grade carcinoma *in situ* of the cervix and an HPV infection but not 29 women who had carcinoma *in situ* and no HPV infection had serum estrone levels twofold higher ($p < 0.05$) than those found in women who did not have cervical carcinoma *in situ* ($n = 45$) (Salazar *et al.*, 2001). [The hypothesis that 16α-hydroxy-estrone is a major factor in estrogen-induced carcinogenesis in general is not supported by recent data (see Sections 4.1 and 4.3 in the monograph on Combined estrogen–progestogen menopausal therapy of this volume), but it may play a role in the HPV-infected cervix. However, in the study by Salazar *et al.* (2001), only serum estrone and not 16α-hydroxy-estrone was measured and other estrogen metabolites have not been considered systematically in the studies reviewed. Therefore, support for the hypothesis that 16α-hydroxyestrone is a major factor in HPV 16-induced cervical carcinogenesis (de Villiers, 2003) is uncertain.]

In transgenic mice that carry the β-galactosidase gene under the control of the HPV 18 long control region (Morales-Peza *et al.*, 2002), ovariectomy suppressed gene expression in the vagina–cervix, but not in the tongue (used as a non-estrogen-responsive control). Treatment with 17β-estradiol, but not progesterone, restored gene expression in the vagina–cervix, and combined treatment with these hormones did not further increase expression. The effect of estrogen was partially blocked by the anti-estrogen tamoxifen. The anti-progestogen RU486 markedly blocked the effect of both hormones combined and also that of 17β-estradiol alone.

In transgenic mice that carry the HPV 16 early region, which contains the *E6* and *E7* genes, under the control of the human keratin 14 promotor (Arbeit *et al.*, 1994), *E6/E7* gene expression was increased by treatment with 17β-estradiol, which ultimately resulted in the development of cervical (and vaginal) squamous-cell carcinomas (Arbeit *et al.*, 1996). These genes were not shown to be estrogen-responsive (Arbeit *et al.*, 1996), and a direct effect of estrogen on their expression is unlikely. In contrast with estrogen-treated wild-type mice, 17β-estradiol caused a substantial increase in proliferating cells in the cervical epithelium in the K14-HPV 16 transgenic mice, an effect that is known to be mediated by the estrogen receptor (Lubahn *et al.*, 1993). When these K14-HPV 16 transgenic mice were compared with other transgenic mice that carry either HPV 16 *E6*, HPV 16 *E7* or HPV 16 *E6/E7* genes under the control of the keratin 14 promotor, the estrogen-induced increase in cell proliferation appeared to be confined to the HPV 16 E7 and the HPV 16 E6/E7 mice, whereas estrogen-induced up-regulation of transgene expression was confined to the HPV 16 E6 mice. After 6 months of treatment with estrogen, the HPV 16, HPV 16 E7 and HPV 16 E6/E7 mice all developed cervical cancer at a high incidence, but no such cancer occurred in the HPV 16 E6 mice (Riley *et al.*, 2003). In another study, continuous treatment with estrogen for 9 months resulted in the development of cervical cancer in 100% of HPV 16 E7 and HPV 16 E6/E7 mice (HPV 16 E6 mice were not studied). However, when the estrogen treatment was discontinued 3 months before the end of the experiment, only the HPV 16 E6/E7 mice developed cervical cancer at a high incidence, whereas the HPV 16 E7 mice had a 50% lower cancer incidence, tumours were smaller and multiplicity was lower (Brake & Lambert, 2005). Estrogen appears to act in these models as a receptor-mediated stimulus of proliferation that is related to the neo-plastic transforming activity of HPV to which genotoxic estrogen metabolites possibly contribute (Arbeit *et al.*, 1996; Riley *et al.*, 2003; Brake & Lambert, 2005). [The results of the discontinuation study by Brake and Lambert (2005) and the observation that *E6* and *E7* expression is enhanced by estrogen via a mechanism that apparently does not involve the estrogen receptor (Arbeit *et al.*, 1996) indicate a complex interaction between *E6* and *E7* in the estrogen-enhanced causation of cervical cancer in these mouse models that carry parts of the HPV genome. In addition to acting as a mitogen via the estrogen receptor, the effects of estrogen probably involve progesterone, progesterone receptors and/or other cellular factors that act on HPV gene expression in a manner that is poorly understood. The effects of progestogens or estrogen–progestogen combinations were not examined in any of these studies.]

4.2.3   *Individual estrogens and progestogens*

(*a*)   *Humans*

Pakarinen *et al.* (1999) studied 28 premenopausal women (mean age, 31–32 years) who had used either 0.03 mg per day levonorgestrel orally, an intrauterine device that released levonorgestrel or an intrauterine device that contained copper for 3 months. The only statistically significant change from baseline was a slight reduction in serum levels of SHBG in the women who took oral levonorgestrel. Levels of serum testosterone and insulin growth factor-binding protein-1 were not changed and no changes occurred in women who used the two intrauterine devices.

(*b*)   *Experimental systems*

No new studies of the estrogens ethinylestradiol or mestranol or the progestogens chlormadinone acetate, ethynodiol diacetate, lynestrenol or norethynodrel that are relevant to the evaluation of the carcinogenic risk of combined contraceptives via the oral or other routes have been published since the last evaluation (IARC, 1999).

(i)   *Estrogens*

17β-Estradiol stimulates the growth of human colon cancer CaCo-2 cells directly *in vitro* via the estrogen receptor which is blocked by anti-estrogens (Di Domenico *et al.*, 1996) and by anti-sense-mediated inhibition of estrogen receptor expression in mouse colon cancer MC-26 cells (Xu & Thomas, 1994). This stimulation appears to be mediated via estrogen receptor-α, since growth is inhibited in colon cancer cells when estrogen receptor-β is expressed (Arai *et al.*, 2000; Nakayama *et al.*, 2000). Moreover, estrogen receptor-β appears to be the predominant form of estrogen receptor in colon cancer and colon cancer cells (Fiorelli *et al.*, 1999; Campbell-Thompson *et al.*, 2001; Witte *et al.*, 2001). Mediation of the stimulatory action of 17β-estradiol on the proliferation of colon cancer cells may also involve a non-genomic mechanism via the protein kinase C path-way (Winter *et al.*, 2000). Male rats treated with colon carcinogens develop more colon cancers than female rats (Di Leo *et al.*, 2001). Treatment of ovariectomized female rats with 17β-estradiol and the colon carcinogen dimethylhydrazine leads to a significant inhibition of the development of colon tumours, from 8.1 ± 1.9 tumours per rat in those treated with carcinogen only to 2.3 ± 1.1 tumours per rat ($p < 0.001$) (Smirnoff *et al.*, 1999). Thus, the available evidence indicates that estrogens inhibit colon carcinogenesis in animal experiments, and experimental studies strongly suggest that the estrogen receptor-β plays an inhibitory role in colon carcinogenesis. These observations support the protective effect of hormonal oral contraceptives and menopausal therapy against colon cancer that has been observed in epidemiological studies (Nanda *et al.*, 1999; Grodstein *et al.*, 1999; Di Leo *et al.*, 2001).

(ii)   *Progestogens*

Cyproterone acetate stimulated the in-vitro production of growth hormone by explants of normal human breast tissue with an estrogen receptor-negative and progesterone receptor-positive phenotype and of insulin-like growth factor I by explants of normal and cancerous human breast tissue with this phenotype (Milewicz *et al.*, 2002).

Recent studies have demonstrated that desogestrel activates the estrogen receptor-α at an activity of about 50% of that of 17β-estradiol but activates the estrogen receptor-β at an activity of only 20% (Rabe *et al.*, 2000). Desogestrel and/or its metabolite 3-keto-desogestrel (etonogestrel) were strongly progestogenic (approximately twofold over progesterone), weakly or not androgenic in animal studies *in vivo* and in-vitro binding assays and weakly or not active on the glucocorticoid receptor (Deckers *et al.*, 2000; Schoonen *et al.*, 2000). The active metabolite of desogestrel, 3-ketodesogestrel, strongly bound to and activated progesterone receptor-A and, to a slightly lesser extent, progesterone receptor-B (Schoonen *et al.*, 1998).

Dienogest has the same degree of progestogenic activity as progesterone; it is anti-estrogenic and anti-androgenic, and binds weakly to progesterone and androgen receptors (Kaufmann *et al.*, 1983; Katsuki *et al.*, 1997a). It has uterotropic effects in rabbits that are stronger than those of norethisterone, medroxyprogesterone acetate and dydrogesterone and are blocked by the anti-progestogen RU486 but does not appear to have anti-mineralocorticoid activity (Katsuki *et al.*, 1997a). Mammary hyperplasia but not neoplasia was observed in preclinical toxicological studies of dienogest in dogs (Hoffmann *et al.*, 1983). Dienogest can inhibit neovascularization, including tumour cell-induced angiogenesis (Nakamura *et al.*, 1999), which raises the possibility that it may counteract tumour progression.

The in-vivo anti-tumour activity and anti-uterotropic activity of dienogest were studied in mice and compared with those of several progestogens. At oral doses of 0.01–1 mg/kg bw per day, dienogest significantly suppressed the 17β-estradiol benzoate-dependent tumour growth of HEC-88nu cells, which express estrogen receptors but not progesterone receptors. These cells were unresponsive to known progestogens such as medroxyprogesterone acetate (100 mg/kg bw per day orally) and norethisterone (100 mg/kg bw per day orally). The suppressive effect of dienogest on tumour growth was not diminished in the presence of excess medroxyprogesterone acetate (100 mg/kg bw per day). Dienogest also suppressed the estradiol-dependent tumour growth of Ishikawa cells (derived from a well-differentiated human endometrial carcinoma) and MCF-7 cells (derived from a human breast carcinoma), both of which express estrogen and progesterone receptors and respond to medroxyprogesterone acetate. However, the minimal effective dose of dienogest (0.01–1 mg/kg per day) was much lower than that of medroxyprogesterone acetate (100 mg/kg per day). Thus dienogest showed potent anticancer activity against hormone-dependent cancers at doses at which other progestogens show no activity. Dienogest showed no anti-uterotropic activity at tumour-suppressive doses (Katsuki *et al.*, 1997b).

Drospirenone is a relatively new progestogen that is used in combined oral contraceptives (Keam & Wagstaff, 2003). It has anti-androgenic and anti-mineralocorticoid effects; it binds strongly to mineralocorticoid receptors, but weakly or not at all to the androgen, glucocorticoid or estrogen (α) receptors (Pollow *et al.*, 1992), with the potential to decrease blood pressure (for reviews see Muhn *et al.*, 1995; Krattenmacher, 2000; Keam & Wagstaff, 2003; Rübig, 2003; Oelkers, 2004).

Studies on the highly progestogenic compound gestodene have demonstrated that its progestogenic activity in an in-vivo system is far lower than those of its in-vitro binding or receptor activation (Deckers *et al.*, 2000; Schoonen *et al.*, 2000; Garcia-Becerra *et al.*, 2004); however, its androgenic activity *in vitro* has been confirmed (Garcia-Becerra *et al.*, 2004) and it appears to have weak binding activity to the glucocorticoid receptor (Schoonen *et al.*, 2000). Its weak estrogenic activity (transactivation of estrogen receptor-mediated gene expression in model cells) appears to derive from its metabolism to the A ring-reduced metabolites, 3β- and 3α,5α-tetrahydrogestodene, and is probably mediated by the activity of 5α-reductase (Lemus *et al.*, 2000, 2001). These metabolites appeared to be selective agonists of estrogen receptor-α but not of estrogen receptor-β (Larrea *et al.*, 2001). The parent compound did not activate estrogen receptors-α or -β (Rabe *et al.*, 2000).

Recent studies have demonstrated that the estrogenic activity (transactivation of estrogen receptor-mediated gene expression in model cells) of levonorgestrel appears to be derived from its metabolism to the A ring-reduced metabolites, 3β- and 3α,5α-levonorgestrel, and is abolished by co-treatment with the pure steroidal anti-estrogen ICI 182,780 (Santillán *et al.*, 2001). Levonorgestrel appears to activate estrogen receptor-β strongly (75–90% of the activity of 17β-estradiol) but estrogen receptor-α is only slightly activated (15–25% of the activity of 17β-estradiol) (Rabe *et al.*, 2000). Its weak androgenic activity was confirmed in androgen receptor-binding and transactivation studies (Garcia-Becerra *et al.*, 2004). Levonorgestrel weakly induced a decrease in insulin growth factor-I and an increase in growth hormone production in primary human breast cancer explants *in vitro* when the explants were progesterone receptor-positive and estrogen receptor-negative, but not in the presence of estrogen receptors or the absence of progesterone receptors (Milewicz *et al.*, 2002).

Studies on norethisterone are summarized in the monograph on Combined estrogen–progestogen menopausal therapy.

4.3   Genetic and related effects

The extensive literature on direct genetic toxicological effects, or the lack of such effects, of the steroid hormones used in combined oral contraceptives has been reviewed previously (IARC, 1979, 1999), and the reader is referred to these tabular and textual considerations of the earlier genotoxicity data. Reports published since the previous evaluations are summarized below. Because many hormones are used in both combined oral contraceptives and hormonal menopausal therapy, synthetic hormones that are used widely in combined oral contraceptives are considered below, but several hormones relevant to this topic are listed exclusively in Section 4.4 of the monograph on Combined estrogen–progestogen menopausal therapy. New evidence has shown that, in aggregate with previous findings, there is a stronger case for the potential of some of these hormones to cause direct genetic damage that could result in genetic alterations of cells.

4.3.1   *Ethinylestradiol*

(a)   *Humans*

Daily oral doses of 0.02 mg ethinylestradiol and 0.075 mg gestodene administered to 30 healthy women in a monthly cycle of 3 weeks with and 1 week without treatment for six consecutive menstrual cycles did not induce micronuclei in the peripheral blood lymphocytes (Loncar *et al.*, 2004).

A significant increase in the number of lymphocytes with DNA fragmentation and an increased frequency of sister chromatid exchange per metaphase was observed in 18 women who took combined oral contraceptives (daily oral doses of 0.02–0.03 mg ethinylestradiol and 0.15 mg desogestrel) for 24 months compared with age-matched untreated controls ($p < 0.005$) (Biri *et al.*, 2002).

In a population-based study of young women (< 45 years of age) in the USA, those who had started using oral contraceptives at least 20 years before the reference date had a twofold increased risk for breast cancer with cyclin D1 overexpression (odds ratio, 2.2; 95% CI, 1.2– 4.0) but not for breast cancer without cyclin D1 overexpression (odds ratio, 1.1; 95% CI, 0.7–1.8) (Terry *et al.*, 2002). The authors suggested that early oral contraceptive use may be associated with the induction of a subset of mammary tumours that overexpress cyclin D1.

Prolonged use of oral contraceptives is more strongly associated with p53-positive breast cancer (odds ratio, 3.1; 95% CI, 1.2–8.1) than p53-negative breast cancer (odds ratio, 1.3; 95% CI, 0.6–3.2) among younger women only (Furberg *et al.*, 2003).

[In the above studies, women who were administered combined oral contraceptives appear to have sustained genetic alterations. It should be recognized that the observed effects of combined oral contraceptives could have been the result of a direct genotoxic effect of the hormonal preparation or could have been an indirect effect of hormonal influences on cellular functions, most notably cell proliferation, mediated by receptor- or non-receptor-linked mechanisms. It is therefore appropriate not to overinterpret these observations as evidence for a direct genotoxic effect.]

(b)   Experimental systems

The tissue- and gender-specific patterns of DNA methylation in the promoter regions of the estrogen receptor and aromatase genes were analysed in adult male and female Japanese Medaka fish (*Oryzias latipes*) exposed to either 0 or 500 ng/L 17α-ethinylestradiol in the water for 14 days. The protein content of the estrogen receptor in exposed fish was significantly increased in all male and female tissues (liver, gonads and brain) compared with controls. Aromatase activity in the exposed fish was significantly increased in the male brain and gonads and female brain compared with controls (Contractor et al., 2004). The changes in DNA methylation of the estrogen receptor and aromatase genes observed indicated that the mechanisms that control gene expression could potentially be altered, as well as gender- and tissue-specific sensitivity. While differences in patterns of DNA methylation did not parallel the changes observed in protein expression, they may impact the regulation of normal gene expression and could be genetically imprinted and transmitted to offspring.

The formation of 8-dihydroxy-2'-deoxyguanosine, an indicator of oxidative DNA damage, has been shown to be increased in the testicular cells of Wistar rats 1 h or 4 h after intraperitoneal injection of 0, 2.8 or 56 mg/kg bw ethinylestradiol *in vivo* and after exposure to 0.1–10 nM 17α-ethinylestradiol for 30 min *in vitro* (Wellejus & Loft, 2002). In the total cell population and in round haploid rat testicular cells, oxidized purines show a bell-shaped concentration–response relationship with maximally increased levels at 10 nM. No significant effects were observed in diploid, S-phase or tetraploid cells. The mRNA level of rat 8-oxo-guanine DNA glycosylase was unaffected by ethinylestradiol (Wellejus et al., 2004).

Siddique et al. (2005) recently analysed the genotoxicity of ethinylestradiol in human lymphocytes by measuring chromosomal aberrations, mitotic index and sister chromatid exchange. Ethinylestradiol was genotoxic at 5 and 10 μM in the presence of a rat liver microsomal fraction (metabolic activation system) with nicotinamide adenine dinucleotide phosphate (NADP). Concomitant treatment with superoxide dismutase increased the frequency of chromosomal aberrations and sister chromatid exchange and decreased the mitotic index compared with levels induced by treatment with ethinylestradiol alone, whereas concomitant treatment with catalase decreased the frequencies of chromosomal aberrations and sister chromatid exchange and increased the mitotic index. Concomitant treatment with catalase in combination with superoxide dismutase also decreased the frequencies of chromosomal aberrations and sister chromatid exchange and increased the mitotic index, which suggests a possible role of reactive oxygen species in the induction of the genotoxic damage. Bukvic et al. (2000) reported that ethinylestradiol and norgestrel (1:5) had an aneuploidogenic effect on cultures of human fibroblasts and lymphocytes. Fluorescent in-situ hybridization (with pancentromeric alphoid probes) analysis of micronuclei from lymphocyte cultures and anaphase preparations from fibroblast cultures supported this conclusion.

In primary rat hepatocytes exposed to ethinylestradiol for 20 h at subtoxic concentrations in the range of 1–50 µM, DNA repair was induced in cells derived from both of two males and one of two females (Martelli *et al.*, 2003).

4.3.2   *Progestogens*

Most progestogens have not been tested systematically for genotoxicity (see Table 20 in the monograph on Combined estrogen–progestogen menopausal therapy and Brambilla & Martelli, 2002). [It should be noted that the negative results for progestogens obtained with the standard battery of genotoxicity tests may be the consequence of using insufficiently sensitive assays, inappropriate target cells and/or suboptimal metabolic activation systems.]

(*a*)   *Cyproterone acetate and some structural analogues*

The genotoxic potential of cyproterone acetate and some of its analogues has been established. Cyproterone acetate is metabolically activated in the liver of female rats to one or more DNA-damaging intermediates that may induce the formation of DNA adducts, DNA repair and increased levels of micronuclei and gene mutations (reviewed by Kasper, 2001; Brambilla & Martelli, 2002; Joosten *et al.*, 2004). Most importantly, cyproterone acetate induced the formation of DNA adducts in primary cultures of human hepatocytes, which indicates that human liver cells can metabolically activate cyproterone acetate to genotoxic intermediates (Werner *et al.*, 1996, 1997). Cyproterone acetate is activated by hepatocytes to reactive species with such a short half-life that they react only with the DNA of the cell in which they are formed. The response is similar in both men and women but is markedly greater in female than in male rats. The promutagenic character of DNA lesions in the liver of female rats is indicated by the increase in the frequency of micronucleated cells, mutations and enzyme-altered preneoplastic foci (reviewed by Brambilla & Martelli, 2002).

Two other synthetic progestogens, chlormadinone acetate and megestrol acetate, and an aldosterone antagonist, potassium canrenoate, share the 17-hydroxy-3-oxopregna-4,6-diene structure with cyproterone acetate. They all induce genotoxic effects that are qualitatively similar to those of cyproterone acetate (Brambilla & Martelli, 2002).

Chlormadinone acetate and megestrol acetate are genotoxic only in the liver of female rats and in primary human hepatocytes from male and female donors (Brambilla & Martelli, 2002). The metabolic activation of these molecules to reactive species and the consequent formation of DNA adducts occur only in intact hepatocytes.

In primary rat hepatocytes exposed for 20 h to subtoxic concentrations ranging from 1 to 50 µM, DNA repair was induced by drospirenone in both of two males and all of three females, by ethinylestradiol in both of two males and one of two females, by oxymetholone in one of two males and one of two females, by norethisterone in one of two males, by progesterone in one of four females and by methyltestosterone in one of four males (Martelli *et al.*, 2003). A few inconclusive responses were observed in rat hepatocytes exposed to progesterone, medroxyprogesterone, norethisterone, methyltestosterone and oxymetholone. The authors of this small study assert that steroid hormones differ in their ability to induce

DNA repair, and that their genotoxicity may be: (*a*) different in rat and human hepatocytes; (*b*) dependent on the sex of the donor; and (*c*) affected by interindividual variability.

In rat hepatocytes, subtoxic concentrations of potassium canrenoate ranging from 10 to 90 μM consistently induced a dose-dependent increase in DNA fragmentation (Martelli *et al.*, 1999; Brambilla & Martelli, 2002). In another study with other steroids, DNA fragmentation was greater in female than in male rat hepatocytes and DNA-damaging potency was decreased in the following order: cyproterone acetate > dienogest > 1,4,6-androstatriene-17β-ol-3-one acetate > dydrogesterone (Mattioli *et al.*, 2004). Under the same experimental conditions, responses in an assay of DNA repair synthesis were positive or inconclusive in hepatocytes from female rats and were consistently negative in those from male rats.

Analysis of sister chromatid exchange and chromosomal aberrations in bone-marrow cells from mice exposed *in vivo* to chlormadinone acetate (5.62 mg/kg bw) showed that this dose is non-genotoxic (Siddique & Afzal, 2004). However, doses of 11.25 and 22.50 mg/kg bw chlormadinone acetate significantly increased the frequency of sister chromatid exchange ($p < 0.001$) and chromosomal aberrations ($p < 0.01$) compared with untreated controls (Siddique & Afzal, 2004). The authors suggested a genotoxic effect of chlormadinone acetate in mouse bone-marrow cells.

Administration of a single high dose of 100 mg/kg bw cyproterone acetate to female *lac*I-transgenic Big Blue™ rats induced a strong initial rise in mutation frequency in the liver over that in controls up to a maximum at 2 weeks after administration accompanied by a corresponding increase in cell proliferation and levels of DNA adducts (Topinka *et al.*, 2004a). The mutation frequency decreased after 2 weeks to one-third of the maximum level and this was maintained for an additional 4 weeks. The levels of DNA adducts in the liver decreased by only 15% during this time, which suggests that most adducts were lost as affected hepatocytes were eliminated. When given as a single dose, 5 mg/kg bw cyproterone acetate did not produce significantly elevated levels of mutation. However, mutation frequencies increased 2.5-fold when female *lac*I-transgenic Big Blue™ rats received repeated daily doses of 5 mg/kg bw cyproterone acetate for 3 weeks (Topinka *et al.*, 2004b).

(*b*)   *Norgestrel*

A study on human lymphocytes showed that norgestrel induced chromosomal aberrations and significant levels of sister chromatid exchange and inhibited lymphocyte proliferation at concentrations of 25 and 50 μg/mL only. In the presence of a metabolic activation system, the values obtained for chromosomal aberrations, sister chromatid exchange and mitotic index were more significant. A time- and dose-dependent genotoxic effect of norgesterol was observed (Ahmad *et al.*, 2001). The authors concluded that norgestrel itself, and possibly its metabolites, are potent mutagens in human lymphocytes.

(*c*)   *Norethisterone*

A study on human lymphocytes that used chromosomal aberrations, sister chromatid exchange and cell-growth kinetics as end-points showed that doses of 20, 40 and 75 μg/mL norethisterone were non-genotoxic either in the presence or in the absence of a metabolic activation system (Ahmad *et al.*, 2001).

Gallmeier *et al.* (2005) applied a novel and particularly sensitive method to screen for DNA damage with special attention to double-strand breaks. They found that norethisterone is probably genotoxic and therefore potentially mutagenic. A *p53*-reporter assay served as a first, high-throughput screening method and was followed by the immuno-fluorescence detection of phosphorylated H2AX (a variant of histone H_2A protein) as a sensitive assay for the presence of double-strand breaks. Norethisterone at concentrations of 2–100 μg/mL activated p53 and induced phosphorylation of H2AX on Ser-139 in the vicinity of double-strand breaks. Phosphorylation of H2AX increased in a dose-dependent manner. Double-strand breaks were not detected with the neutral comet assay, a less sensitive method than H2AX phosphorylation. The authors suggested that, since norethisterone induced double-strand breaks in their experiments, this both complements and adds a new aspect to the existing literature on its genotoxic potential. However, they noted that, since the effective concentrations of norethisterone in these assays were approximately 100–1000-fold higher than therapeutic doses, the significance of these findings with regard to human exposure has yet to be determined.

In-vitro studies that analysed gene expression of isolated normal endometrial epithelial cells treated with estradiol and norethisterone acetate showed upregulation of the *Wnt-7a* gene; with estradiol only, *Wnt-7a* was expressed at very low levels (Oehler *et al.*, 2002). *Wnt* genes are a large family of developmental genes that are associated with cellular responses such as carcinogenesis.

5.   Summary of Data Reported and Evaluation

5.1   Exposure data

The first oral hormonal contraceptives that were found to inhibit both ovulation and implantation were developed in the 1950s and included both estrogen and progestogen. Since that time, changes in component ingredients, doses used and the temporal sequencing of exposure to hormones have occurred with emerging technologies and in an effort to reduce adverse effects. The dominant trends in recent years have been towards the use of lower doses of estrogen, the use of progestogens that are less androgenic, the multiplication of product formulations and the continuing development of novel delivery systems. In current preparations, ethinylestradiol is the most common estrogen, although a variety of other estrogens is also available. An even greater range of progestogens is used. The estrogen and progestogen components are usually given together orally in a monthly cycle, e.g. 21 days of constant or varying doses followed by 7 days without hormones. Combined hormonal contraceptives can also be administered by injection, transdermal patch and vaginal device. In addition to their regular use for contraception, other common indications for these products include emergency contraception, and the treatment of acne and menstrual disorders. Some commonly used formulations, doses, routes of administration and schedules of exposure are new and their possible long-term adverse effects have not been evaluated.

Worldwide, more than 100 million women — an estimated 10% of all women of reproductive age — currently use combined hormonal contraceptives, a large majority of which are in the form of oral preparations. Current use of these drugs is greatest in developed countries (16%) and is lower in developing countries (6%). Rates of 'ever use' higher than 80% have been reported for some developed countries. In developing countries, 32% of women were estimated to have ever used hormonal contraception. Overall, the use of combined hormonal contraception is increasing, but there is extreme variability between countries. In many countries, these preparations are mainly used by women of younger age and higher level of education, and who have greater access to health care.

5.2   Human carcinogenicity data

Breast cancer

More than 10 cohort studies and 60 case–control studies that included over 60 000 women with breast cancer reported on the relationship between the oral use of combined hormonal contraceptives and the risk for this disease. The totality of the evidence suggested an increase in the relative risk for breast cancer among current and recent users. This effect was noted particularly among women under 35 years of age at diagnosis who had begun using contraceptives when young (< 20 years), whereas the increased risk declined sharply with older age at diagnosis. By 10 years after cessation of use, the risk in women who had used combined hormonal contraceptives appeared to be similar to that in women who had never used them. Important known risk factors did not appear to account for the association. The possibility that the association seen for current and recent users is due to detection bias was not ruled out, but it was considered to be unlikely that this would explain the association observed in young women.

Endometrial cancer

Four cohort studies and 21 case–control studies reported on the relationship between the oral use of combined hormonal contraceptives and the risk for endometrial cancer. The results of these studies consistently showed that the risk for endometrial cancer in women who had taken these medications is approximately halved. The reduction in risk was generally greater with longer duration of use of combined hormonal contraceptives and persisted for at least 15 years after cessation of use, although the extent of the protective effect may wane over time. Few data were available on the more recent, low-dose formulations.

Cervical cancer

Five cohort and 16 case–control studies of the oral use of combined hormonal contraceptives and invasive cervical cancer had been reviewed previously. The Working Group at that time could not rule out biases related to sexual behaviour, screening and other factors as possible explanations for the observed association with increasing duration of use.

Since then, two cohort and seven case–control studies have provided new information on invasive or in-situ carcinoma and oral use of combined hormonal contraceptives; all but the three most recent studies were summarized in a meta-analysis of published data. The totality of the evidence indicated that, overall, the risk for cervical cancer increased with increasing duration of use of combined hormonal contraceptives, and was somewhat greater for in-situ than for invasive cancer. The relative risk appeared to decline after cessation of use. The results were broadly similar regardless of adjustment for the number of sexual partners, cervical screening, tobacco smoking and the use of barrier contraceptives. The association was found in studies conducted in both developed and developing countries. The possibility that the observed association is due to detection bias was not ruled out, but it was considered to be unlikely that this would explain the increase in risk. Studies in which information on human papillomavirus infection — the main cause of cervical cancer — was available suggested that the prevalence of the infection was not increased among users of combined hormonal contraceptives, and the association with cervical cancer was also observed in analyses that were restricted to human papillomavirus-positive cases and controls.

Ovarian cancer

Data from an additional three cohort and 20 case–control studies that were new or had been updated since the last evaluation showed that women who had ever used combined hormonal contraceptives orally had an overall reduced risk for ovarian cancer and an inverse relationship was observed with duration of use. The reduced risk appeared to persist for at least 20 years after cessation of use. The effect of combined hormonal contraceptives on the reduction of risk for ovarian cancer is not confined to any particular type of oral formulation nor to any histological type of ovarian cancer, although it was less consistent for mucinous than for other types in several studies.

Liver cancer

Long-term oral use of combined hormonal contraceptives was associated with an increase in the risk for hepatocellular carcinoma in all nine case–control studies conducted in populations that had low prevalences of hepatitis B viral infection and chronic liver disease — which are major causes of liver cancer — and in analyses in which women with such infections were excluded. Three cohort studies showed no significant association between the oral use of combined hormonal contraceptives and the incidence of or mortality from liver cancer, but the expected number of cases was very small, which resulted in low statistical power. Few data were available for the more recent, low-dose formulations. In the three case–control studies conducted in populations that had a high prevalence of infection with hepatitis viruses, no statistically significant increase in the risk for hepatocellular carcinoma was associated with the oral use of combined hormonal contraceptives, but little information was available on long-term use.

Cutaneous melanoma

Four cohort and 16 case–control studies provided information on the oral use of combined hormonal contraceptives and the risk for cutaneous malignant melanoma. No consistent evidence for an association was found with respect to current use, duration of use, time since last use or age at first use. The few studies that suggested an increase in risk may reflect the possibility that women who took oral contraceptives may have had more contacts with the medical system and were thus more likely to have had pigmented lesions removed.

Colorectal cancer

Seven cohort and 13 case–control studies provided information on the oral use of combined hormonal contraceptives and the risk for colorectal cancer. Most studies did not show an increase in risk in women who had ever used contraceptives or in relation to duration of use. The results were generally similar for colon and rectal cancer when examined separately, and two case–control studies showed a significant reduction in risk.

5.3   Animal carcinogenicity data

The data evaluated in this section showed a consistent carcinogenic effect of several estrogen–progestogen combinations across different animal models in several organs. The evidence of carcinogenicity for one of the newer progestogens studied, dienogest, was not satisfactory for an evaluation.

Estrogen–progestogen combinations

In female and male mice, the incidence of pituitary adenoma was increased by administration of mestranol plus chlormadinone acetate, mestranol plus ethynodiol diacetate, ethinylestradiol plus ethynodiol diacetate, mestranol plus norethisterone, ethinylestradiol plus norethisterone (females only) and mestranol plus norethynodrel. The latter combination also increased the incidence of pituitary adenomas in female rats.

The incidence of malignant mammary tumours was increased in female and male mice by ethinylestradiol plus megestrol acetate, in female and male rats by ethinylestradiol plus ethynodiol diacetate and in female rats by mestranol plus norethisterone and mestranol plus norethynodrel. The incidence of benign mammary tumours was increased in male rats by ethinylestradiol plus norethisterone acetate, in intact and castrated male mice by ethinylestradiol plus chlormadinone acetate and in castrated male mice by mestranol plus norethynodrel. Ethinylestradiol plus norethisterone acetate did not cause tumour formation in any tissue in one study in female monkeys.

In female mice, the incidence of malignant non-epithelial uterine tumours was increased by ethinylestradiol plus ethynodiol diacetate and the incidence of vaginal or cervical tumours was increased by norethynodrel plus mestranol. In female mice treated with 3-methylcholanthrene to induce genital tumours, ethinylestradiol plus lynestrenol, ethinylestradiol plus norgestrel and mestranol plus norethynodrel increased the incidence of uterine tumours; however, this occurred only at the highest doses of ethinylestradiol plus lynestrenol and ethinylestradiol plus norgestrel that were tested. Lower doses inhibited tumorigenesis induced by 3-methylcholanthrene alone.

In female rats, the incidence of hepatocellular carcinomas was increased by ethinylestradiol plus norethisterone acetate; this combination and mestranol plus norethisterone also increased the incidence of liver adenomas in male rats. Liver foci, which are putative preneoplastic lesions, were induced in female rats by mestranol plus norethynodrel. In female rats initiated for hepatocarcinogenesis with N-nitrosodiethylamine, mestranol plus norethynodrel increased the formation of altered hepatic foci.

In one study, subcutaneous administration of levonorgestrel with ethinylestradiol or estradiol to female rabbits induced deciduosarcomas in several organs (uterus, spleen, ovary, liver and lung).

Estrogens

The incidence of pituitary adenomas was increased by ethinylestradiol and mestranol in female and male mice and by ethinylestradiol in female rats.

The incidence of malignant mammary tumours in female and male mice and female rats was increased by ethinylestradiol and mestranol; however, mestranol did not increase the incidence of mammary tumours in female dogs in a single study.

Ethinylestradiol increased the incidence of cervical tumours in female mice.

In female and male mice, ethinylestradiol increased the incidence of hepatocellular adenomas. In female rats, ethinylestradiol and mestranol increased the numbers of altered hepatic foci. In rats, ethinylestradiol increased the incidence of adenomas in females and males and that of hepatocellular carcinomas in females, whereas mestranol increased the incidence of hepatic nodules and carcinomas combined in females.

The incidence of microscopic malignant kidney tumours was increased in male hamsters exposed to ethinylestradiol.

In female mice initiated for liver carcinogenesis and exposed to unleaded gasoline, ethinylestradiol increased the number of altered hepatic foci; however, when given alone after the liver carcinogen, it reduced the number of such foci.

In female rats initiated for liver carcinogenesis, ethinylestradiol and mestranol increased the number of altered hepatic foci and the incidence of adenomas and carcinomas. Ethinylestradiol also increased the incidence of kidney adenomas, renal-cell carcinomas and liver carcinomas in male rats initiated with N-nitrosoethyl-N-hydroxyethylamine. In female hamsters initiated with N-nitrosobis(2-oxopropyl)amine, ethinylestradiol increased the incidence of renal tumours and the multiplicity of dysplasias.

In female rabbits, subcutaneous administration of ethinylestradiol alone was associated with the proliferation of hepatic bile duct cells.

In female mice, subcutaneous injection of ethinylestradiol alone was associated with the development of uterine adenocarcinomas. In male hamsters, subcutaneous implantation of estradiol alone was associated with the development of renal tumours of unspecified histology.

Oral administration of ethinylestradiol to *p53*-deficient female mice in combination with an intraperitoneal injection of the known carcinogen *N*-ethyl-*N*-nitrosourea increased the incidence of uterine atypical hyperplasias and stromal sarcomas.

Subcutaneous injection of 2-hydroxy- and 4-hydroxyestradiol induced uterine adenocarcinomas in female mice and subcutaneous implantation of estradiol induced renal tumours in male hamsters.

In female mice initiated with *N*-ethyl-*N'*-nitro-*N*-nitrosoguanidine, subcutaneous implantation of estradiol, estrone, estriol, 16β-hydroxyestrone diacetate, 16α-hydroxyestrone and 17-epiestrol increased the incidence of endometrial adenocarcinomas.

Progestogens

The incidence of pituitary adenomas was increased by norethisterone in female mice and by norethynodrel in female and male mice and male rats.

The incidence of malignant mammary tumours was increased in female mice by lynestrenol, megestrol acetate and norethynodrel. In female rats, lynestrenol and norethisterone slightly increased the incidence of malignant mammary tumours. Norethisterone also slightly increased the incidence of malignant mammary tumours in male rats, while norethynodrel increased the incidence of both benign and malignant mammary tumours in male rats. In female dogs, chlormadinone acetate, lynestrenol and megestrol acetate increased the incidence of benign and malignant mammary tumours; however, lynestrenol had a protective effect at a low dose but enhanced tumour incidence at two higher doses. Levonorgestrel did not increase the incidence of mammary tumours in one study in dogs.

In female mice treated with 3-methylcholanthrene to induce uterine tumours, norethynodrel further increased the tumour incidence.

Megestrol acetate increased the incidence of liver adenomas in female mice. Cyproterone acetate increased the incidence of liver adenomas and hepatocellular carcinomas in female and male mice, but at levels that exceeded the maximum tolerated dose. In rats, the incidence of liver adenomas was increased by norethisterone acetate (females and males), norethisterone (males), norethynodrel and cyproterone acetate (females and males). The numbers of altered hepatic foci in female rats were also increased by norethisterone acetate and cyproterone acetate. In male mice treated with chlormadinone acetate, ethynodiol diacetate, lynestrenol, norethisterone or norethisterone acetate, the incidence of liver adenomas was increased. In female rats treated with *N*-nitrosodiethylamine to initiate hepatocarcinogenesis, norethynodrel increased the number of altered hepatic foci. Norethynodrel alone was shown to increase the incidence of hepatocarcinomas in male rats.

Levonorgestrel in combination with *N*-nitrosobis(2-oxopropyl)amine did not increase the incidence of renal dysplastic lesions or tumours in female hamsters.

Oral administration of dienogest induced mammary gland proliferation in female dogs but not in female rats or monkeys.

5.4   Other relevant data

Absorption, distribution, metabolism and excretion

Estrogenic and progestogenic compounds in oral contraceptives are readily absorbed and undergo metabolism to varying extents by bacterial enzymes, enzymes in the intestinal mucosa and especially enzymes in the liver. The metabolism typically involves reduction, hydroxylation and conjugation. The so-called 'first-pass' through the liver reduces the overall bioavailability of oral contraceptives. Peak concentration levels in the systemic circulation are observed between 0.5 and 4 h after intake. Hydroxylated metabolites are usually conjugated as glucuronides or sulfates and are eliminated rapidly with half-lives of 8–24 h.

The formulations of combined hormonal contraceptives continue to evolve, especially with the introduction of new progestogens. In general, the chemical structure of a progestogen determines its relative binding affinities for progesterone and other steroid receptors, as well as sex hormone-binding globulin, which determine its biological effects. The logic involved in the development of newly synthesized progestogens, such as dienogest and drospirenone, is that they be devoid of estrogenic, androgenic and antagonist effects.

Estrogens are discussed in the monograph on Combined estrogen–progestogen menopausal therapy.

Receptor-mediated effects

Exposure to combined hormonal contraceptives increases the proliferation of human breast epithelial cells, as observed in biopsies and fine-needle aspirate samples collected during small randomized studies. Combined hormonal contraceptives have atrophic and anti-proliferative effects on the endometrium that are apparently independent of the regimen and the progestogen used. Ethinylestradiol plus levonorgestrel induces ovarian epithelial cell apoptosis in intact monkeys. Estrogens or progestogens may enhance human papillomavirus gene expression in the human cervix via progesterone receptor mechanisms and hormone-response elements in the viral genome. In-vitro studies support this concept, and mechanisms other than those that are receptor-mediated may be involved. Experiments in transgenic mouse models that express human papillomavirus 16 genes in the cervix showed that estrogens can cause cervical cancer, probably via receptor-mediated processes. This effect was diminished after cessation of treatment with estrogens. Colon carcinogenesis in animal models is inhibited by estrogens and there is adequate evidence to suggest that estrogens have inhibitory effects on colon cancer cells via estrogen receptor-β. Various studies document the possibility of complex interactions of combined hormonal contraceptives with hormonal systems. No data were available to the Working Group on the effects of time since cessation of treatment or duration of treatment.

Genetic and related effects

There is additional evidence to support the conjecture that certain estrogens function as directly acting genotoxins. These findings give further credence to the hypothesis that certain estrogens are carcinogenic through direct genotoxic effects in addition to their presumed action via a receptor-mediated mechanism. Some of the more recent genotoxicity data suggest that some progestogens used in combined hormonal contraceptives may also act as direct genotoxins. Few data were available on the effects of combined exposures to estrogens and progestogens.

5.5   Evaluation

There is *sufficient evidence* in humans for the carcinogenicity of combined oral estrogen–progestogen contraceptives. This evaluation was made on the basis of increased risks for cancer of the breast among current and recent users only, for cancer of the cervix and for cancer of the liver in populations that are at low risk for hepatitis B viral infection.

There is *evidence suggesting lack of carcinogenicity* in humans for combined oral estrogen–progestogen contraceptives in the endometrium, ovary and colorectum. There is convincing evidence in humans for their protective effect against carcinogenicity in the endometrium and ovary.

There is *sufficient evidence* in experimental animals for the carcinogenicity of the combinations of ethinylestradiol plus ethynodiol diacetate, mestranol plus norethynodrel, ethinylestradiol plus levonorgestrel and estradiol plus levonorgestrel.

There is *sufficient evidence* in experimental animals for the carcinogenicity of the estrogens ethinylestradiol and mestranol.

There is *sufficient evidence* in experimental animals for the carcinogenicity of the progestogens norethynodrel and lynestrenol.

There is *limited evidence* in experimental animals for the carcinogenicity of the combinations of ethinylestradiol plus megestrol acetate, mestranol or ethinylestradiol plus chlormadinone acetate, mestranol plus ethynodiol diacetate, mestranol plus lynestrenol, mestranol or ethinylestradiol plus norethisterone and ethinylestradiol plus norgestrel.

There is *limited evidence* in experimental animals for the carcinogenicity of the progestogens chlormadinone acetate, cyproterone acetate, ethynodiol diacetate, megestrol acetate, norethisterone acetate and norethisterone.

There is *inadequate evidence* in experimental animals for the carcinogenicity of the progestogens levonorgestrel, norgestrel and dienogest.

Overall evaluation

Combined oral estrogen-progestogen contraceptives are *carcinogenic to humans (Group 1)*. There is also convincing evidence in humans that these agents confer a protective effect against cancer of the endometrium and ovary.

6. References

Adam, S.A., Sheaves, J.K., Wright, N.H., Mosser, G., Harris, R.W. & Vessey, M.P. (1981) A case–control study of the possible association between oral contraceptives and malignant melanoma. *Br. J. Cancer*, **44**, 45–50

Adami, H.-O., Bergström, R., Persson, I. & Sparén, P. (1990) The incidence of ovarian cancer in Sweden, 1960–1984. *Am. J. Epidemiol.*, **132**, 446–452

Ahmad, M.E., Shadab, G.G.H.A., Azfer, M.A. & Afzal, M. (2001) Evaluation of genotoxic potential of synthetic progestins norethindrone and norgestrel in human lymphocytes in vitro. *Mutat. Res.*, **494**, 13–20

Ali, M.M. & Cleland, J. (2005) Sexual and reproductive behaviour among single women aged 15–24 in eight Latin American countries: A comparative analysis. *Soc. Sci. Med.*, **60**, 1175–1185

Althuis, M.D., Brogan, D.R., Coates, R.J., Daling, J.R., Gammon, M.D., Malone, K.E., Schoenberg, J.B. & Brinton, L.A. (2003) Hormonal content and potency of oral contraceptives and breast cancer risk among young women. *Br. J. Cancer*, **88**, 50–57

Arai, N., Ström, A., Rafter, J.J. & Gustafsson, J.-A. (2000) Estrogen receptor beta mRNA in colon cancer cells: Growth effects of estrogen and genistein. *Biochem. biophys. Res. Commun.*, **270**, 425–431

Arbeit, J.M., Münger, K., Howley, P.M. & Hanahan, D. (1994) Progressive squamous epithelial neoplasia in K14-human papillomavirus type 16 transgenic mice. *J. Virol.*, **68**, 4358–4368

Arbeit, J.M., Howley, P.M. & Hanahan, D. (1996) Chronic estrogen-induced cervical and vaginal squamous carcinogenesis in human papillomavirus type 16 transgenic mice. *Proc. natl Acad. Sci. USA*, **93**, 2930–2935

Archer, D.F. (1999) Endometrial histology during use of a low-dose estrogen–desogestrel oral contraceptive with a reduced hormone-free interval. *Contraception*, **60**, 151–154

Archer, D.F., Timmer, C.J. & Lammers, P. (1994) Pharmacokinetics of a triphasic oral contraceptive containing desogestrel and ethinyl estradiol. *Fertil. Steril.*, **61**, 645–651

Auborn, K.J., Woodworth, C., DiPaolo, J.A. & Bradlow, H.L. (1991) The interaction between HPV infection and estrogen metabolism in cervical carcinogenesis. *Int. J. Cancer*, **49**, 867–869

Baan, R., Straif, K., Grosse, Y., Secretan, B., El Ghissassi, F., Bouvard, V., Altieri, A., Cogliano, V. & the WHO International Agency for Research on Cancer Monograph Working Group (2007) Carcinogenicity of alcoholic beverages. *Lancet Oncol.*, **8**, 292–293

Back, D.J., Breckenridge, A.M., Crawford, F.E., McIver, M., Orme, M.L., Rowe, P.H. & Smith, E. (1978) Kinetics of norethindrone in women. II. Single-dose kinetics. *Clin. Pharmacol. Ther.*, **24**, 448–53

Back, D.J., Bates, M., Breckenridge, A.M., Hall, J.M., McIver, M., Orme, M.L., Park, B.K. & Rowe, P.H. (1981) The pharmacokinetics of levonorgestrel and ethynylestradiol in women — Studies with ovran and ovranette. *Contraception*, **23**, 229–239

Back, D.J., Grimmer, S.F.M., Shenoy, N. & Orme, M.L'E. (1987) Plasma concentrations of 3-keto-desogestrel after oral administration of desogestrel and intravenous administration of 3-keto-desogestrel. *Contraception*, **35**, 619–626

Beard, C.M., Hartmann, L.C., Atkinson, E.J., O'Brien, P.C., Malkasian, G.D., Keeney, G.L. & Melton, L.J., III. (2000) The epidemiology of ovarian cancer: A population-based study in Olmsted County, Minnesota, 1935–1991. *Ann. Epidemiol.*, **10**, 14–23

Beral, V., Ramcharan, S. & Faris, R. (1977) Malignant melanoma and oral contraceptive use among women in California. *Br. J. Cancer*, **36**, 804–809

Beral, V., Evans, S., Shaw, H. & Milton, G. (1984) Oral contraceptive use and malignant melanoma in Australia. *Br. J. Cancer*, **50**, 681–685

Beral, V., Hannaford, P. & Kay, C. (1988) Oral contraceptive use and malignancies of the genital tract. Results from the Royal College of General Practitioners' Oral Contraception Study. *Lancet*, **ii**, 1331–1335

Beral, V., Hermon, C., Kay, C., Hannaford, P., Darby, S. & Reeves, G. (1999) Mortality associated with oral contraceptive use: 25 year follow up of cohort of 46 000 women from Royal College of General Practitioners' oral contraception study. *Br. med. J.*, **318**, 96–100

Bergink, W., Assendorp, R., Kloosterboer, L., van Lier, W., Voortman, G. & Qvist, I. (1990) Serum pharmacokinetics of orally administered desogestrel and binding of contraceptive progestogens to sex hormone-binding globulin. *Am. J. Obstet. Gynecol.*, **163**, 2132–2137

Berrington, A., Jha, P., Peto, J., Green, J. & Hermon, C. for the UK National Case–Control Study of Cervical Cancer (2002) Oral contraceptives and cervical cancer (Letter to the Editor). *Lancet*, **360**, 410

Bhat, H.K., Calaf, G., Hei, T.K., Loya, T. & Vadgama, J.V. (2003) Critical role of oxidative stress in estrogen-induced carcinogenesis. *Proc. natl Acad. Sci. USA*, **100**, 3913–3918

Biri, A., Civelek, E., Karahalil, B. & Sardas, S. (2002) Assessment of DNA damage in women using oral contraceptives. *Mutat. Res.*, **521**, 113–119

Blackburn, R.D., Cunkelman, J.A. & Zlidar, V.M. (2000) *Oral Contraceptives — An Update* (Population Reports, Series A, No. 9), Baltimore, MD, Johns Hopkins University School of Public Health, Population Information Program

Blode, H., Wuttke, W., Loock, W., Roll, G. & Heithecker, R. (2000) A 1-year pharmacokinetic investigation of a novel oral contraceptive containing drospirenone in healthy female volunteers. *Eur. J. Contracept. reprod. Health Care*, **5**, 256–264

Bongaarts, J. & Johansson, E. (2000) Future trends in contraception in the developing world: Prevalence and method mix. *Stud. Fam. Plann.*, **33**

Booth, M., Beral, V. & Smith, P. (1989) Risk factors for ovarian cancer: A case–control study. *Br. J. Cancer*, **60**, 592–598

Bosetti, C., Negri, E., Trichopoulos, D., Franceschi, S., Beral, V., Tzonou, A., Parazzini, F., Greggi, S. & La Vecchia, C. (2002) Long-term effects of oral contraceptives on ovarian cancer risk. *Int. J. Cancer*, **102**, 262–265

Bostick, R.M., Potter, J.D., Kushi, L.H., Sellers, T.A., Steinmetz, K.A., McKenzie, D.R., Gapstur, S.M. & Folsom, A.R. (1994) Sugar, meat, and fat intake, and non-dietary risk factors for colon cancer incidence in Iowa women (United States). *Cancer Causes Control*, **5**, 38–52

Boyd, R.A., Zegarac, E.A., Posvar, E.L. & Flack, M.R. (2001) Minimal androgenic activity of a new oral contraceptive containing norethindrone acetate and graduated doses of ethinyl estradiol. *Contraception*, **63**, 71–76

Brake, T. & Lambert, P.F. (2005) Estrogen contributes to the onset, persistence, and malignant progression of cervical cancer in a human papillomavirus-transgenic mouse model. *Proc. natl Acad. Sci. USA*, **102**, 2490–2495

Brambilla, G. & Martelli, A. (2002) Are some progestins genotoxic liver carcinogens? *Mutat. Res.*, **512**, 155–163

Bray, F., Loos, A.H., Tognazzo, S. & La Vecchia, C. (2005) Ovarian cancer in Europe: Cross-sectional trends in incidence and mortality in 28 countries, 1953–2000. *Int. J. Cancer*, **113**, 977–990

Brinton, L.A., Daling, J.R., Liff, J.M., Schoenberg, J.B., Malone, K.E., Stanford, J.L., Coates, R.J., Gammon, M.D., Hanson, L. & Hoover, R.N. (1995) Oral contraceptives and breast cancer risk among younger women. *J. natl Cancer Inst.*, **87**, 827–835

Brinton, L.A., Brogan, D.R., Coates, R.J., Swanson, C.A., Potischman, N. & Stanford, J.L. (1998) Breast cancer risk among women under 55 years of age by joint effects of usage of oral contraceptives and hormone replacement therapy. *Menopause*, **5**, 145–151

Bukvic, N., Susca, F., Bukvic, D., Fanelli, M. & Guanti, G. (2000) 17 alpha Ethinylestradiol and norgestrel in combination induce micronucleus increases and aneuploidy in human lymphocyte and fibroblast cultures. *Teratog. Carcinog. Mutag.*, **20**, 147–159

Burkman, R., Schlesselman, J.J. & Zieman, M. (2004) Safety concerns and health benefits associated with oral contraception. *Am. J. Obstet. Gynecol.*, **190**, S5–22

Campbell-Thompson, M., Lynch, I.J. & Bhardwaj, B. (2001) Expression of estrogen receptor (ER) subtypes and ERbeta isoforms in colon cancer. *Cancer Res.*, **61**, 632–640

Carol, W., Klinger, G., Jager, R., Kasch, R. & Brandstadt, A. (1992) Pharmacokinetics of ethinylestradiol and levonorgestrel after administration of two oral contraceptive preparations. *Exp. clin. Endocrinol.*, **99**, 12–17

CASH (Cancer and Steroid Hormone) (1986) Oral-contraceptive use and the risk of breast cancer. The Cancer and Steroid Hormone Study of the Centers for Disease Control and the National Institute of Child Health and Human Development. *New Engl. J. Med.*, **315**, 405–411

CASH (Cancer and Steroid Hormone) (1987a) Combination oral contraceptive use and the risk of endometrial cancer. The Cancer and Steroid Hormone Study of the Centers for Disease Control and the National Institute of Child Health and Human Development. *J. Am. med. Assoc.*, **257**, 796–800

CASH (Cancer and Steroid Hormone) (1987b) The reduction in risk of ovarian cancer associated with oral contraceptive use. The Cancer and Steroid Hormone Study of the Centers for Disease Control and the National Institute of Child Health and Human Development. *New Engl. J. Med.*, **316**, 650–655

Castle, P.E., Wacholder, S., Lorincz, A.T., Scott, D.R., Sherman, M.E., Glass, A.G., Rush, B.B., Schussler, J.E. & Schiffman, M. (2002) A prospective study of high-grade cervical neoplasia risk among human papillomavirus-infected women. *J. natl Cancer Inst.*, **94**, 1406–1414

Castoria, G., Barone, M.V., Di Domenico, M., Bilancio, A., Ametrano, D., Migliaccio, A. & Auricchio, F. (1999) Non-transcriptional action of oestradiol and progestin triggers DNA synthesis. *EMBO J.*, **18**, 2500–2510

Cavalcanti, S.M.B., Zardo, L.G., Passos, M.R.L. & Oliveira, L.H.S. (2000) Epidemiological aspects of human papillomavirus infection and cervical cancer in Brazil. *J. Infect.*, **40**, 80–87

Chan, W.-K., Klock, G. & Bernard, H.-U. (1989) Progesterone and glucocorticoid response elements occur in the long control regions of several human papillomaviruses involved in anogenital neoplasia. *J. Virol.*, **63**, 3261–3269

Chatterton, R.T., Jr, Geiger, A.S., Mateo, E.T., Helenowski, I.B. & Gann, P.H. (2005) Comparison of hormone levels in nipple aspirate fluid of pre- and postmenopausal women: Effect of oral contraceptives and hormone replacement. *J. clin. Endocrinol. Metabol.*, **90**, 1686–1691

Chen, Y.-H., Huang, L-H. & Chen, T.-M. (1996) Differential effects of progestins and estrogens on long control regions of human papillomavirus types 16 and 18. *Biochem. biophys.Res. Commun.*, **224**, 651–659

Chiaffarino, F., Pelucchi, C., Parazzini, F., Negri, E., Franceschi, S., Talamini, R., Conti, E., Montella, M. & La Vecchia, C. (2001) Reproductive and hormonal factors and ovarian cancer. *Ann. Oncol.*, **12**, 337–341

Chie, W.C., Li, C.Y., Huang, C.S., Chang, K.J., Yen, M.L. & Lin, R.S. (1998) Oral contraceptives and breast cancer risk in Taiwan, a country of low incidence of breast cancer and low use of oral contraceptives. *Int. J. Cancer*, **77**, 219–223

Chute, C.G., Willett, W.C., Colditz, G.A., Stampfer, M.J., Rosner, B. & Speizer, F.E. (1991) A prospective study of reproductive history and exogenous estrogens on the risk of colorectal cancer in women. *Epidemiology*, **2**, 201–207

Claus, E.B., Stowe, M. & Carter, D. (2003) Oral contraceptives and the risk of ductal breast carcinoma in situ. *Breast Cancer Res. Treat.*, **81**, 129–136

Colditz, G.A. for the Nurses' Health Study Research Group (1994) Oral contraceptive use and mortality during 12 years of follow-up: The Nurses' Health Study. *Ann. intern. Med.*, **120**, 821–826

Collaborative Group on Hormonal Factors in Breast Cancer (1996a) Breast cancer and hormonal contraceptives: Collaborative reanalysis of individual data on 53 297 women with breast cancer and 100 239 women without breast cancer from 54 epidemiological studies. *Lancet*, **347**, 1713–1727

Collaborative Group on Hormonal Factors in Breast Cancer (1996b) Breast cancer and hormonal contraceptives: Further results. *Contraception*, **54** (Suppl.), 1S–106S

Collaborative MILTS Project Team (1997) Oral contraceptives and liver cancer. *Contraception*, **56**, 275–284

Contractor, R.G., Foran, C.M., Li, S. & Willett, K.L. (2004) Evidence of gender- and tissue-specific promoter methylation and the potential for ethinylestradiol-induced changes in Japanese Medaka (*Oryzias latipes*) estrogen receptor and aromatase genes. *J. Toxicol. environ Health*, **A67**, 1–22

Coutinho, E.M., Athayde, C., Dantas, C., Hirsch, C. & Barbosa, I. (1999) Use of a single implant of elcometrine (ST-1435), a nonorally active progestin, as a long acting contraceptive for postpartum nursing women. *Contraception*, **59**, 115–122

Cramer, D.W., Hutchison, G.B., Welch, W.R., Scully, R.E. & Knapp, R.C. (1982) Factors affecting the association of oral contraceptives and ovarian cancer. *New Engl. J. Med.*, **307**, 1047–1051

Cramer, D.W., Greenberg, E.R., Titus-Ernstoff, L., Liberman, R.F., Welch, W.R., Li, E. & Ng, W.G. (2000) A case–control study of galactose consumption and metabolism in relation to ovarian cancer. *Cancer Epidemiol. Biomarkers Prev.*, **9**, 95–101

Deacon, J.M., Evans, C.D., Yule, R., Desai, M., Binns, W., Taylor, C. & Peto, J. (2000) Sexual behaviour and smoking as determinants of cervical HPV infection and of CIN3 among those infected: A case–control study nested within the Manchester cohort. *Br. J. Cancer*, **88**, 1565–1572

Deckers, G.H., Schoonen, W.G.E.J. & Kloosterboer, H.J. (2000) Influence of the substitution of 11-methylene, Δ^{15}, and/or 18-methyl groups in norethisterone on receptor binding, transactivation assays and biological activities in animals. *J. ster. Biochem. mol. Biol.*, **74**, 83–92

Dezarnaulds, G. & Fraser, I.S. (2002) Vaginal ring delivery of hormone replacement therapy — A review. *Expert Opin. Pharmacother.*, **4**, 201–212

Di Domenico, M., Castoria, G., Bilancio, A., Migliaccio, A. & Auricchio, F. (1996) Estradiol activation of human colon carcinoma-derived caco-2 cell growth. *Cancer Res.*, **56**, 4516–4521

Di Leo, A., Linsalata, M., Cavallini, A., Messa, C. & Russo, F. (1992) Sex steroid hormone receptors, epidermal growth factor receptor, and polyamines in human colorectal cancer. *Dis. Colon Rectum*, **35**, 305–309

Di Leo, A., Messa, C., Cavallini, A. & Linsalata, M. (2001) Estrogens and colorectal cancer. *Curr. Drug Targets imm. endocr. metab. Disorders*, **1**, 1–12

Duell, E.J. & Holly, E.A. (2005) Reproductive and menstrual risk factors for pancreatic cancer: A population-based study of San Francisco Bay area women. *Am. J. Epidemiol.*, **161**, 741–747

Dumeaux, V., Alsaker, E. & Lund, E. (2003) Breast cancer and specific types of oral contraceptives: A large Norwegian cohort study. *Int. J. Cancer*, **105**, 844–850

Dumeaux, V., Lund, E. & Hjartaker, A. (2004) Use of oral contraceptives, alcohol, and risk for invasive breast cancer. *Cancer Epidemiol. Biomarkers Prev.*, **13**, 1302–1307

Edmondson, H.A., Henderson, B. & Benton, B. (1976) Liver-cell adenomas associated with use of oral contraceptives. *New Engl. J. Med.*, **294**, 470–472

Elwood, J.M., Whitehead, S.M., Davison, J., Stewart, M. & Galt, M. (1990) Malignant melanoma in England: Risks associated with naevi, freckles, social class, hair colour, and sunburn. *Int. J. Epidemiol.*, **19**, 801–810

Fanchin, R., de Ziegler, D., Bergeron, C., Righini, C., Torrisi, C. & Frydman, R. (1997) Transvaginal administration of progesterone. *Obstet. Gynecol.*, **90**, 396–401

Fernandez, E., La Vecchia, C., Franceschi, S., Braga, C., Talamini, R., Negri, E. & Parazzini, F. (1998) Oral contraceptive use and risk of colorectal cancer. *Epidemiology*, **9**, 295–300

Feskanich, D., Hunter, D.J., Willett, W.C., Spiegelman, D., Stampfer, M.J., Speizer, F.E. & Colditz, G.A. (1999) Oral contraceptive use and risk of melanoma in premenopausal women. *Br. J. Cancer*, **81**, 918–923

Fiorelli, G., Picariello, L., Martineti, V., Tonelli, F. & Brandi, M.L. (1999) Functional estrogen receptor β in colon cancer cells. *Biochem. biophys. Res. Commun.*, **261**, 521–527

Forman, D., Doll, R. & Peto, R. (1983) Trends in mortality from carcinoma of the liver and the use of oral contraceptives. *Br. J. Cancer*, **48**, 349–354

Forman, D., Vincent, T.J. & Doll, R. (1986) Cancer of the liver and the use of oral contraceptives. *Br. med. J.*, **292**, 1357–1361

Fotherby, K. (1990) Potency and pharmacokinetics of gestagens. *Contraception*, **41**, 533–550

Franceschi, S., La Vecchia, C., Helmrich, S.P., Mangioni, C. & Tognoni, G. (1982) Risk factors for epithelial ovarian cancer in Italy. *Am. J. Epidemiol.*, **115**, 714–719

Franceschi, S., Parazzini, F., Negri, E., Booth, M., La Vecchia, C., Beral, V., Tzonou, A. & Trichopoulos, D. (1991a) Pooled analysis of 3 European case–control studies of epithelial ovarian cancer. III. Oral contraceptive use. *Int. J. Cancer*, **49**, 61–65

Franceschi, S., Bidoli, E., Talamini, R., Barra, S. & La Vecchia, C. (1991b) Colorectal cancer in northeastern Italy: Reproductive, menstrual and female hormone-related factors. *Eur. J. Cancer*, **27**, 604–608

Fraser, I.S. (2000) Forty years of combined oral contraception: The evolution of a revolution. *Med. J. Austr.*, **173**, 541–544

Fu, H., Darroch, J.E., Haas, T. & Ranjit, N. (1999) Contraceptive failure rates: New estimates from the 1995 National Survey of Family Growth. *Fam. Plann. Perspect.*, **31**, 56–63

Furberg, H., Millikan, R.C., Geradts, J., Gammon, M.D., Dressler, L.G., Ambrosone, C.B. & Newman, B. (2003) Reproductive factors in relation to breast cancer characterized by p53 protein expression (United States). *Cancer Causes Control*, **14**, 609–618

Furner, S.E., Davis, F.G., Nelson, R.L. & Haenszel, W. (1989) A case–control study of large bowel cancer and hormone exposure in women. *Cancer Res.*, **49**, 4936–4940

Gago-Dominguez, M., Castelao, J.E., Yuan, J.-M., Ross, R.K. & Yu, M.C. (1999) Increased risk of renal cell carcinoma subsequent to hysterectomy. *Cancer Epidemiol. Biomarkers Prev.*, **8**, 999–1003

Gallagher, R.P., Elwood, J.M., Hill, G.B., Coldman, A.J., Threlfall, W.J. & Spinelli, J.J. (1985) Reproductive factors, oral contraceptives and risk of malignant melanoma: Western Canada Melanoma Study. *Br. J. Cancer*, **52**, 901–907

Gallmeier, E., Winter, J.M., Cunningham, S.C., Kahn, S.R. & Kern, S.E. (2005) Novel genotoxicity assays identify norethindrone to activate p53 and phosphorylate H2AX. *Carcinogenesis*, **26**, 1811–1820

Gallo, M.F., Nanda, K., Grimes, D.A. & Schulz, K.F. (2004) 20 mcg Versus > 20 mcg estrogen combined oral contraceptives for contraception (review). *Cochrane Database Syst. Rev.*, **4**, Art. No. CD003989

Gallus, S., Bosetti, C., Franceschi, S., Levi, F., Simonato, L., Negri, E., & La Vecchia, C. (2001) Oesophageal cancer in women: Tobacco, alcohol, nutritional and hormonal factors. *Br. J. Cancer*, **85**, 341–345

Garcia-Becerra, R., Cooney, A.J., Borja-Cacho, E., Lemus, A.E., Pérez-Palacios, G. & Larrea, F. (2004) Comparative evaluation of androgen and progesterone receptor transcription selectivity indices of 19-nortestosterone-derived progestins. *J. ster. Biochem. mol. Biol.*, **91**, 21–27

Gefeller, O., Hassan, K. & Wille, L. (1998) Cutaneous malignant melanoma in women and the role of oral contraceptives. *Br. J. Dermatol.*, **138**, 122–124

Gemer, O., Moscovici, O., Ben-Horin, C.L., Linov, L., Peled, R. & Segal S. (2004) Oral contraceptives and liver hemangioma: A case–control study. *Acta obstet. gynaecol. scand.*, **83**, 1199–1201

Glaser, S.L., Clarke, C.A., Nugent, R.A., Stearns, C.B. & Dorfman, R.F. (2003) Reproductive factors in Hodgkin's disease in women. *Am. J. Epidemiol.*, **158**, 553–563

Gnagy, S., Ming, E.E., Devesa, S.S., Hartge, P. & Whittemore, A.S. (2000) Declining ovarian cancer rates in U.S. women in relation to parity and oral contraceptive use. *Epidemiology*, **11**, 102–105

Godard, B., Foulkes, W.D., Provencher, D., Brunet, J.S., Tonin, P.N., Mes-Masson, A.M., Narod, S.A. & Ghadirian, P. (1998) Risk factors for familial and sporadic ovarian cancer among French Canadians: A case–control study. *Am. J. Obstet. Gynecol.*, **179**, 403–410

Goebelsmann, U., Hoffman, D., Chiang, S. & Woutersz, T. (1986) The relative bioavailability of levonorgestrel and ethinyl estradiol administered as a low-dose combination oral contraceptive. *Contraception*, **34**, 341–351

Goldzieher, J.W. & Brody, S.A. (1990) Pharmacokinetics of ethinyl estradiol and mestranol. *Am. J. Obstet. Gynecol.*, **163**, 2114–2119

Grabrick, D.M., Hartmann, L.C., Cerhan, J.R., Vierkant, R.A., Therneau, T.M., Vachon, C.M., Olson, J.E., Couch, F.J., Anderson, K.E., Pankratz, V.S. & Sellers, T.A. (2000) Risk of breast cancer with oral contraceptive use in women with a family history of breast cancer. *J. Am. med. Assoc.*, **284**, 1791–1798

Green, A. & Bain, C. (1985) Hormonal factors and melanoma in women. *Med. J. Austr.*, **142**, 446–448

Green, J., Berrington de Gonzalez, A., Smith, J.S., Franceschi, S., Appleby, P., Plummer, M. & Beral, V. (2003) Human papillomavirus infection and use of oral contraceptives. *Br. J. Cancer*, **88**, 1713–1720

Greer, J.B., Modugno, F., Allen, G.O. & Ness, R.B. (2005) Androgenic progestins in oral contraceptives and the risk of epithelial ovarian cancer. *Obstet. Gynecol.*, **105**, 731–740

Greggi, S., Parazzini, F., Paratore, M.P., Chatenoud, L., Legge, F., Mancuso, S. & La Vecchia, C. (2000) Risk factors for ovarian cancer in central Italy. *Gynecol. Oncol.*, **9**, 50–54

Grodstein, F., Newcomb, P.A. & Stampfer, M.J. (1999) Postmenopausal hormone therapy and the risk of colorectal cancer: A review and meta-analysis. *Am. J. Med.*, **106**, 574–582

Guengerich, F.P. (1988) Oxidation of 17 alpha-ethynylestradiol by human liver cytochrome P-450. *Mol. Pharmacol.*, **33**, 500–508

Hammond, G.L., Rabe, T. & Wagner, J.D. (2001) Preclinical profiles of progestins used in formulations of oral contraceptives and hormone replacement therapy. *Am. J. Obstet. Gynecol.*, **185**, S24–S31

Hammouda, D., Muñoz, N., Herrero, R., Arslan, A., Bouhadet, A., Oublil, M., Djedeat, B., Fontanière, B., Snijders, P., Meijer, C. & Franceschi, S. (2005) Cervical carcinoma in Algiers, Algeria: Human papillomavirus and lifestyle factors. *Int. J. Cancer*, **113**, 483–489

Hannaford, P. & Elliot, A. (2005) Use of exogenous hormones by women and colorectal cancer: Evidence from the Royal College of General Practitioners' Oral Contraception Study. *Contraception*, **71**, 95–98

Hannaford, P.C., Villard-Mackintosh, L., Vessey, M.P. & Kay, C.R. (1991) Oral contraceptives and malignant melanoma. *Br. J. Cancer*, **63**, 430–433

Hannaford, P.C., Croft, P.R. & Kay, C.R. (1994) Oral contraception and stroke. Evidence from the Royal College of General Practitioners' Oral Contraception Study. *Stroke*, **25**, 935–942

Hannaford, P.C., Kay, C.R., Vessey, M.P., Painter, R. & Mant, J. (1997) Combined oral contraceptives and liver disease. *Contraception*, **55**, 145–151

Harlow, B.L., Weiss, N.S., Roth, G.J., Chu, J. & Daling, J.R. (1988) Case–control study of borderline ovarian tumors: Reproductive history and exposure to exogenous female hormones. *Cancer Res.*, **48**, 5849–5852

Harris, R., Whittemore, A.S., Itnyre, J. & the Collaborative Ovarian Cancer Group (1992) Characteristics relating to ovarian cancer risk: Collaborative analysis of 12 US case–control studies. III. Epithelial tumors of low malignant potential in white women. *Am. J. Epidemiol.*, **136**, 1204–1211

Hartge, P., Schiffman, M.H., Hoover, R., McGowan, L., Lesher, L. & Norris, H.J. (1989) A case–control study of epithelial ovarian cancer. *Am. J. Obstet. Gynecol.*, **161**, 10–16

Haselkorn, T., Stewart, S.L. & Horn-Ross, P.L. (2003) Why are thyroid cancer rates so high in Southeast Asian women living in the United States? The Bay Area Thyroid Cancer Study. *Cancer Epidemiol. Biomarkers Prev.*, **12**, 144–150

Hasenack, H.G., Bosch, A.M.G. & Käär, K. (1986) Serum levels of 3-keto-desogestrel after oral administration of desogestrel and 3-keto-desogestrel. *Contraception*, **33**, 591–596

Heimdal, K., Skovlund, E. & Moller, P. (2002) Oral contraceptives and risk of familial breast cancer. *Cancer Detect. Prev.*, **26**, 23–27

Helmrich, S.P., Rosenberg, L., Kaufman, D.W., Miller, D.R., Schottenfeld, D., Stolley, P.D. & Shapiro, S. (1984) Lack of an elevated risk of malignant melanoma in relation to oral contraceptive use. *J. natl Cancer Inst.*, **72**, 617–620

Henderson, B.E., Casagrande, J.T., Pike, M.C., Mack, T., Rosario, I. & Duke, A. (1983a) The epidemiology of endometrial cancer in young women. *Br. J. Cancer*, **47**, 749–756

Henderson, B., Preston-Martin, S., Edmonson, H.A., Peters, R.L. & Pike, M.C. (1983b) Hepatocellular carcinoma and oral contraceptives. *Br. J. Cancer*, **48**, 437–440

Hendrickse, C.W., Jones, C.E., Donovan, I.A., Neoptolemos, J.P. & Baker, P.R. (1993) Oestrogen and progesterone receptors in colorectal cancer and human colonic cancer cell lines. *Br. J. Surg.*, **80**, 636–640

Heuner, A., Kuhnz, W., Heger-Mahn, D., Richert, K. & Humpel, M. (1995) A single-dose and 3-month clinical-pharmacokinetic study with a new combination oral contraceptive. *Adv. Contracept.*, **11**, 207–225

Hildreth, N.G., Kelsey, J.L., LiVolsi, V.A., Fischer, D.B., Holford, T.R., Mostow, E.D., Schwartz, P.E. & White, C. (1981) An epidemiologic study of epithelial carcinoma of the ovary. *Am. J. Epidemiol.*, **114**, 398–405

Hoffmann, H., Hillesheim, H.G., Güttner, J., Stade, K., Merbt, E.-M., & Holle, K. (1983) Long term toxicological studies on the progestin STS 557. *Exp. clin. Endocrinol.*, **81**, 179–196

Holly, E.A., Weiss, N.S. & Liff, J.M. (1983) Cutaneous melanoma in relation to exogenous hormones and reproductive factors. *J. natl Cancer Inst.*, **70**, 827–831

Holly, E.A., Cress, R.D. & Ahn, D.K. (1995) Cutaneous melanoma in women. III. Reproductive factors and oral contraceptive use. *Am. J. Epidemiol.*, **141**, 943–950

Holman, C.D., Armstrong, B.K. & Heenan, P.J. (1984) Cutaneous malignant melanoma in women: Exogenous sex hormones and reproductive factors. *Br. J. Cancer*, **50**, 673–680

van Hooff, M.H.A., Hirasing, R.A., Kaptein, M.B.M., Koppenaal, C., Voorhorst, F.J. & Schoemaker, J. (1998) The use of oral contraception by adolescents for contraception, menstrual cycle problems or acne. *Acta obstet. gynaecol. scand.*, **77**, 898–904

Hsing, A.W., Hoover, R.N., McLaughlin, J.K., Co-Chien, H.T., Wacholder, S., Blot, W.J. & Fraumeni, J.F. (1992) Oral contraceptives and primary liver cancer among young women. *Cancer Causes Control*, **3**, 43–48

Hulka, B.S., Chambless, L.E., Kaufman, D.G., Fowler, W.C., Jr & Greenberg, B.G. (1982) Protection against endometrial carcinoma by combination-product oral contraceptives. *J. Am. med. Assoc.*, **247**, 475–477

Humpel, M., Wendt, H., Dogs, G., Weiss, C., Rietz, S. & Speck, U. (1977) Intraindividual comparison of pharmacokinetic parameters of d-norgestrel, lynestrenol and cyproterone acetate in 6 women. *Contraception*, **16**, 199–215

Humpel, M., Wendt, H., Pommerenke, G., Weiss, C. & Speck, U. (1978) Investigations of pharma-cokinetics of levonorgestrel to specific consideration of a possible first-pass effect in women. *Contraception*, **17**, 207–220

Hümpel, M., Täuber, U., Kuhnz, W., Pfeffer, M., Brill, K., Heithecker, R., Louton, T. & Steinberg, B. (1990) Comparison of serum ethinyl estradiol, sex-hormone-binding globulin, corticoid-binding globulin and cortisol levels in women using two low-dose combined oral contra-ceptives. *Horm. Res.*, **33**, 35–39

IARC (1979) *IARC Monographs on the Evaluation of the Carcinogenic Risk of Chemicals to Humans*, Vol. 21, *Sex Hormones (II)*, Lyon

IARC (1988) IARC Monographs on the Evaluation of Carcinogenic Risks to Humans, Vol. 44, Alcohol Drinking, Lyon

IARC (1994) IARC Monographs on the Evaluation of Carcinogenic Risks to Humans, Vol. 59, Hepatitis Viruses, Lyon

IARC (1999) *IARC Monographs on the Evaluation of Carcinogenic Risks to Humans*, Vol. 72, *Hormonal Contraception and Post-menopausal Hormonal Therapy*, Lyon

IARC (2004) IARC Monographs on the Evaluation of Carcinogenic Risks to Humans, Vol. 83, Tobacco Smoke and Involuntary Smoking, Lyon

IARC (2007) *IARC Monographs on the Evaluation of the Carcinogenic Risk of Chemicals to Humans*, Vol. 90, *Human Papillomaviruses*, Lyon

IMS Health (2005) *IMS Health MIDAS*, June 2005

Iribarren, C., Haselkorn, T., Tekawa, I.S. & Friedman, G.D. (2001) Cohort study of thyroid cancer in a San Francisco Bay area population. *Int. J. Cancer*, **93**, 745–750

Isaksson, E., von Schoultz, E., Odlind, V., Soderqvist, G., Csemiczky, G., Carlström, K., Skoog, L. & von Schoultz, B. (2001) Effects of oral contraceptives on breast epithelial proliferation. *Breast Cancer Res. Treat.*, **65**, 163–169

Ishikawa, T., Inoue, S., Kakinuma, C., Kuwayama, C., Hamada, Y. & Shibutani, Y. (2000) Growth-stimulating effect of dienogest, a synthetic steroid, on rodent, canine, and primate mammary glands. *Toxicology*, **151**, 91–101

Jacobs, E.J., White, E. & Weiss, N.S. (1994) Exogenous hormones, reproductive history, and colon cancer (Seattle, Washington, USA). *Cancer Causes Control*, **5**, 359–366

Jain, M.G., Rohan, T.E. & Howe, G.R. (2000) Hormone replacement therapy and endometrial cancer in Ontario, Canada. *J. clin. Epidemiol.*, **53**, 385–391

Jänne, O.A., Zook, B.C., Didolkar, A.K., Sundaram, K. & Nash, H.A. (2001) The roles of estrogen and progestin in producing deciduosarcoma and other lesions in the rabbit. *Toxicol. Pathol.*, **29**, 417–421

Jick, S.S., Walker, A.M. & Jick, H. (1993) Oral contraceptives and endometrial cancer. *Obstet. Gynecol.*, **82**, 931–935

Jick, H., Jick, S.S., Gurewich, V., Myers, M.W. & Vasilakis, C. (1995) Risk of idiopathic cardio-vascular death and nonfatal venous thromboembolism in women using oral contraceptives with differing progestagen components. *Lancet*, **346**, 1589–1593

John, E.M., Whittemore, A.S., Harris, R., Itnyre, J. & Collaborative Ovarian Cancer Group (1993) Characteristics relating to ovarian cancer risk: Collaborative analysis of seven US case–control studies. Epithelial ovarian cancer in black women. *J. natl Cancer Inst.*, **85**, 142–147

Joosten, H.F.P., van Acker, F.A.A., van den Dobbelsteen, D.J., Horbach, G.J.M.J. & Krajnc, E.I. (2004) Genotoxicity of hormonal steroids. *Toxicol. Lett.*, **151**, 113–134

Junod, S.W. & Marks, L. (2002) Women's trials: The approval of the first oral contraceptive pill in the United States and Great Britain. *J. Hist. Med. allied Sci.*, **57**, 117–160

Kalandidi, A., Tzonou, A., Lipworth, L., Gamatsi, I., Filippa, D. & Trichopoulos, D. (1996) A case–control study of endometrial cancer in relation to reproductive, somatometric, and lifestyle variables. *Oncology*, **53**, 354–359

Kampman, E., Bijl, A.J., Kok, C. & van't Veer, P. (1994) Reproductive and hormonal factors in male and female colon cancer. *Eur. J. Cancer Prev.*, **3**, 329–336

Kampman, E., Potter, J.D., Slattery, M.L., Caan, B.J. & Edward S. (1997) Hormone replacement therapy, reproductive history, and colon cancer: A multicenter, case–control study in the United States. *Cancer Causes Control*, **8**, 146–158

Karagas, M.R., Stukel, T.A., Dykes, J., Miglionico, J., Greene, M.A., Carey, M., Armstrong, B., Elwood, J.M., Gallagher, R.P., Green, A., Holly, E.A., Kirkpatrick, C.S., Mack, T., Østerlind, A., Rosso, S. & Swerdlow, A.J. (2002) A pooled analysis of 10 case–control studies of melanoma and oral contraceptive use. *Br. J. Cancer*, **86**, 1085–1092

Kasper, P. (2001) Cyproterone acetate: A genotoxic carcinogen? *Pharmacol. Toxicol.*, **88**, 223–231

Katsuki, Y., Sasagawa, S., Takano, Y., Shibutani, Y., Aoki, D., Udagawa, Y. & Nozawa, S. (1997a) Animal studies on the endocrinological profile of dienogest, a novel synthetic steroid. *Drugs exp. clin. Res.*, **23**, 45–62

Katsuki, Y., Shibutani, Y., Aoki, D. & Nozawa, S. (1997b) Dienogest, a novel synthetic steroid, overcomes hormone-dependent cancer in a different manner than progestins. *Cancer*, **79**, 169–176

Kaufman, D.W., Shapiro, S., Slone, D., Rosenberg, L., Miettinen, O.S., Stolley, P.D., Knapp, R.C., Leavitt, T., Jr, Watring, W.G., Rosenshein, N.B., Lewis, J.L., Jr, Schottenfeld, D. & Engle, R.L., Jr (1980) Decreased risk of endometrial cancer among oral-contraceptive users. *New Engl. J. Med.*, **303**, 1045–1047

Kaufmann, G., Schlegel, J., Eychenne, B. & Schubert, K. (1983) Receptor binding of STS 557. *Exp. clin. Endocrinol.*, **81**, 222–227

Kay, C.R. (1981) Malignant melanoma and oral contraceptives (Letter to the Editor). *Br. J. Cancer*, **44**, 479

Kazmi, S.M., Visconti, V., Plante, R.K., Ishaque, A. & Lau, C. (1993) Differential regulation of human progesterone receptor A and B form-mediated *trans*-activation by phosphorylation. *Endocrinology*, **133**, 1230–1238

Keam, S.J. & Wagstaff, A.J. (2003) Ethinylestradiol/drospirenone: A review of its use as an oral contraceptive. *Treat. Endocrinol.*, **2**, 49–70

Kelsey, J.L., Livolsi, V.A., Holford, T.R., Fischer, D.B., Mostow, E.D., Schwartz, P.E., O'Connor, T. & White, C. (1982) A case–control study of cancer of the endometrium. *Am. J. Epidemiol.*, **116**, 333–342

Ketting, E. (1988) The relative reliability of oral contraceptives; findings of an epidemiological study. *Contraception*, **37**, 343–348

Kew, M.C., Song, E., Mohammed, A. & Hodkinson, J. (1990) Contraceptive steroids as a risk factor for hepatocellular carcinoma: A case–control study in South African black women. *Hepatology*, **11**, 298–302

Kirkpatrick, C.S., White, E. & Lee, J.A. (1994) Case–control study of malignant melanoma in Washington State. II. Diet, alcohol, and obesity. *Am. J. Epidemiol.*, **139**, 869–880

Kopera, H. (1985) [Unintended effects of oral contraceptives. II. Progesterone-induced effects, drug-drug interactions]. *Wien. med. Wochenschr.*, **135**, 415–419 (in German)

Koumantaki, Y., Tzonou, A., Koumantakis, E., Kaklamani, E., Aravantinos, D. & Trichopoulos, D. (1989) A case–control study of cancer of endometrium in Athens. *Int. J. Cancer*, **43**, 795–799

Krattenmacher, R. (2000) Drospirenone: Pharmacology and pharmacokinetics of a unique progestogen. *Contraception*, **62**, 29–38

Kreiger, N., Lacroix, J. & Sloan, M. (2001) Hormonal factors and pancreatic cancer in women. *Ann. Epidemiol.*, **11**, 563–567

Kreuzer, M., Gerken, M., Heinrich, J., Kreienbrock, L. & Wichmann, H.-E. (2003) Hormonal factors and risk of lung cancer among women? *Int. epidemiol. Assoc.*, 32, 263–271

Kuhl, H. (1996) Comparative pharmacology of newer progestogens. *Drugs*, **51**, 188–215

Kuhl, H., Jung-Hoffmann, C. & Heidt, F. (1988a) Serum levels of 3-keto-desogestrel and SHBG during 12 cycles of treatment with 30 µg ethinylestradiol and 150 µg desogestrel. *Contraception*, **38**, 381–390

Kuhl, H., Jung-Hoffmann, C. & Heidt, F. (1988b) Alterations in the serum levels of gestodene and SHBG during 12 cycles of treatment with 30 micrograms ethinylestradiol and 75 micrograms gestodene. *Contraception*, **38**, 477–486

Kuhnz, W., Humpel, M., Schutt, B., Louton, T., Steinberg, B. & Gansau, C. (1990a) Relative bio-availability of ethinyl estradiol from two different oral contraceptive formulations after single oral administration to 18 women in an intraindividual cross-over design. *Horm. Res.*, **33**, 40–44

Kuhnz, W., Pfeffer, M. & Al Yacoub, G. (1990b) Protein binding of the contraceptive steroids gestodene, 3-keto-desogestrel and ethinylestradiol in human serum. *J. ster. Biochem.*, **35**, 313–318

Kuhnz, W., Sostarek, D., Gansau, C., Louton, T. & Mahler, M. (1991) Single and multiple administration of a new triphasic oral contraceptive to women: Pharmacokinetics of ethinyl estradiol and free and total testosterone levels in serum. *Am. J. Obstet. Gynecol.*, **165**, 596–602

Kuhnz, W., Al Yacoub, G. & Fuhrmeister, A. (1992) Pharmacokinetics of levonorgestrel and ethinylestradiol in 9 women who received a low-dose oral contraceptive over a treatment period of 3 months and, after a wash-out phase, a single oral administration of the same contraceptive formulation. *Contraception*, **46**, 455–469

Kuhnz, W., Baumann, A., Staks, T., Dibbelt, L., Knuppen, R. & Jutting, G. (1993) Pharmacokinetics of gestodene and ethinylestradiol in 14 women during three months of treatment with a new tri-step combination oral contraceptive: Serum protein binding of gestodene and influence of treatment on free and total testosterone levels in the serum. *Contraception*, **48**, 303–322

Kuhnz, W., Staks, T. & Jutting, G. (1994a) Pharmacokinetics of levonorgestrel and ethinylestradiol in 14 women during three months of treatment with a tri-step combination oral contraceptive: Serum protein binding of levonorgestrel and influence of treatment on free and total testosterone levels in the serum. *Contraception*, **50**, 563–579

Kuhnz, W., Blode, H. & Mahler, M. (1994b) Systemic availability of levonorgestrel after single oral administration of a norgestimate-containing combination oral contraceptive to 12 young women. *Contraception*, **49**, 255–263

Kuhnz, W., Heuner, A., Humpel, M., Seifert, W. & Michaelis, K. (1997) In vivo conversion of norethisterone and norethisterone acetate to ethinyl etradiol in postmenopausal women. *Contraception*, **56**, 379–385

Kuiper, G.G.J.M., Enmark, E., Pelto-Huikko, M., Nilsson, S. & Gustafsson, J.A. (1996) Cloning of a novel estrogen receptor expressed in rat prostate and ovary. *Proc. natl Acad. Sci. USA*, **93**, 5925–5930

Kuiper, G.G.J.M., Carlsson, B., Grandien, K., Enmark, E., Häggblad, J., Nilsson, S. & Gustafsson, J.-A. (1997) Comparison of the ligand binding specificity and transcript tissue distribution of estrogen receptors alpha and beta. *Endocrinology*, **138**, 863–870

Kumar, N., Koide, S.S., Tsong, Y.-Y. & Sundaram, K. (2000) Nestorone®: A progestin with a unique pharmacological profile. *Steroids*, **65**, 629–636

Kumle, M., Weiderpass, E., Braaten, T., Persson, I., Adami, H.-O. & Lund, E. (2002) Use of oral contraceptives and breast cancer risk: The Norwegian–Swedish Women's Lifestyle and Health Cohort Study. *Cancer Epidemiol. Biomarkers Prev.*, **11**, 1375–1381

Kumle, M., Alsaker, E. & Lund, E. (2003) [Use of oral contraceptives and risk of cancer, a cohort study.] *Tidsskr. Nor. Laegeforen.*, **123**, 1653–1656 (in Norwegian)

Kumle, M., Weiderpass, E., Braaten, T., Adami, H.-O. & Lund, E. (2004) Risk for invasive and borderline epithelial ovarian neoplasias following use of hormonal contraceptives: The Norwegian–Swedish Women's Lifestyle and Health Cohort Study. *Br. J. Cancer*, **90**, 1386–1391

Kune, G.A., Kune, S. & Watson, L.F. (1990) Oral contraceptive use does not protect against large bowel cancer. *Contraception*, **41**, 19–25

Lacey, J.V., Brinton, L.A., Abbas, F.M., Barnes, W.A., Gravitt, P.E., Greenberg, M.D., Green, S.M., Hadjimichael, O.C., McGowan, L., Mortel, R., Schwartz, P.E., Silverberg, S.G. & Hildesheim, A. (1999) Oral contraceptives as risk factors for cervical adenocarcinomas and squamous cell carcinomas. *Cancer Epidemiol. Biomarkers Prev.*, **8**, 1079–1085

Langholz, B., Richardson, J., Rappaport, E., Waisman, J., Cockburn, M. & Mack, T. (2000) Skin characteristics and risk of superficial spreading and nodular melanoma (United States). *Cancer Causes Control*, **11**, 741–750

Larrea, F., Garcia-Becerra, R., Lemus, A.E., Garcia, G.A., Pérez-Palacios, G., Jackson, K.J., Coleman, K.M., Dace, R., Smith, C.L. & Cooney, A.J. (2001) A-ring reduced metabolites of 19-nor synthetic progestins as subtype selective agonists for ER alpha. *Endocrinology*, **142**, 3791–3799

La Vecchia, C., Decarli, A., Fasoli, M., Franceschi, S., Gentile, A., Negri, E., Parazzini, F. & Tognoni, G. (1986) Oral contraceptives and cancers of the breast and of the female genital tract. Interim results from a case–control study. *Br. J. Cancer*, **54**, 311–317

La Vecchia, C., Negri, E., Levi, F., Decarli, A. & Boyle, P. (1998) Cancer mortality in Europe: Effects of age, cohort of birth and period of death. *Eur. J. Cancer*, **34**, 118–141

La Vecchia, C., Ron, E., Franceschi, S., Dal Maso, L., Mark, S.D., Chatenoud, L., Braga, C., Preston-Martin, S., McTiernan, A., Kolonel, L., Mabuchi, K., Jin, F., Wingren, G., Galanti, M.R., Hallquist, A., Lund, E., Levi, F., Linos, D. & Negri, E. (1999) A pooled analysis of case–control studies of thyroid cancer. III. Oral contraceptives, menopausal replacement therapy and other female hormones. *Cancer Causes Control*, **10**, 157–166

Lê, M.G., Cabanes, P.A., Desvignes, V., Chanteau, M.F., Mlika, N. & Avril, M.F. (1992) Oral contraceptive use and risk of cutaneous malignant melanoma in a case–control study of French women. *Cancer Causes Control*, **3**, 199–205

Lemus, A.E., Santillán, R., Damián-Matsumura, P., Garcia, G.A., Grillasca, I. & Pérez-Palacios, G. (2001) In vitro metabolism of gestodene in target organs: Formation of A-ring reduced derivatives with oestrogenic activity. *Eur. J. Pharmacol.*, **417**, 249–256

Lemus, A.E., Zaga, V., Santillán, R., Garcia, G.A., Grillasca, I., Damián-Matsumura, P., Jackson, K.J., Cooney, A.J., Larrea, F. & Pérez-Palacios, G. (2000) The oestrogenic effects of gestodene, a potent contraceptive progestin, are mediated by its A-ring reduced metabolites. *J. Endocrinol.*, **165**, 693–702

Lepescheux, L., Secchi, J., Gaillard-Kelly, M. & Miller, P. (2001) Effects of 17 beta-estradiol and tri-megestone alone, and in combination, on the bone and uterus of ovariectomized rats. *Gynecol. Endocrinol.*, **15**, 312–320

Levi, F., La Vecchia, C., Gulie, C., Negri, E., Monnier, V., Franceschi, S., Delaloye, J.F. & De Grandi, P. (1991) Oral contraceptives and the risk of endometrial cancer. *Cancer Causes Control*, **2**, 99–103

Levi, F., Pasche, C., Lucchini, F. & La Vecchia, C (2003) Oral contraceptives and colorectal cancer. *Dig. Liver Dis.*, **35**, 85–87

Levi, F., Lucchini, F., Negri, E., Boyle, P. & La Vecchia, C. (2004) Cancer mortality in Europe, 1995–1999, and an overview of trends since 1960. *Int. J. Cancer*, **110**, 155–169

Lew, R.A., Sober, A.J., Cook, N., Marvell, R. & Fitzpatrick, T.B. (1983) Sun exposure habits in patients with cutaneous melanoma: A case–control study. *J. Dermatol. surg. Oncol.*, **9**, 981–986

Loncar, D., Milosevic-Djordjevic, O., Zivanovic, A., Grujicic, D. & Arsenijevic, S. (2004) Effect of a low-dose ethinylestradiol and gestodene in combination on the frequency of micronuclei in human peripheral blood lymphocytes of healthy women in vivo. *Contraception*, **69**, 327–331

Lubahn, D.B., Moyer, J.S., Golding, T.S., Couse, J.F., Korach, K.S. & Smithies, O. (1993) Altera-tion of reproductive function but not prenatal sexual development after insertional disruption of the mouse estrogen receptor gene. *Proc. natl Acad. Sci. USA*, **90**, 11162–11166

Lüdicke, F., Johannisson, E., Helmerhorst, F.M., Campana, A., Foidart, J.-M. & Heithecker, R. (2001) Effect of a combined oral contraceptive containing 3 mg of drospirenone and 30 µg of ethinyl estradiol on the human endometrium. *Fertil. Steril.*, **76**, 102–107

Lundberg, V., Tolonen, H., Stegmayr, B., Kuulasmaa, K. & Asplund, K. (2004) Use of oral contra-ceptives and hormone replacement therapy in the WHO MONICA project. *Maturitas*, **48**, 39–49

Mack, W.J., Preston-Martin, S., Bernstein, L., Qian, D. & Xiang, M. (1999) Reproductive and hormonal risk factors for thyroid cancer in Los Angeles County females. *Cancer Epidemiol. Biomarkers Prev.*, **8**, 991–997

Madeleine, M.M., Daling, J.R., Schwartz, S.M., Shera, K., McKnight, B., Carter, J.J., Wipf, G.C., Critchlow, C.W., McDougall, J.K., Porter, P. & Galloway, D.A. (2001) Human papillomavirus and long-term oral contraceptive use increase the risk of adenocarcinoma *in situ* of the cervix. *Cancer Epidemiol. Biomarkers Prev.*, **10**, 171–177

Magnusson, C.M., Persson, I.R., Baron, J.A., Ekbom, A., Bergstrom, R. & Adami, H.-O. (1999) The role of reproductive factors and use of oral contraceptives in the aetiology of breast cancer in women aged 50 to 74 years. *Int. J. Cancer*, **80**, 231–236

Mant, J.W.F. & Vessey, M.P. (1995) Trends in mortality from primary liver cancer in England and Wales 1975–92: Influence of oral contraceptives. *Br. J. Cancer*, **72**, 800–803

Marchbanks, P.A., McDonald, J.A., Wilson, H.G., Folger, S.G., Mandel, M.G., Daling, J.R., Bernstein, L., Malone, K.E., Ursin, G., Strom, B.L., Norman, S.A. & Weiss, L.K. (2002) Oral contraceptives and the risk of breast cancer. *New Engl. J. Med.*, **346**, 2025–2032

Martelli, A., Mattioli, F., Carrozzino, R., Ferraris, E., Marchese, M., Angiola, M. & Brambilla, G. (1999) Genotoxicity testing of potassium canrenoate in cultured rat and human cells. *Muta-genesis*, **14**, 463–472

Martelli, A., Mattioli, F., Angiola, M., Reimann, R. & Brambilla, G. (2003) Species, sex and inter-individual differences in DNA repair induced by nine sex steroids in primary cultures of rat and human hepatocytes. *Mutat. Res.*, **536**, 69–78

Martinez, M.E., Grodstein, F., Giovannucci, E., Colditz, G.A., Speizer, F.E., Hennekens, C., Rosner, B., Willett, W.C. & Stampfer, M.J. (1997) A prospective study of reproductive factors, oral contraceptive use, and risk of colorectal cancer. *Cancer Epidemiol. Biomarkers Prev.*, **6**, 1–5

Mattioli, F., Garbero, C., Gosmar, M., Manfredi, V., Carrozzino, R., Martelli, A. & Brambilla, G. (2004) DNA fragmentation, DNA repair and apoptosis induced in primary rat hepatocytes by dienogest, dydrogesterone and 1,4,6-androstatriene-17beta-ol-3-one acetate. *Mutat. Res.*, **564**, 21–29

McGuire, J.L., Phillips, A., Hahn, D.W., Tolman, E.L., Flor, S. & Kafrissen, M.E. (1990) Pharmacologic and pharmacokinetic characteristics of norgestimate and its metabolites. *Am. J. Obstet. Gynecol.*, **163**, 2127–2131

McGuire, V., Felberg, A., Mills, M., Ostrow, K.L., DiCioccio, R., John, E.M., West, D.W. & Whittemore, A.S. (2004) Relation of contraceptive and reproductive history to ovarian cancer risk in carriers and noncarriers of BRCA1 gene mutations. *Am. J. Epidemiol.*, **160**, 613–618

Meirik, O., Fraser, I.S. & d'Arcangues, C. for the WHO Consultation on Implantable Contraceptives for Women (2003) Implantable contraceptives for women. *Hum. Rep. Update*, **9**, 49–59

Milewicz, T., Kolodziejczyk, J., Krzysiek, J., Basta, A., Sztefko, K., Kurek, S., Stachura, J. & Gregoraszczuk, E.L. (2002) Cyproterone, norethindrone, medroxyprogesterone and levo-norgestrel are less potent local human growth hormone and insulin-like growth factor I secretion stimulators than progesterone in human breast cancer explants expressing the estrogen receptor. *Gynecol. Endocrinol.*, **16**, 319–329

Mills, P.K., Riordan, D.G. & Cress, R.D. (2004) Epithelial ovarian cancer risk by invasiveness and cell type in the Central Valley of California. *Gynecol. Oncol.*, **95**, 215–225

Mitsumori, K., Shimo, T., Onodera, H., Takagi, H., Yasuhara, K., Tamura, T., Aoki, Y., Nagata, O. & Hirose, M. (2000) Modifying effects of ethinylestradiol but not methoxychlor on N-ethyl-N-nitrosourea-induced uterine carcinogenesis in heterozygous *p53*-deficient CBA mice. *Toxicol. Sci.*, **58**, 43–49

Modan, B., Hartge, P., Hirsh-Yechezkel, G., Chetrit, A., Lubin, F., Beller, U., Ben-Baruch, G., Fishman, A., Menczer, J., Ebbers, S.M., Tucker, M.A., Wacholder, S., Struewing, J.P., Friedman, E., Piura, B. & the National Israel Ovarian Cancer Study Group (2001) Parity, oral contraceptives, and the risk of ovarian cancer among carriers and noncarriers of a BRCA1 or BRCA2 mutation. *New Engl. J. Med.*, **345**, 235–240

Modugno, F., Ness, R.B. & Wheeler, J.E. (2001) Reproductive risk factors for epithelial ovarian cancer according to histologic type and invasiveness. *Ann. Epidemiol.*, **11**, 568–574

Modugno, F., Ness, R.B., Allen, G.O., Schildkraut, J.M., Davis, F.G. & Goodman, M.T. (2004) Oral contraceptive use, reproductive history, and risk of epithelial ovarian cancer in women with and without endometriosis. *Am. J. Obstet. Gynecol.*, **191**, 733–740

Moerman, C.J., Bueno de Mesquita, H.B. & Runia, S. (1994) Smoking, alcohol consumption and the risk of cancer of the biliary tract; a population-based case–control study in The Netherlands. *Eur. J. Cancer Prev.*, **3**, 427–436

Molano, M., van den Brule, A., Plummer, M., Weiderpass, E., Posso, H., Arslan, A., Meijer, C.J.L.M., Muñoz, N., Franceschi, S. & the HPV Study Group (2003) Determinants of clearance of human papillomavirus infections in Colombian women with normal cytology: A population-based, 5-year follow-up study. *Am. J. Epidemiol.*, **158**, 486–494

Monsonego, J., Magdelenat, H., Catalan, F., Coscas, Y., Zerat, L. & Sastre, X. (1991) Estrogen and progesterone receptors in cervical human papillomavirus related lesions. *Int. J. Cancer*, **48**, 533–539

Morales-Peza, N., Auewarakul, P., Juarez, V., Garcia-Carranca, A. & Cid-Arregui, A. (2002) *In vivo* tissue-specific regulation of the human papillomavirus type 18 early promoter by estrogen, progesterone, and their antagonists. *Virology*, **294**, 135–140

Moreno, V., Bosch, F.X., Muñoz, N., Meijer, C.J.L.M., Shah, K.V. Walboomers, J.M.M., Herrero, R. & Franceschi, S. (2002) Effect of oral contraceptives on risk of cervical cancer in women with human papillomavirus infection: The IARC multicentric case–control study. *Lancet*, **359**, 1085–1092

Mosselman, S., Polman, J. & Dijkema, R. (1996) ER beta: Identification and characterization of a novel human estrogen receptor. *FEBS Lett.*, **392**, 49–53

Moyer, D.L. & Felix, J.C. (1998) The effects of progesterone and progestins on endometrial proliferation. *Contraception*, **57**, 399–403

Muhn, P., Krattenmacher, R. Beier, S., Elger, W. & Schillinger, E. (1995) Drospirenone: A novel progestogen with antimineralocorticoid and antiandrogenic activity. Pharmacological characterization in animal models. *Contraception*, **51**, 99–110

Nakamura, M., Katsuki, Y., Shibutani, Y. & Oikawa, T. (1999) Dienogest, a synthetic steroid, suppresses both embryonic and tumor-cell-induced angiogenesis. *Eur. J. Pharmacol.* **386**, 33–40

Nakayama, Y., Sakamoto, H., Satoh, K. & Yamamoto, T. (2000) Tamoxifen and gonadal steroids inhibit colon cancer growth in association with inhibition of thymidylate synthase, survivin and telomerase expression through estrogen receptor beta mediated system. *Cancer Lett.*, **161**, 63–71

Naldi, L., Altieri, A., Imberti, G.L., Giordano, L., Gallus, S. & La Vecchia, C. on behalf of the Oncology Study Group of the Italian Group for Epidemiologic Research in Dermatology (GISED) (2005) Cutaneous malignant melanoma in women. Phenotypic characteristics, sun exposure, and hormonal factors: A case–control study from Italy. *Ann. Epidemiol.*, **15**, 545–550

Nanda, K., Bastian, L.A., Hasselblad, V. & Simel, D.L. (1999) Hormone replacement therapy and the risk of colorectal cancer: A meta-analysis. *Obstet. Gynecol.* **93**, 880–888

Narod, S.A., Risch, H., Moslehi, R., Dorum, A., Neuhausen, S., Olsson, H., Provencher, D., Radice, P., Evans, G., Bishop, S., Brunet, J.-S. & Ponder, B.A.J. for the Hereditary Ovarian Cancer Clinical Study Group (1998) Oral contraceptives and the risk of hereditary ovarian cancer. *New Engl. J. Med.*, **339**, 424–428

Narod, S.A., Dube, M.P., Klijn, J., Lubinski, J., Lynch, H.T., Ghadirian, P., Provencher, D., Heimdal, K., Moller, P., Robson, M., Offit, K., Isaacs, C., Weber, B., Friedman, E., Gershoni-Baruch, R., Rennert, G., Pasini, B., Wagner, T., Daly, M., Garber, J.E., Neuhausen, S.L., Ainsworth, P., Olsson, H., Evans, G., Osborne, M., Couch, F., Foulkes, W.D., Warner, E., Kim-Sing, C., Olopade, O., Tung, N., Saal, H.M., Weitzel, J., Merajver, S., Gauthier-Villars, M., Jernstrom, H., Sun, P. & Brunet, J.-S. (2002) Oral contraceptives and the risk of breast cancer in BRCA1 and BRCA2 mutation carriers. *J. natl Cancer Inst.*, **94**, 1773–1779

Nelson, R.A., Levine, A.M. & Bernstein, L. (2001) Reproductive factors and risk of intermediate- or high-grade B-cell non-Hodgkin's lymphoma in women. *J. clin. Oncol.*, **19**, 1381–1387

Ness, R.B., Grisso, J.A., Klapper, J., Schlesselman, J.J., Silberzweig, S., Vergona, R., Morgan, M., Wheeler, J.E. & the SHARE Study Group (2000) Risk of ovarian cancer in relation to estrogen and progestin dose and use characteristics of oral contraceptives. *Am. J. Epidemiol.*, **152**, 233–241

Ness, R.B., Grisso, J.A., Vergona, R., Klapper, J., Morgan, M. & Wheeler, J.E. for the Study of Health and Reproduction (SHARE) Study Group (2001) Oral contraceptives, other methods of contraception, and risk reduction for ovarian cancer. *Epidemiology*, **12**, 307–312

Neuberger, J., Forman, D., Doll, R. & Williams, R. (1986) Oral contraceptives and hepatocellular carcinoma. *Br. med. J.*, **292**, 1355

Newbold, R.R. & Liehr, J.G. (2000) Induction of uterine adenocarcinoma in CD-1 mice by catechol estrogens. *Cancer Res.*, **60**, 235–237

Newbold, R.R., Bullock, B.C. & McLachlan, J.A. (1990) Uterine adenocarcinoma in mice following developmental treatment with estrogens: A model for hormonal carcinogenesis. *Cancer Res.*, **50**, 7677–7681

Newcomb, P.A. & Trentham-Dietz, A. (2003) Patterns of postmenopausal progestin use with estrogen in relation to endometrial cancer (United States). *Cancer Causes Control*, **14**, 195–201

Newcomer, L.M., Newcomb, P.A., Trentham-Dietz, A., Longnecker, M.P. & Greenberg, E.R. (2003) Oral contraceptive use and risk of breast cancer by histologic type. *Int. J. Cancer*, **106**, 961–964

Newfield, L., Bradlow, H.L., Sepkovic, D.W. & Auborn, K. (1998) Estrogen metabolism and the malignant potential of human papillomavirus immortalized keratinocytes. *Proc. Soc. exp. Biol. Med.*, **217**, 322–326

Nichols, H.B., Trentham-Dietz, A., Hampton, J.M. & Newcomb, P.A. (2005) Oral contraceptive use, reproductive factors, and colorectal cancer risk: Findings from Wisconsin. *Cancer Epidemiol. Biomarkers Prev.*, **14**, 1212–1218

Nonogaki, H., Fujii, S., Konishi, I., Nanbu, Y., Ozaki, S., Ishikawa, Y. & Mori, T. (1990) Estrogen receptor localization in normal and neoplastic epithelium of the uterine cervix. *Cancer*, **66**, 2620–2627

Norman, S.A., Berlin, J.A., Weber, A.L., Strom, B.L., Daling, J.R., Weiss, L.K., Marchbanks, P.A., Bernstein, L., Voigt, L.F., McDonald, J.A., Ursin, G., Liff, J.M., Burkman, R.T., Malone, K.E., Simon, M.S., Folger, S.G., Deapen, D., Wingo, P.A. & Spirtas, R. (2003) Combined effect of oral contraceptive use and hormone replacement therapy on breast cancer risk in postmenopausal women. *Cancer Causes Control*, **14**, 933–943

Odlind, V., Weiner, E., Victor, A. & Johansson, E.D.B. (1979) Plasma levels of norethindrone after single oral dose administration of norethindrone and lynestrenol. *Clin. Endocrinol.*, **10**, 29–38

Oehler, M.K., MacKenzie, I.Z., Wallwiener, D., Bicknell, R. & Rees, M.C.P. (2002) Wnt-7a is upregulated by norethisterone in human endometrial epithelial cells: A possible mechanism by which progestogens reduce the risk of estrogen-induced endometrial neoplasia. *Cancer Lett.*, **186**, 75–81

Oelkers, W. (2004) Drospirenone, a progestogen with antimineralocorticoid properties: A short review. *Mol. cell. Endocrinol.*, **217**, 255–261

Oettel, M., Bervoas-Martin, E.W., Golbs, S., Hobe, G., Kaufmann, G., Mathieu, M., Moore, C., Puri, C., Ritter, P., Reddersen, G., Schön, R., Strauch, G. & Zimmermann, H. (1995) A 19-nor-progestin without a 17α-ethinyl group. I. Dienogest from a pharmacokinetic point of view. *Drugs Today*, **31**, 499–516

Olshan, A.F., Smith, J., Cook, M.N., Grufferman, S., Pollock, B.H., Stram, D.O., Seeger, R.C., Look, A.T., Cohn, S.L., Castleberry, R.P. & Bondy, M.L. (1999) Hormone and fertility drug use and the risk of neuroblastoma: A report from the Children's Cancer Group and the Pediatric Oncology Group. *Am. J. Epidemiol.*, **150**, 930–938

Oosterbaan, H.P. (1999) An open-label study of the effects of a 24-day regimen of gestodene 60 µg/ethinylestradiol 15 µg on endometrial histological findings in healthy women. *Eur. J. Contracept. reprod. Health Care*, **4**, 3–8

Orme, M., Back, D.J., Ward, S. & Green, S. (1991) The pharmacokinetics of ethynylestradiol in the presence and absence of gestodene and desogestrel. *Contraception*, **43**, 305–316

Østerlind, A., Tucker, M.A., Stone, B.J. & Jensen, O.M. (1988) The Danish case–control study of cutaneous malignant melanoma. III. Hormonal and reproductive factors in women. *Int. J. Cancer*, **42**, 821–824

Pakarinen, P., Lahteenmaki, P. & Rutanen, E.-M. (1999) The effect of intrauterine and oral levonorgestrel administration on serum concentrations of sex hormone-binding globulin, insulin and insulin-like growth factor binding protein-1. *Acta obstet. gynaecol. scand.*, **78**, 423–428

Palmer, J.R., Rosenberg, L., Kaufman, D.W., Warshauer, M.E., Stolley, P. & Shapiro, S. (1989) Oral contraceptive use and liver cancer. *Am. J. Epidemiol.*, **130**, 878–882

Palmer, J.R., Rosenberg, L., Strom, B.L., Harlap, S., Zauber, A.G., Warshauer, E.M. & Shapiro, S. (1992) Oral contraceptive use and risk of cutaneous malignant melanoma. *Cancer Causes Control*, **3**, 547–554

Palmer, J.R., Driscoll, S.G., Rosenberg, L., Berkowitz, R.S., Lurain, J.R., Soper, J., Twiggs, L.B., Gershenson, D.M., Kohorn, E.I., Berman, M., Shapiro, S. & Rao, R.S. (1999) Oral contraceptive use and risk of gestational trophoblastic tumors. *J. natl Cancer Inst.*, **91**, 635–640

Parazzini, F., La Vecchia, C., Negri, E., Bocciolone, L., Fedele, L. & Franceschi, S. (1991a) Oral contraceptives use and the risk of ovarian cancer: An Italian case–control study. *Eur. J. Cancer*, **27**, 594–598

Parazzini, F., Restelli, C., La Vecchia, C., Negri, E., Chiari, S., Maggi, R. & Mangioni, C. (1991b) Risk factors for epithelial ovarian tumours of borderline malignancy. *Int. J. Epidemiol.*, **20**, 871–877

Parazzini, F., La Vecchia, C., Negri, E. & Villa, A. (1994) Estrogen replacement therapy and ovarian cancer risk. *Int. J. Cancer*, **57**, 135–136

Parazzini, F., Cipriani, S., Mangili, G., Garavaglia, E., Guarnerio, P., Ricci, E., Benzi, G., Salerio, B., Polverino, G. & La Vecchia, C. (2002) Oral contraceptives and risk of gestational trophoblastic disease. *Contraception*, **65**, 425–427

Parazzini, F., Chiaffarino, F., Negri, E., Surace, M., Benzi, G., Franceschi, S., Fedele, L. & La Vecchia, C. (2004) Risk factors for different histological types of ovarian cancer. *Int. J. Gynecol. Cancer*, **14**, 431–436

Parkin, D.M., Srivatanakul, P., Khlat, M., Chenvidhya, D., Chotiwan, P., Insiripong, S., L'Abbé, K.A. & Wild, C.P. (1991) Liver cancer in Thailand. I. A case–control study of cholangiocarcinoma. *Int. J. Cancer*, **48**, 323–328

Parslov, M., Lidegaard, O., Klintorp, S., Pedersen, B., Jonsson, L., Eriksen, P.S. & Ottesen, B. (2000) Risk factors among young women with endometrial cancer: A Danish case–control study. *Am. J. Obstet. Gynecol.*, **182**, 23–29

Persson, I., Schmidt, M., Adami, H.-O., Bergstrom, R., Pettersson, B. & Sparen, P. (1990) Trends in endometrial cancer incidence and mortality in Sweden, 1960–84. *Cancer Causes Control*, **1**, 201–208

Peters, R.K., Pike, M.C., Chang, W.W.L. & Mack, T.M. (1990) Reproductive factors and colon cancers. *Br. J. Cancer*, **61**, 741–748

Pettersson, B., Adami, H.-O., Bergström, R. & Johansson, E.D.B. (1986) Menstruation span — A time-limited risk factor for endometrial carcinoma. *Acta Obstet. Gynecol. Scand.*, **65**, 247–255

Piccinino, L.J. & Mosher, W.D. (1998) Trends in contraceptive use in the United States: 1982–1995. *Fam. Plann. Perspect.*, **30**, 4–10

Piérard-Franchimont, C., Gaspard, U., Lacante, P., Rhoa, M., Slachmuylders, P. & Piérard, G.E. (2000) A quantitative biometrological assessment of acne and hormonal evaluation in young women using a triphasic low-dose oral contraceptive containing gestodene. *Eur. J. Contracept. reprod. Health Care*, **5**, 275–286

Pietras, R.J., Nemere, I. & Szego, C.M. (2001) Steroid hormone receptors in target cell membranes. *Endocrine*, **14**, 417–427

Pihan, G.A., Purohit, A., Wallace, J., Knecht, H., Woda, B., Quesenberry, P. & Doxsey, S.J. (1998) Centrosome defects and genetic instability in malignant tumors. *Cancer Res.*, **58**, 3974–3985

Pike, M.C., Pearce, C.L., Peters, R., Cozen, W., Wan, P. & Wu, A.H. (2004) Hormonal factors and the risk of invasive ovarian cancer: A population-based case–control study. *Fertil. Steril.*, **82**, 186–195

Pollow, K., Juchem, M., Elger, W., Jacobi, N., Hoffmann, G. & Mobus, V. (1992) Dihydrospirore-none (ZK30595): A novel synthetic progestagen — characterization of binding to different receptor proteins. *Contraception*, **46**, 561–574

Polychronopoulou, A., Tzonou, A., Hsieh, C., Kaprinis, G., Rebelakos, A., Toupadaki, N. & Trichopoulos, D. (1993) Reproductive variables, tobacco, ethanol, coffee and somatometry as risk factors for ovarian cancer. *Int. J. Cancer*, **55**, 402–407

Potter, J.D. & McMichael, A.J. (1983) Large bowel cancer in women in relation to reproductive and hormonal factors: A case–control study. *J. natl Cancer Inst.*, **71**, 703–709

Purdie, D., Green, A., Bain, C., Siskind, V., Ward, B., Hacker, N., Quinn, M., Wright, G., Russell, P. & Susil, B. for the Survey of Women's Health Group (1995) Reproductive and other factors and risk of epithelial ovarian cancer: An Australian case–control study. *Int. J. Cancer*, **62**, 678–684

Purdie, D.M., Siskind, V., Bain, C.J., Webb, P.M. & Green, A.C. (2001) Reproduction-related risk factors for mucinous and nonmucinous epithelial ovarian cancer. *Am. J. Epidemiol.*, **153**, 860–864

Rabe, T., Bohlmann, M.K., Rehberger-Schneider, S. & Prifti, S. (2000) Induction of estrogen receptor-alpha and -beta activities by synthetic progestins. *Gynecol. Endocrinol.*, **14**, 118–126

Ramcharan S., Pellegrin, F.A., Ray, R. & Hsu, J.P. (1981) *The Walnut Creek Contraceptive Study. A Prospective Study of the Side Effects of Oral Contraceptives*, Vol. III (NIH Publ. No. 81-564), Bethesda, MD, National Institutes of Health

Razandi, M., Pedram, A., Park, S.T. & Levin, E.R. (2003) Proximal events in signaling by plasma membrane estrogen receptors. *J. biol. Chem.*, **278**, 2701–2712

Richardson, H., Abrahamowicz, M., Tellier, P.-P., Kelsall, G., du Berger, R., Ferenczy, A., Coutlée, F. & Franco, E.L. (2005) Modifiable risk factors associated with clearance of type-specific cervical human papillomavirus infections in a cohort of university students. *Cancer Epidemiol. Biomarkers*, **14**, 1149–1156

Riley, R.R., Duensing, S., Brake, T., Munger, K., Lambert, P.F. & Arbeit, J.M. (2003) Dissection of human papillomavirus E6 and E7 function in transgenic mouse models of cervical carcinogenesis. *Cancer Res.*, **63**, 4862–4871

Riman, T., Dickman, P.W., Nilsson, S., Correia, N., Nordlinder, H., Magnusson, C.M. & Persson, I.R. (2001) Risk factors for epithelial borderline ovarian tumors: Results of a Swedish case–control study. *Gynecol. Oncol.*, **83**, 575–585

Riman, T., Dickman, P.W., Nilsson, S., Correia, N., Nordlinder, H., Magnusson, C.M. & Persson, I.R. (2002) Risk factors for invasive epithelial ovarian cancer: Results from a Swedish case–control study. *Am. J. Epidemiol.*, **156**, 363–373

Risch, H.A., Weiss, N.S., Lyon, J.L., Daling, J.R. & Liff, J.M. (1983) Events of reproductive life and the incidence of epithelial ovarian cancer. *Am. J. Epidemiol.*, **117**, 128–139

Risch, H.A., Marrett, L.D. & Howe, G.R. (1994) Parity, contraception, infertility, and the risk of epithelial ovarian cancer. *Am. J. Epidemiol.*, **140**, 585–597

Risch, H.A., Marrett, L.D., Jain, M. & Howe, G.R. (1996) Differences in risk factors for epithelial ovarian cancer by histologic type. Results of a case–control study. *Am. J. Epidemiol.*, **144**, 363–372

Rodriguez, G.C., Walmer, D.K., Cline, M., Krigman, H., Lessey, B.A., Whitaker, R.S., Dodge, R. & Hughes, C.L. (1998) Effect of progestin on the ovarian epithelium of macaques: Cancer prevention through apoptosis? *J. Soc. gynecol. Invest.*, **5**, 271–276

Rodriguez, G.C., Nagarsheth, N.P., Lee, K.L., Bentley, R.C., Walmer, D.K., Cline, M., Whitaker, R.S., Isner, P., Berchuck, A., Dodge, R.K. & Hughes, C.L. (2002) Progestin-induced apoptosis in the Macaque ovarian epithelium: Differential regulation of transforming growth factor-beta. *J. natl Cancer. Inst.*, **94**, 50–60

Rooks, J.B., Ory, H.W., Ishak, K.G., Strauss, L.T., Greenspan, J.R., Hill, A.P. & Tyler, C.W. (1979) Epidemiology of hepatocellular adenoma. The role of oral contraceptive use. *J. Am. med. Assoc.*, **242**, 644–648

Rosenberg, L., Shapiro, S., Slone, D., Kaufman, D.W., Helmrich, S.P., Miettinen, P.S., Stolley, P.D., Rosenshein, N.B., Schottenfeld, D. & Engle, R.L., Jr (1982) Epithelial ovarian cancer and combination oral contraceptives. *J. Am. med. Assoc.*, **247**, 3210–3212

Rosenberg, L., Palmer, J.R., Zauber, A.G., Warshauer, M.E., Lewis, J.L., Jr, Strom, B.L., Harlap, S. & Shapiro, S. (1994) A case–control study of oral contraceptive use and invasive epithelial ovarian cancer. *Am. J. Epidemiol.*, **139**, 654–661

Rosenblatt, K.A., Thomas, D.B. & The WHO Collaborative Study of Neoplasia and Steroid Contraceptives (1991) Hormonal content of combined oral contraceptives in relation to the reduced risk of endometrial carcinoma. *Int. J. Cancer*, **49**, 870–874

Rosenblatt, K.A., Carter, J.J., Iwasaki, L.M., Galloway, D.A. & Stanford, J.L. (2004) Contraceptive methods and induced abortions and their association with the risk of colon cancer in Shanghai, China. *Eur. J. Cancer*, **40**, 590–593

Ross, J., Hardee, K., Mumford, E. & Eid, S. (2002) Contraceptive method choice in developing countries. *Int. Fam. Plann. Perspect.*, **28**, 32–40

Rossing, M.A., Voigt, L.F., Wicklund, K.G., Williams, M. & Daling, J.R. (1998) Use of exogenous hormones and risk of papillary thyroid cancer (Washington, United States). *Cancer Causes Control*, **9**, 341–349

Royar, J., Becher, H. & Chang-Claude, J. (2001) Low-dose oral contraceptives: Protective effect on ovarian cancer risk. *Int. J. Cancer*, **95**, 370–374

Rübig, A. (2003) Drospirenone: A new cardiovascular-active progestin with antialdosterone and antiandrogenic properties. *Climacteric*, **6** (Suppl. 3), 49–54

Russo, I.H. & Russo, J. (1996) Mammary gland neoplasia in long-term rodent studies. *Environ. Health Perspect.*, **104**, 938–967

Sager, G., Orbo, A., Jaeger, R. & Engström, C. (2003) Non-genomic effects of progestins — Inhibition of cell growth and increased intracellular levels of cyclic nucleotides. *J. ster. Biochem. mol. Biol.*, **84**, 1–8

Sakoda, L.C. & Horn-Ross, P.L. (2002) Reproductive and menstrual history and papillary thyroid cancer risk: The San Francisco Bay Area Thyroid Cancer Study. *Cancer Epidemiol. Biomarkers Prev.*, **11**, 51–57

Salazar, E.L., Mercado, E., Sojo, I. & Salcedo, M. (2001) Relationship between estradiol 16 alpha-hydroxylation and human papillomavirus infection in cervical cell transformation. *Gynecol. Endocrinol.*, **15**, 335–340

Salazar-Martinez, E., Lazcano-Ponce, E.C., Gonzalez Lira-Lira, G., Escudero-De Los, R.P., Salmeron-Castro, J. & Hernandez-Avila, M. (1999) Reproductive factors of ovarian and endometrial cancer risk in a high fertility population in Mexico. *Cancer Res.*, **59**, 3658–3662

Salmen, T., Heikkinen, A.-M., Mahonen, A., Kroger, H., Komulainen, M., Pallonen, H., Saarikoski, S., Honkanen, R. & Maenpää, P.H. (2003) Relation of aromatase gene polymorphism and hormone replacement therapy to serum estradiol levels, bone mineral density, and fracture risk in early postmenopausal women. *Ann. Med.*, **35**, 282–288

Santillán, R., Pérez-Palacios, G., Reyes, M., Damian-Matsumura, P., Garcia, G.A., Grillasca, I. & Lemus, A.E. (2001) Assessment of the oestrogenic activity of the contraceptive progestin levonorgestrel and its non-phenolic metabolites. *Eur. J. Pharmacol.*, **427**, 167–174

dos Santos Silva, I. & Swerdlow, A.J. (1995) Recent trends in incidence of and mortality from breast, ovarian and endometrial cancers in England and Wales and their relation to changing fertility and oral contraceptive use. *Br. J. Cancer*, **72**, 485–492

Sarkar, N.N. (2003) Steroidal contraceptive vaginal rings. *Int. J. clin. Pract.*, **57**, 392–395

Schiff, D., Suman, V.J., Yang, P., Rocca, W.A. & O'Neill, B.P. (1998) Risk factors for primary central nervous system lymphoma. *Cancer*, **82**, 975–982

Schildkraut, J.M., Calingaert, B., Marchbanks, P.A., Moorman, P.G. & Rodriguez, G.C. (2002) Impact of progestin and estrogen potency in oral contraceptives on ovarian cancer risk. *J. natl Cancer Inst.*, **94**, 32–38

Schindler, A.E., Campagnoli, C., Druckmann, R., Huber, J., Pasqualini, J.R., Schweppe, K.W. & Thijssen, J.H.H. (2003) Classification and pharmacology of progestins. *Maturitas*, **46** (Suppl. 1), 7–16

Schlesselman, J.J., Stadel, B.V., Korper, M., Yu, W. & Wingo, P.A. (1992) Breast cancer detection in relation to oral contraception. *J. clin. Epidemiol.*, **45**, 449–459

Schoonen, W.G.E.J., Dijkema, R., de Ries, R.J.H., Wagenaars, J.L., Joosten, J.W.H., de Gooyer, M.E., Deckers, G.H. & Kloosterboer, H.J. (1998) Human progesterone receptor A and B isoforms in CHO cells. II. Comparison of binding, transactivation and ED_{50} values of several synthetic (anti)progestagens *in vitro* in CHO and MCF-7 cells and *in vivo* in rabbits and rats. *J. Ster. Biochem. mol. Biol.*, **64**, 157–170

Schoonen, W.G.E.J., Deckers, G., de Gooijer, M.E., de Ries, R., Mathijssen-Mommers, G., Hamersma, H. & Kloosterboer, H.J. (2000) Contraceptive progestins. Various 11-substituents combined with four 17-substituents: 17alpha-Ethynyl, five- and six-membered spiromethylene ethers or six-membered spiromethylene lactones. *J. ster. Biochem. mol. Biol.*, **74**, 109–123

Schüz, J., Kaletsch, U., Meinert, R., Kaatsch, P., Spix, C. & Michaelis, J. (2001) Risk factors for neuroblastoma at different stages of disease. Results from a population-based case–control study in Germany. *J. clin. Epidemiol.*, **54**, 702–709

Seeger, H., Wallwiener, D. & Mueck, A.O. (2003) The effect of progesterone and synthetic pro-gestins on serum- and estradiol-stimulated proliferation of human breast cancer cells. *Horm. Metab. Res.*, **35**, 76–80

Shampo, M.A. & Kyle, R.A. (2004) John Rock: Pioneer in the development of oral contraceptives. *Mayo Clin. Proc.*, **79**, 844

Shapiro, S., Rosenberg, L., Hoffman, M., Truter, H., Cooper, D., Rao, S., Dent, D., Gudgeon, A., van Zyl, J., Katzenellenbogen, J. & Baillie, R. (2000) Risk of breast cancer in relation to the use of injectable progestogen contraceptives and combined estrogen/progestogen contra-ceptives. *Am. J. Epidemiol.*, **151**, 396–403

Shapiro, S., Rosenberg, L., Hoffman, M., Kelly, J.P., Cooper, D.D., Carrara, H., Denny, L.E., du Toit, G., Allan, B.R., Stander, J.A. & Williamson, A.L. (2003) Risk of invasive cancer of the cervix in relation to the use of injectable progestogen contraceptives and combined estrogen/progestogen oral contraceptives (South Africa). *Cancer Causes Control*, **14**, 485–495

Shenfield, G.M. (1993) Oral contraceptives. Are drug interactions of clinical significance? *Drug Saf.*, **9**, 21–37

Shields, T.S., Brinton, L.A., Burk, R.D., Wang, S.S., Weinstein, S.J., Ziegler, R.G., Studentsov, Y.Y., McAdams, M. & Schiffman, M. (2004) A case–control study of risk factors for invasive cervical cancer among US women exposed to oncogenic types of human papillomavirus. *Cancer Epidemiol. Biomarkers Prev.*, **13**, 1574–1582

Shields-Botella, J., Duc, I., Duranti, E., Puccio, F., Bonnet, P., Delansorne, R. & Paris, J. (2003) An overview of nomegestrol acetate selective receptor binding and lack of estrogenic action on hormone-dependent cancer cells. *J. ster. Biochem. mol. Biol.*, **87**, 111–122

Shu, X.O., Brinton, L.A., Gao, Y.T. & Yuan, J.M. (1989) Population-based case–control study of ovarian cancer in Shanghai. *Cancer Res.*, **49**, 3670–3674

Shu, X.O., Brinton, L.A., Zheng, W., Gao, Y.T., Fan, J. & Fraumeni, J.F., Jr (1991) A population-based case–control study of endometrial cancer in Shanghai, China. *Int. J. Cancer*, **49**, 38–43

Siddique, Y.H. & Afzal, M. (2004) Evaluation of genotoxic potential of synthetic progestin chlor-madinone acetate. *Toxicol. Lett.*, **153**, 221–225

Siddique, Y.H., Beg, T. & Afzal, M. (2005) Genotoxic potential of ethinylestradiol in cultured mammalian cells. *Chem.-biol. Interact.*, **151**, 133–141

Silins, I., Wang, X., Tadesse, A., Jansen, K.U., Schiller, J.T., Avall-Lundqvis, E., Frankendal, B. & Dillner, J. (2004) A population-based study of cervical carcinoma and HPV infection in Latvia. *Gynecol. Oncol.*, **93**, 484–492

Singh, S., Poulsom, R., Hanby, M.A., Rogers, L.A., Wright, N.A., Sheppard, M.C. & Langman, M.J.S. (1998) Expression of oestrogen receptor and oestrogen-inducible genes pS2 and ERD5 in large bowel mucosa and cancer. *J. Pathol.*, **184**, 153–160

Sisenwine, S.F., Kimmel, H.B., Liu, A.L. & Ruelius, H.W. (1975a) Excretion and stereoselective biotransformations of *dl*-, *d*- and *l*-norgestrel in women. *Drug Metab. Dispos.*, **3**, 180–188

Sisenwine, S.F., Kimmel, H.B., Liu, A.L. & Ruelius, H.W. (1975b) The presence of *dl*-, *d*- and *l*-norgestrel and their metabolites in the plasma of women. *Contraception*, **12**, 339–353

Siskind, V., Green, A., Bain, C. & Purdie, D. (2000) Beyond ovulation: Oral contraceptives and epithelial ovarian cancer. *Epidemiology*, **11**, 106–110

Sitruk-Ware, R. (2002) Progestogens in hormonal replacement therapy: New molecules, risks, and benefits. *Menopause*, **9**, 6–15

Sitruk-Ware, R. (2004a) New progestogens: A review of their effects in perimenopausal and post-menopausal women. *Drugs Aging*, **21**, 865–883

Sitruk-Ware, R. (2004b) Pharmacological profile of progestins. *Maturitas*, **47**, 277–283

Skinner, H.G., Michaud, D.S., Colditz, G.A., Giovannucci, E.L., Stampfer, M.J., Willett, W.C. & Fuchs, C.S. (2003) Parity, reproductive factors, and the risk of pancreatic cancer in women. *Cancer Epidemiol. Biomarkers Prev.*, **12**, 433–438

Slattery, M.L., Samowitz, W.S. & Holden, J.A. (2000) Estrogen and progesterone receptors in colon tumors. *Am. J. clin. Pathol.*, **113**, 364–368

Smirnoff, P., Liel, Y., Gnainsky, J., Shany, S. & Schwartz, B. (1999) The protective effect of estrogen against chemically induced murine colon carcinogenesis is associated with decreased CpG island methylation and increased mRNA and protein expression of the colonic vitamin D receptor. *Oncol. Res.*, **11**, 255–264

Smith, M.A., Fine, J.A., Barnhill, R.L. & Berwick, M. (1998) Hormonal and reproductive influences and risk of melanoma in women. *Int. epidemiol. Assoc.*, **27**, 751–757

Smith, J.S., Green, J., Berrington de Gonzalez, A., Appleby, P., Peto, J., Plummer, M., Franceschi, S. & Beral, V. (2003) Cervical cancer and use of hormonal contraceptives: A systematic review. *Lancet*, **361**, 1159–1167

Song, R.X., Santen, R.J., Kumar, R., Adam, L., Jeng, M.-H., Masamura, S. & Yue, W. (2002) Adaptive mechanisms induced by long-term estrogen deprivation in breast cancer cells. *Mol. cell. Endocrinol.*, **193**, 29–42

Song, R.X., Barnes, C.J., Zhang, Z., Bao, Y., Kumar, R. & Santen, R.J. (2004) The role of Shc and insulin-like growth factor 1 receptor in mediating the translocation of estrogen receptor ? to the plasma membrane. *Proc. natl Acad. Sci. USA*, **101**, 2076–2081

Stanczyk, F.Z. (2003) All progestins are not created equal. *Steroids*, **68**, 879–890

Stanczyk, F.Z. & Roy, S. (1990) Metabolism of levonorgestrel, norethindrone, and structurally related contraceptive steroids. *Contraception*, **42**, 67–96

Stanczyk, F.Z., Mroszczak, E.J., Ling, T., Runkel, R., Henzl, M., Miyakawa, I. & Goebelsmann, U. (1983) Plasma levels and pharmacokinetics of norethindrone and ethinylestradiol administered in solution and as tablets to women. *Contraception*, **28**, 241–251

Stanczyk, F.Z., Lobo, R.A., Chiang, S.T. & Woutersz, T.B. (1990) Pharmacokinetic comparison of two triphasic oral contraceptive formulations containing levonorgestrel and ethinylestradiol. *Contraception*, **41**, 39–53

Stanford, J.L., Brinton, L.A., Berman, M.L., Mortel, R., Twiggs, L.B., Barrett, R.J., Wilbanks, G.D. & Hoover, R.N. (1993) Oral contraceptives and endometrial cancer: Do other risk factors modify the association? *Int. J. Cancer*, **54**, 243–248

Sturdee, D.W., Rantala, M.L., Colau, J.C., Zahradnik, H.P., Riphagen, F.E. & Multicenter MLS Investigators (2004) The acceptability of small intrauterine progestogen-releasing system for continuous combined hormone therapy in early postmenopausal women. *Climacteric*, **7**, 404–411

Sulak, P.J. (2004) Contraceptive redesign: New progestins/new regimens. *J. Fam. Pract.*, **Suppl.**, S3–S8

Sutter-Dub, M.-T. (2002) Rapid non-genomic and genomic responses to progestogens, estrogens, and glucocorticoids in the endocrine pancreatic B cell, the adipocyte and other cell types. *Steroids*, **67**, 77–93

Swerdlow, A.J., English, J., MacKie, R.M., O'Doherty, C.J., Hunter, J.A.A., Clark, J. & Hole, D.J. (1986) Benign melanocytic naevi as a risk factor for malignant melanoma. *Br. med. J.*, **292**, 1555–1559

Taioli, E. & Wynder, E.L. (1994) Re: Endocrine factors and adenocarcinoma of the lung in women. *J. natl Cancer Inst.*, **86**, 869–870

Takahashi, M., Shimomoto, T., Miyajima, T.K., Yoshida, M., Katashima S., Uematsu, F., Maekawa, A. & Nakae, D. (2004) Effects of estrogens and metabolites on endometrial carcinogenesis in young adult mice initiated with *N*-ethyl-*N'*-nitro-*N*-nitrosoguanidine. *Cancer Lett.*, **211**, 1–9

Tarone, R.E. & Chu, K.C. (2000) Age-period-cohort analyses of breast-, ovarian-, endometrial- and cervical-cancer mortality rates for Caucasian women in the USA. *J. Epidemiol. Biostat.*, **5**, 221–231

Tauber, U., Tack, J.W. & Matthes, H. (1989) Single dose pharmacokinetics of gestodene in women after intravenous and oral administration. *Contraception*, **40**, 461–479

Tavani, A., Negri, E., Parazzini, F., Franceschi, S. & La Vecchia, C. (1993) Female hormone utilisation and risk of hepatocellular carcinoma. *Br. J. Cancer*, **67**, 635–637

Tavani, A., Ricci, E., La Vecchia, C., Surace, M., Benzi, G., Parazzini, F. & Franceschi, S. (2000) Influence of menstrual and reproductive factors on ovarian cancer risk in women with and without family history of breast or ovarian cancer. *Int. J. Epidemiol.*, **29**, 799–802

Tavani, A., Bosetti, C., Dal Maso, L., Giordano, L., Franceschi, S. & La Vecchia, C. (2004) Influence of selected hormonal and lifestyle factors on familial propensity to ovarian cancer. *Gynecol. Oncol.*, **92**, 922–926

Teichmann, A. (2003) Pharmacology of estradiol valerate/dienogest. *Climacteric*, **6** (Suppl. 2), 17–23

Terry, M.B., Gammon, M.D., Schoenberg, J.B., Brinton, L.A., Arber, N. & Hibshoosh, H. (2002) Oral contraceptive use and cyclin D1 overexpression in breast cancer among young women. *Cancer Epidemiol. Biomarkers Prev.*, **11**, 1100–1103

Tessaro, S., Beria, J.U., Tomasi, E. & Barros, A.J. (2001) [Oral contraceptive and breast cancer: A case–control study]. *Rev. Saude publica*, **35**, 32–38 (in Spanish)

Thomas, D.B., Ray, R.M., Koetsawang, A., Kiviat, N., Kuypers, J., Qin, Q., Ashley, R.L. & Koetsawang, S. (2001a) Human papillomaviruses and cervical cancer in Bangkok. I. Risk factors for invasive cervical carcinomas with human papillomavirus types 16 and 18 DNA. *Am. J. Epidemiol.*, **153**, 723–731

Thomas, D.B., Qin, Q., Kuypers, J., Kiviat, N., Ashley, R.I., Koetsawang, A., Ray, R.M. & Koetsawang, S. (2001b) Human papillomaviruses and cervical cancer in Bangkok. II. Risk factors for *in situ* and invasive squamous cell cervical carcinomas. *Am. J. Epidemiol.*, **153**, 732–739

Thomas, D.B., Ray, R.M., Qin, Q. & the WHO Collaborative Study of Neoplasia and Steroid Contraceptives (2002) Risk factors for progression of squamous cell cervical carcinoma *in situ* to invasive cervical cancer: Results of a multinational study. *Cancer Causes Control*, **13**, 683–690

Tofteng, C.L., Kindmark, A., Brandstrom, H., Abrahamsen, B., Petersen, S., Stiger, F., Stilgren, L.S., Jensen, J.E.B., Vestergaard, P., Langdahl, B.L. & Mosekilde, L. (2004) Polymorphisms in the *CYP19* and *AR* genes — Relation to bone mass and longitudinal bone changes in postmenopausal women with or without hormone replacement therapy: The Danish Osteoporosis Prevention Study. *Calcif. Tissue int.*, **74**, 25–34

Topinka, J., Oesterle, D., Reimann, R. & Wolff, T. (2004a) No-effect level in the mutagenic activity of the drug cyproterone acetate in rat liver. Part I. Single dose treatment. *Mutat. Res.*, **550**, 89–99

Topinka, J., Oesterle, D., Reimann, R. & Wolff, T. (2004b) No-effect level in the mutagenic activity of the drug cyproterone acetate in rat liver. Part II. Multiple dose treatment. *Mutat. Res.*, **550**, 101–108

Trapido, E.J. (1983) A prospective cohort study of oral contraceptives and cancer of the endometrium. *Int. J. Epidemiol.*, **12**, 297–300

Troisi, R., Schairer, C., Chow, W.-H., Schatzkin, A., Brinton, L.A. & Fraumeni, J.F., Jr (1997) A prospective study of menopausal hormones and risk of colorectal cancer (United States). *Cancer Causes Control*, **8**, 130–138

Tsukada, T., Tomooka, Y., Takai, S., Ueda, Y., Nishikawa, S., Yagi, T., Tokunaga, T., Takeda, N., Suda, Y., Abe, S., Matsuo, I., Ikawa, Y. & Aizawa, S. (1993) Enhanced proliferative potential in culture of cells from p53-deficient mice. *Oncogene*, **8**, 3313–3322

Tuba, Z., Bardin, C.W., Dancsi, A., Francsics-Czinege, E., Molnar, C., Csorgei, J., Falkay, G., Koide, S.S., Kumar, N., Sundaram, K., Dukat-Abrok, V. &. Balogh, G. (2000) Synthesis and biological activity of a new progestogen, 16-methylene-17alpha-hydroxy-18-methyl-19-norpregn-4-ene-3,20-dione acetate. *Steroids*, **65**, 266–274

Tung, K.H., Goodman, M.T., Wu, A.H., McDuffie, K., Wilkens, L.R., Kolonel, L.N., Nomura, A.M., Terada, K.Y., Carney, M.E. & Sobin, L.H. (2003) Reproductive factors and epithelial ovarian cancer risk by histologic type: A multiethnic case–control study. *Am. J. Epidemiol.*, **158**, 629–638

Tzonou, A., Day, N.E., Trichopoulos, D., Walker, A., Saliaraki, M., Papapostolou, M. & Polychronopoulou, A. (1984) The epidemiology of ovarian cancer in Greece: A case–control study. *Eur. J. Cancer clin. Oncol.*, **20**, 1045–1052

United Nations (2004a) *World Population Monitoring 2002, Reproductive Rights and Reproductive Health* (ST/ESA/SER.A/215), New York, Department of Economic and Social Affairs, Population Division

United Nations (2004b) *Press Release: Majority of World's Couples of Reproductive Age are Using Contraception* (DEV/2469; POP/902), New York, Department of Public Information [http:// www.un.org/esa/population/publications/contraceptive2003/WallChart_CP2003_pressrelease. htm]

United Nations (2004c) *World Contraceptive Use 2003* (United Nations Publication, Sales No. E. Ø4.XIII.2), New York, Department of Economic and Social Affairs, Population Division

Ursin, G., Ross, R.K., Sullivan-Halley, J., Hanisch, R., Henderson, B. & Bernstein, L. (1998) Use of oral contraceptives and risk of breast cancer in young women. *Breast Cancer Res. Treat.*, **50**, 175–184

Ursin, G., Wu, A.H., Hoover, R.N., West, D.W., Nomura, A.M., Kolonel, L.N., Pike, M.C. & Ziegler, R.G. (1999) Breast cancer and oral contraceptive use in Asian–American women. *Am. J. Epidemiol.*, **150**, 561–567

Vall Mayans, M., Calvet, X., Bruix, J., Bruguera, M., Costa, J., Estève, J., Bosch, F.X., Bru, C. & Rodés, J. (1990) Risk factors for hepatocellular carcinoma in Catalonia, Spain. *Int. J. Cancer*, **46**, 378–381

Van Hoften, C., Burger, H., Peeters, P.H., Grobbee, D.E., Van Noord, P.A. & Leufkens, H.G. (2000) Long-term oral contraceptive use increases breast cancer risk in women over 55 years of age: The DOM cohort. *Int. J. Cancer*, **87**, 591–594

Van Vliet, H.A.A.M., Grimes, D.A., Helmerhorst, F.M. & Schulz, K.F. (2006a) Biphasic versus monophasic oral contraceptives for contraception (Review). *Cochrane Database Syst. Rev.*, **3**, Art. No. CD002032

Van Vliet, H.A.A.M., Grimes, D.A., Lopez, L.M., Schulz, K.F. & Helmerhorst, F.M. (2006b) Triphasic versus monophasic oral contraceptives for contraception. *Cochrane Database Syst. Rev.*, **3**, Art. No. CD003553

Van Vliet, H.A.A.M., Grimes, D.A., Helmerhorst, F.M. & Schulz, K.F. (2006c) Biphasic versus triphasic oral contraceptives for contraception (review). *Cochrane Database Syst. Rev.*, **3**, Art. No. CD003283

Vegeto, E., Shahbaz, M.M., Wen, D.X., Goldman, M.E., O'Malley, B.W. & McDonnell, D.P. (1993) Human progesterone receptor A form is a cell- and promoter-specific repressor of human progesterone receptor B function. *Mol. Endocrinol.*, **7**, 1244–1255

Vessey, M.P. & Painter, R. (1995) Endometrial and ovarian cancer and oral contraceptives — Findings in a large cohort study. *Br. J. Cancer*, **71**, 1340–1342

Vessey, M.P., Villard Mackintosh, L., McPherson, K. & Yeates, D. (1989) Mortality among oral contraceptive users: 20 year follow up of women in a cohort study. *Br. med. J.*, **299**, 1487–1491

Vessey, M., Painter, R. & Yeates, D. (2003) Mortality in relation to oral contraceptive use and cigarette smoking. *Lancet*, **362**, 185–191

de Villiers, E.-M. (2003) Relationship between steroid hormone contraceptives and HPV, cervical intraepithelial neoplasia and cervical carcinoma. *Int. J. Cancer*, **103**, 705–708

Voigt, L.F., Deng, Q. & Weiss, N.S. (1994) Recency, duration, and progestin content of oral contraceptives in relation to the incidence of endometrial cancer (Washington, USA). *Cancer Causes Control*, **5**, 227–233

Waetjen, L.E. & Grimes, D.A. (1996) Oral contraceptives and primary liver cancer: Temporal trends in three countries. *Obstet. Gynecol.*, **88**, 945–949

Waliszewski, P., Blaszczyk, M., Wolinska-Witort, E., Drews, M., Snochowski, M. & Hurst, R.E. (1997) Molecular study of sex steroid receptor gene expression in human colon and in colorectal carcinomas. *J. surg. Oncol.*, **64**, 3–11

Walker, G.R., Schlesselman, J.J. & Ness, R.B. (2002) Family history of cancer, oral contraceptive use, and ovarian cancer risk. *Am. J. Obstet. Gynecol.*, **186**, 8–14

van Wayenburg, C.A.M., van der Schouw, Y.T., van Noord, P.A.H. & Peeters, P.H.M. (2000) Age at menopause, body mass index, and the risk of colorectal cancer mortality in the Dutch Diagnostisch Onderzoek Mammacarcinoom (DOM) cohort. *Epidemiology*, **11**, 304–308

Weiderpass, E., Adami, H.-O., Baron, J.A., Magnusson, C., Lindgren, A. & Persson, I. (1999) Use of oral contraceptives and endometrial cancer risk (Sweden). *Cancer Causes Control*, **10**, 277–284

Weiss, N.S. & Sayvetz, T.A. (1980) Incidence of endometrial cancer in relation to the use of oral contraceptives. *New Engl. J. Med.*, **302**, 551–554

Weiss, N.S., Lyon, J.L., Liff, J.M., Vollmer, W.M. & Daling, J.R. (1981a) Incidence of ovarian cancer in relation to the use of oral contraceptives. *Int. J. Cancer*, **28**, 669–671

Weiss, N.S., Daling, J.R. & Chow, W.H. (1981b) Incidence of cancer of the large bowel in women in relation to reproductive and hormonal factors. *J. natl Cancer Inst.*, **67**, 57–60

Wellejus, A. & Loft, S. (2002) Receptor-mediated ethinylestradiol-induced oxidative DNA damage in rat testicular cells. *FASEB J.*, **16**, 195–201

Wellejus, A., Bornholdt, J., Vogel, U.B., Risom, L., Wiger, R. & Loft, S. (2004) Cell-specific oxidative DNA damage induced by estrogen in rat testicular cells in vitro. *Toxicol. Lett.*, **150**, 317–323

Werner, S., Kunz, S., Wolff, T. & Schwarz, L.R. (1996) Steroidal drug cyproterone acetate is activated to DNA-binding metabolites by sulfonation. *Cancer Res.*, **56**, 4391–4397

Werner, S., Kunz, S., Beckurts, T., Heidecke, C.-D., Wolff, T. & Schwarz, L.R. (1997) Formation of DNA adducts by cyproterone acetate and some structural analogues in primary cultures of human hepatocytes. *Mutat. Res.*, **395**, 179–187

Westerdahl, J., Olsson, H., Måsbäck, A., Ingvar, C. & Jonsson, N. (1996) Risk of malignant melanoma in relation to drug intake, alcohol, smoking and hormonal factors. *Br. J. Cancer*, **73**, 1126–1131

White, E., Malone, K.E., Weiss, N.S. & Daling, J.R. (1994) Breast cancer among young U.S. women in relation to oral contraceptive use. *J. natl Cancer Inst.*, **86**, 505–514

Whittemore, A.S., Balise, R.R., Pharoah, P.D., Dicioccio, R.A., Oakley-Girvan, I., Ramus, S.J., Daly, M., Usinowicz, M.B., Garlinghouse-Jones, K., Ponder, B.A., Buys, S., Senie, R., Andrulis, I., John, E., Hopper, J.L. & Piver, M.S. (2004) Oral contraceptive use and ovarian cancer risk among carriers of BRCA1 or BRCA2 mutations. *Br. J. Cancer*, **91**, 1911–1915

Whittemore, A.S., Harris, R., Itnyre, J. & the Collaborative Ovarian Cancer Group (1992) Characteristics relating to ovarian cancer risk: Collaborative analysis of 12 US case–control studies. II. Invasive epithelial ovarian cancers in white women. *Am. J. Epidemiol.*, **136**, 1184–1203

WHO (1995) Venous thromboembolic disease and combined oral contraceptives: Results of international multicentre case–control study. World Health Organization Collaborative Study of Cardiovascular Disease and Steroid Hormone Contraception. *Lancet*, **346**, 1575–1582

WHO Collaborative Study of Neoplasia and Steroid Contraceptives (1988) Endometrial cancer and combined oral contraceptives. *Int. J. Epidemiol.*, **17**, 263–269

WHO Collaborative Study of Neoplasia and Steroid Contraceptives (1989a) Epithelial ovarian cancer and combined oral contraceptives. *Int. J. Epidemiol.*, **18**, 538–545

WHO Collaborative Study of Neoplasia and Steroid Contraceptives (1989b) Combined oral contraceptives and liver cancer. *Int. J. Cancer*, **43**, 254–259

WHO Collaborative Study of Neoplasia and Steroid Contraceptives (1989c) Combined oral contraceptives and gallbladder cancer. *Int. J. Epidemiol.*, **18**, 309–314

Wiegratz, I. & Kuhl, H. (2004) Progestogen therapies: Differences in clinical effects? *Trends Endocrinol. Metab.*, **15**, 277–285

Wiegratz, I., Kutschera, E., Lee, J.H., Moore, C., Mellinger, U., Winkler, U.H. & Kuhl, H. (2003) Effect of four different oral contraceptives on various sex hormones and serum-binding globulins. *Contraception*, **67**, 25–32

Wildemeersch, D., Batar, I., Affandi, B., Andrade, A., Shangchun, W., Jing, H. & Xiaoming, C. (2003) The 'frameless' intrauterine system for long-term reversible contraception: A review of 15 years of clinical experience. *J. obstet. gynaecol. Res.*, **29**, 164–173

Willett, W.C., Bain, C., Hennekens, C.H., Rosner, B. & Speizer, F.E. (1981) Oral contraceptives and risk of ovarian cancer. *Cancer*, **48**, 1684–1687

Winter, D.C., Taylor, C., O'Sullivan, G.C. & Harvey, B.J. (2000) Mitogenic effects of oestrogen mediated by a non-genomic receptor in human colon. *Br. J. Surg.*, **87**, 1684–1689

Witte, D., Chirala, M., Younes, A., Li, Y. & Younes, M. (2001) Estrogen receptor beta is expressed in human colorectal adenocarcinoma. *Hum. Pathol.*, **32**, 940–944

Wittenberg, J., Cook, L.S., Rossing, M.A. & Weiss, N.S. (1999) Reproductive risk factors for mucinous and non-mucinous epithelial ovarian cancer. *Epidemiology*, **10**, 761–763

Wu, M.L., Whittemore, A.S., Paffenbarger, R.S., Jr, Sarles, D.L., Kampert, J.B., Grosser, S., Jung, D.L., Ballon, S., Hendrickson, M. & Mohle-Boetani, J. (1988) Personal and environmental characteristics related to epithelial ovarian cancer. I. Reproductive and menstrual events and oral contraceptive use. *Am. J. Epidemiol.*, **128**, 1216–1227

Wu-Williams, A.H., Lee, M., Whittemore, A.S., Gallagher, R.P., Jiao, D., Zheng, S., Zhou, L., Wang, X., Chen, K., Jung, D., Teh, C.-Z., Ling, C., Xu, J.Y. & Paffenbarger, R.S., Jr (1991) Reproductive factors and colorectal cancer risk among Chinese females. *Cancer Res.*, **51**, 2307–2311

Xu, X. & Thomas, M.L. (1994) Estrogen receptor-mediated direct stimulation of colon cancer cell growth in vitro. *Mol. cell. Endocrinol.*, **105**, 197–201

Yen, S., Hsieh, C.C. & MacMahon, B. (1987) Extrahepatic bile duct cancer and smoking, beverage consumption, past medical history, and oral-contraceptive use. *Cancer*, **59**, 2112–2116

Ylitalo, N., Sorensen, P., Josefsson, A., Frisch, M., Sparen, P., Ponten, J., Gyllensten, U., Melbye, M. & Adami, H.-O. (1999) Smoking and oral contaceptives as risk factors for cervical carcinoma *in situ*. *Int. J. Cancer*, **81**, 357–365

Yu, M.C., Tong, M.J., Govindarajan, S. & Henderson, B.E. (1991) Nonviral risk factors for hepatocellular carcinoma in a low-risk population, the non-Asians of Los Angeles County, California. *J. natl Cancer Inst.*, **83**, 1820–1826

Yu, M.W., Chang, H.C., Chang, S.C., Liaw, Y.F., Lin, S.M., Liu, C.J., Lee, S.D., Lin, C.L., Chen, P.J., Lin, S.C. & Chen, C.J. (2003) Role of reproductive factors in hepatocellular carcinoma: Impact on hepatitis B- and C-related risk. *Hepatology*, **38**, 1393–1400

Yue, W., Berstein, L.M., Wang, J.-P., Clark, G.M., Hamilton, C.J., Demers, L.M. & Santen, R.J. (2001) The potential role of estrogen in aromatase regulation in the breast. *J. ster. Biochem. mol. Biol.*, **79**, 157–164

Yuzpe, A.A. (2002) Oral contraception: Trends over time. *J. reprod. Med.*, **47**, 967–973

Zanetti, R., Franceschi, S., Rosso, S., Bidoli, E. & Colonna, S. (1990) Cutaneous malignant melanoma in females: The role of hormonal and reproductive factors. *Int. J. Epidemiol.*, **19**, 522–526

Zaridze, D., Mukeria, A. & Duffy, S.W. (1992) Risk factors for skin melanoma in Moscow. *Int. J. Cancer*, **52**, 159–161

Zatonski, W.A., Lowenfels, A.B., Boyle, P., Maisonneuve, P., Bueno de Mesquita, H.B., Ghadirian, P., Jain, M., Przewozniak, K., Baghurst, P., Moerman, C.J., Simard, A., McMichael, A.J., Hsieh, C.C. & Walker, A.M. (1997) Epidemiologic aspects of gallbladder cancer: A case–control study of the SEARCH Program of the International Agency for Research on Cancer. *J. natl Cancer Inst.*, **89**, 1131–1138

Zivaljevic, V., Vlajinac, H., Jankovic, R., Marinkovic, J., Dzodic, R., Sipeti Grujii, S., Paunovic, I., Diklic, A. & Zivaljevic, B. (2003) Case–control study of female thyroid cancer — Menstrual, reproductive and hormonal factors. *Eur. J. Cancer Prev.*, **12**, 63–66

Zlidar, V.M., Gardner, R., Rutstein, S.O., Morris, L., Goldberg, H. & Johnson, K. (2003) *New Survey Findings: The Reproductive Revolution Continues* (Population Reports, Series M, No. 17), Baltimore, Johns Hopkins Bloomberg School of Public Health, The INFO Project [http://www.infoforhealth.org/pr/m17/]

COMBINED ESTROGEN–PROGESTOGEN MENOPAUSAL THERAPY

COMBINED ESTROGEN–PROGESTOGEN
MENOPAUSAL THERAPY

These substances were considered by a previous Working Group, in June 1998 (IARC, 1999), under the title 'Post-menopausal hormonal therapy'. Since that time, new data have become available, and these have been incorporated into the monograph and taken into consideration in the present evaluation.

1. Exposure Data

1.1 Introduction

Estrogen–progestogen menopausal therapy involves the co-administration of an estrogen and a progestogen to peri- or menopausal women. While it is indicated most clearly for control of menopausal symptoms, the use of estrogens with or without progestogens has expanded to include the treatment or prevention of a range of chronic conditions that are associated with ageing. Such widespread, long-term use was often perceived as a 'replacement', in that it physiologically reconstituted vital functions that were lost with menopausal ovarian failure. This pattern was propitiated by the 'medicalization' of the menopause, which was perceived as pathological rather than as an expected and natural event in life. Evidence from the Women's Health Initiative, which showed a clearly harmful effect of the use of estrogen–progestogen combinations, has modified this attitude; as a result, use of the term 'replacement' has diminished. Patterns of exposure are also changing rapidly as the use of hormonal therapy declines, the indications are restricted and the duration of the therapy is reduced.

Combined estrogen–progestogen formulations are available for oral and transdermal administration, although separate administration of each component is still frequent. Progestogens are available orally, while estrogen may be administered orally, transdermally or transvaginally. The timing of exposure to these hormones may be continuous (both estrogen and progestogen at set daily doses), sequential (estrogen daily with progestogen for the last 10–14 days of the cycle) or cyclical (as with sequential, but including 7 days without hormonal exposure).

Chemical and physical data and information on the production and use of individual ingredients used in formulations of combined estrogen–progestogen therapy are given in Annex 1. Trade names and composition of combined products used in hormonal meno-pausal therapy are presented in Annex 4.

1.2   Historical overview

The earliest forms of hormone used for the treatment of the effects of natural ovarian failure or surgical removal of the ovaries were natural extracts of ovarian tissue, placenta and urine from pregnant women. These extracts contained both estrogen and progestogen, as well as other substances. Experiments in the late nineteenth century demonstrated the clinical benefit of injecting these extracts to alleviate menopausal symptoms, particularly in women who had premature natural or surgically induced menopause (IARC, 1999).

The identification and purification of ovarian hormones in the late 1920s and 1930s enabled wider clinical use of hormonal menopausal therapy. Esterone, estriol and proges-terone were identified in 1929, followed by estradiol in 1936 (IARC, 1979). Progesterone was isolated in crystalline form in 1934. Although the use of estrogen and progesterone injections was reported in the 1930s (Hirvonen, 1996), for several subsequent decades, menopausal symptoms were treated mainly with estrogen alone rather than with combined estrogen–progestogen therapy. The extraction of conjugated estrogens from the urine of pregnant mares led to the marketing in 1943 of Premarin, the first orally active and readily available estrogen (IARC, 1999).

Further developments followed the production of the orally active progestogens, nore-thisterone (also known as norethindrone in the USA) in 1950 and norethynodrel in 1952, which were ultimately used in combined oral hormonal contraceptives (see the monograph on 'Combined estrogen–progestogen contraceptives'). During the 1960s and early 1970s, hormonal menopausal therapy was most common in the USA and usually comprised estrogen therapy without a progestogen (Davis et al., 2005). Estrogen–progestogen therapy was used by some clinicians, particularly in Europe, primarily for better control of uterine bleeding during treatment (IARC, 1999). Doses in hormonal menopausal therapy at that time were relatively high compared with current standards, and 1.25 mg conjugated equine estrogens were reportedly used in the USA (Pasley et al., 1984). Use of hormonal meno-pausal therapy increased through the 1960s until the mid-1970s, particularly in women who experienced natural menopause.

An association between estrogen therapy and endometrial cancer described in 1975 (Smith et al., 1975; Ziel & Finkle, 1975) led to a rapid decline in levels of estrogen use, and by 1980 reached those noted in the mid-1960s (Kennedy et al., 1985). Many clinicians and researchers advocated that a progestogen be added to estrogen when treating meno-pausal women with a uterus to offset the proliferating action of estrogen with the differen-tiating action of progestogen. Studies that began in 1979 (Thom et al., 1979; Whitehead et al., 1981) demonstrated that progestogens attenuated the risk for endometrial cancer associated with the use of estrogen alone. In the early 1980s, the use of combined estrogen–

progestogen became more common, while greater attention to endometrial monitoring was recommended for users of estrogen only (American College of Physicians, 1992).

Ultimately, prescriptions for menopausal estrogens began to rise again with a significant increase in the use of combined estrogen–progestogen that continued throughout the 1990s. However, regional differences persisted; for example, combined therapy remained less common in the USA compared with the United Kingdom (Kennedy *et al.*, 1985; Townsend, 1998).

As use expanded in the 1980s and 1990s, the menopause was increasingly defined as a hormone deficiency that could be treated through 'replacement' of the missing hormones. Not only was estrogen established as a preventive therapy for osteoporosis in oophorectomised women (Aitken *et al.*, 1973; Lindsay *et al.*, 1980), but it was suggested that 'hormone replacement therapy' could reduce the risk for a range of related conditions, including cognitive decline (Campbell & Whitehead, 1977) and cardiovascular disease (Ross *et al.*, 1981; Greendale *et al.*, 1999). A variety of social and medical factors stimulated an increase in use, including evidence of supporting benefits, corporate promotion of hormonal therapy (Palmlund, 1997) and increasing interest in women's health issues.

Estrogen–progestogen therapy became increasingly used for longer periods by older women and for indications far removed from menopausal symptoms. Combined therapy also became the norm for women with a uterus whereas estrogen therapy alone was largely limited to women who had surgically induced menopause. Use continued to increase despite reports of a greater risk for breast cancer associated with hormonal therapy (Hoover *et al.*, 1976; Colditz *et al.*, 1993), perhaps because of uncertainties in the estimation of the magnitude of this risk (Grady *et al.*, 1992).

During this time, prevalence of current use remained lower in non-white women and lower socioeconomic groups (Stafford *et al.*, 1998). Increase in the use of hormonal therapy was greater outside of than within the USA (IARC, 1999).

In response to the increase in use of concomitant estrogens and progestogens, a number of combined formulations were developed in the mid-1990s, including both continuous combinations (fixed daily dose of estrogen and progestogen) and cyclical combinations (fixed daily dose of estrogen with a progestogen component on a given number of days per month). Intermittent administration of progestogen, as with the cyclical formulations, generally results in withdrawal uterine bleeding, whereas continuous administration does not. A transdermal patch that contained estrogen and progestogen was marketed in 1998.

There were some indications that the benefit of hormonal therapy was uncertain, and observational studies that suggested this benefit were unable to rule out confounding. The assumptions that were fundamental to the expansion of hormonal therapy came under particular scrutiny following the publication of the Heart and Estrogen/Progestin Replacement Study (HERS) in 1998. HERS showed no protective effect against recurrent events of cardiovascular disease in women with known cardiovascular problems who were randomized to conjugated equine estrogens and medroxyprogesterone (Hulley *et al.*, 1998). The initial suggestion of a temporal pattern of early harm and later benefit that emerged in this study was not confirmed on further follow-up (Grady *et al.*, 2002a). As a result of dampened enthusiasm for hormonal therapy, levels of use peaked in 2000 and plateaued in subsequent years (Hersh *et al.*, 2004).

A more dramatic change in patterns of practice followed the results of the Women's Health Initiative (WHI) trial in July 2002. Women with no history of known cardiovascular disease were randomized to receive combined hormonal therapy. Contrary to expectations based on observational data, WHI showed that rates of cardiovascular events were higher in women exposed to conjugated equine estrogens and medroxyprogesterone than in those exposed to placebo (Rossouw *et al.*, 2002; Manson *et al.*, 2003; Majumdar *et al.*, 2004). In addition, it was reported that conjugated equine estrogens and medroxyprogesterone increased the risk for other adverse events (Chlebowski *et al.*, 2003; Rapp *et al.*, 2003; Shumaker *et al.*, 2003; Wassertheil-Smoller *et al.*, 2003) that were not offset by reduced risks for fractures and colorectal cancer. Furthermore, overall quality of life was not improved by treatment compared with placebo (Hays *et al.*, 2003a). While the results were not as dramatic, publication of the second WHI trial that involved administration of estrogen alone (Women's Health Initiative Steering Committee, 2004) reinforced a new consensus on the increase in adverse vascular outcomes associated with hormonal menopausal therapy.

Although some doubts were raised regarding the reliability and generalizability of the WHI results (Shapiro, 2003; Strickler, 2003), practice patterns changed tremendously. Prescriptions in the USA fell by 50% during the 18 months that followed the results of the WHI (Hersh *et al.*, 2004; Majumdar *et al.*, 2004). Internationally, similar reductions occurred in western Europe and most of the Western Pacific (Table 1). The decline in the use of hormonal therapy was particularly marked for combined estrogen–progestogen therapy.

Use has begun to shift towards lower-dose formulations (e.g. 0.30 mg conjugated equine estrogens and 1.5 mg medroxyprogesterone). Simultaneously, there is less use of hormonal menopausal therapy among older women. Patterns of use will probably change further as numerous professional organizations continue to recommend the use of lower doses, shorter durations of use and limiting use to more severe menopausal symptoms (US Preventive Service Task Force, 2002; North American Menopause Society, 2004; Wathen *et al.*, 2004).

1.3   Preparations of estrogen–progesterone menopausal therapy

A variety of products are available for use in combined estrogen–progestogen menopausal therapy, either as individual estrogen and progestogen components that can be co-administered or as a combined product. The use of individual components may allow better tailoring compared with combined products. A number of combined formulations are described in Annex 4.

Available estrogen products can be defined by their estrogen form, dose and mode of delivery. The most common estrogens available for hormonal menopausal therapy are conjugated equine estrogen, conjugated plant-based estrogen, estradiol and ethinylestradiol. A range of three to five different doses are often available for each product, varying from low-dose (0.3–0.5 mg orally) to high-dose (2.5–5 mg). Estrogen products are available in oral form, transdermal patches and intravaginal rings. These products can be used either for estrogen-only therapy (e.g. in women who have had a hysterectomy) or in conjunction with a progestogen to provide combined hormonal therapy.

Table 1. Trends in sales of combined estrogen–progestogen menopausal therapy products for selected years (millions of standard units[a])

Regions[b]	1994	1999	2004
Africa	21.0	29.9	27.7
South Africa	20.0	28.9	26.7
West Africa	1.1	1.0	1.1
Eastern Mediterranean	8.9	21.5	27.7
Europe	1 269.5	1 858.3	1 078.4
Eastern Europe	36.2	184.8	159.8
Western Europe	1 233.3	1 673.5	918.6
North America	39.7	1 089.4	421.8
South America	100.2	284.5	190.4
South East Asia	20.0	36.9	67.5
India	0	0	1.2
Korea	7.8	16.8	43.9
Rest of South East Asia	10.5	17.3	20.5
Western Pacific	100.8	219.7	107.0
Australia/New Zealand	17.5	75.8	34.3
China/Hong Kong	0.8	10.8	4.5
Japan	67.6	54.6	36.9
Taiwan, China	4.6	58.5	24.3
Rest of Western Pacific	10.4	20.0	7.1
Total	1 560.1	3 550.2	1 920.6

From IMS Health (2005)

[a] Standard units are sales in terms of standard dose units; the standard dose unit for oral products is one tablet or capsule

[b] *West Africa* includes: Benin, Burkina, Cameroon, Congo, Gabon, Guinea, Ivory Coast, Mali, Senegal, Togo;

Eastern Mediterranean includes: Egypt, Jordan, Kuwait, Lebanon, Morocco, Saudi Arabia, Tunisia, United Arab Emirates;

Eastern Europe includes: Belarus, Bulgaria, Czech Republic, Estonia, Hungary, Latvia, Lithuania, Poland, Russian Federation, Slovakia, Slovenia, Ukraine;

Western Europe includes: Austria, Belgium, Denmark, Finland, France, Germany, Greece, Ireland, Israel, Italy, Luxembourg, Netherlands, Norway, Portugal, Spain, Sweden, Switzerland, Turkey, UK;

North America includes: Canada, Central America (Costa Rica, El Salvador, Guatemala, Honduras, Nicaragua, Panama), Mexico, Puerto Rico, USA;

Rest of South East Asia includes: Indonesia, Pakistan, Thailand;

South America includes: Argentina, Brazil, Chile, Colombia, Dominican Republic, Ecuador, Peru, Uruguay, Venezuela;

Rest of Western Pacific includes: Malaysia, Philippines, Singapore.

A range of progestogens are available for use in combined hormonal therapy. Those most commonly used are medroxyprogesterone acetate, norethisterone and levonorgestrel. Several doses of each progestogen are usually available. For example, medroxyprogesterone acetate is often available in doses of 1.5, 2.5, 5 and 10 mg. While oral forms predominate, progestogens also are available as a vaginal pessary, a systemically absorbed vaginal gel, a transdermal patch and an intrauterine device. Administration of progestogen may follow one of three types of schedule. In continuous combined therapy, the same dose of both estrogen and progestogen is administered each day. In sequential therapy, 10–14 days of progestogen is provided per cycle in addition to daily estrogen. In cyclical therapy, a cycle consists of estrogen alone, followed by progestogen with estrogen and then 5–7 days with no hormones.

Combined oral products that contain both estrogen and progestogen provide greater convenience to users, as only one rather than two tablets are taken. The various preparations available differ in their estrogen component, their progestogen component, the dose of these components, and the schedule and mode of drug administration. Despite the potential for a plethora of combinations, a relatively small number are manufactured. Continuous dose schedules during which the same doses are taken on a daily basis are most common. Less commonly, progestogens may be delivered for only a portion of a monthly cycle (e.g. Premphase). Combined products are frequently available at two dose levels. Oral forms of combined therapy predominate, but a combined transdermal patch and a vaginal ring are also available.

The selection of a specific regimen for menopausal therapy depends on the preferences and needs of each women. Further, evidence regarding long-term risk may motivate physicians to recommend a specific formulation. A number of the products available for hormonal menopausal therapy have only recently been introduced and their long-term effects have not been evaluated fully.

1.4   Patterns of use

A number of studies have provided information on patterns of use of hormonal menopausal therapy, most of which is related to women in developed countries and does not differentiate between use of estrogen alone or in combination with progestogen. Data from individual studies are summarized in Table 2. Most of the available information reflects use in the late 1990s when hormonal therapy had reached its peak. Another set of studies examined more recent use and provided an indication of the extent to which use has declined since the results of the WHI Study.

1.4.1   *Patterns of use in 1990–2000*

Table 2 summarizes the prevalence of current use of estrogen–progestogen menopausal therapy during the years 1997–2003. The section below details those studies that provide additional information on patterns of use during this period.

Table 2. Selected studies of the prevalence of current use of estrogen–progestogen menopausal therapy, 1997–2003

Reference	Country	Year(s) of study	Age group (years)	Prevalence of current use		Comments
				Combined estrogen–progestogen therapy	Any current hormonal therapy	
Pre-2002						
MacLaren & Woods (2001)	USA	1998	40–65	NR	39%	
Progetto Menopausa Italia Study (2001)	Italy	1997–99	45–75	NR	8.5%	
Banks et al. (2002) (EPIC)	Denmark	1993–97	50–64	NR	29.0%	
	Germany				38.6–40.7%	2 centres
	Greece				2.1%	
	Italy				4.4–11.5%	2 centres
	Netherlands				14.3%	
	Spain				4.5–11.5%	2 centres
	United Kingdom				28.1–30.3%	2 centres
Benet Rodriguez et al. (2002)	Spain	1989–99	≥ 40	NR	> 3.19%	Detail by 5-year age group and by year
Merom et al. (2002)	Israel	1998	45–74	NR	16.8%	
Million Women Study Collaborators (2002)	United Kingdom	1996–2000	50–64	17%	33%	
Mueller et al. (2002)	Germany	1985 1990 1995	45–64	0.1% 4.0% 13.9%	3.0% 8.8% 22.6%	
Bakken et al. (2004)	Norway	1996–98	Postmenopausal 45–54	24%	35%	

Table 2 (contd)

Reference	Country	Year(s) of study	Age group (years)	Prevalence of current use		Comments
				Combined estrogen–progestogen therapy	Any current hormonal therapy	
Buist et al. (2004)	USA	1999	40–80	14.6%	27.2%	
Heng et al. (2004)	Singapore	1994–97	45–69	NR	21%	Ever use
Hersch et al. (2004)	USA	1995	50–74	16%	33%	
		2001	50–74		42%	
Lundberg et al. (2004)	20 countries	1989–97	45–64	NR	0–56%	
Manzoli et al. (2004)	Italy	1999–2001	50–70	2.9%	6.9%	
Rachoń et al. (2004)	Poland	April 2002	45–64	[9.3%]	12%	
Carney et al. (2006)	USA	1996–99	> 40	13%	43%	
Post-2002						
Strothmann & Schneider (2003)	France	2003	45–75	NR	23%	
	Germany				19%	
	Spain				5%	
	United Kingdom				19%	
Bilgrami et al. (2004)	New Zealand	December 2002	45–64	3%	11%	
Buist et al. (2004)	USA	December 2002	40–80	8%	17%	
MacLennan et al. (2004)	Australia	2003	> 50	7%	19%	

NR, not reported

Based on sales data, Jolleys and Olesen (1996) compared the use of hormonal therapy in the USA and Europe and found three strata of prevalence of use: the USA were in the highest stratum (20% of women); the United Kingdom and Scandinavian countries were in the intermediate group (9–16%); and continental Europe had the lowest prevalence (< 5%). The authors noted that use in France, however, was increasing towards levels found in the intermediate group. A later review on the use of hormonal therapy and risk for cancer by Beral *et al.* (1999) estimated that at least 20 million women in developed countries were currently using hormonal therapy.

Based on sales data, Benet-Rodriguez *et al.* (2002) estimated that prevalence of the use of hormonal therapy among women aged 40 years or over increased from 0.7% in 1989 to 3.4% in 1999. In 1998, prevalence was highest in the age group 50–54 years (10.8%) and was below 1% in women over 65 years of age.

Buist *et al.* (1999) examined patterns of long-term use of hormonal therapy in women aged 50–80 years in Seattle, WA, USA. Long-term users (> 10 years) and short-term users were significantly younger than never users. Compared with never users, long-term users were also more likely to be married, to have had surgically induced menopause, to have experienced menopausal symptoms, to see their family doctor and have mammograms and were less likely to smoke. Estrogen alone was the predominant therapy; combined therapy was more common among short-term (< 10 years) users than among long-term users.

Donker *et al.* (2000) reported on first-time users of hormonal therapy in a survey in the Netherlands. The number of prescriptions for such therapy increased from 2 to 3% between 1995 and 1998. Between 1987–88 and 1995–98, sequential therapy was prescribed more frequently than continuous therapy, but there has been a gradual shift from sequential to continuous therapy in the last few years. There was also a trend in prescriptions from estrogen towards combinations of estrogen and progestogen.

MacLaren and Woods (2001) found that, among peri- or postmenopausal women aged 40–65 years in the USA, use of hormonal therapy was lower among women who experienced natural menopause (31%) than among those who had surgically induced menopause (56%). The median duration of use was 5 years, and 25% reported taking hormones for 10 years or more.

In a study of over 40 000 women aged 45–75 years in Italy (Progetto Menopausa Italia Study Group, 2001), 12% were ever users, among whom 74% were current users. Mean duration of use was approximately 20 months in both current and former users. Ever users were more likely to have a higher education, be nulliparous, have had an early menopause, have ever used oral contraceptives and have a history of osteoporosis, and less likely to have cardiovascular disease or diabetes.

The EPIC [European Prospective Investigation into Cancer and Nutrition] Working Group (Banks *et al.*, 2002) examined the patterns of use of hormonal therapy in women aged 50–64 years in several European countries. Current use varied from 2% in Greece to 41% in Heidelberg, Germany, and ever-use varied from 7 to 55%, respectively. In all centres (except in Germany), the most frequent duration of use among ever users was less than 1 year; long-term use (> 10 years) varied from 26% in Denmark to 2% in southern Italy.

Merom *et al.* (2002) examined Israeli women aged 45–74 years in 1998 who had had a natural menopause, among whom 17% were current users and 13% were past users. The prevalence of current use was higher among post- than among perimenopausal women (15% versus 7%). The rates of current and ever use were highest in the 55–59-year age group and lowest in the 70–74-year age group. Current users were more likely to be more highly educated, to work outside the home and be married (compared with divorcees or widows), to have used contraceptives, to make regular visits to a gynaecologist, to be lean, to have regular physical activity and ever to have smoked.

The Million Women Study Collaborators (2002) examined patterns of use in women in the United Kingdom aged 50–64 years in 1996–2000. Of this cohort, 50% had ever used hormonal therapy, of whom 33% reported current use and 17% reported past use. Average age at initiation of therapy was 49.1 years; 38% started at 45–49 years and 37% started at 50–54 years of age. The most common duration of treatment was 1–4 years (37%) followed by 5–9 years (33%); the mean duration of use was 4.9 years.

Mueller *et al.* (2002) reported trends in use of hormonal therapy in Germany in 1984–95, based on a survey of women aged 45–64 years who were included in the WHO Monitoring Trends and Determinants in Cardiovascular Disease (MONICA) study. The highest prevalence of use (29.8%) was among women aged 55–59 years. Use of combined hormonal therapy increased from almost non-existent levels in 1985 to 4.0% in 1990 and 13.9% in 1995.

Ekström *et al.* (2003) examined patterns of use of hormonal therapy in women aged 45, 50, 55 and 60 years in Sweden and found that 50–52% of women aged 55 and 60 years had ever used hormonal therapy; the mean length of treatment was 4.4 years. Current users were more likely to be on antidepressive medication and/or cardiovascular drugs, to report psychological and physical menopausal symptoms and to have visited a psychotherapist.

Bakken *et al.* (2004) reported on over 35 000 postmenopausal women aged 45–64 years from the Norwegian Women and Cancer (NOWAC) cohort study, among whom 80% of ever-users of hormones were current users.

From a sample of women in the USA, Haas *et al.* (2004) found that use of hormones in 1997 was highest among white women (53%) and lowest among African-American, Latina, Chinese and Philipina women (30–34%); it was also much higher among women who had had a hysterectomy (60% versus 36%).

By 2001 in the USA, almost half (42%) of all postmenopausal women under the age of 65 years were being treated with hormonal therapy (Hersh *et al.*, 2004). It was reported that 38% of users were taking combined therapy, either as a single preparation or as separate estrogen and progestogen components.

Based on a sample population for a case–control study, Newcomb *et al.* (2002) reported that 25–28% of all postmenopausal women in the USA had ever used hormonal therapy in 1992–95. Of these users, 30% had used combined therapy.

Bromley *et al.* (2004) reported on the proportion of women who used hormonal therapy from 1992 to 1998. Women who started hormonal therapy during this period were less likely to have a history of a range of diseases but were more likely to have a history of osteoporosis, hysterectomy, hyperlipidaemia and prior oral contraceptive use than non-users.

Lundberg *et al.* (2004) reported data collected from the MONICA study. Prevalence of current use in women aged 45–64 years varied enormously from 0% in Moscow, Russian Federation, to 42% in Newcastle, Australia, and Canada. Low prevalence of use (< 10%) was noted for central, eastern and southern Europe, the Russian Federation and China, while the highest prevalence of use was reported in populations in western and northern Europe, North America and Australia. Ever use in Perth, Australia, was estimated at 66% of women aged 50–54 years. Regional differences within the same country were generally modest compared with inter-country variations. The highest prevalence was in the age group 45–49 years in 12 populations, in the age group 50–54 years in nine populations and in the age group 55–59 years in four populations.

Rachon *et al.* (2004) examined use of hormonal therapy among Polish women over 45 years of age in April 2002. Overall current use was 12% in women aged 45–64 years and was 16% in the age group 45–54 years; ever use was in the range of 25 and 20% for women aged 45–54 years and 55–64 years, respectively. Women with a medium or higher level of education were more likely to be current users than those who had had a basic education.

Fournier *et al.* (2005) reported that, among women born between 1925 and 1950 and followed-up between 1990 and 2000, users were more likely than non-users to have had an early menarche, an early menopause, to be parous, to have a personal history of benign breast disease, to have no familial history of breast cancer in first-degree relatives, to be lean, to have a higher level of education, to have used oral contraceptives and to have used oral progestogens before the menopause.

1.4.2   *Recent trends in hormonal menopausal therapy*

Large and rapid changes in the use of combined hormonal menopausal therapy took place in 2002 as a consequence of the publication of the results of the WHI. International data (IMS Health, 2005) suggest that sales of combined hormonal therapy (estrogen and progestogens in a single preparation) declined substantially worldwide (Table 1). Decreases between 1999 and 2004 were noted in Europe (42% decline), North America (61%), South America (33%) and the western Pacific (51%). Increased or stable sales of combined hormonal therapy were noted in Africa, the eastern Mediterranean and South-East Asia during the same period.

In the USA, overall use of hormonal therapy fell by about 38% and that of combined estrogen–progestogen therapy by 58% between 2001 and the first half of 2003 (Hersh *et al.*, 2004) (Figure 1). As use continued to decrease 18 months after the WHI results (Rossouw *et al.*, 2002), sales of Prempro (conjugated equine estrogens plus methoxyprogesterone acetate) had fallen by 80% (Majumdar *et al.*, 2004). Haas *et al.* (2004) found similar time trends from survey data.

Figure 1. Annual number of US prescriptions for hormonal therapy by formulation, 1995–July 2003

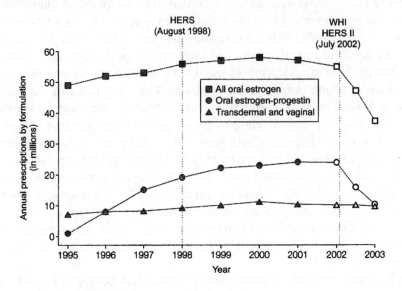

Modified from Hersh *et al.* (2004)
HERS, Heart and Estrogen/Progestin Replacement Study; WHI, Women's Health Initiative
Data for January to June 2002, July to December 2002 and January to July 2003 are included (open symbols).
Data are from the National Prescription Audit Plus, IMS Health.

Strothmann and Schneider (2003) analysed data from France, Germany, Spain and the United Kingdom in women aged 45–75 years in 2003 and found that in all four countries the number of former users was relatively similar to that of current users.

Bilgrami *et al.* (2004) presented data from New Zealand. Based on survey information, current use of hormone therapy dropped from 15% in June 2002 to 11% in December 2002. The majority of women who had stopped using hormonal therapy specifically identified the results of the WHI trial as their reason. Further data from the New Zealand Pharmacy Management Agency (Metcalfe, 2004) showed a decline of 65% in use of hormonal therapy between 2001 and 2004. Examination of monthly data showed a continued decline through to March 2005.

MacLennan *et al.* (2004a) specifically examined changes in use patterns in Australia and found that prevalence of current use had declined from 22.5% in 2000 to 14.4% in 2003 among women aged > 40 years. Over the same period, duration of use decreased by an average of 10 months among current users. Unlike in studies in the 1990s, the number of past users exceeded the number of current users.

No data were available to the Working Group on changes in use in developing countries.

2. Studies of Cancer in Humans

2.1   Breast cancer

2.1.1   *Background*

In the previous evaluation (IARC, 1999), most of the epidemiological evidence derived from studies that assessed the use of estrogen alone in relation to subsequent risk for breast cancer. The evidence related to combined therapy with estrogen plus a progestogen was considered to be insufficient to reach any firm conclusion. However, in relation to hormonal menopausal therapy with estrogen alone, the evidence was summarized as follows.

A pooled analysis from 51 studies and a review that included 15 cohort studies and 23 case–control studies showed a small increase in risk for ever use, which increased with longer duration of use (5 years or more), and an increased risk in current and recent users. Some information was available on women who used and then stopped using menopausal estrogen therapy; based on this evidence, the increased risk appeared to disappear several years after cessation of use. There was also evidence to suggest that the increase in risk was predominantly for small, localized tumours of the breast. The data were, however, insufficient to determine whether the risk varied with type of compound or the dose of various compounds used.

This evaluation relied heavily on the pooled analysis from the collaborative group in Oxford (Collaborative Group on Hormonal Factors in Breast Cancer, 1997), which had compiled and re-analysed the original data of 51 studies, 22 of which provided information on the hormonal constituents of the preparations. In the re-analysis, data on hormonal constituents were available for 4640 women; 12% (557) of these women had received combined estrogens and progestogens, and 249 women with breast cancer had used combined treatment. The results showed that, among women who were currently using combined therapy, the relative risk was 1.2 (95% confidence interval [CI], 0.8–1.5; based on 136 exposed cases) for less than 5 years of use and 1.5 (95% CI, 0.9–2.2; based on 58 exposed cases) for more than 5 years of use.

These limited data did not provide a firm basis for any conclusion regarding the effects of the use of combined estrogen–progestogen therapy on the risk for breast cancer. Subsequently, many studies, including clinical trials, have assessed the risk for breast cancer in relation to the use of combined hormonal therapy by menopausal women.

2.1.2   *Randomized clinical trials* (Table 3)

The WHI investigators conducted two large, randomized, double-blind, placebo-controlled trials that evaluated the effects of estrogen alone and estrogen plus progestogen on the prevention of chronic disease in 27 347 postmenopausal women aged 50–79 years (Women's Health Initiative Study Group, 1998; Anderson *et al.*, 2003; Stefanick *et al.*, 2003). The incidence of coronary heart disease was the primary outcome and the incidence of invasive breast cancer was the primary safety outcome. Both trials were interrupted prematurely because of adverse effects.

In these two trials, postmenopausal women were recruited between 1993 and 1998 from 40 US clinical centres mainly by mass mailing (Hays *et al.*, 2003b). All women had baseline mammograms and clinical breast examinations. A total of 16 608 eligible women with a uterus at baseline were randomized in equal proportions to treatment with continuous combined conjugated equine estrogens (0.625 mg per day) plus medroxyprogesterone acetate (2.5mg per day) in a single tablet or to a matching placebo. A total of 10 739 women who had had a hysterectomy were randomized with equal probability to conjugated equine estrogens (0.625 mg per day) or placebo. The intervention period was planned to end in 2005, giving a projected mean follow-up of 8.5 years. Participants were followed every 6 months; annual visits to the clinic and mammography were required. Designated outcomes were ascertained by self-reporting at every 6-month contact and documented by medical records that were locally and centrally adjudicated. These outcome procedures were performed by study staff who were blinded to treatment assignment. Vital status was known for 96.7 and 94.7% of the participants in the estrogen plus progestogen (mean follow-up, 5.6 years) and estrogen alone trials (mean follow-up, 6.8 years), respectively (Chlebowski *et al.*, 2003; Anderson *et al.*, 2004).

In May 2002, the Independent Data and Safety Monitoring Board recommended that the estrogen plus progestogen trial be stopped on the basis of an adverse effect on the incidence of breast cancer and an overall assessment that risks exceeded benefits. The protocol-specified weighted log-rank statistic for breast cancer (p-value = 0.001) had crossed the pre-defined monitoring boundary for adverse effects (p-value = 0.02) (Rossouw *et al.*, 2002). The weights in this log-rank statistic were defined by time since randomization, and rose linearly from 0 at time of randomization to 1 at year 10 and thereafter; this effectively down-weighted early differences that were thought to be less probably related to treatment. For simplicity, the initial publication presented unweighted hazard ratios for comparisons of all outcomes, based on the locally adjudicated data available on outcomes at the time that the trial was stopped. These analyses did not acknowledge the anticipated time-dependent effect for breast cancer.

The final unweighted hazard ratio of estrogen plus progestogen for invasive breast cancer was 1.24 (95% CI, 1.04–1.50; weighted p = 0.003; 349 cases) (Chlebowski *et al.*, 2003). There was a statistically significant interaction with time since randomization that suggested an effect of duration of exposure. In women who took estrogen plus progestogen, tumours were slightly larger, and more likely to be node-positive and to be at regional

Table 3. Randomized clinical trials of combined hormone therapy and the risk for breast cancer[a]

Reference, name of trial	Country	Age at recruit-ment	Size of trial	Period of trial	Mean duration of follow-up (years)	No. of exposed women	No. (%) of women using placebo	Total no. of breast cancer cases	Histological type of breast cancer	Cases in exposed women	Cases in placebo women	Hazard ratio (95% CI), treated versus placebo
Hulley *et al.* (2002), HERS	USA	44–79	2 763	1993–2000	4.1	1 380	1 383	88	Invasive	34	25	1.38 (0.82–2.31)
Chlebowski *et al.* (2003), WHI	USA	50–79	16 608	1993–98	5.6	8 506	8 102	822	Invasive + *in situ*	245	185	1.24 (1.02–1.50)
									Invasive	199	150	1.24 (1.01–1.54)
									In situ	46	37	1.18 (0.77–1.82)

CI, confidence interval; HERS, Heart and Estrogen/Progestin Replacement Study; WHI, Women's Health Initiative
[a] In both studies, the treated group received 0.625 mg conjugated equine estrogens and 2.5 mg of medroxyprogesterone acetate.

or advanced stages than those diagnosed in women who took placebo. The incidence of in-situ cancers was not significantly elevated (hazard ratio, 1.18; 95% CI, 0.77–1.82; weighted p = 0.09; 84 cases). Mammography rates were high (≥ 88.6% in each year) and did not differ between groups (Chlebowski et al., 2003). Limitations of the study included the proportion of women who discontinued study medications (42% for estrogen plus progestogen and 38% for placebo), the proportion who initiated hormonal therapy outside of the trial (6% versus 11%, respectively) and the proportion of women for whom unblinding of clinical gynaecologists was required (40% versus 7%), primarily to manage vaginal bleeding (Rossouw et al., 2002).

The HERS was a randomized, double-blind, placebo-controlled trial designed to test the effects of continuous combined hormonal therapy (0.625 mg conjugated equine estrogens plus 2.5 mg medroxyprogesterone acetate daily) for the prevention of recurrent coronary heart disease among 2763 women aged 44–79 years with a uterus and with documented coronary disease at enrolment. The trial ended after a mean duration of follow-up of 4.1 years and reported no overall effect on coronary heart disease. No significant effect was found on the incidence of breast cancer (relative risk, 1.38; 95% CI, 0.82–2.31; 88 cases) (Hulley et al., 2002).

2.1.3   Cohort studies (Table 4)

Persson et al. (1999) assessed the use of combined hormonal menopausal therapy and subsequent risk for breast cancer in a prospective study of 10 472 women in Sweden. Information on use of hormonal therapy was obtained at recruitment to the study through prescription records in pharmacies. The cohort was followed for over 6 years by linkage to the Swedish Cancer Registry, and 198 women were registered with incident breast cancer during that time. The relative risk associated with ever use of combined hormonal menopausal therapy was not specified. However, the relative risk for 1–6 years of use at entry to the study was 1.4 (95% CI, 0.9–2.3) compared with never use or use for less than 1 year, and that associated with use for more than 6 years was 1.7 (95% CI, 1.1–2.6). These results were adjusted for age, length of follow-up, age at first full-term pregnancy, body mass index, education and age at menopause. The results also showed that the estimated relative risks were higher for recent or current use than for past use. Recent or current use was associated with a relative risk of 2.8 (95% CI, 0.8–10.0) and use in the past with a relative risk of 1.9 (95% CI, 0.6–6.1).

In a cohort study in the USA, Schairer et al. (2000) investigated whether the use of combined hormonal menopausal therapy increased the risk for breast cancer. The cohort of 46 355 postmenopausal women was recruited from a mammography screening programme and followed for 10 years. During follow-up, 2082 women were diagnosed with breast cancer. Ever use of combined hormonal menopausal therapy was associated with a relative risk of 1.3 (95% CI, 1.0–1.6), but the increase in risk was largely restricted to current users or use within the last 4 years (relative risk, 1.4; 95% CI, 1.1–1.8). These results were adjusted for age, mammography screening, age at menopause, body mass index and level of

Table 4. Cohort studies of the use of combined hormone therapy and the risk for breast cancer

Reference	Country	Age at recruit-ment (years)	Size of cohort	Period of cohort	Average of follow-up (years)	Total no. of cases	Histo-logical diagnosis	Sub-sites	Hormone therapy (type/regimen)	No. of cases	Relative risk (95% CI)	Comments
Person et al. (1999)	Sweden	65 (mean)	10 472	1987–93	5.7	198	Invasive		Never	48	1.0	Adjusted for age, follow-up time, age at first full-term pregnancy, body mass index, education, menopausal age/status
									1–6 years	28	1.4 (0.9–2.3)	
									≥ 6 years	44	1.7 (1.1–2.6)	
Schairer et al. (2000)	USA	Not specified	46 355	1980–95	10.2	2802	All	All	Never	761	1.0	Adjusted for age, education, body mass index, age at menopause, mammographic screening
									Ever	101	1.3 (1.0–1.6)	
							Invasive	Ductal/lobular	Never	145	1.0	
									Ever	33	[1.73[a]]	
							Invasive	Ductal only	Never	128	1.0	
									Ever	26	[1.55[a]]	
Beral et al. (2003)	UK	50–64	1 084 110	1996–2001	2.6	9364	Invasive		Never	2894	1.0	Adjusted for age, region, socio-economic status, body mass index, alcoholic beverage consumption, ever use of oral contraceptives, time since menopause, parity
									Current	1934	2.00 (1.91–2.09)	
									Duration[b]			
									< 1 year	97	1.45 (1.19–1.78)	
									1–4 years	582	1.74 (1.60–1.89)	
									5–9 years	850	2.17 (2.03–2.33)	
									≥ 10 years	362	2.31 (2.08–2.56)	
									All continuous combined			
									< 5 years	243	1.57 (1.37–1.79)	
									≥ 5 years	388	2.40 (2.15–2.67)	
									All sequential combined			
									< 5 years	403	1.77 (1.59–1.97)	
									≥ 5 years	778	2.12 (1.95–2.30)	

Table 4 (contd)

Reference	Country	Age at recruitment (years)	Size of cohort	Period of cohort	Average of follow-up (years)	Total no. of cases	Histological diagnosis	Sub-sites	Hormone therapy (type/regimen)	No. of cases	Relative risk (95% CI)	Comments
Jernström et al. (2003a)	Sweden	50–64	6 586	1995–2000	4.1	101	NR		Never	2422	1.0	Adjusted for age at entry and time of follow-up; continuous combined formula only
									Ever	NR	3.3 (1.9–5.6)	
									Duration			
									≤ 2 years	NR	3.7 (1.8–7.4)	
									3–4 years	NR	2.2 (0.84–5.9)	
									> 4 years	NR	3.7 (1.8–7.7)	
Olsson et al. (2003)	Sweden	25–65	29 508	1990–92	Not specified	556	NR		Never		1.0	Adjusted for age, age at menarche, age at first full-term pregnancy, parity, age at menopause, family history of breast cancer
									Ever combined continuous therapy	622	2.45 (1.61–3.71)	
									Never		1.0	
									Ever combined sequential therapy	655	1.22 (0.74–2.00)	
Bakken et al. (2004)	Norway	45–64	31 451	1996–98	Not specified	331	NR	All	Never	130	1.0	Adjusted for age, body mass index, age at menarche, ever use of oral contraceptives, time since menopause, family history of breast cancer, mammography, parity, age at first delivery
									Current	116	2.5 (1.9–3.2)	
									Ever use			
									< 5 years	63	2.3 (1.7–3.2)	
									≥ 5 years	51	2.8 (2.0–4.0)	
									Sequential regimen			
									< 5 years	19	1.7 (1.0–2.8)	
									≥ 5 years	14	2.2 (1.3–3.8)	
									Continuous regimen			
									< 5 years	44	2.6 (1.9–3.7)	
									≥ 5 years	37	3.2 (2.2–4.6)	

Table 4 (contd)

Reference	Country	Age at recruitment (years)	Size of cohort	Period of cohort	Average of follow-up (years)	Total no. of cases	Histological diagnosis	Sub-sites	Hormone therapy (type/regimen)	No. of cases	Relative risk (95% CI)	Comments
Stahlberg et al. (2004)	Denmark	≥ 45	10 874	1993–99	Not specified	244	In situ/invasive		Never	110	1.0	Adjusted for age at menopause, age at menarche, parity, age at first birth, use of oral contraceptives, history of benign breast disease, smoking, night work, body mass index, height, physical activity, alcoholic beverage intake
									Current	75	2.70 (1.96–3.73)	
									Continuous	23	4.16 (2.56–6.75)	
									< 5 years	4	1.96 (0.72–5.36)	
									5–9 years	6	4.96 (2.16–11.39)	
									≥ 10 years	10	6.78 (3.41–13.48)	
									Current cyclical	52	1.94 (1.26–3.00)	
									< 5 years	10	1.58 (0.79–3.17)	
									5–9 years	9	2.47 (1.23–4.95)	
									≥ 10 years	10	2.18 (1.09–4.33)	
Tjønneland et al. (2004)	Denmark	50–60	23 618	1993–97	4.8	423	Invasive	Lobular only	Never	15	1.0	Adjusted for parity, age at first birth, history of benign breast tumour surgery, education, alcoholic beverage consumption, body mass index
									Current	41	3.53 (1.94–6.41)	
								Ductal only	Never	109	1.0	
									Current	158	2.10 (1.64–2.7)	
Ewertz et al. (2005)	Denmark	50–67	48 812	1989–2002	10	869	NR		Never	561	1.0	Adjusted for age, age at first birth, parity
									Sequential progestogen-derived progestogen	6	0.57 (0.26–1.28)	
									Sequential testosterone-derived progestogen	80	1.52 (1.21–1.93)	
									Continuous testosterone-derived progestogen	13	0.99 (0.57–1.72)	

Table 4 (contd)

Reference	Country	Age at recruit-ment (years)	Size of cohort	Period of cohort	Average of follow-up (years)	Total no. of cases	Histo-logical diagnosis	Sub-sites	Hormone therapy (type/ regimen)	No. of cases	Relative risk (95% CI)	Comments
Fournier et al. (2005)	France	52.8 (mean)	54 548	Non-specified	5.8	NR	Invasive		Never Current use	NR 323	1.0 1.3 (1.1–1.5)	Adjusted for time since menopause, body mass index, age at menopause, parity, age at first full-term pregnancy, family history of breast cancer, personal history of benign breast disease, use of oral contraceptives, mammography screening

NR, not reported
[a] No confidence intervals were provided.
[b] Data on duration missing for 43 women

education. When the data were stratified by body mass index, no increased risk related to the use of hormonal therapy was observed in women with an index > 24.4. However, in women with an index of 24.4 or less, the relative risk associated with 5 years of use or more was 2.0 (95% CI, 1.3–3.0). Thus, hormonal therapy that comprised estrogen plus a progestogen exerted its effects primarily, if not solely, among lean women. The investigators also studied the effect of duration of combined therapy and histological subtypes of breast cancer. The results suggested a similar increase in risk with increasing duration of use for ductal and lobular carcinoma, but the number of cases within the subtypes of breast cancer was small and the results should be interpreted with caution.

Risk for breast cancer and the use of hormonal menopausal therapy was also evaluated in the Million Women Study (Beral *et al.*, 2003). More than a million women in the United Kingdom between 50 and 64 years of age were recruited into the study between 1996 and 2001 and provided detailed information on their use of hormonal menopausal therapy. They were followed up for cancer incidence and death. Half of the women had used some type of hormonal menopausal therapy and nearly 150 000 women were current users of combined hormonal therapy. During 2.6 years of follow-up, 9364 women were diagnosed with invasive breast cancer, and current users were more likely than never users to develop the disease. The relative risk for current compared with never use of combined hormonal therapy at the time of recruitment was 2.00 (95% CI, 1.91–2.09), but the association varied according to duration of use. Among current users, use for 1–4 years was associated with a relative risk of 1.74 (95% CI, 1.60–1.89; 582 exposed cases) compared with never users, and use for 10 years or more was associated with a relative risk of 2.31 (95% CI, 2.08–2.56; 362 exposed cases). In relation to past use, the relative risk was 1.04 (95% CI, 0.94–1.16). The relative risks were adjusted for age, region of residence, socioeconomic status, body mass index, alcoholic beverage consumption, ever use of oral contraceptives, time since menopause and parity. Little variation in the associations was observed among women who used different preparations of combined regimens. Thus, among women who had used a treatment containing medroxyprogesterone acetate for less than 5 years, the relative risk was 1.60 (95% CI, 1.33–1.93), and that for women who had taken it for 5 years or more was 2.42 (95% CI, 2.10–2.80). Similarly, treatment for less than 5 years with a therapy containing norethisterone was associated with a relative risk of 1.53 (95% CI, 1.35–1.75); when use of norethisterone lasted for 5 years or more, the relative risk was 2.10 (95% CI, 1.89–2.34). Different modes of administration were also compared and broadly similar relative risks related to daily (relative risk, 1.57; 95% CI, 1.37–1.79) and cyclical (relative risk, 1.77; 95% CI, 1.59–1.97) use of combined hormonal therapy were found. Among women with a body mass index < 25, the relative risk for breast cancer associated with the use of combined hormonal therapy was 2.31 (95% CI, 2.12–2.53) and that in women with a body mass index of ≥ 25 was 1.78 (95% CI, 1.64–1.94). An attempt was made to assess the association between use of hormonal menopausal therapy and mortality from breast cancer, but, at the time of publication, the data did not allow reliable estimates of this. However, in a letter (Banks *et al.*, 2004), it was reported that, for all types combined, current users had a 30% higher risk for mortality from breast cancer than never users (relative risk, 1.30; 95% CI, 1.11–1.53).

The association of the use of combined hormonal menopausal therapy with an increased risk for breast cancer was assessed in a prospective study in southern Sweden (Jernström et al., 2003a) in a cohort of 6586 women aged 50–64 years at baseline. During 4 years of follow-up by linkage to the Swedish Cancer Registry, 101 women were registered with incident breast cancer. Ever use of combined hormonal menopausal therapy was associated with a relative risk of 3.3 (95% CI, 1.9–5.6) compared with never use. In relation to duration of use, the relative risk associated with use for 2 years or less (relative risk, 3.7; 95% CI, 1.8–7.4) was not substantially different from that associated with use for 5 years or more (relative risk, 3.7; 95% CI, 1.8–7.7).

Another prospective study, conducted in the same region in Sweden as the above study, was based on more than 29 000 women (Olsson et al., 2003). The women were followed up by linkage to the Swedish Cancer Registry, and 556 cases of breast cancer were registered. The analyses focused on the duration of use of combined hormonal menopausal therapy and whether the mode of administration had different effects on the risk for breast cancer. The relative risk associated with daily ever use of combined hormonal menopausal therapy was 2.45 (95% CI, 1.61–3.71), and sequential administration was associated with a relative risk of 1.22 (95% CI, 0.74–2.00) compared with never users. The relative risk increased with recency and duration of use. Compared with never users, those who reported daily use of combined preparations for 4 years or more had a relative risk of 4.60 (95% CI, 2.39–8.84) and those who had taken combined sequential therapy for 4 years or more had a relative risk of 2.23 (95% CI, 0.90–5.56). These results were adjusted for age, age at menarche, age at first full-term pregnancy, parity, age at menopause and family history of breast cancer.

In the NOWAC Study, the association between use of combined hormonal menopausal therapy and the risk for breast cancer was assessed in a prospective follow-up of 31 451 postmenopausal women who were aged 45–64 years at entry (Bakken et al., 2004). Information on the use of hormonal menopausal therapy was collected at recruitment by self-administered questionnaires; during follow-up by linkage to the Norwegian Cancer Registry, 331 women were registered with incident breast cancer. The association for ever use versus never use of combined preparations was not reported, but current users of combined hormonal therapy at study entry had a relative risk of 2.5 (95% CI, 1.9–3.2; 116 exposed cases) compared with never users. For current users of combined therapy for less than 5 years, the relative risk was 2.3 (95% CI, 1.7–3.2; 63 exposed cases); for longer duration of use, the relative risk was 2.8 (95% CI, 2.0–4.0; 51 exposed cases). These results were adjusted for age, body mass index, age at menarche, ever use of oral contraceptives, time since menopause, family history of breast cancer, history of mammography screening and age at first birth. The investigators also studied the effect of daily versus sequential use of progestogens in the combined treatment. Daily treatment for less than 5 years was associated with a relative risk of 2.6 (95% CI, 1.9–3.7; 44 exposed cases); for longer duration of daily treatment, the relative risk was 3.2 (95% CI, 2.2–4.6; 37 exposed cases) compared with the risk of never users. In comparison, the relative risk associated with a cyclical regimen was 1.7 (95% CI, 1.0–2.8; 19 exposed cases) for less than 5 years of use and 2.2 (95% CI, 1.3–3.8; 14 exposed cases) for 5 years or more.

A cohort study from Denmark investigated whether different progestogens in combined hormonal menopausal therapy exert different effects on the risk for breast cancer (Stahlberg et al., 2004). Brands of combined hormonal menopausal therapy were coded as containing either 'progesterone-like' (typically medroxyprogesterone acetate) or 'testosterone-like' (typically norethisterone or levonorgestrel) progestogens. More than 23 000 nurses received a questionnaire in 1993, of whom nearly 20 000 responded and returned information on their use of combined hormonal menopausal therapy. After exclusions, 10 874 women were eligible for breast cancer follow-up through the Danish Cancer Registry and, among these, 244 women were registered with incident breast cancer during 6 years of follow-up. The association with ever use or with past use of combined hormonal therapy was not specified in the report. However, the relative risk associated with current use at entry to the study was 2.70 (95% CI, 1.96–3.73) compared with the risk of never users. Among current users of combined treatment with 'testosterone-like' progestogens, the relative risk was also increased. When these progestogens were administered daily, the relative risk was 4.16 (95% CI, 2.56–6.75) and when they were given less than daily (termed cyclically or sequentially), the relative risk was 1.94 (95% CI, 1.26–3.00) compared with never users. The report did not provide details on the number of days during a cycle that sequential treatment was given.

Another Danish cohort study (The Diet, Cancer and Health Study) assessed type of hormonal menopausal therapy used in relation to the risk for breast cancer, and specified the association according to histological subtypes (Tjønneland et al., 2004). Among 23 618 women with information on hormonal therapy who were assumed to be postmenopausal, 423 incident cases of breast cancer were identified through the Danish Cancer Registry over a median follow-up of 4.8 years. The results for ever use or past use were not reported. However, the effects of daily and cyclical regimens of combined preparations were compared, and whether these modes of administration exterted different effects on the risk for lobular and ductal breast carcinoma was examined. In relation to lobular carcinoma, rates of breast cancer associated with the use of daily and cyclical regimens were essentially identical, whereas the risk for ductal carcinoma was slightly higher when the progestogens were administered daily compared with sequentially.

In a cohort of 48 812 Danish women who were aged 50–67 years at baseline, Ewertz et al. (2005) linked information from the Danish Prescription Database to information on incident cases of breast cancer registered by the Danish Cancer Registry during 10 years of follow-up. Altogether, 869 women were registered with breast cancer during the study period. The effects of different progestogens were studied: combined therapy that contained either levonorgestrel, norethisterone, norgestimate, desogestrel or gestodene was classified as combined treatment with 'testosterone-derived' progestogens, and treatment containing medroxyprogesterone [acetate] as combined treatment with 'progesterone-derived' progestogens. Results related to ever use versus never use of combined preparations were not reported, but the association with current use was specified for various types of combined regimens. Current cyclical use of estrogen plus a progesterone-derived progestogen was associated with a relative risk of 0.57 (95% CI, 0.26–1.28; six exposed cases). Current daily use of estrogen plus a testosterone-derived progestogen was associated with a relative risk of 0.99 (95% CI, 0.57–1.72; 13 exposed cases); among current users of cyclical regimens of estrogen plus a testosterone-derived progestogen, the relative risk was 1.52 (95% CI, 1.21–1.93; 80 exposed cases). These results were adjusted for age, age at first birth and parity.

Fournier *et al.* (2005) assessed the use of different types of hormonal menopausal therapy in relation to risk for breast cancer among 54 548 French women; 948 primary invasive breast cancers were diagnosed during 5.8 years of follow-up. Average use of combined hormonal menopausal therapy was 2.8 years. The association for ever use versus never use with breast cancer was not specified in the report, but women who were current users of combined hormonal therapy had a relative risk of 1.3 (95% CI, 1.1–1.5) compared with never users. The main aim of this study was to examine the effects of different types of progestogens that were used in the combined treatment. Current use of treatment that contained micronized progesterone (only given transdermally) was associated with a relative risk of 0.9 (95% CI, 0.7–1.2; 55 exposed cases). In contrast, current use of synthetic progestogens was associated with a relative risk of 1.4 (95% CI, 1.2–1.7; 268 exposed cases). These results were adjusted for a range of factors, including age, age at menopause, body mass index, parity, age at first birth, family history of breast cancer and previous use of oral contraceptives.

2.1.4   *Case-control studies* (Table 5)

A large population-based case–control study in Sweden (Magnusson *et al.*, 1999) included 3345 women aged 50–74 years who had been diagnosed with invasive breast cancer and 3454 controls of similar age. The main objective was to assess whether the use of combined hormonal therapy is associated with risk for breast cancer, with particular reference to long duration of use. For ever use of combined therapy, the relative risk for breast cancer was 1.63 (95% CI, 1.37–1.94) compared with never use. Risk increased with duration of use: the relative risk for 2–5 years of use was 1.40 (95% CI, 1.01–1.94), that for 5–10 years of use was 2.43 (95% CI, 1.72–3.44) and that for 10 or more years of use was 2.95 (95% CI, 1.84–4.72). These results were adjusted for age, parity, age at first birth, age at menopause, body mass index and height. The results from two sub-analyses were also presented; however, these analyses did not include only women who had exclusively used combined treatment, but also women who had used estrogen-only treatment at some time. The results suggested that combined preparations that contain testosterone-derived progestogens may confer higher risk (relative risk, 1.68; 95% CI, 1.39–2.03; 324 exposed cases) than combined therapy that contains progesterone-derived progestogens (relative risk, 1.14; 95% CI, 0.69–1.88; 32 exposed cases). The results also showed that

Table 5. Case–control studies of the use of combined hormone therapy and the risk for breast cancer

Reference, location	Study period	Age (years)	Histology	Sub-site	Therapy (type/regimen)	Cases	Controls	Odds ratio	95% CI	Duration Years	Odds ratio	95% CI	Time since last use Years	Odds ratio	95% CI
Magnusson et al. (1999), Sweden	1993–95	50–74	Invasive	All	Never	1738	2201	1.0							
					Ever	409	295	1.63	1.37–1.94	> 2–5	1.40	1.01–1.94			
										> 5–10	2.43	1.72–3.44			
										> 10	2.95	1.84–4.72			
					E + T[a]	324	229	1.68	1.39–2.03	≤ 5	1.33	1.05–1.68			
										> 5	2.74	1.99–3.78			
					Cyclic	102	76	1.48	1.08–2.04	> 2–5	1.34	0.71–2.54			
										> 5–10	1.89	0.88–4.09			
					Continuous	139	124	1.41	1.09–1.83	> 2–5	1.26	0.76–2.09			
										> 5–10	2.89	1.66–5.00			
					E + P[b]	32	34	1.14	0.69–1.88	≤ 5	1.41	0.80–2.51			
										> 5	0.79	0.26–2.39			
Li, C.I. et al. (2000), USA (King County, WA)	1988–90	50–64	Invasive and in situ	All	Never	180	187	1.0							
				Ductal	Ever	35	55	0.70	0.50–1.20	NR			Current	0.70	0.50–1.10
				Lobular	Ever	12	55	2.50	1.10–4.60	NR			Current	2.60	1.10–5.80
			Invasive	All	Never	159	187	1.0							
				Ductal	Ever	30	55	0.70	0.40–1.20	NR			Current	0.70	0.40–1.10
				Lobular	Ever	9	55	2.60	1.00–6.70	NR			Current	2.60	0.80–5.80
Ross et al. (2000), USA (Los Angeles, CA)	1987–96	55–72	Invasive and in situ	All	Never	873	784			1.0		NR			
					Ever	425	324	NR		NR		NR			
					Cyclical	218	166			1–5	1.19	NR			
						75	48			> 5–10	1.58	NR			
						27	14			> 10	1.79	NR			
					Daily	59	58			1–5	0.88	NR			
						23	18			> 5–10	1.28	NR			
						23	20			> 10	1.23	NR			

Table 5 (contd)

Reference, location	Study period	Age (years)	Histology	Sub-site	Therapy (type/regimen)	Cases	Controls	Odds ratio	95% CI	Duration			Time since last use		
										Years	Odds ratio	95% CI	Years	Odds ratio	95% CI
Kirsh & Kreiger (2002), Canada	1995–96	20–74	Invasive	All	Never	272	283	1.0		<1	0.86	0.26–2.82			
					Ever	48	33	1.22	0.72–2.06	1–4	0.96	0.39–2.39			
										5–9	0.84	0.31–2.24			
										≥10	3.48	1.00–12.1			
Newcomb et al. (2002), USA (New Hampshire, Wisconsin, Massachusetts)	1992–94	50–79	Invasive	All	Never	3827	4132	1.0		<5	1.36	1.07–1.73	Current	1.39	1.12–1.71
					Ever	315	286	1.43	1.18–1.74	≥5	1.57	1.15–2.14	<5	1.71	0.92–3.18
													≥5	2.38	0.82–6.87
				Ductal	Ever	208	286	1.43	1.14–1.79						
				Lobular	Ever	32	286	2.01	1.25–3.22						

Table 5 (contd)

Reference, location	Study period	Age (years)	Histology	Sub-site	Therapy (type/regimen)	Cases	Controls	Odds ratio	95% CI	Duration — Years	Odds ratio	95% CI	Time since last use — Years	Odds ratio	95% CI
Weiss et al. (2002); Daling et al. (2002), USA (Atlanta, GA; Detroit, MI; Philadelphia, PA; Los Angeles, CA; Seattle, WA)	1994–98	35–64	Invasive	All	Never	672	655	1.0							
					Ever	689	630	[1.13]		2–<5	1.3	0.96–1.63	Current	1.22	0.99–1.50
										≥5	1.2	0.92–1.48	≥0.5	0.76	0.60–0.97
					Sequential	287	267	[1.05]		2–<5	1.1	0.73–1.58	Current	0.91	0.67–1.24
										≥5	1	0.69–1.32	≥0.5	1.07	0.80–1.41
					Continuous	419	352	[1.20]		2–<5	1.20	0.88–1.65	Current	1.29	1.02–1.64
										≥5	1.4	0.98–1.85	≥0.5	0.78	0.57–1.06
			Ductal		Never	515	655	1.0							
					Ever	448	534	1.00	0.80–1.30	2–<5	1.00	0.80–1.30	≥5	0.70	0.50–1.10
										≥5	1.00	0.80–1.30	>0–0.5	1.20	0.90–1.50
					Sequential	230	284	1.00	0.80–1.30	0.5–<5	1.00	0.80–1.40	≥5	0.90	0.60–1.40
										≥5	1.00	0.70–1.30	>0–0.5	0.90	0.70–1.30
					Continuous	268	280	1.20	0.90–1.50	0.5–<5	1.20	0.90–1.50	≥5	0.70	0.40–1.30
										≥5	1.20	0.90–1.50	>0–0.5	1.30	1.00–1.70
			Lobular		Never	75	655	1.0							
					Ever	112	534	1.80	1.20–2.60	0.5–<5	1.60	1.00–2.40	≥5	0.90	0.40–2.10
										≥5	2.00	1.30–3.20	>0–0.5	2.20	1.40–3.30
					Sequential	53	284	1.40	0.90–2.20	0.5–<5	1.30	0.80–2.30	≥5	1.30	0.60–2.70
										≥5	1.50	0.80–2.60	>0–0.5	1.40	0.80–2.50
					Continuous	75	280	2.20	1.40–3.50	0.5–<5	2.10	1.30–3.30	≥5	1.60	0.60–4.10
										≥5	2.50	1.40–4.30	>0–0.5	2.40	1.50–3.80

Table 5 (contd)

Reference, location	Study period	Age (years)	Histology	Sub-site	Therapy (type/regimen)	Cases	Controls	Odds ratio	95% CI	Duration Years	Odds ratio	95% CI	Time since last use Years	Odds ratio	95% CI
Li et al. (2003), USA (3-county Puget Sound, WA)	1997–99	65–79	Invasive	All	Never	284	339	1.0		0.5–<5	1.30	0.80–2.20	Current	1.9	1.6–2.6
					Ever	136	964	1.80	1.30–2.50	5–<15	2.00	1.30–3.20			
					Sequential	80	55	1.80	1.20–2.70						
					Continuous	159	116	1.60	1.20–2.20						
				Ductal	Never	199	339	1.0		<5	1.40	0.8–2.5	Former	2.00	1.1–3.7
					Ever	89	96	1.60	1.10–2.30	5–<15	1.60	1.0–2.7	Current	1.70	1.2–2.4
										≥15	1.90	1.1–3.2	0.5–<5	1.30	0.8–2.3
													5–<15	1.70	1.1–2.7
					Sequential	52	55	1.70	1.10–2.60						
					Continuous	102	116	1.50	1.10–2.00						
				Lobular	Never	47	339	1.0		<5	1.40	0.8–2.5	Former	2.00	0.7–5.7
					Ever	29	96	2.50	1.40–4.30	5–<15	3.40	1.7–7.0	Current	3.10	1.9–5.2
										≥15	2.40	1.1–5.5	0.5–<5	1.30	0.5–3.6
													5–<15	4.60	2.5–8.5
					Sequential	19	55	2.80	1.50–5.40						
					Continuous	40	116	2.70	1.60–4.40						

CI, confidence interval; NR, not reported
[a] Estrogen + testosterone-like progestogen
[b] Estrogen + progesterone-like progestogen

the positive association between the use of hormonal menopausal therapy and risk for breast cancer may be confined to women with a body mass index lower than 27 kg/m^2.

Li, C.I. *et al.* (2000) conducted a case–control study in the USA that involved 537 women who had breast cancer and were 50–64 years of age and 492 controls selected at random from the population. The aim of the study was to investigate whether the use of combined hormonal menopausal therapy has different effects on different histological subtypes of breast cancer. For women who had used combined hormonal therapy for at least 6 months, the relative risk for ductal breast carcinoma was 0.7 (95% CI, 0.5–1.2; 35 exposed cases) and that for lobular breast carcinoma was 2.5 (95% CI, 1.1–4.6; 12 exposed cases). Using a likelihood ratio test, the difference between these two estimates of relative risk was statistically significant ($p = 0.007$). The relative risk associated with current use of combined hormonal therapy for at least 6 months was 2.6 (95% CI, 1.1–5.8) for lobular breast carcinoma compared with the risk in never users. These results were adjusted for age and type of menopause (natural or surgical). In comparison, there was no increase in the risk for ductal breast carcinoma (relative risk, 0.7; 95% CI, 0.5–1.1) related to current use of combined hormonal menopausal therapy. A similar comparison between the estimates suggested that the difference was statistically significant ($p < 0.03$).

The specific aim of a case–control study in the USA (Ross *et al.*, 2000) was to investigate whether daily administration of combined hormonal therapy exerts a different effect on risk for breast cancer than sequential administration. The study included 1897 post-menopausal women with breast cancer and 1637 postmenopausal population controls. The age range of the participants was 55–72 years. The relative risk for ever use versus never use of combined preparations was not reported, but the risk for breast cancer increased with duration of use. For every 5 years of use of combined therapy, the relative risk was 1.24 (95% CI, 1.07–1.45). The risk related to combined regimens with cyclical pro-gestogens was slightly higher than that found for regimens in which progestogens were given daily, but the difference was not statistically significant: for 5 years of use, the odds ratio for the cyclical regimen was 1.38 (95% CI, 1.13–1.68; 320 exposed cases) versus 1.09 (95% CI, 0.88–1.35; 105 exposed cases) for the daily regimen. These results were adjusted for age, age at menarche, family history of breast cancer, age at first full-term pregnancy, parity, age at menopause, previous use of oral contraceptives, body weight and consumption of alcoholic beverages.

A population-based case–control study in Canada on data from the Enhanced Cancer Surveillance Project (Kirsh & Kreiger, 2002) included 320 incident cases of breast cancer and 316 controls (with information or hormonal therapy use) who were frequency-matched by age. A self-administered questionnaire was used to collect information on the use of combined hormonal menopausal therapy between 1995 and 1997. Long duration of use (10 years or longer) of combined estrogen–progestogen therapy was associated with an increased risk (odds ratio, 3.48; 95% CI, 1.00–12.11) compared with never use.

Another large case–control study in the USA (Newcomb *et al.*, 2002) investigated the type and duration of use of combined hormonal menopausal therapy in relation to the risk for breast cancer. The study included 5298 postmenopausal cases of breast cancer aged

50–79 years of age and 5571 control women who were randomly selected from population lists. The relative risk for ever use versus never use of combined regimens was 1.43 (95% CI, 1.18–1.74; 315 exposed cases). Women who used regimens with daily progestogens had a relative risk of 1.45 (95% CI, 1.06–1.99; 115 exposed cases), but the association was similar for women who used the different types of sequential therapy. The relative risk for breast cancer increased with duration of use: the increase per year of combined treatment was approximately 4% (relative risk, 1.04; 95% CI, 1.01–1.08) and that for recent use for more than 5 years was 1.57 (95% CI, 1.15–2.14).

The association between the use of combined hormonal menopausal therapy and the risk for breast cancer was also studied in the CARE [Contraceptive and Reproductive Experience] multicentre case–control study in the USA. Weiss et al. (2002) included 1870 post-menopausal women with breast cancer aged 35–64 years and 1953 controls identified by random-digit dialling. Current users for 5 or more years of daily combined hormonal menopausal therapy were at increased risk for breast cancer (odds ratio, 1.54; 95% CI, 1.10–2.17) compared with never users. Among current users, increasing duration of use was associated with increasing risk (p for trend = 0.01). Whether different regimens of combined hormonal menopausal therapy may have different effects on different histological subtypes of breast cancer was also studied within the same study (Daling et al., 2002). Cases were 1749 post-menopausal women under 65 years of age with a diagnosis of breast cancer; the 1953 controls were those included in the study of Weiss et al. (2002). The aim was to assess whether combined hormonal therapy increases the risk for lobular breast carcinoma. The tumours were grouped into three histological categories: 1386 patients had ductal carcinoma, 148 had lobular carcinoma and 115 women were diagnosed with a mixture of these histological subtypes. Another 100 patients were divided among less prevalent histological types of breast cancer. The association with ever use (≥ 6 months) versus never use of combined menopausal therapy was not reported, but current daily use of combined treatment was associated with an increased risk for invasive lobular disease (odds ratio, 2.2; 95% CI, 1.4–3.5; 75 exposed cases). The relative risks were adjusted for age, race, study site and age at menopause.

A case–control study in the USA (Li et al., 2003) assessed duration and patterns of use of combined hormonal therapy in relation to histological subtypes and hormonal receptor status of breast cancer. The study included 975 women aged 65–79 years who had invasive breast cancer classified according to histology and hormone receptor status and 1007 population controls. For women who had ever used combined hormonal therapy only, the relative risk for breast cancer was 1.8 (95% CI, 1.3–2.5) compared with the risk in never users. When examined by histological subtype, ever users of combined hormonal menopausal therapy had an increased risk for both invasive ductal carcinoma (relative risk, 1.6; 95% CI, 1.1–2.3; 89 exposed cases) and invasive lobular carcinoma (relative risk, 2.5; 95% CI, 1.4–4.3; 29 exposed cases). The increased risk for lobular carcinoma was greater in women who had used combined therapy for a relatively long time. For lobular carcinoma, the relative risk for use for between 5 and 15 years was 3.4 (95% CI, 1.7–7.0) and that for use for longer than 15 years was 2.4 (95% CI, 1.1–5.5). Both current and former use for at least 6 months were associated with an increased risk for all histological sub-types. With regard to different hormone receptor properties, the results showed that, among ever users, the relative risk for estrogen and progesterone receptor-positive tumours was 2.0 (95% CI, 1.5–2.7). The risk increased with duration of use, but did not differ according to whether progestogens were given sequentially (relative risk, 1.8; 95% CI, 1.2–2.7) or daily (relative risk, 1.6; 95% CI, 1.2–2.2). In relation to estrogen or progesterone receptor-negative breast cancer, no increase in risk was found, but low statistical power related to hormone receptor-negative disease limited the ability of the study to evaluate this subtype of breast cancer reliably.

2.2   Endometrial cancer

Postmenopausal women who use estrogen-only therapy are at an increased risk for endometrial cancer, and the risk increases with increasing duration of use (IARC, 1999). To counteract this risk, many women use combined estrogen–progestogen regimens. At the time when the previous evaluation on this topic was made, only four published studies provided information on the effects of the combined regimens on the risk for endometrial cancer, and the limited available evidence suggested that the addition of progestogens reduced the elevated risk associated with estrogen.

2.2.1   Descriptive studies

Using data from the Southern California Kaiser Foundation Health Plan, Ziel et al. (1998) reported patterns of prescription of hormonal menopausal therapy among women aged over 45 years in 1971–93 and related them to trends in the incidence of endometrial cancer. Use of combined estrogen–progestogen regimens began to increase during the mid-1980s. A log-linear model fitted to the data indicated that, since about 1984, the prescription of progestogens together with estrogens was negatively associated with the incidence rates of endometrial cancer. The authors concluded that their observation was consistent with the hypothesis that progestogens administered in conjunction with estrogens can protect against much of the increased risk for endometrial cancer associated with the use of estrogens alone.

2.2.2   Randomized trials

In a trial in which 168 institutionalized women were randomized to receive estrogen–progestogen menopausal therapy or placebo, no case of endometrial cancer occurred in the treated group and one case occurred in those who received placebo (Nachtigall et al., 1979).

The HERS randomized 2763 women with previous coronary heart disease to either placebo or a daily regimen of 0.625 mg conjugated equine estrogen and 2.5 mg medroxy-progesterone acetate. The women were then followed up for 4.1 years on average (Hulley *et al.*, 1998). During the follow-up period, two endometrial cancers were diagnosed in the treated group and four were diagnosed in the placebo group to give a relative risk of 0.49 (95% CI, 0.09–2.68) for use of continuous combined therapy compared with placebo.

In the WHI Trial, 16 608 women who had not had a hysterectomy were randomized to receive placebo or a daily regimen of 0.625 mg conjugated equine estrogen and 2.5 mg medroxyprogesterone acetate. After an average follow-up of 5.6 years, Anderson *et al.* (2003) reported that 27 incident cases of endometrial cancer had occurred among those randomized to continuous combined hormonal therapy and 31 cases among those randomized to placebo. The relative risk was 0.81 (95% CI, 0.48–1.36) for the use of continuous combined therapy compared with placebo.

2.2.3   *Cohort studies*

Cohort studies that presented relative risk estimates for endometrial cancer associated with the use of estrogen–progestogen menopausal therapy published from 1999 onwards are summarized in Table 6.

Hammond *et al.* (1979) followed up approximately 600 women, approximately half of whom had used either estrogen-only or estrogen–progestogen preparations and half of whom had not used hormones. No cases of endometrial cancer were observed among the 72 women who received estrogen–progestogen therapy, whereas three cases were observed among women who did not. No person–years or age-adjusted relative risks were reported.

Gambrell (1986) reported that the incidence of endometrial cancer among women who had used combined hormonal therapy (eight cases in 16 327 woman–years) was lower than that among women who did not use any hormonal therapy (nine cases in 4480 woman–years). No age-adjusted relative risks were reported.

Persson *et al.* (1999) updated their earlier report on the follow-up of a cohort of Swedish women who had used hormonal menopausal therapy (Persson *et al.*, 1989). The cohort had initially been identified through pharmacy records; in 1987–88, the women were mailed a follow-up questionnaire requesting further details on their use of hormonal therapy and other personal characteristics. The 8438 women who replied were linked to the National Swedish Cancer Registry; 66 endometrial cancers were identified in the cohort up to December 1993. In comparison with the population rates in the Uppsala health care region, the relative risk for endometrial cancer associated with use of estrogen–progestogen therapy was 1.4 (95% CI, 0.9–2.3; six exposed cases) for 1–6 years of use and 1.7 (95% CI, 1.1–2.6; 11 exposed cases) for more than 6 years of use. There was no significant difference according to duration of use. Estimates of relative risk were not given according to the number of days per month that progestogens were added to estrogen therapy or by time since last use of the therapy.

Pukkala *et al.* (2001) linked prescription records for hormonal menopausal therapy to cancer registry data in Finland and compared incidence rates of endometrial cancer in users of combined therapy with those in the general population in Finland. Among 78 549 women who were taking progestogens added to estrogen therapy for 10–12 days every month, the

Table 6. Cohort studies of the use of estrogen–progestogen menopausal therapy use and risk for endometrial cancer by number of days that progestogens were added to estrogen therapy per month, duration of use and type of progestogen

Reference, location	Study period	Age range (years)	Source population	Type/measure of combined therapy	No. of cases	Relative risk (95% CI)	Comments
Persson et al. (1999), Sweden	1987–93	65 (median)	8438 women	None	12	1.0	Adjusted for age, length of follow-up, age at first full-term pregnancy, body mass index, education, menopausal age/status
				Any progestogen added to estrogen			
				Duration			
				≤ 6 years	6	1.4 (0.9–2.3)	
				> 6 years	11	1.7 (1.1–2.6)	
Pukkala et al. (2001), Finland	1994–97	Any age	94 505 women	Progestogens 14 days every 3 months	61	2.0 (1.6–2.6)	Standardized incidence ratios, using the female Finnish population
				Progestogens 10–12 days per month	141	1.3 (1.1–1.6)	
Bakken et al. (2004), Norway	1991–NR	45–64	67 336 women	None	45	1.0	Adjusted for age, body mass index, smoking, ever use of oral contraceptives, time since menopause, parity, age at last birth
				Any	11	0.7 (0.4–1.4)	

Table 6 (contd)

Reference, location	Study period	Age range (years)	Source population	Type/measure of combined therapy	No. of cases	Relative risk (95% CI)	Comments
Beral et al. (2005), United Kingdom	1996–2002	50–65	716 738 women	None	773	1.0	Adjusted for age, region of residence, socioeconomic status, body mass index, alcoholic beverage consumption, ever use of oral contraceptives, time since menopause, parity
				Progestogens, every day/month			
				Any	73	0.71 (0.59–0.90)	
				Duration			
				< 5 years	28	0.55 (0.37–0.80)	
				≥ 5 years	44	0.90 (0.66–1.22)	
				Type of progestogen			
				Norethisterone	46	0.76 (0.57–1.03)	
				Medroxyprogesterone acetate	27	0.63 (0.43–0.93)	
				Progestogens, 10–14 days/ month			
				Any	242	1.05 (0.90–1.22)	
				Duration			
				< 5 years	95	0.90 (0.72–1.12)	
				≥ 5 years	140	1.17 (0.97–1.41)	
				Type of progestogen			
				Norgestrel	183	1.09 (0.93–1.29)	
				Norethisterone	53	0.93 (0.70–1.23)	

CI, confidence interval; NR, not reported

standardized incidence ratio (SIR) for endometrial cancer was 1.3 (95% CI, 1.1–1.6; 141 cases); among 15 956 women who used progestogens added to estrogen for 14 days every 3 months, the standardized incidence ratio was 2.0 (95% CI, 1.6–2.6; 61 cases).

Bakken *et al.* (2004) followed 67 336 Norwegian women aged 45–64 years who were recruited in 1991–97. Information on use of hormonal therapy was obtained from self-completed questionnaires and incident cancers were determined by linkage to data from the Cancer Registry of Norway. Among 7268 women who were using estrogen–progestogen menopausal therapy at the time of recruitment, 11 incident endometrial cancers were diagnosed. The associated relative risk was 0.7 (95% CI, 0.4–1.4), adjusted for age, body mass index, tobacco smoking, use of oral contraceptives, time since menopause, parity and age at first birth. Estimates of relative risk were not given according to the number of days per month that progestogens were added to estrogen therapy or by time since last use of the therapy.

In 1996–2001, the Million Women Study Collaborators (Beral *et al.*, 2005) recruited over a million women in the United Kingdom aged 50–65 years through the National Health Service Breast Screening Programme. Information was collected on the last formulation of hormonal therapy used and the total duration of use of such therapy or any type of hormonal therapy. This self-reported information showed 97% agreement with prescription records on whether combined or estrogen-only menopausal therapy was currently used (Banks *et al.*, 2001). At recruitment, 716 738 members of the cohort were postmenopausal and had not had a hysterectomy or previous diagnosis of cancer. Follow-up of these women via national cancer registries over an average of 3.4 years identified 1320 women with incident endometrial cancer. Compared with never users of hormonal therapy (773 cases), the relative risks for endometrial cancer were 0.71 (95% CI, 0.56–0.90; 73 exposed cases) for any use of continuous estrogen–progestogen therapy and 1.05 (95% CI, 0.91–1.22; 242 exposed cases) for any use of cyclical estrogen–progestogen therapy (usually including progestogens for 10–14 days per month). The relative risks were adjusted for age, region of residence, socioeconomic status, body mass index, alcoholic beverage consumption, ever use of oral contraceptives, time since menopause and parity. The difference between the effects of continuous and cyclical estrogen–progestogen therapy was highly significant ($p = 0.006$). Most women were current or recent users of these therapies at the time of recruitment into the study and, although there was no significant difference in the findings between current and past users, there was limited power to detect any difference, since the average time since last use was only 1–3 years among former users. Among women who had last used a combined therapy (both continuous and cyclical), there were no significant differences according to duration of use or the constituent progestogen. Nine factors that could potentially modify the effects of hormonal therapy on endometrial cancer were examined, and only body mass index consistently showed a significant interaction. Among women with body mass indices of < 25, 25–29 and ≥ 30 kg/m², respectively, the relative risks for endometrial cancer were 1.07 (95% CI, 0.73–1.56), 0.88 (95% CI, 0.60–1.30) and 0.28 (95% CI, 0.14–0.55) for use of continuous combined therapy and 1.54 (95% CI, 1.20–1.99), 1.07 (95% CI, 0.82–1.40) and 0.67 (95% CI, 0.49–0.91) for use of cyclical combined therapy.

2.2.4   *Case–control studies*

The case–control studies that presented relative risk estimates for endometrial cancer associated with the use of estrogen–progestogen menopausal therapy are summarized in Table 7.

A multicentre study was conducted with 300 menopausal women who had been diagnosed with endometrial cancer at seven US hospitals located in five different areas of the country and 207 age-, race- and residence-matched control women from the general population (Brinton & Hoover, 1993). Use of any estrogen–progestogen therapy for 3 months or longer was reported by 11 (4%) of the case women and nine (5%) of the control women (odds ratio, 1.8; 95% CI, 0.6–4.9 adjusted for age, parity, weight and years of oral contraceptive use).

Jick *et al.* (1993) studied women who were members of a large health maintenance organization in western Washington State, USA. Women with endometrial cancer were identified from the tumour registry of the organization and control women were other members; both groups included only women who used the pharmacies of the organization and who had previously completed a questionnaire sent to all female members for a study of mammography. Use of hormonal menopausal therapy was ascertained from the pharmacy database. Relative to women who had never or briefly (≤ 6 months) used menopausal hormones, those who had used any estrogen–progestogen therapy within the previous year had a non-significant increased risk (odds ratio, 1.9; 95% CI, 0.9–3.8; 18 cases), after adjustment for age, calendar year, age at menopause, body mass and history of oral contraceptive use. Former users (last use ≥ 1 year earlier) had no significant increase in risk (odds ratio, 0.9; 95% CI, 0.3–3.4; six incident cases), but the statistical power to compare current and past users was limited.

Beresford *et al.* (1997) expanded the study population originally investigated by Voigt *et al.* (1991) and evaluated the risk for endometrial cancer among women who had used estrogen–progestogen therapy exclusively. Women who had been diagnosed with endometrial cancer in 1985–91 were identified from a population-based cancer registry and their characteristics were compared with control women from the general population in western Washington State, USA. The analysis included 394 cases and 788 controls. Relative to women who had never or briefly (≤ 6 months) used menopausal hormones, women who had used only estrogen–progestogen therapy had a borderline increased risk for endometrial cancer (odds ratio, 1.4; 95% CI, 1.0–1.9), after adjustment for age, body mass and county of residence. For women who had used estrogen–progestogen therapy for ≤ 10 days per cycle for at least 5 years, the odds ratio was 3.7 (95% CI, 1.7–8.2; five exposed cases); among women who had used combined therapy with progestogens added cyclically for more than 10 days each month for at least 5 years, the relative risk was 2.5 (95% CI, 1.1–5.5). Statistical power to compare current and past users was limited. Using data from the same study population, McKnight *et al.* (1998) reported that the relative risk associated with the use of cyclical progestogens added for 10–24 days per month was 2.6 (95% CI, 1.3–5.5; 14 exposed cases) among women who had never used estrogen-only previously,

Table 7. Case–control studies of estrogen–progestogen therapy and endometrial cancer risk, by number of days progestogen was added per cycle, duration, and type of progestogen

Reference, location	Study period	Age range (years)	Source of controls	Type/measure of combined therapy	No. of subjects Cases	No. of subjects Controls	Adjusted odds ratio (95% CI)	Comments
Brinton & Hoover (1993), USA (seven hospitals in five areas)	1987–90	20–74	General population	No use Any use for ≥ 3 months[a]	222 11	176 9	1.0 1.8 (0.6–4.9)	Adjusted for age, parity, weight, years of oral contraceptive use
Jick et al. (1993), USA (Washington State)	1989–89	50–64	Members of health maintenance organization	No use or use ≤ 6 months Current/recent Duration (years) < 3 ≥ 3	97 18 NR NR	606 83 NR NR	1.0 1.9 (0.9–3.8) 2.2 (0.7–7.3) 1.3 (0.5–3.4)	Adjusted for age, calendar year, age at menopause, body mass index, oral contraceptive use
Beresford et al. (1997), USA (Washington State)	1985–91	45–74	General population	No use or use ≤ 6 months Any use *Progestogen ≤ 10 days/month* Duration (months) 6–35 36–59 ≥ 60 *Progestogen > 10 days/month* Duration (months) 6–35 36–59 ≥ 60 *Progestogen every day/month*	337 67 12 3 15 10 5 12 9	685 134 14 7 12 31 23 16 33	1.0 1.4 (1.0–1.9) 2.1 (0.9–4.7) 1.4 (0.3–5.4) 3.7 (1.7–8.2) 0.8 (0.4–1.8) 0.6 (0.2–1.6) 2.5 (1.1–5.5) 0.6 (0.3–1.3)	Adjusted for age, body mass index, country of residence

Table 7 (contd)

Reference, location	Study period	Age range (years)	Source of controls	Type/measure of combined therapy	No. of subjects		Adjusted odds ratio (95% CI)	Comments
					Cases	Controls		
Pike et al. (1997), USA (California)	1987–93	50–74	General population (neighbours)	*Any use, progestogen < 10 days/month*[b]				Adjusted for age at menarche, time to regular cycle, parity, weight, duration of breast feeding, amenorrhoea, tobacco smoking, oral contraceptive use, age at menopause
				Duration (months)				
				0	759	744	1.0	
				1–24	35	22	1.4 (NR)	
				25–60	12	12	1.5 (NR)	
				≥60	27	13	3.5 (NR)	
				Any use, progestogen ≥ 10 days/month				
				Duration (months)				
				0	754	703	1.0	
				1–24	37	30	1.0 (NR)	
				25–60	19	25	0.7 (NR)	
				≥60	23	33	1.1 (NR)	
				Any use, progestogen every day/month				
				Duration (months)				
				0	739	710	1.0	
				1–24	45	41	1.1 (NR)	
				25–60	25	15	1.4 (NR)	
				≥60	24	25	1.3 (NR)	
Weiderpass et al. (1999), Sweden	1994–95	50–74	General population	No use	573	2798	1.0	Adjusted for age, age at menopause, parity, age at last birth, body mass index and duration of previous menopausal hormone use
				Any use[a]	119	477	1.3 (1.0–1.7)	
				Progestogen ~10 days/month, ever	90	300	2.0 (1.4–2.7)	
				Duration (years)				
				<5	38	191	1.5 (1.0–2.2)	
				≥5	40	78	2.9 (1.8–4.6)	
				Progestogen, every day/month, ever	41	237	0.7 (0.4–1.0)	
				Duration (years)				
				<5	32	162	0.8 (0.5–1.3)	
				≥5	2	53	0.2 (0.1–0.8)	

Table 7 (contd)

Reference, location	Study period	Age range (years)	Source of controls	Type/measure of combined therapy	No. of subjects		Adjusted odds ratio (95% CI)	Comments
					Cases	Controls		
Jain et al. (2000), Canada (Ontario)	1994–98	> 48	Property assessment list of the Ontario Ministry of Finance	No use	292	316	1.0	Adjusted for age, weight, menarche age, age at menopause, period disorders, education, parity, smoking and physical activity
				Ever use of combined therapy	128	136	1.37 (0.99–1.89)	
				Progestogen for ~10 days/month, ever	65	87	1.05 (0.71–1.56)	
				Duration (years)				
				< 3	18	40	0.57 (0.31–1.06)	
				≥ 3	47	47	1.49 (0.93–2.40)	
				Progestogen every day/month only	15	14	1.51 (0.67–3.42)	
Mizunuma et al. (2001), Japan	1995–97	62.0 (mean)	63 hospitals	Never use of therapy	934	1188	1.0	Adjusted for age, parity, body mass index, height
				Ever use of combined therapy				
				Duration (months)				
				< 12	6	6	0.9 (0.3–3.0)	
				≥ 12	2	6	0.6 (0.1–3.1)	
Newcomb & Trentham-Dietz (2003), USA (Wisconsin)	1991–94	40–79	Medicare beneficiaries	No use	402	1667	1.0	Adjusted for age, parity, body mass index, tobacco smoking, oral contraceptive use
				Ever use of any combined therapy	48	166	1.69 (1.15–2.47)	
				Progestogen added for				
				< 10 days/month	8	21	2.43 (1.00–5.92)	
				10–21 days/month	14	71	1.10 (0.59–2.07)	
				> 21 days/month	20	62	2.26 (1.27–4.00)	
				Progestogen for ≤ 21 days/month Medroxyprogesterone acetate				
				< 10 mg	6	24	1.29 (0.49–3.36)	
				> 10 mg	10	54	1.11 (0.53–2.32)	
				Progestogen for > 21 days/month Medroxyprogesterone acetate				
				< 10 mg	12	45	1.68 (0.82–3.43)	
				> 10 mg	2	8	5.75 (1.75–18.9)	

CI, confidence interval; NR, not reported

[a] Women taking estrogen only included

[b] Use of estrogen only and other combined therapy adjusted for in the analysis

but only 0.21 (95% CI, 0.07–0.66; four exposed cases and controls) among women who had used estrogen-only therapy previously. In a study that included the same study subjects, Hills *et al.* (2000) reported that the relative risk associated with the use of progestogens added to estrogen on a daily basis was 0.6 (95% CI, 0.3–1.3; nine exposed cases, 33 exposed controls).

Pike *et al.* (1997) identified 833 women with endometrial cancer from a population-based cancer registry in Los Angeles County, CA, USA, and matched them to control women of similar age and race (white) who lived in the same neighbourhood as the matched case or to 791 women randomly identifed from the US Health Care Financing Administration computer tapes. The risk for endometrial cancer was investigated among women who had used estrogen–progestogen with progestogen added for fewer than 10 days per cycle, for ≥ 10 days per cycle and continuously. The relative risks were [1.9 (95% CI, 1.3–2.6)] for fewer than 10 days per cycle and [0.96 (95% CI, 0.69–1.34)] for ≥ 10 days per month [the referent group for each analysis was women who had never used that type of therapy]. The odds ratios for every additional 5 years of use were 1.9 (95% CI, 1.3–2.7) and 1.1 (95% CI, 0.8–1.4), respectively, after adjustment for age at menarche, time to regular cycles, parity, weight, duration of breast-feeding, amenorrhoea, tobacco smoking, duration of oral contraceptive use and age at menopause. No significant increase in the odds ratio was found for daily use of progestogens together with estrogens (relative risk, 1.23; 95% CI, 0.88–1.71; 94 exposed cases, 81 exposed controls); for every additional 5 years of use, the odds ratio increased by 1.1 (95% CI, 0.8–1.4). No comparisons were made between current and past users of these therapies.

Weiderpass *et al.* (1999) conducted a population-based case–control study in Sweden of 709 women aged 50–74 years who were diagnosed with endometrial cancer in 1994–95 and 3368 matched controls. When users of estrogen–progestogen menopausal therapy were compared with never users of any type of therapy, the overall relative risk for endometrial cancer was 1.3 (95% CI, 1.0–1.7; 119 exposed cases, 477 exposed controls). All analyses were adjusted by age, age at menopause, parity, age at last birth, body mass index and duration of previous use of various types of menopausal hormones. The odds ratio was 2.0 (95% CI, 1.4–2.7) for use of progestogens added cyclically for an average of 10 days each month and 0.7 (95% CI, 0.4–1.0) for use of continuous combined therapy. Among the users of therapy with progestogens added cyclically, the relative risk was significantly higher in women who had used hormonal therapy for more than 5 years (odds ratio, 2.9; 95% CI, 1.8–4.6) than in those who had used them for shorter durations (odds ratio, 1.5; 95% CI, 1.0–2.2). Among users of continuous combined therapy, the risk was lower in women who had used the therapy for more than 5 years (odds ratio, 0.2; 95% CI, 0.1–0.8) than in those who had used them for shorter durations (odds ratio, 0.8; 95% CI, 0.5–1.3). There were no significant differences in risk according to the specific progestogenic constituent of the therapy.

Jain *et al.* (2000) conducted a population-based case–control study in Ontario, Canada, on 512 women with endometrial cancer and 513 controls. Cases identified through the Ontario Cancer Registry were diagnosed between 1994 and 1998. Controls were identified from property assessment lists maintained by the Ontario Ministry of Finances. Subjects were interviewed at home. For women who reported that they had used estrogen–progestogen menopausal therapy compared with those who had never used any type of therapy, the relative risk for endometrial cancer was 1.37 (95% CI, 0.99–1.89). All analyses were adjusted by age, education, parity, weight, age at menarche, tobacco smoking, past oral contraceptive use, education, and calorie intake and expenditure. Among the users of combined therapy, there were no significant differences according to duration of use, recency of use or the number of days each month that progestogens were added to estrogen therapy but statistical power to compare such patterns of use was limited.

Mizunuma *et al.* (2001) conducted a hospital-based case–control study in Japan of 1025 women who were diagnosed with endometrial cancer in 1995–97 and 1267 matched controls from 63 hospitals. Women who used estrogens with progestin for ≥ 12 months had an odds ratio of 0.6 (95% CI, 0.11–3.11), and those who used estrogens without progestin for ≥ 12 months had an odds ratio of 2.6 (95% CI, 0.23–28.2). Among the users of combined therapy, there were no significant differences according to duration of use; data on risk were not given according to the number of days per month that progestogens were added to estrogen therapy.

Newcomb and Trentham-Dietz (2003) conducted a population-based case–control study in Wisconsin, USA, of 591 women aged 40–79 years who were diagnosed with endometrial cancer in 1991–94 and 2045 matched controls. For ever use of any type of estrogen–progestogen menopausal therapy compared with never use, the odds ratio for endometrial cancer was 1.69 (95% CI, 1.15–2.47). All analyses were adjusted for age, parity, body mass index, tobacco smoking and past oral contraceptive use. For progestogens added cyclically for fewer than 10 days each month, the odds ratio for endometrial cancer was 2.43 (95% CI, 1.00–5.92); for progestogens added cyclically for 10–21 days each month, the relative risk was 1.10 (95% CI, 0.59–2.07); and for daily use of progestogens, the relative risk was 2.26 (95% CI, 1.27–4.00). There were no significant differences in risk according to recency of use, duration of use or the dose of progestogen used, but the power to detect such differences was low.

2.2.5   *Overview*

Two randomized trials, four cohort studies and eight case–control studies have reported relative risks for endometrial cancer associated with the use of combined estrogen–progestogen therapy. Most investigators found that the fewer days each month that progestogens were added to estrogen therapy, the higher was the relative risk for endometrial cancer. Figure 2 summarizes the overall findings. Five of eight studies, including the Million Women Study, reported risks below unity for the addition of progestogen every day. Five of six studies on progestogens added for 10–24 days per month and all four studies on progestogens added for < 10 days per month reported an increased risk for endometrial cancer (Million Women Study Collaborators, 2005).

Figure 2. Summary of published studies on the relation between use of combined estrogen–progestogen hormonal therapy and endometrial cancer, according to the number of days per month that progestogens are added to estrogen therapy

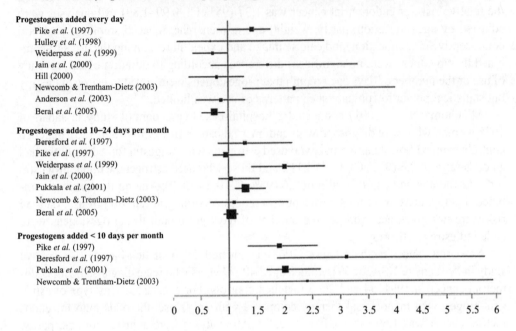

Adapted from Million Women Study Collaborators (2005)

Among the eight studies that reported on the effect of progestogens added to estrogen therapy on a daily basis, only one (Newcomb & Trentham-Dietz, 2003) found that the risk for endometrial cancer was significantly higher in never users of any type of hormonal therapy.

Overall, no consistent trend was found with increasing duration of use of continuous combined therapy (Table 8), and no significant differences were found according to the specific type of progestogen used (Beral *et al.*, 2005) or according to progestogen dose (Newcomb & Trentham-Deitz, 2003).

In the seven studies that reported on the effect of progestogens added to estrogens for 10–21 days per month, all found that the risk for endometrial cancer was similar to or slightly higher than that seen in never users of any type of hormonal therapy (Table 9). Five of the seven studies presented results separately according to duration of use of the therapy and, in every study, the relative risk tended to be higher with longer use. Among users of hormonal therapy with progestogens added for 10–21 days per month, no significant differences were found according to the specific type of progestogen used (Beral *et al.*, 2005).

Table 8. Summary of results on the association of endometrial cancer with the daily addition of progestogens to estrogen therapy

Reference, location	Exposure category	No. of cases	No. of controls/ population at risk	Relative risk/ odds ratio (95% CI)
Observational studies				
Pike et al. (1997), USA	No use	739	710	1.0
	Any use	94	81	1.07 (0.80–1.43)
	Duration ≥ 5 years	24	33	1.34 (NR)
Weiderpass et al. (1999), Sweden	Never	641	3 014	1.0
	Ever	41	237	0.7 (0.4–1.0)
	Duration ≥ 5 years	2	32	0.2 (0.1–0.8)
Hill et al. (2000), USA	No use of any hormonal therapy	392	793	1.0
	Ever continuous hormonal therapy	9	33	0.6 (0.3–1.3)
Jain et al. (2000), Canada	No use	292	316	1.0
	Exclusive use of continuous hormonal therapy	15	14	1.51 (0.67–3.42)
Newcomb & Threntham-Dietz (2003), USA	No use	402	1 667	1.0
	Any use	20	62	2.26 (1.27–4.00)
Beral et al. (2005), United Kingdom	Never users	763	395 786	1.0
	Any use	73	69 577	0.71 (0.56–0.90)
	Duration ≥ 5 years	44	33 600	0.90 (0.66–1.22)
Randomized trials				
Hulley et al. (1998), USA	Placebo[a]	2		1.0
	Estrogen-progestin[a]	4		0.49 (0.09–2.68)
Anderson et al. (2003), USA	Placebo[b]	27		1.0
	Estrogen-progestin[b]	31		0.81 (0.48–1.36)

CI, confidence interval; NR, not reported

[a] 2763 women were randomized.

[b] 16 608 women were randomized.

All four studies that reported on the risk for endometrial cancer associated with use of combined hormonal therapy with progestogens added for less than 10 days per month found an increased risk for endometrial cancer associated with such use, although the risk was lower than that associated with the use of estrogen-only therapy (Beresford et al., 1997; Pike et al., 1997; Pukkala et al., 2001; Newcomb & Trentham-Dietz, 2003). The two studies that reported results according to duration of use found that the risk tended to be higher with longer use (Table 10).

Table 9. Summary of results from studies of endometrial cancer and the addition of progestogens cyclically to estrogen therapy for 10–21 days each month

Reference, location	Exposure category	No. of cases	No. of controls/ population at risk	SIR/odds ratio (95% CI)
Beresford et al. (1997), USA	Never	270	593	1.0
	Any use	25	64	1.3 (0.8–2.2)
	Duration ≥ 5 years	12	16	2.5 (1.1–5.5)
Pike et al. (1997), USA	No use	754	703	1.0
	Any use	79	88	1.07 (0.82–1.41)
	Duration > 5 years	23	33	1.09 [NR]
Weiderpass et al. (1999)[a], Sweden	Never	597	2 963	1.0
	Ever	90	300	2.0 (1.4–2.7)
	Duration ≥ 5 years	40	78	2.9 (1.8–4.6)
Jain et al. (2000)[b], Canada	No use	292	316	1.0
	Any use	65	87	1.05 (0.71–1.56)
	Duration ≥ 3 years	47	47	1.49 (0.93–2.40)
Pukkala et al. (2001), Finland	Any use	141	105[c]	1.3 (1.1–1.6)
Newcomb & Threntham-Dietz (2003), USA	No use	402	1 667	1.0
	Any use	14	71	1.10 (0.59–2.07)
Beral et al. (2005), United Kingdom	No use	763	395 785	1.0
	Any use	242	145 486	1.05 (0.91–1.22)
	Duration ≥ 5 years	140	75 000	1.17 (0.97–1.41)

CI, confidence interval; NR, not reported; SIR, standardized incidence ratio
[a] The average duration of use of progestogens was about 10 days each month.
[b] All but six cases used progestogens for 10 or more days each month.
[c] Expected number of cases, based on incidence rates of endometrial cancer in Finland

Taken together, the results are consistent with the view that the addition of progestogens to estrogen therapy lessens the risk associated with the use of estrogens alone, and that the greater the number of days per month that progestogens are added, the greater is the reduction in risk. The addition of progestogens for less than 10 days per month is associated with a clear increase in the risk for endometrial cancer. To reduce the rates of endometrial cancer in menopausal women to levels that are found in never users of hormonal therapy, progestogens may need to be added to estrogens most of the time and possibly on a daily basis. Since the use of combined estrogen–progestogen therapy began relatively recently, there is as yet little information on the effects of combined estrogen–progestogen therapy on the risk for endometrial cancer many years after cessation of use.

Table 10. Summary of results of studies of endometrial cancer and the addition of progestogens to estrogen therapy cyclically for < 10 days each month

Reference, location	Exposure category	No. of cases	No. of controls/ population at risk	Relative risk/ odds ratio (95% CI)
Beresford *et al.* (1997), USA	Never	270	593	1.0
	Any use	25	26	3.1 (1.7–5.7)
	Duration ≥ 5 years	15	12	3.7 (1.7–8.2)
Pike *et al.* (1997), USA	No use	759	744	1.0
	Any use	74	49	1.9 (1.3–2.6)
	Duration > 5 years	27	13	3.49 (NR)
Pukkala *et al.* (2001), Finland	Any use	61	30	2.0 (1.6–2.6)
Newcomb & Threntham-Dietz (2003), USA	No use	402	1667	1.0
	Any use	8	21	2.4 (1.0–5.9)

CI, confidence interval; NR, not reported

2.3   Cervical cancer

Persistent infection by certain types of human papillomavirus (HPV) is generally considered to be a necessary cause of cervical cancer (IARC, 2007). However, only a small proportion of women who are infected by these viruses develop a cervical neoplasm, which clearly indicates that co-factors probably play an etiological role. Since the uterine cervix is responsive to estrogens and progestogens, these hormones could act to modify the carcinogenic potential of an HPV infection. Combined estrogen–progestogen hormonal therapy at menopause is one exogenous source of these hormones. Their possible role in cervical carcinogenesis has not been studied adequately in humans. Combined estrogen–progestogen hormonal therapy has not been widely used for a sufficiently long period of time for adequate epidemiological study of the risk for cervical cancer in relation to long-term use or to use a long time after initial or most recent exposure.

2.3.1   *HPV infection*

Two randomized trials have provided some initial information of relevance (Smith *et al.*, 1997; Anderson *et al.*, 2003). In a study from Iowa, USA, among women who were enrolled in the Postmenopausal Estrogen/Progestin Intervention trial (Smith *et al.*, 1997), 105 women aged 45–64 years were initially tested for nine high-risk types of HPV DNA (16, 18, 31, 33, 35, 39, 45, 51, 52) in cervical scrapings on enrolment and two years later using polymerase chain reaction (PCR)-based technology. Table 11 shows the results at

Table 11. Summary of results from a randomized trial of estrogen and estrogen–progestogen combinations that show percentages of women who were HPV-positive or HPV-negative at baseline and who were HPV-positive after 2 years of treatment

Treatment	HPV-negative at baseline			HPV-positive at baseline		
	Total no. of women	HPV-positive at 2 years		Total no. of women	HPV-positive at 2 years	
		No.	%		No.	%
Placebo	17	3	17.6	5	1	20.0
CEE[a]	12	3	25.0	8	3	37.5
CEE + progestogen (all combinations)	36	7	19.4	27	7	25.9
CEE/2.5 MPA[b]	11	2	18.2	8	3	37.5
CEE/10 MPA[c]	12	2	16.7	10	2	20.0
CEE/200 MP[d]	13	3	23.1	9	2	22.2
Any hormone treatment	48	10	20.8	35	10	28.6

From Smith *et al.* (1997)
CEE, conjugated equine estrogens; HPV, human papillomavirus; MP, micronized progesterone; MPA, medroxyprogesterone acetate
[a] CEE, 0.625 mg daily
[b] 0.625 mg CEE plus 2.5 mg MPA daily
[c] 0.625 mg CEE daily plus 10 mg MPA daily on days 1–12 of cycle
[d] 0.625 mg CEE daily plus 200 mg MP daily on days 1–12 of cycle

2 years in women who initially tested HPV-positive or HPV-negative. Among women who initially tested negative for HPV DNA, the percentage that became positive was not significantly higher in any of the treatment groups than in the placebo group. The treatment groups included one estrogen-only group and three estrogen–progestogen groups. When these three groups were combined, the percentage that were HPV DNA-positive after 2 years of follow-up was also not statistically significantly different in the combined group than in the placebo group. Thus, the incidence of HPV (or recrudescence of existing infection missed on enrolment) was apparently not influenced by estrogen–progestogen treatment. Among women who were initially positive for HPV DNA, the percentage that remained positive at 2 years did not vary significantly by treatment, and the percentage in the three estrogen–progestogen groups combined was not significantly different from that in the placebo group. In any individual woman, the type of HPV at 2 years was not always the same as the type at baseline. The infections at 2 years thus represented a mixture of new and persistent infections. The results did not provide evidence to suggest that estrogen–progestogen therapy alters the risk for either new or persistent infection. Five women were found 2 years after enrolment to have an abnormal Papanicolaou (Pap) smear; four had

atypical cells of undetermined significance and one had atypical squamous cells. No such cells occurred in women with a positive HPV DNA test at baseline or concurrently with a suspicious Pap smear; their relevance to cervical carcinoma and the sensitivity of the HPV DNA assays used were therefore questioned. Abnormal Pap smears were not associated with treatment group. At baseline, the prevalence of HPV DNA was 22.7% in the placebo group and varied from 40.0 to 45.5% in the four treatment groups, suggesting that women in the placebo group may have been at lower risk for HPV infection than those in the treatment groups. If this were the case, it would bias the results towards higher rates of HPV being observed in the treatment groups than in the placebo group at follow-up, and this, in addition to chance, could explain the slightly higher rates of HPV in some of the treatment groups than in the placebo group as shown in Table 11. [However, this study was of low statistical power, so that true differences in rates of HPV infection among study groups could have been missed. Larger studies of longer duration will be needed to determine more definitively whether estrogen–progestogen therapy alters the risk for acquisition or persistence of HPV.]

2.3.2 Cervical neoplasia

Table 12 summarizes results relevant to cervical cancer from the WHI (Anderson et al., 2003). Between October 1993 and October 1998, women who had not had a hysterectomy aged 50–79 years in 40 participating clinics in the USA were randomized to either treatment

Table 12. Summary of results from a randomized trial of estrogen–progestogen combination showing percentages of women at follow-up with LGSIL, HGSIL and cervical cancer

Treatment	Total no. of women[a]	Results of Pap smears						Reported cervical cancer[b,c]	
		LGSIL		HGSIL		Cancer[b]			
		No.	%	No.	%	No.	%	No.	%[d]
Placebo	7599	420	5.5	29	0.4	3	0.04	8	0.02
CEE/MPA[e]	7950	619	7.8	25	0.3	2	0.03	5	0.01

From Anderson et al. (2003)
CEE, conjugated equine estrogen; HGSIL, high-grade squamous intrepithelial lesion; LGSIL, low-grade squamous intraepithelial lesion; MPA, medroxyprogesterone acetate
[a] 503 women in the placebo group and 556 women in the estrogen–progestogen group with no follow-up smears excluded
[b] Whether in situ or invasive not stated in published report
[c] Not stated whether reported cervical cancer cases include those detected at Papanicolaou smear screening.
[d] Annualized %
[e] 0.625 mg CEE plus 0.25 mg MPA daily

with 0.625 mg conjugated equine estrogens plus 2.5 mg medroxyprogesterone acetate daily (n = 8506) or placebo (n = 8102). Most women had Pap smears every 3 years. After a mean follow-up period of 5.6 years, the incidence of cervical cancer as reported from the 40 parti-cipating clinics did not differ significantly between the treatment and placebo groups (hazard ratio, 1.4; 95% CI, 0.5–4.4). It was not indicated whether the cancers were invasive or *in situ*. There were significantly (p < 0.001) more low-grade squamous intraepithelial lesions in the treatment group (7.8%) than in the placebo group (5.5%), but the relationship of these lesions to cervical neoplasia is uncertain. Furthermore, this may result from more women in the treatment group having had Pap smears as part of a clinical evaluation for vaginal bleeding than those in the placebo group. There was no significant difference in rates of high-grade squamous intraepithelial lesions (HSIL) or of cervical cancer (presumably carcinoma *in situ*) detected by Pap smears in the two groups of women. Although this study provides little cause for concern that combined continuous estrogen–progestogen therapy for over 5 years alters the risk for cervical cancer, the statistical power to detect an alteration in risk of any type of cervical carcinoma was low, and the duration of follow-up was too short to determine whether risk is increased a long time after initial or last use. The increased risk for HSIL in the treated group warrants further investigation.

2.3.3   *Overview*

There is little evidence from these two randomized trials to suggest that combined estrogen–progestogen therapy alters the risk for persistent HPV infection, HSIL or cervical cancer, but both studies were of limited statistical power to detect true increases in risks in women who are exposed to these treatments.

2.4   Ovarian cancer

2.4.1   *Background*

Major findings of cohort and case–control studies published before the last evaluation (IARC, 1999), including two meta-analyses (Garg *et al.*, 1998; Coughlin *et al.*, 2000), and a re-analysis of individual data on hormonal therapy and risk for ovarian cancer indicate that long-term use of hormonal therapy is associated with a moderate, but consistent excess risk for ovarian cancer (IARC, 1999; Negri *et al.*, 1999; Bosetti *et al.*, 2001). In a meta-analysis of 10 published studies (nine case–control, one cohort), the overall risk for invasive ovarian cancer for ever users of hormonal therapy was 1.15 (95% CI, 1.05–1.27), with no difference in risk for hospital-based and population-based case–control studies (Garg *et al.*, 1998). Another meta-analysis of 15 studies (Coughlin *et al.*, 2000), however, found no significant overall association (relative risk, 1.1; 95%, CI, 0.9–1.7). The studies that have been published since the last evaluation (IARC, 1999) are summarized below.

2.4.2   Controlled clinical trials

The WHI, a randomized, controlled primary prevention trial, included 8506 women aged 50–79 years who were treated with combined hormonal therapy and 8102 untreated women (Writing Group for the Women's Health Initiative Investigators, 2002). In the group that received combined hormonal therapy, 20 cases of ovarian cancer occurred versus 12 in the placebo group, which corresponded to a multivariate relative risk of 1.58 (95% CI, 0.77–3.24). Nine deaths from ovarian cancer occurred in the combined hormonal therapy group versus three in the placebo group (relative risk, 2.70; 95% CI, 0.73–10.00) (Anderson et al., 2003).

2.4.3   Cohort studies

One cohort study (Pukkala et al., 2001) provided data on combined hormonal therapy and ovarian cancer. In this Finnish record linkage study, 15 956 women who received long-cycle hormonal therapy (with added progestogen every 2nd or 3rd month) and 78 549 who used monthly cycle therapy were identified from the medical reimbursement register of the national Social Insurance Institution (between 1994 and 1997). Cancer incidence was ascertained through the files of the population-based country-wide Finnish Cancer Registry. By the end of follow-up, 23 cases of ovarian cancer in the long-cycle cohort and 104 in the monthly cycle cohort were observed, to yield SIRs of 1.0 (95% CI, 0.63–1.5) and 1.1 (95% CI, 0.93–1.4), respectively.

A cohort study based on the Breast Cancer Detection Demonstration Project included 329 incident cases of ovarian cancer (Lacey et al., 2002). Compared with never use of any type of hormonal therapy, the relative risk for exclusive use of combined hormonal therapy was 1.1 (95% CI, 0.64–1.7; 18 cases), in the absence of any duration–risk relation (relative risk for ≥ 2 years of use, 0.80; 95% CI, 0.35–1.8). The relative risk for use of combined hormonal therapy after that of estrogen-only therapy was 1.5 (95% CI, 0.91–2.4; based on 21 cases).

2.4.4   Case–control studies (Table 13)

In a population-based study of 793 incident cases of epithelial ovarian cancer diagnosed between 1990 and 1999 in Queensland, New South Wales and Victoria, Australia, and 855 controls (Purdie et al., 1999), the relative risk adjusted for age, education, area of residence, body mass index, hysterectomy, tubal sterilization, use of talc, tobacco smoking, oral contraceptive use, parity and family history of breast or ovarian cancer was 1.34 (95% CI, 0.83–2.17) for the use of estrogens and progestogens in combination. There was no consistent relation with duration of use, time since last use or any other time factor.

In a case–control study from Sweden of 193 epithelial borderline cases, Riman et al. (2001) reported an odds ratio of 0.98 (95% CI, 0.57–1.68) for estrogens with cyclic progestogens and 0.87 (95% CI, 0.46–1.64) for estrogens and continuous progestogens compared with never users. None of the trends in risk with duration of use were significant.

Table 13. Case–control studies of the use of combined hormonal therapy and the risk for ovarian cancer

Reference, location	No. of cases	No. of controls	Odds ratio[a] (95% CI) Ever use	Longest use (duration)	Current/recent use
Purdie et al. (1999), Australia	793	855	1.34 (0.83–2.17)	1.33 (0.88–2.00) (> 3 years)	1.24 (0.73–2.09)
Riman et al. (2001), Sweden (borderline neoplasms)	193	3899	0.98 (0.57–1.68) sequential 0.87 (0.46–1.64) continuous	0.91 (0.44–2.03) (≥ 2 years) 0.89 (0.35–2.28) (≥ 2 years)	–
Riman et al. (2002), Sweden (invasive neoplasms)	655	3899	1.41 (1.15–1.72)	2.03 (1.30–3.17) (≥ 10 years)	–
Sit et al. (2002), USA	484	926	1.06 (0.74–1.52) conjugated estrogens 1.08 (0.59–2.00) non-conjugated estrogens	–	–
Glud et al. (2004), Denmark	376	1111	1.14 (1.01–1.28)[b] 1.00 (0.95–1.06)[c]	–	–
Pike et al. (2004), USA	477	660	– –	0.90 (0.55–1.48)[d] (≥ 5 years) 1.13 (0.15–8.3)[e]	–

CI, confidence interval
[a] Reference category was never use of combined hormonal therapy.
[b] Per additional gram of estrogen intake
[c] Per additional gram of progestogen intake
[d] Natural menopause
[e] Hysterectomy

In the same study that included 655 cases of ovarian cancer and 3899 controls aged 50–74 years, the odds ratio was 1.41 (95% CI, 1.15–1.72) for ever use of combined hormone therapy (Riman *et al.*, 2002). For longest use (≥ 10 years), the odds ratio was 2.03 (95% CI, 1.30–3.17). There was no consistent pattern for time since last use. Adjustment was made for age, parity, body mass index, age at menopause, hysterectomy and duration of oral contraceptive use. The results were similar for serous, mucinous and endometrioid ovarian cancers. No information was presented on sequential or combined hormonal therapy.

A study conducted between 1994 and 1998 in Delaware Valley, USA, included 484 cases of ovarian cancer aged 45 years or over and 926 community controls frequency-matched by age and area of residence (Sit *et al.*, 2002). Adjustment was made for age, parity, oral contraceptive use, family history of ovarian cancer and history of tubal ligation. The hormonal therapy formulation was classified as estrogen plus progestogen or estrogen alone. The relative risk was 1.06 (95% CI, 0.74–1.52) for progestogen with conjugated estrogens and 1.08 (95% CI, 0.59–2.00) for progestogen with non-conjugated estrogens.

A nationwide case–control study was conducted in Denmark between 1995 and 1999 and included 376 cases of ovarian cancer and 1111 population controls (Glud *et al.*, 2004). The results were presented in terms of groups of estrogen or progestogen intake, with adjustment for parity, use of oral contraceptives, family history of ovarian cancer and infertility. The odds ratio per additional gram of intake was 1.14 (95% CI, 1.01–1.28) for estrogens and 1.00 (95% CI, 0.95–1.06) for progestogens and was similar for estrogen only (odds ratio, 1.05; 95% CI, 0.97–1.14) and combined estrogen–progestogen therapies (odds ratio, 1.08; 95% CI, 1.01–1.16). There was no relationship with duration of use independent from cumulative dose.

A case–control study was conducted between 1992 and 1998 in Los Angeles County, CA, USA, on 477 cases of invasive epithelial ovarian cancer and 660 populations controls aged 18–74 years (Pike *et al.*, 2004). Participation rates were approximately 80% of cases and 70% of controls approached. Multivariate relative risks were adjusted for age, ethnicity, socioeconomic status, education, family history of ovarian cancer, tubal ligation, use of talc, nulliparity, age at last birth, menopausal status, age at menopause and use of oral contraceptives. Among women with natural menopause, the odds ratios per 5 years of use were 1.16 (95% CI, 0.92–1.48) for estrogen-only therapy and 0.97 (95% CI, 0.77–1.23) for combined hormonal therapy. Corresponding values for women with surgical menopause were 1.11 (95% CI, 0.92–1.35) and 1.30 (95% CI, 0.63–2.67).

2.5   Liver cancer

Persson *et al.* (1996) studied cancer risks after hormonal menopausal therapy in a population-based cohort of 22 579 women aged 35 years or more who lived in the Uppsala health care region in Sweden. Women who had ever received a prescription for hormonal menopausal therapy between 1977 and 1980 were identified and followed until 1991; information on use of hormones was obtained from pharmacy records. The expected numbers of cases were calculated from national incidence rates. There was no information on tobacco smoking or alcoholic beverage consumption. There were 43 cancers of the hepatobiliary tract that comprised 14 hepatocellular carcinomas, five cholangiocarcinomas, 23 gallbladder cancers and one unclassified. The expected number was 73.2, to give an SIR of 0.6 (95% CI, 0.4–0.8) for any type of hormonal menopausal therapy. The SIRs for treatment with estradiol combined with levonorgestrel were 0.6 (95% CI, 0.1–2.3) for hepatocellular carcinoma, 0.7 (95% CI, 0.0–3.8) for cholangiocarcinoma and zero (six cases expected) for gallbladder cancer. There was no information on infection with hepatitis viruses.

2.6   Colorectal cancer

2.6.1   Background

The previous monograph (IARC, 1999) reported details from three cohort studies and one case–control study on the use of combinations of estrogens and progestogens. Since then, new data have been published on the risks and benefits of estrogen plus progestogen treatment in menopausal women, including two randomized trials (the WHI Trial and the HERS Follow-up Study) (Hulley et al., 2002; Writing Group for the Women's Health Initiative Investigators, 2002), one cohort study (Pukkala et al., 2001) and two case–control studies (Jacobs et al., 1999; Prihartono et al., 2000). Other studies have focused on estrogen only or did not provide separate information for estrogen only and combined hormonal therapy (Paganini-Hill, 1999; Csizmadi et al., 2004; Hannaford & Elliot, 2005; Nichols et al., 2005).

2.6.2   Randomized trials

Two large randomized clinical trials have been published that provided information on combined hormonal therapy and colorectal cancer (Table 14).

The HERS was a randomized trial of the use of estrogen plus progestogen in which 2763 menopausal women under 80 years of age at baseline who had coronary artery disease and no prior hysterectomy were recruited at 20 outpatient and community settings between 1993 and 2000 in the USA (Hulley et al., 2002). Of these, 1380 women were allocated to the treatment group (0.625 mg per day conjugated estrogens plus 2.5 mg per day medroxyprogesterone acetate) and 1383 to the placebo group. After a mean of 4.1 years of follow-up, 11 cases of colon cancer were observed in the combined hormonal therapy group versus 16 in the placebo group, which corresponded to a relative risk of 0.69 (95% CI, 0.32–1.49) (Hulley et al., 2002).

The WHI Study was a randomized, controlled, primary prevention trial (that was planned to continue for 8.5 years) in which 16 608 menopausal women aged 50–79 years who had a uterus at baseline were recruited at 40 clinical centres between 1993 and 1998 in the USA. Of these, 8506 women were allocated to the treatment group (0.625 mg per day conjugated estrogens plus 2.5 mg per day medroxyprogesterone acetate) and 8102 to the placebo group (Writing Group of the Women's Health Initiative, 2002). At the end of

Table 14. Randomized clinical trials on the association between the use of combined hormonal therapy and the risk for colorectal cancer

Reference, location	Participants Outcome No. cases/group size	Relative risk (95% CI)	Comments
Chlebowski et al. (2004), USA	Healthy postmenopausal women with intact uterus Colorectal cancer Treatment group: 43/8506 Placebo group: 72/8102	0.56 (0.38–0.81)	WHI study; treatment: 0.625 mg/day conjugated estrogens plus 2.5 mg/day medroxy-progesterone acetate; multi-centre study; terminated early
Hulley et al. (2002), USA	Postmenopausal women with previous heart disease Colon cancer Treatment group: 11/1380 Placebo group: 16/1383	0.69 (0.32–1.49)	HERS; treatment: 0.625 mg/day conjugated estrogens plus 2.5 mg/day medroxy-progesterone acetate; multi-centre study; terminated early

CI, confidence interval; HERS, Heart and Estrogen/Progestin Replacement Study; WHI, Women's Health Initiative

active intervention (mean follow-up, 5.6 years), 43 cases of invasive colorectal cancer were observed in the combined hormonal therapy group versus 72 in the placebo group (relative risk, 0.56; 95% CI, 0.38–0.81) (Chlebowski et al., 2004). The reduction in the risk for colorectal cancer in the hormonal therapy group was largely confined to local disease (relative risk, 0.26; 95% CI, 0.13–0.53), rather than regional or metastatic disease (relative risk, 0.87; 95% CI, 0.54–1.41). Within the category of regional or metastatic disease, the cancers in the hormonal therapy group were associated with a greater number of positive nodes than the corresponding types of cancer in the placebo group (Chlebowski et al., 2004).

2.6.3 Cohort studies (Table 15)

In addition to the three cohort studies reviewed previously (IARC, 1999), one cohort study (Pukkala et al., 2001) provided new data on the potential association between the use of combined hormonal therapy and the risk for colorectal cancer. In this Finnish record linkage study, 15 956 women who took long-cycle hormonal therapy (administered orally on a 3-month basis: 70 days 2 mg estradiol valerate, 14 days 2 mg estradiol valerate plus 20 mg medroxyprogesterone acetate and 7-day tablet-free period) and 78 549 who took monthly or short-cycle (11 days 2 mg estradiol valerate, 10 days 2 mg estradiol vale-rate and 0.25 mg levonorgestrel and 7-day tablet-free period) hormonal therapy were identified from the medical reimbursement register of the national Social Insurance Institution (between 1994 and 1997); cancer incidence was ascertained through the files of the population-based country-wide Finnish Cancer Registry. SIRs were computed by

Table 15. Cohort studies on the association between the use of combined hormonal therapy and the risk for colorectal cancer

Reference, location	No. cases (or deaths)/cohort size	Follow-up (years)	Relative risk (95% CI) (ever versus never use)	Comments
Risch & Howe (1995), Canada	230/32 973	14	Colon, 1.07 (0.58–1.99) Rectum, 1.16 (0.53–2.52)	Linkage study (cancer registry–drug database); age-adjusted
Persson et al. (1996), Sweden	295/22 597	13	Colon, 0.6 (0.4–1.0) Rectum, 0.8 (0.4–1.3)	Relative risk for incident cancer (age-adjusted); no effect among 5573 hormone users (fixed combined brand); relative risk for mortality from colon cancer adjusted for age, 0.6 (95% CI, 0.2–1.1)
Troisi et al. (1997), USA	313/33 779	7.7	Colon, 1.4 (0.7–2.5)	Relative risk adjusted for age (unaltered when adjusted for education, body mass index, parity or use of oral contraceptives); no differences right/left colon; no trend with duration of use
Pukkala et al. (2001), Finland	11/15 956[a] 50/78 549[b]	5	Colon, 0.67 (0.34–1.20) Colon, 0.85 (0.63–1.10)	Linkage study (Social Insurance Institution drug database and Cancer Registry); relative risk adjusted for age; recency and duration of use not assessed

CI, confidence interval

[a] Long cycle (2 or 3-month) administration of combined hormonal therapy

[b] Short cycle (1-month) administration of combined hormonal therapy

comparing the observed number of cases in the assembled cohort with those expected using national incidence rates. By the end of follow-up, 11 cases of colon cancer were observed in the long-cycle cohort and 50 cases in the monthly cycle cohort, to yield an age-adjusted SIR for colon cancer of 0.67 (95% CI, 0.34–1.20) and 0.85 (95% CI, 0.63–1.10), respectively (Pukkala *et al.*, 2001).

2.6.4   *Case–control studies* (Table 16)

Since the previous evaluation (IARC, 1999), a nested case–control study of more than 1400 women aged 55–79 years who were enrolled from the Group Health Cooperative, a health maintenance organization in Washington State, USA, has been published (Jacobs *et al.*, 1999). Between 1984 and 1993, 341 incident cases of colon cancer and 1679 controls matched by age and length of enrolment in the cooperative were identified. From the records of prescriptions for progestogen tablets, the authors identified 268 cases and 1294 controls who had used combined hormonal therapy during a 5-year period (progestogen-only users and estrogen-only users excluded). The age-adjusted odds ratio for colon

Table 16. Case–control studies on the association between the use of combined hormonal therapy and the risk for colorectal cancer

Reference, location	No. cases/ controls	Odds ratio (95% CI)[a]	Comments
Newcomb & Storer (1995), USA	694/1622	Colon, 0.54 (0.28–1.0)[a] Rectum, 1.1 (0.51–2.5)[a]	Adjustment for age, alcoholic beverage consumption, body mass index, family history of cancer, sigmoidoscopy
Jacobs *et al.* (1999), USA	268/1294	Colon < 180 tablets[b], 0.59 (0.28–1.24) ≥ 180 tablets[b], 1.04 (0.59–1.82)	Nested case–control study in a health maintenance organization; adjustment for age; further adjustment for smoking, height, weight, body mass index, oral contraceptive use, parity, age at first birth, age at menopause and hysterectomy status did not alter the odds ratios.
Prihartono *et al.* (2000), USA	404/404	Colon Last use < 1 year, 0.9 (0.4–2.2) Duration ≥ 5 years, 0.7 (0.2–2.5)	Adjusted for fat, fruit and vegetable intake, physical activity, body mass index, history of screening for colorectal cancer

CI, confidence interval

[a] Ever use versus never use

[b] Progestogen tablet counts: assuming 100% compliance and 10 progestogen tablets per month, consumption of < 180 tablets is equivalent to 1.5 years of use and consumption of ≥ 180 tablets is equivalent to ≥ 1.5 years of consumption.

cancer was 0.59 (95% CI, 0.28–1.24) for those who consumed less than 180 progestogen tablets [assuming 100% compliance and 10 progestogen tablets per month, consumption of 180 tablets is equivalent to 1.5 years of use] and 1.04 (95% CI, 0.59–1.82) for those who consumed > 180 tablets [or used combined hormonal therapy for more than 1.5 years] compared with never users. Adjustment for other covariates did not substantially change these estimates. Duration of use and analysis of colon subsite was not presented for users of combined hormonal therapy.

Prihartono *et al.* (2000) conducted a matched population-based case–control study among women aged 20–69 years in Massachusetts, USA, between 1992 and 1994, and included 515 incident cases of colon cancer (out of 1847 potential eligible cases) and 515 matched controls. The final analysis was restricted to pairs of women with natural menopause or who had had a hysterectomy (404 cases, 404 matched controls). Recent use (interval since last use, < 1 year) of combined hormonal therapy showed an odds ratio of 0.9 (95% CI, 0.4–2.2; 13 exposed cases, 15 exposed controls). Longer duration of use (> 5 years) of combined hormonal therapy showed an odds ratio of 0.7 (95% CI, 0.2–2.5; seven exposed cases, nine exposed controls). The odds ratio was adjusted for fat, fruit and vegetable intake, physical activity, body mass index and history of screening for colorectal cancer.

2.7   Lung cancer

The large population-based mortality study in Sweden (Persson *et al.*, 1996) found no association with lung cancer in users of combined hormonal therapy, and a similar study in Finland found non-significant associations for long (SIR, 1.2; 95% CI, 0.69–1.9) or monthly (SIR, 0.75; 95% CI, 0.53–1.0) cycles of hormonal therapy (Pukkala *et al.*, 2001).

A case–control study in Texas, USA, in which 60 cases of lung cancer and 78 controls reported use of combined hormonal therapy reported a multivariate odds ratio of 0.61 (95% CI, 0.40–0.92) (Schabath *et al.*, 2004).

The HERS (Hulley *et al.*, 2002) and WHI (Writing Group for the Women's Health Initiative Investigators, 2002) trials showed a hazard ratio of 1.39 (95% CI, 0.84–2.28) and 1.04 (95% CI, 0.71–1.53) for lung cancer, respectively.

2.8   Other cancers

Data on other cancers were inadequate for an evaluation as nearly all studies failed to report the type of hormonal therapy used.

3. Studies of Cancer in Experimental Animals

Only one study on the carcinogenicity of conjugated equine estrogens plus progestogens was reviewed in the previous monograph (IARC, 1999; Sakamoto *et al.*, 1997a).

3.1   Oral administration

3.1.1   *Mouse*

In a study to compare estrogen therapy with combined estrogen–progestogen therapy that used conjugated equine estrogens or conjugated equine estrogens plus medroxyprogesterone acetate, three groups of 14 female SHN mice (a strain that has a high spontaneous rate of mammary tumours and uterine adenomyosis), 71 days [about 10 weeks] of age, were fed 0 (controls) or 1.875 mg/kg of diet conjugated equine estrogens (Premarin®) with or without 7.5 mg/kg of diet medroxyprogesterone acetate (Provera®) for 230 days. Based upon a daily dietary intake of 2–3 g per mouse weighing 20–30 g, the daily intakes of conjugated equine estrogens and medroxyprogesterone acetate were calculated to be 0.19 and 0.75 mg/kg bw per day, respectively. Mice were killed 20 days after the appearance of a palpable mammary tumour or at 300 days of age. The significance of differences was evaluated by the χ^2 test. The incidence of mammary tumours [of unspecified histopathology] did not differ in the three groups (control, 4/14; estrogen alone, 6/14; estrogen–progestogen, 5/14). However, treatment with estrogen–progestogen shortened the latent period of mammary tumorigenesis by 44 days ($p < 0.05$ versus controls; not statistically significantly different from estrogen only). Treatment with estrogen–progestogen completely suppressed the development of uterine adenomyosis (0/14 versus 5/14 controls or 6/14 estrogen only-treated mice, $p < 0.01$) (Sakamoto *et al.*, 1997b). [These results are somewhat confounded by the potential influence of endogenous ovarian hormones that are reduced in the post-menopausal state. Endogenous estradiol levels in controls (3.91 ± 1.16 pg/mL) were significantly lower ($p < 0.01$) than those in estrogen only-treated (28.15 ± 2.91 pg/mL) and estrogen–progestogen-treated (20.15 ± 1.37 pg/mL) mice. However, the levels in hormone-treated mice were physiological and did not exceed that observed on day 1 of the estrus cycle (Raafat *et al.* 1999).]

3.1.2   *Monkey*

In one study, ovariectomized cynomolgus monkeys (*Macaca fascicularis*), 5–13 years of age, were treated for 2.5 years with either conjugated equine estrogen alone (Premarin®) (equivalent to 0.625 mg per woman per day; 22 animals) or in combination with medroxyprogesterone acetate (Cycrin®) (equivalent to 2.5 mg per woman per day; 21 animals) in the diet or were untreated (26 animals). Determination of serum hormone levels of estradiol and medroxyprogesterone acetate confirmed the completeness of ovariectomy. The experiment was terminated at the end of the treatment phase. Mammary gland atrophy was seen in control animals. Eighty-six per cent (18/21) of the estrogen–progestogen-treated animals had mammary hyperplasia, defined as greater mammary gland development than that seen in animals with normal cycles ($p = 0.0065$). Forty-one per cent (9/22) of the animals given estrogen only had mammary hyperplasia. No neoplasms were observed (Cline *et al.*, 1996).

In a subsequent, similar study, a progestogen-only group was added and the treatments were administered in the diet for 3 years. Ovariectomies were carried out 3 months before the start of treatments. The treatment groups were controls (no treatment; 27 animals), conjugated equine estrogen-treated (0.625 mg per woman per day equivalent; 27 animals), medroxyprogesterone acetate-treated (2.5 mg per woman per day equivalent; 26 animals) and estrogen–progestogen-treated (0.625 mg per woman per day equivalent conjugated equine estrogen plus 2.5 mg per woman per day equivalent medroxyprogesterone acetate; 26 animals); mean age at the end of the study was 7.5 years. The effective number of control animals was 20. Mammary gland lobuloalveolar hyperplasia was increased with estrogen-only treatment (effective number of animals, 25) and the effect was further increased with estrogen–progestogen treatment (effective number of animals, 26) [incidence not provided]; this development exceeded that usually seen in premenopausal animals with normal cycles. Progestogen-alone treatment (effective number of animals, 19) did not increase hyperplasia. No neoplasms, ductal hyperplasia or atypia were observed (Cline *et al.*, 1998).

In a third study (Cline *et al.*, 2002a) designed to assess the effect of tibolone, a similar experimental protocol and the same doses were used as those described by Cline *et al.* (1996). Twenty-eight to 31 ovariectomized monkeys (6–8 years of age) per group were treated for 2 years. Mammary lobuloalveolar hyperplasia was observed in 19/30 (63%) control, 27/28 (96%, $p < 0.001$) estrogen only-treated and 28/29 (97%, $p < 0.001$) estrogen–progestogen-treated animals. No neoplasms were observed.

3.2   Administration with a known carcinogen

Rat

7,12-Dimethylbenz[*a*]anthracene

Female Sprague-Dawley rats, 48 days [about 7 weeks] of age, were divided into four groups of seven rats per group and were administered: 7,12-dimethylbenz[*a*]anthracene (DMBA) alone (as a single intravenous injection of 5 mg); DMBA and were oophorectomized; DMBA plus conjugated estrogens (Premarin®) at a concentration of 1.875 mg/kg of diet and were oophorectomized; or DMBA plus Premarin® plus medroxyprogesterone acetate (Proveza®) at a concentration of 7.5 mg/kg of diet and were oophorectomized. The animals were autopsied at 285 days [about 41 weeks] of age. Mammary tumours were found in 6/7 rats given DMBA, 0/7 given DMBA plus oophorectomy, 5/7 given DMBA plus Premarin® plus oophorectomy and 5/7 given Premarin® plus medroxyprogesterone acetate plus oophorectomy. Thus, oophorectomy completely inhibited mammary tumour development, but conjugated estrogen with or without medroxyprogesterone acetate markedly stimulated mammary carcinogenesis in the ovariectomized rats (Sakamoto *et al.*, 1997a).

4. Other Data Relevant to an Evaluation of Carcinogenicity and its Mechanisms

4.1 Absorption, distribution, metabolism and excretion

The distribution of progestogens is described in the monograph on Combined estrogen–progestogen contraceptives. That of estrogens is described below.

4.1.1 *Humans*

Little more has been discovered about the absorption and distribution of estrone, estradiol and estriol products and conjugated equine estrogens in humans since the previous evaluation (IARC, 1999). Greater progress has been made in the identification and characterization of the enzymes that are involved in estrogen metabolism and excretion. The various metabolites and the responsible enzymes, including genotypic variations, are described below (see Figures 3 and 4). Sulfation and glucuronidation are the main metabolic reactions of estrogens in humans.

(*a*) *Metabolites*

(i) *Estrogen sulfates*

Several members of the sulfotransferase (SULT) gene family can sulfate hydroxysteroids, including estrogens. The importance of SULTs in estrogen conjugation is demonstrated by the observation that a major component of circulating estrogen is sulfated, i.e. estrone sulfate (reviewed by Pasqualini, 2004). In addition to the parent hormones, estrone and estradiol, SULTs can also conjugate their respective catechols and also methoxyestrogens (Spink *et al.*, 2000; Adjei & Weinshilboum, 2002). The resulting sulfated metabolites are more hydrophilic and can be excreted.

In postmenopausal breast cancers, levels of estrone sulfate can reach 3.3 ± 1.9 pmol/g tissue, which is five to nine times higher than the corresponding plasma concentration (equating gram of tissue with millilitre of plasma) (Pasqualini *et al.*, 1996). In contrast, levels of estrone sulfate in premenopausal breast tumours are two to four times lower than those in plasma. Since inactive estrone sulfate can serve as a source for biologically active estradiol, it is of interest that various progestogens caused a significant decrease in the formation of estradiol when physiological concentrations of estrone sulfate were incubated with breast cancer cells MCF-7 and T47D (reviewed by Pasqualini, 2003).

Figure 3. Pathways of the metabolism and redox cycling of estradiol, estriol and estrone

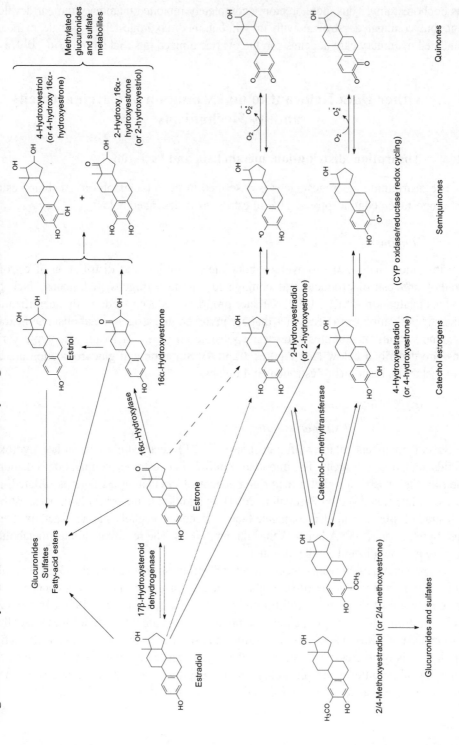

Modified from Yager & Liehr (1996)

Figure 4. The estrogen metabolism pathway is regulated by oxidizing phase I and conjugating phase II enzymes

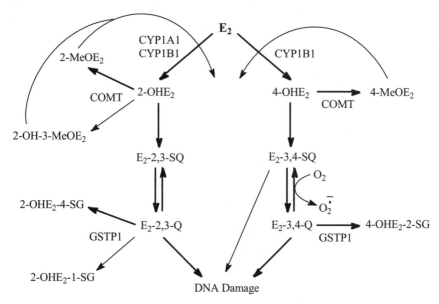

Adapted from Dawling *et al.* (2003)

COMT, catechol-*O*-methyltransferase; CYP, cytochrome P450; E_2, estradiol; GSH, glutathione; GST, glutathione *S*-transferase; $MeOE_2$, methoxyestradiol; OH, hydroxy; OHE_2, hydroxyestradiol; Q, quinone; SG, *S*-glutathione (oxidized); SQ, semiquinone

CYP1A1 and CYP1B1 catalyse the oxidation of E_2 to the catechol estrogens $2\text{-}OHE_2$ and $4\text{-}OHE_2$. The catechol estrogens are either methylated by COMT to methoxyestrogens ($2\text{-}MeOE_2$, $2\text{-}OH\text{-}3\text{-}MeOE_2$, $4\text{-}MeOE_2$) or further oxidized to semiquinones ($E_2\text{-}2,3\text{-}SQ$, $E_2\text{-}3,4\text{-}SQ$) and quinones ($E_2\text{-}2,3\text{-}Q$, $E_2\text{-}3,4\text{-}Q$). The methoxyestrogens exert feedback inhibition on CYP1A1 and CYP1B1, as indicated by the curved arrows, and reduce the formation of oxidative E_2 metabolites. The estrogen quinones are either conjugated by GSTP1 to GSH-conjugates ($2\text{-}OHE_2\text{-}1\text{-}SG$, $2\text{-}OHE_2\text{-}4\text{-}SG$, $4\text{-}OHE_2\text{-}2\text{-}SG$) or they form quinone–DNA adducts (e.g. $4\text{-}OHE_2\text{-}N7\text{-}guanine$) or oxidative DNA adducts via quinone–semiquinone redox cycling (e.g. 8-OH-deoxyguanosine). The same pathway applies to estrone. The thicker arrows indicate preferential reactions.

(ii)   *Estrogen glucuronides*

Estradiol and estrone and their respective catechols are recognized as substrates by various isoforms of the uridine-5′ diphosphate (UDP)-glucuronyltransferase (UGT) enzyme family. Several isoforms were more active towards catechol estrogens than towards the parent hormones (Albert *et al.*, 1999; Turgeon *et al.*, 2001). The resulting glucuronidated metabolites are more hydrophilic and can be excreted in bile and urine.

(iii)   *Estrogen fatty acid esters*

Several steroids, including estradiol, have been shown to undergo esterification to long-chain fatty acids in a number of mammalian tissues (Hochberg, 1998). The responsible enzyme, fatty acyl-coenzyme A (CoA):estradiol-17β-acyltransferase, has a pH optimum of

5–5.5, which distinguishes it from the related enzyme, acyl-CoA:cholesterol acyltransferase (optimal pH ~7.0) (Xu et al., 2001a,b). The fatty acyl-CoA:estradiol-17β-acyltransferase shows specificity for the D-ring, especially the C-17β group of the estrogen molecule. The vicinity of a bulky 16α-hydroxy group appears to hamper the accessibility to the C-17β hydroxyl, which results in a reduced rate (28%) of esterification of estriol compared with estradiol (Pahuja et al., 1991). The D-ring esterification of estradiol has two effects: (i) the bulky fatty acid moiety prevents the binding of estradiol fatty acid to the estrogen receptor; and (ii) the fatty acid moiety shields the D-ring from oxidative metabolism to estrone. Thus, estradiol fatty acid may play a role in the action of estrogen by affecting the intracellular equilibrium between estrone and estradiol.

In the circulation, estradiol fatty acids are mainly bound by plasma lipoproteins; the majority (54%) are recovered in the high-density lipoprotein (HDL) and 28% in the low-density lipoprotein (LDL) fractions (Vihma et al., 2003a). They are present in very small amounts in the blood of premenopausal women, although their concentration increases 10-fold during pregnancy, from 40 pmol/L in early pregnancy to 400 pmol/L in late pregnancy (Vihma et al., 2001). Treatment of postmenopausal women with either oral or transdermal estradiol for 12 weeks resulted in a differential effect on serum estradiol fatty acids and non-esterified estradiol. Both types of application led to similar median concentrations of free (non-protein-bound) estradiol but only the oral therapy caused an increase (27%) in median serum estradiol fatty acid (Vihma et al., 2003b). The change during treatment in serum concentrations of estradiol fatty acid, but not those of non-esterified estradiol correlated positively with enhanced forearm blood flow responses in vivo. These data suggest that an increase in serum estradiol fatty acid may contribute to the effects of oral treatment with estradiol, compared with those of an equipotent transdermal dose.

(iv)	*Oxidative metabolism*

Estradiol and estrone undergo extensive oxidative metabolism via the action of several cytochrome P450 (CYP) monooxygenases. Each CYP favours the hydroxylation of specific carbons, altogether, the CYP enzymes can hydroxylate virtually all carbons in the steroid molecule, with the exception of the inaccessible angular carbons 5, 8, 9, 10 and 13 (Badawi et al., 2001; Lee et al., 2001, 2002, 2003a,b; Kisselev et al., 2005). The generation of hydroxyl and keto functions at specific sites of the steroid nucleus markedly affects the biological properties of the respective estrogen metabolites, i.e. different hydroxylation reactions yield estrogenic, non-estrogenic or carcinogenic metabolites. Quantitatively and functionally, the most important reactions occur at carbons 2, 4 and 16.

Catechol estrogens

2- and 4-Hydroxyestrone, -estradiol and -estriol have been shown to serve a physiological function, to have some hormonal activity and to be substrates in the oxidative estrogen metabolism pathway. In their physiological function, they mediate the activation of dormant blastocysts for implantation into the receptive uterus. Specifically, 4-hydroxyestradiol produced in the uterus from estradiol mediates blastocyst activation for implantation in a paracrine manner. This effect is not mediated by the estrogen receptor but via prostaglandin synthesis (Paria *et al.*, 1998, 2000). The oxidative metabolism of estrogens to catechol estrogens is generally thought to terminate the estrogenic signal, although catechol estrogens retain some binding affinity to the estrogen receptor. Treatment of MCF-7 cells with 2- and 4-hydroxyestradiol increased the rate of cell proliferation and the expression of estrogen-inducible genes such as the progesterone receptor (*PR*) gene and *pS2*. Relative to estradiol, 2- and 4-hydroxyestradiol increased proliferation rate, level of PR protein and *pS2* mRNA expression by 36 and 76%, 10 and 28% and 48 and 79%, respectively (Schütze *et al.*, 1993, 1994).

Catechol estrogens occupy a key position in the oxidative pathway of estrogen metabolism (see Figures 3 and 4). They are products as well as substrates of CYP1A1 and CYP1B1 (Hachey *et al.*, 2003; Dawling *et al.*, 2004). Specifically, CYP1A1 converts estradiol firstly to 2-hydroxyestradiol and then to the estradiol-2,3-semiquinone and estradiol quinone. CYP1B1 converts estradiol firstly to 2- as well as to 4-hydroxyestradiol and then to the corresponding semiquinones and quinones. Estrone is metabolized in a similar manner by CYP1A1 and CYP1B1 (Lee *et al.*, 2003a). The catechol estrogens also serve as substrates for catechol-*O*-methyltransferase (COMT), which catalyses *O*-methylation by forming monomethyl ethers at the 2-, 3- and 4-hydroxyl groups. Conjugated equine estrogens are also substrates for COMT (Yao *et al.*, 2003). COMT generated two products from 2-hydroxyestrogens, but only one product from 4-hydroxyestrogens (Dawling *et al.*, 2001; Lautala *et al.*, 2001; Goodman *et al.*, 2002). With 2-hydroxyestradiol and 2-hydroxyestrone, COMT catalysed the methylation of the 2- and 3-hydroxy groups, which resulted in the formation of 2-methoxyestradiol and 2-hydroxy-3-methoxyestradiol and 2-methoxyestrone and 2-hydroxy-3-methoxyestrone, respectively. In contrast, for 4-hydroxyestradiol and 4-hydroxyestrone, methylation occurred only at the 4-hydroxyl group, which resulted in the formation of 4-methoxyestradiol and 4-methoxyestrone, respectively. 3-Methoxy-4-hydroxyestradiol and -estrone were not produced by COMT.

The observation that catechol estrogens are carcinogenic in animal experiments (IARC, 1999) has prompted studies in human tissues. Examination of microsomal estradiol hydroxylation in human breast cancer showed significantly higher 4-hydroxy-:2-hydroxyestradiol ratios in tumour tissue than in adjacent normal breast tissue (Liehr & Ricci, 1996), while the breast cancer tissue samples contained fourfold higher levels of 4-hydroxyestradiol than normal tissue from benign breast biopsies (Rogan *et al.*, 2003). Comparison of intra-tissue concentrations of estrogens (estrone, estradiol, estriol), hydroxyestrogens (16α-hydroxyestrone, 2-hydroxyestrone, 2-hydroxyestradiol, 4-hydroxyestrone, 4-hydroxyestradiol) and methoxyestrogens (2-methoxyestrone, 2-methoxyestradiol, 4-methoxyestrone, 4-methoxyestradiol) in normal and malignant breast revealed the highest concentration of 4-hydroxyestradiol in malignant tissue (Castagnetta *et al.*, 2002). The concentration (1.6 nmol/g tissue) determined by combined high performance liquid chromatography (HPLC) and gas chromatography–mass spectrometry (GC–MS) was more than twice as high as that of any other compound. [The Working Group noted that such high levels in neoplastic mammary tissue suggests a mechanistic role of 4-hydroxyestradiol in tumour development; see also Section 4.4.]

16α-Hydroxyestrogens

An analysis of 15 CYP isozymes showed that CYP1A1, 3A4, 3A5 and 2C8 catalysed the 16α-hydroxylation of both estrone and estradiol (Badawi *et al.*, 2001; Lee *et al.*, 2003a,b). In contrast, CYP3A7 distinguished the two estrogen substrates with > 100 times higher maximum velocity of the enzyme:Michaelis-Menten constant (V_{max}:K_m) ratio for the 16α-hydroxylation of estrone than that of estradiol. The difference in reaction rates is most probably due to the difference in structure at the C-17 position of estrone and estradiol. The presence of the 17-ketogroup in estrone appears to be essential for recognition of the substrate and 16α-hydroxylation by CYP3A7 (Lee *et al.*, 2003b).

Similarly to catechol estrogens, 16α-hydroxylated estrogens are hormonally active, chemically reactive and potentially mutagenic. 16α-Hydroxyestrone possesses the unique property of binding covalently to the estrogen receptor and other nuclear proteins, such as histones. Mechanistically, a Schiff base is formed from 16α-hydroxyestrone by a reaction with amino groups in proteins. The Schiff base, in turn, undergoes Heyns rearrangement to result in the formation of a stable 16-keto-17β-amino estrogen adduct (Miyairi *et al.*, 1999).

Bradlow *et al.* (1996) proposed that increased formation of 16α-hydroxyestrone and estriol may be associated with an increased risk for developing breast cancer. They presented the hypothesis that the ratio of the two urinary metabolites 2-hydroxy-estrone:16α-hydroxyestrone is inversely correlated with the risk for breast cancer. They chose the numerator 2-hydroxyestrone to reflect the 'good' C-2 hydroxylation and the denominator 16α-hydroxyestrone to reflect the 'bad' C-16α hydroxylation pathways of estrogen metabolism. Enzyme immunoassays for simultaneous quantitation of 2- and 16α-hydroxyestrone levels in urine have been developed and improved to correlate with results obtained by GC–MS (Falk *et al.*, 2000). The enzyme immunoassay has been applied to the analysis of blood samples from premenopausal women. Current users of oral contraceptives had a significantly lower plasma 2-hydroxyestrone:16α-hydroxyestrone ratio than non-users ($p = 10^{-21}$) (Jernstrom *et al.*, 2003b).

Results from epidemiological studies on the association between 2- and 16α-hydroxylation and breast cancer are inconsistent. Several case–control studies found an increased risk for breast cancer associated with a lower 2-hydroxyestrone:16α-hydroxyestrone ratio (Ho *et al.*, 1998; Zheng *et al.*, 1998), while other groups did not observe a difference in this ratio between controls and patients (Ursin *et al.*, 1999). All of these studies measured metabolites after the diagnosis of breast cancer, which raises the possibility that the results may have been affected by the tumour. Two prospective studies addressed this issue but also yielded inconsistent results. The first was carried out in women on the island of Guernsey, United Kingdom. Urine samples were collected and stored in the 1970s when all women were healthy. Almost 20 years later, Meilahn *et al.* (1998) analysed the samples and reported a median of 1.6 for the 2-hydroxyestrone:16α-hydroxyestrone ratio in 42 post-menopausal women who had developed breast cancer and 1.7 in 139 matched control subjects. Compared with women in the lowest tertile category of 2:16α-hydroxyestrone ratio, women in the highest tertile had an odds ratio for breast cancer of 0.71, but the 95% CI was wide and was not statistically significant (95% CI, 0.29–1.75). Analysis of premenopausal women in the Guernsey cohort showed no difference between cases and controls. The second prospective study of Italian women had a shorter average follow-up of 5.5 years (Muti *et al.*, 2000). The odds ratio in postmenopausal women was 1.31 (95% CI, 0.53–3.18). In the premenopausal group, women in the highest quintile of the 2:16α-hydroxyestrone ratio had an adjusted odds ratio of 0.55 (95% CI, 0.23–1.32). A third type of epidemiological study examined urinary metabolites in women of different ethnic groups that are known to have different rates of breast cancer. One study examined healthy postmenopausal women randomly selected from the Singapore Chinese Health Study (67 subjects) and the Los Angeles Multiethnic Cohort Study (58 subjects). Although the incidence of breast cancer is substantially lower in Singaporean women than among American women, there were no significant differences between the groups in urinary 16α-hydroxyestrone levels or 2:16α-hydroxyestrone ratios (Ursin *et al.*, 2001). Finally, no differences were found in premenopausal women with or without a family history of breast cancer (Ursin *et al.*, 2002).

(v)   *Methoxyestrogens*

Methoxyestrogens are methyl ether metabolites of catechol estrogens produced by COMT. In addition, 2-methoxyestradiol is not just a by-product of estrogen metabolism but is also endowed with antiproliferative activity. It has been shown to inhibit the proliferation of both hormone-dependent and hormone-independent breast cancer cells (LaVallee *et al.*, 2003). The antiproliferative effect is not limited to breast cancer cells but extends to leukaemia, and pancreatic and lung cancer cells (Schumacher *et al.*, 1999; Huang *et al.*, 2000). Human xenograft studies in animal models have demonstrated the oral bioavailability and a high therapeutic index of methoxyestrogens with no sign of systemic toxicity. These features and their broad antitumour activity against a variety of tumour cells have led to the current testing of methoxyestrogens as potential therapeutic agents in clinical trials (Pribluda *et al.*, 2000; Schumacher & Neuhaus, 2001). Several synthetic analogues were equally as effective as 2-methoxyestradiol or were even more potent than the endogenous compound (Wang *et al.*, 2000; Brueggemeier *et al.*, 2001; Tinley *et al.*, 2003).

The antiproliferative effect of 2-methoxyestradiol appears to be concentration-dependent and to involve several mechanisms. At nano- and micromolar concentrations, 2-methoxyestradiol disrupted microtubule function, induced apoptosis and inhibited angiogenesis (Klauber *et al.*, 1997; Yue *et al.*, 1997; Huang *et al.*, 2000; LaVallee *et al.*, 2003). At concentrations $\geq 1\ \mu M$, it caused chromosome breaks and aneuploidy (Tsutsui *et al.*, 2000).

Methoxyestrogens are also substrates for CYP1A1 and CYP1B1, which catalyse their *O*-demethylation to catechol estrogens, and thus effectively reverse the COMT reaction by which they were formed (Dawling *et al.*, 2003). Specifically, both CYP1A1 and CYP1B1 demethylated 2-methoxy- and 2-hydroxy-3-methoxyestradiol to 2-hydroxyestradiol, and CYP1B1 additionally demethylated 4-methoxyestradiol to 4-hydroxyestradiol. Thus, CYP1A1 and CYP1B1 recognize as substrates both the parent hormone estradiol and the methoxyestrogens, 2-methoxy-, 2-hydroxy-3-methoxy- and 4-methoxyestradiol. Kinetic analysis showed that estradiol and the methoxyestrogens are alternate substrates, each of which is catalysed by the same enzyme but by a different type of reaction (Dawling *et al.*, 2003). Because they are converted to identical catechol estrogen products, each inhibits formation of 2- and 4-hydroxyestradiol from the other substrate in a non-competitive manner. It has been proposed that methoxyestrogens exert feedback inhibition on CYP1A1 and CYP1B1, which affects the entire oxidative metabolic pathway of estrogen in several ways. First, CYP1A1 and CYP1B1 generate catechol estrogen substrates for COMT and, at the same time, compete with COMT by converting the catechol estrogens to estrogen quinones. In turn, the methoxyestrogens generated by COMT are alternate substrates for CYP1A1 and CYP1B1 and inhibit oxidation of the parent hormone estradiol (and most probably also that of the catechol estrogens). Second, the inhibition occurs at a strategic point in the pathway where it branches into 2- and 4-hydroxycatechol estrogens. This may be important in view of the apparent difference in carcinogenicity of these two substances (Liehr & Ricci, 1996; Cavalieri *et al.*, 2000). Third, all three products of the COMT-mediated reaction (i.e. 2-methoxy-, 2-hydroxy-3-methoxy- and 4-methoxyestradiol) act as inhibitors, and thereby maximize the feedback regulation (Dawling *et al.*, 2003). Fourth, the feedback regulation occurs at the step in the pathway that precedes the conversion to estrogen semiquinones and quinones, and thereby reduces the formation of reactive oxygen species during semiquinone–quinone redox cycling and the potential for estrogen-induced DNA damage (Dawling *et al.*, 2003).

(vi)   *Estrogen–glutathione conjugates*

The labile estrogen quinones react with a variety of physiological compounds, including amino acids such as lysine and cysteine and the tripeptide, glutathione (γ-glutamyl-cysteinyl-glycine, GSH) (Cao *et al.*, 1998). MS analysis of the GSH–estrogen isomers revealed that the catechol estrogen attachment is at the cysteine moiety of GSH, and the cysteine sulfur binds to an A-ring carbon vicinal to the catechol carbons, i.e. C-1 or C-4 in 2-hydroxyestradiol and C-2 in 4-hydroxyestradiol (Ramanathan *et al.*, 1998). Thus, the point of attachment of the -*S*-glutathione (-SG) moiety is always directly adjacent to an oxygen-bearing carbon, in line with all other known quinone–GSH conjugates (Bolton *et al.*, 2000).

GSH is the most abundant intracellular non-protein thiol and is found at concentrations that range from 0.1 to 10 mM. In an in-vitro study, Hachey *et al.* (2003) used 0.1 mM GSH and recombinant, purified glutathione *S*-transferase P1 (GSTP1) and estradiol and observed a faster rate of estrogen quinone conjugation in the presence of GSTP1 than in the absence of the enzyme. 2-Hydroxyestradiol and 4-hydroxyestradiol did not form conjugates with GSH alone or in the presence of GSTP1. These data indicate that the enzymatic conversion of catechol estrogens to estrogen quinones by CYP1B1 is a necessary step for the subsequent GSH conjugation reaction. The enzymatic reaction with GSTP1 yielded only mono-conjugates, i.e. 2-hydroxyestradiol-1-SG, 2-hydroxyestradiol-4-SG and 4-hydroxyestradiol-2-SG. There was no evidence of bis-conjugates, such as 2-hydroxy-estradiol-1,4-bisSG and 4-hydroxyestradiol-1,2-bisSG. GSTP1 is also a target for equine catechol estrogens (Yao *et al.*, 2002). Equine catechol significantly decreased GSH levels and the activity of GSTP1-1 in human breast cancer cells.

All GSH conjugates are catabolized via the mercapturic acid pathway. First, the gluta-myl moiety is removed from the GSH conjugate by transpeptidation, which is catalysed by γ-glutamyl transpeptidase. The resulting cysteinylglycine conjugate is then hydrolysed by cysteinyl-glycine dipeptidase to yield the cysteine conjugate. The final step entails acety-lation to the *N*-acetylcysteine conjugate, a mercapturic acid compound. Estrogen–GSH conjugates are excreted in the urine mostly as *N*-acetylcysteine conjugates but also as cysteine conjugates (Todorovic *et al.*, 2001). Thus, estrogen quinones are detoxified in tissues by GST-mediated GSH conjugation and the resultant GSH conjugates are cata-bolized to *N*-acetylcysteine conjugates that are readily excreted.

(b)   Enzymes

(i)   CYP1A1

Although other CYP enzymes, such as CYP1A2 and CYP3A4, are involved in hepatic and extrahepatic hydroxylation of estrogen, CYP1A1 and CYP1B1 display the highest level of expression in breast tissue (reviewed by Jefcoate *et al.*, 2000; Lee *et al.*, 2003a). The human gene for CYP1A1 is polymorphic. Apart from the wild-type (*CYP1A1*1*), 10 alleles have been described in different populations. However, several are very rare and of unknown functional significance (Karolinska Institutet, 2007). The most common alleles that result in amino acid substitutions are *CYP1A1*2* (462Ile → Val) and *CYP1A1*4* (461Thr → Asn). Kisselev *et al.* (2005) expressed and purified CYP1A1.1, CYP1A1.2 and CYP1A1.4 proteins and performed enzymatic assays of estrogen hydroxylation in reconsti-tuted CYP1A1 systems. All three CYP1A1 isoforms catalysed the hydroxylation of estradiol and estrone to 2-, 15α-, 6α- and barely detectable 4-hydroxylated estrogen metabolites. The CYP1A1.2 variant had a significantly higher catalytic activity, especially for 2-hydroxylation. The catalytic efficiencies for 2-hydroxyestradiol and 2-hydroxyestrone were 5.7- and 12-fold higher, respectively, compared with the wild-type enzyme. Several studies found no overall association between the risk for breast cancer and the polymorphisms in codons 461 and 462 (Huang *et al.*, 1999; reviewed by Mitrunen & Hirvonen, 2003).

In addition to genetic variation, there is a striking interindividual variation in *CYP1A1* expression. For example, Goth-Goldstein *et al.* (2000) measured *CYP1A1* mRNA expression in 58 non-tumour breast specimens from 26 breast cancer patients and 32 cancer-free individuals by reverse transcription-PCR. *CYP1A1* expression varied between speci-mens by ~400-fold and was independent of *CYP1A1* genotype and age of the patient.

A second study used quantitative immunoblotting of normal and malignant breast tissues and observed ~150-fold differences in CYP1A1 protein expression between individuals (El-Rayes *et al.*, 2003). Attempts to explain such a high degree of interindividual variation in CYP1A1 expression have focused primarily on genetic polymorphisms within the *CYP1A1* gene with inconsistent results. Since the expression of CYP1A1 is induced via the aryl hydrocarbon receptor (AhR), Smart and Daly (2000) extended the investigation to the *AhR* gene, and observed that *AhR*-mediated induction of CYP1A1 appears to be influenced by the 1721G → A (554Arg → Lys) polymorphism in exon 10 of the *AhR* gene. The 554Arg residue lies close to the transactivation domain of the AhR protein. Individuals who had at least one copy of the variant 1721A allele showed significantly higher levels of CYP1A1 activity compared with individuals who were negative for the polymorphism ($p = 0.0001$). Levels of 3-methylcholanthrene-induced CYP1A1 activity in lymphocytes also varied by sex: women exhibited significantly lower activity than men (Smart & Daly, 2000). The authors suggested that interindividual variation in levels of CYP1A1 activity appears to be associated more with regulatory factors than with polymorphisms in the *CYP1A1* gene.

(ii)   *CYP1B1*

CYP1B1 is the main enzyme that converts estradiol to 4-hydroxyestradiol (Jefcoate *et al.*, 2000). Since animal studies have implicated 4-hydroxyestradiol in the development of cancer, the expression of CYP1B1 in hormone-responsive tissues such as the breast has attracted interest. Murray *et al.* (2001) performed several immunohistochemical studies of CYP1B1 expression in the breast. Breast cancer tissue but not normal breast tissue expressed CYP1B1. Forty-six of 60 (77%) invasive breast cancers showed cytoplasmic staining of tumour cells, which ranged from strong in 10 to moderate in 12 and weak in 24 cases. There was no relationship between the presence of CYP1B1 and the histological type or grade of the tumour, the presence of lymph node metastasis or estrogen receptor status (McFadyen *et al.*, 1999). Immunohistochemical analysis of CYP1B1 expression also revealed cytoplasmic staining in a wide range of other cancers of different histo-genetic types, including cancers of the colon, oesophagus, lung, brain and testis. Similar to the breast, no immunostaining occurred in corresponding normal tissues (Murray *et al.*, 1997). These findings contradict the observation that normal human mammary epithelial cells isolated and cultured from reduction mammoplasty tissue of seven individual donors expressed significant levels of CYP1B1 (< 0.01–1.4 pmol/mg microsomal protein) as determined by immunoblot analysis (Larsen *et al.*, 1998). The discrepancy between the studies regarding the presence of CYP1B1 protein in normal mammary epithelium may be due to the use of different antibodies, to the induction of CYP1B1 as a result of the iso-lation of the mammary epithelial cells from mammoplasty tissue or to their in-vitro culture over 6 days (Murray *et al.*, 2001).

Several polymorphisms have been identified in the *CYP1B1* gene, four of which are associated with amino acid substitutions: 48Arg → Gly, 119Ala → Ser, 432Val → Leu and 453Asn → Ser (Stoilov *et al.*, 1998; McLellan *et al.*, 2000). There is considerable ethnic variation in the frequency of these polymorphisms. For example, the 432Val allele is present in approximately 70% of African-Americans, 40% of Caucasians and less than 20% of Chinese (Bailey et al., 1998; Tang et al., 2000).

Several investigators have examined the effect of CYP1B1 polymorphisms on enzyme function (Shimada et al., 1999; Hanna et al., 2000; Li, D.N. et al., 2000; McLellan et al., 2000; Lewis et al., 2003). Although all studies analysed the 4- and 2-hydroxylation of estradiol by CYP1B1, a comparison of the results needs to take into account differences in expression systems (bacteria, yeast), assay conditions (microsomal membranes, purified proteins) and the type of analysis of estrogen metabolites (HPLC, GC–MS). Some studies also provided an incomplete definition of constructs, i.e. only two or three of the four amino acids were listed. For these reasons, the results are inconsistent, although it appears that there is at best a two- to threefold difference in catalytic activity between wild-type CYP1B1 and any variant isoform.

Several studies have examined the association of CYP1B1 polymorphisms with the risk for breast and endometrial cancer. Two case–control studies that involved 1355 Caucasian and African-American women found no association with the risk for breast cancer (Bailey et al., 1998; De Vivo et al., 2002). Another case–control study of 186 Asian cases of breast cancer and 200 Asian controls found that women with the 432Leu/Leu genotype had a 2.3-fold (95% CI, 1.2–4.3) elevated risk for breast cancer compared with women with the 432Val/Val genotype (Zheng et al., 2000). Sasaki et al. (2003) examined 113 Japanese patients with endometrial cancer and 202 healthy controls. Women who had the homozygous 119Ser/Ser and 432Val/Val genotypes had relative risks for endometrial cancer of 3.32 (95% CI, 1.38–8.01) and 2.49 (95% CI, 1.10–5.66) compared with those who had wild-type CYP1B1. McGrath et al. (2004) examined codons 432 and 453 in women who had endometrial cancer within the Nurses' Health Study (222 cases, 666 controls). Carriers of the 453Ser allele had a significantly decreased risk for endometrial cancer (odds ratio, 0.62; 95% CI, 0.42–0.91), and there was no association with the 432Val → Leu polymorphism. A case–control study of postmenopausal Swedish women (689 cases, 1549 controls) examined polymorphisms at codons 119, 432 and 453 and found no evidence for an association between CYP1B1 genotype and risk for endometrial cancer (Rylander-Rudqvist et al., 2004). However, two studies observed an association of the 432Val/Val genotype with expression of estrogen receptor in breast cancer patients (Bailey et al., 1998; De Vivo et al., 2002). Another study noted a significant association between the 119Ser/Ser genotype and expression of estrogen receptors α and β in endometrial cancer patients (Sasaki et al., 2003). One study of postmenopausal women found that carriers of the 432Leu and 453Ser alleles had modestly higher plasma levels of estradiol but similar levels of estrone and estrone sulfate (De Vivo et al., 2002), while another study found no such association (Tworoger et al., 2004). The 432Leu → Val polymorphism was also investigated in relation to other cancers and showed no association with lung cancer but increased risks for ovarian cancer associated with the 432Leu allele and for prostate cancer associated with the 432Val allele (Tang et al., 2000; Watanabe et al., 2000; Goodman, M.T. et al., 2001).

(iii)   Catechol-O-methyltransferase (COMT)

The enzymatic activity of recombinant, purified COMT has been determined for methylation of the catechol estrogen substrates 2- and 4-hydroxyestradiol and 2- and 4-hydroxyestrone (Dawling et al., 2001; Lautala et al., 2001; Goodman et al., 2002). COMT catalysed the formation of monomethyl ethers at the 2-, 3- and 4-hydroxyl groups. Dimethyl ethers were not observed. The rates of methylation of 2-hydroxyestradiol and 2-hydroxyestrone yielded typical hyperbolic patterns, whereas those of 4-hydroxyestradiol and 4-hydroxyestrone exhibited a sigmoid curve pattern (Dawling et al., 2001). Thus, COMT interacts differently with the 2- and 4-hydroxyestrogen substrates. Methylation of 2-hydroxyestrogen substrates exhibits Michaelis-Menten saturation kinetics and yields two products, i.e. 2- and 3-methoxyestrogens. In contrast, the methylation of 4-hydroxyestrogen substrates displays sigmoid saturation kinetics that indicates cooperative binding and yields only a single product, i.e. 4-methoxyestrogen. The main structural difference between 2- and 4-hydroxy catechol estrogens is the proximity of the 4-hydroxyl group to the B-ring of the steroid. The 2- and 3-hydroxyl groups in 2-hydroxyestrogen appear to be similar in reactivity, whereas the 3- and 4-hydroxyl groups in 4-hydroxyestrogen differ in reactivity to the point that, in the latter, only the 4-hydroxyl group becomes methylated.

Dawling et al. (2001) compared the enzymatic activity of wild-type (108Val) COMT with that of the common variant (108Met). The 108Met variant, unlike wild-type COMT, was thermolabile, and led to two- to threefold lower levels of production of methoxyestrogen. These results differ from those of Goodman et al. (2002) but are in agreement with two other studies (Lachman et al., 1996; Syvänen et al., 1997). Dawling et al. (2001) developed an enzyme-linked immunosorbent assay to quantify COMT in breast cancer cell lines and determined that ZR-75 and MCF-7 cells contain similar amounts of COMT, but differ in genotype and enzymatic activity. The catalytic activity of variant COMT in MCF-7 cells was two- to threefold lower than that of wild-type COMT in ZR-75 cells. Since COMT is expressed ubiquitously, it appears that the COMT genotype significantly affects levels of catechol estrogens throughout the body. However, Goodman et al. (2002) found no difference between breast cancer cell lines of different COMT genotypes (MCF-10A and ZR-75-1 with high activity allele COMT[HH], and NCF-7 and T47D with low activity allele COMT[LL]), except for the formation of 2-methoxyestradiol.

Immunohistochemical analysis of benign and malignant breast tissue revealed the presence of COMT in the cytoplasm of all epithelial cells. Immunoreactive COMT was also observed in the nucleus of some benign and malignant epithelial cells. There was no correlation between histopathology and the number of cells with nuclear COMT, size of foci that contained such cells or intensity of nuclear COMT immunostaining. Staining of both intra- and interlobular stromal cells was always of a much lower intensity than that of epithelial cells in the same tissue sections (Weisz et al., 2000).

Several epidemiological studies have examined the association of COMT genotype with the risk for breast cancer. A meta-analysis of 13 studies published through to July 2004 did not support the hypothesis that the low-activity variant of COMT, as a single factor, leads to increased risk for breast cancer (Wen et al., 2005). However, Goodman, J.E. et al.

(2001) observed an association between the risk for breast cancer, *COMT* genotype and micronutrients in the folate metabolic pathway. These micronutrients (i.e. cysteine, homocysteine, folate, vitamin B12, pyridoxal 5′-phosphate) are known to influence levels of the methyl donor *S*-adenosylmethionine, and *S*-adenosylhomocysteine, a COMT inhibitor that is generated by the demethylation of *S*-adenosylmethionine. High-activity homozygous *COMT*1* cases of breast cancer had significantly lower levels of homocysteine ($p = 0.05$) and cysteine ($p = 0.04$) and higher levels of pyridoxal 5′-phosphate ($p = 0.02$) than homozygous *COMT*1* controls. In contrast, low-activity homozygous *COMT*2* cases had higher levels of homocysteine ($p = 0.05$) than low-activity homozygous *COMT*2* controls. An increase in the number of *COMT*2* alleles was significantly associated with an increased risk for breast cancer in women with levels of folate below the median (p for trend $= 0.05$) or levels of homocysteine above the median (p for trend $= 0.02$). No association was seen between vitamin B12, *COMT* genotype and risk for breast cancer (Goodman, J.E. *et al.*, 2001). These findings are consistent with a role of certain folate pathway micronutrients in the mediation of the association between *COMT* genotype and the risk for breast cancer. At the same time, these results illustrate the complex interaction of genetic and nutritional factors in the development of breast cancer. Equally complex is the interaction of the *COMT* genotype with other risk factors such as mammographic density (Hong *et al.*, 2003).

Lavigne *et al.* (2001) examined the effect of estrogen metabolism on oxidative DNA damage (8-hydroxy-2′-deoxyguanosine [8-OH-dG]) in 2,3,7,8-tetrachlorodibenzo-*para*-dioxin-pretreated MCF-7 cells exposed to estradiol with and without Ro41-0960, a specific inhibitor of COMT. Administration of the COMT inhibitor blocked the formation of 2-methoxyestradiol and, at the same time, increased the levels of 2-hydroxyestradiol and 8-OH-dG. During inhibition of COMT, increased oxidative DNA damage was detected in MCF-7 cells exposed to concentrations of estradiol as low as 0.1 µM, whereas, when COMT was not inhibited, no increase in 8-OH-dG was detected at concentrations of estradiol ≤ 10 µM. These results demonstrate that COMT activity is protective against oxidative DNA damage associated with catechol estrogen metabolites. In the absence of COMT activity and methoxyestrogens, a linear relation was observed between levels of 2- plus 4-hydroxyestradiol and 8-OH-dG. However, this relationship did not remain under experimental conditions that allowed limited formation of methoxyestrogens (when cells were treated with a lower concentration of COMT inhibitor), i.e. 8-OH-dG levels were lower than those expected for a given concentration of 2- plus 4-hydroxyestradiol in the presence of 2-methoxyestradiol. The authors suggested that 2-methoxyestradiol may reduce the formation of 8-OH-dG.

(iv)   *Glutathione* S-*transferases*

Hachey *et al.* (2003) determined that GSTP1 and CYP1B1 are coordinated in sequential reactions, i.e. 4- and 2-hydroxyestradiol did not form GSH conjugates in the presence of GSTP1 unless they were first oxidized by CYP1B1 to their corresponding quinones. CYP1B1 metabolized estradiol to two products, 4- and 2-hydroxyestradiol, and further to estradiol-3,4-quinone and estradiol-2,3-quinone, while GSTP1 formed three products, 4-hydroxyestradiol-2-SG, 2-hydroxyestradiol-4-SG, and 2-hydroxyestradiol-1-SG, the last of which in smaller amounts. The rate of conjugation was in the order 4-hydroxyestradiol-2-SG > 2-hydroxyestradiol-4-SG >> 2-hydroxyestradiol-1-SG, which indicated a difference in the regiospecific reactivity of the two quinones. Estradiol-2,3- and estradiol-3,4-quinones are products of CYP1B1- and substrates of GSTP1-mediated reactions but also react non-enzymatically with other nucleophiles, as indicated by a 10-fold concentration gap between catechol estrogens and GSH–estrogen conjugates. It has been suggested that, although both reactions are coordinated qualitatively in terms of product formation and substrate utilization, the quantitative gap would enable the accumulation of estrogen quinones and their potential for DNA damage.

Based on protein levels, GSTP1 is the most important member of the GST family expressed in breast tissue (Kelley et al., 1994; Alpert et al., 1997). However, two other GST isoforms, GSTM1 and GSTA1, are also expressed in mammary epithelium, although at lower levels. About 50% of Caucasian and 30% of African women possess the GSTM1 null genotype and therefore completely lack GSTM1 expression in all tissues including the breast (Garte et al., 2001). GSTs are known to have selective as well as overlapping substrate specificities. It is unknown at present whether GSTM1 and GSTA1 are capable of conjugating estrogen quinones similarly to GSTP1 (Hachey et al., 2003).

The GSTP1 gene also possesses two polymorphisms in codons 104 (Ile → Val) and 113 (Ala → Val) that are associated with altered catalytic activity towards polycyclic aromatic hydrocarbons (Hu et al., 1997; Ji et al., 1999). It is unknown at present whether the GSTP1-mediated conjugation of estrogen quinones varies between the GSTP1 wild-type and its variants.

Several epidemiological studies found no overall association between polymorphism in GSTP1 codon 104 and the risk for breast cancer (reviewed by Mitrunen & Hirvonen, 2003). The polymorphic allele in codon 113 showed a tendency for an increased risk in one study and a protective effect in another (Krajinovic et al., 2001; Maugard et al., 2001). A comprehensive review of 15 studies of GSTM1 published through to 2002 found no overall evidence for an association of the GSTM1 null genotype with risk for breast cancer (Mitrunen & Hirvonen, 2003).

(v)   Uridine-5′ diphosphate (UDP)-glucuronosyltransferases

The UDP-glucuronosyltransferase (UGT) superfamily currently consists of 16 functional genes that are organized into two families of enzymes, UGT1 and UGT2 (King et al., 2000; Tukey & Strassburg, 2000). The study of UGTs was initiated by the hypothesis that UGT-mediated estrogen conjugation reduces catechol estrogen levels and thereby decreases the risk for breast cancer (Raftogianis et al., 2000). Similarly to the sulfotransferase (SULT) superfamily, several UGT isoforms are capable of estrogen conjugation, i.e. UGT1A1, -1A3, -1A7, -1A8, -1A9, -1A10, -2B4, -2B7, -2B11 and -2B15 (Lévesque et al., 1999; King et al., 2000; Turgeon et al., 2001). Although a comprehensive study of all known UGTs has not yet been performed, individual studies indicate that, of those tested,

UGT1A1, -1A3, -1A8, -1A9 and -2B7 have the highest activity toward estrogens (Albert et al., 1999; Tukey & Strassburg, 2000; Turgeon et al., 2001; Vallée et al., 2001). The parent hormones, estradiol and estrone, and their respective catechols are recognized as substrates, but individual isoforms display distinct differences in substrate specificity and conjugation efficiency. Comparison of UGT1A3 and -2B7 showed regioselective conjugation of estradiol, i.e. UGT1A3 only conjugated the C-3 hydroxyl group of the A-ring, whereas UGT2B7 conjugated the 17β-hydroxyl in the D-ring, to yield estradiol-3 and 17β-glucuronides, respectively (Gall et al., 1999). Several isoforms, including UGT1A1, -1A9 and -2B7, were more active towards the catechol estrogens than the parent hormones. In contrast, comparison of catechol estrogen substrates revealed that UGT1A1 and -1A3 were more active toward 2-hydroxyestradiol, while UGT1A9 and -2B7 conjugated 4-hydroxy-estradiol more efficiently (Cheng et al., 1998; Albert et al., 1999). Although the catechols derived from estradiol and estrone are generally metabolized with similar efficiencies, UGT2B7 displayed seven- to 12-fold higher activity (1320 pmol/min/mg microsomal protein) towards 4-hydroxyestrone than 4-hydroxyestradiol, in spite of similar apparent K_m values (Cheng et al., 1998; Turgeon et al., 2001). The highest activity was recorded for the UGT1A9-mediated conjugation of 4-hydroxyestradiol (2500 pmol/min/mg) (Albert et al., 1999).

Few studies have examined UGT expression in breast tissue, and have usually been limited to the detection of the transcript. Of the isoforms with the highest activity toward estrogen conjugation, UGT1A9 mRNA was detectable in breast tissue whereas UGT1A1 mRNA was not detected (Albert et al., 1999; Vallée et al., 2001). UGT2B7 appears to be the only isoform that has been examined for both transcript and protein. UGT2B7 transcript was present in normal mammary tissue, but not in T47D and ZR-75 breast cancer cells (Turgeon et al., 2001). A detailed immunohistochemical study (Gestl et al., 2002) demonstrated expression of UGT2B7 protein in normal mammary epithelium obtained from either reduction mammoplasties or tissue distant from invasive cancer in mastectomy specimens. In contrast, expression of UGT2B7 protein was significantly reduced in malignant cells. The observed difference in UGT2B7 expression between benign and malignant cells is consistent with the hypothesis that UGT-mediated conjugation of catechol estrogens prevents the formation of potentially carcinogenic estrogen quinones. Based on the efficiency of estrogen conjugation and expression in breast tissue, UGT1A9 and -2B7 may be considered to be the predominant isoforms in mammary metabolism of estrogen.

To date, polymorphisms have been described in seven of the 16 functional human UGT genes, namely UGT1A1, -1A6, -1A7, -1A8, -2B4, -2B7 and -2B15 (Lévesque et al., 1999; Huang et al., 2002; Miners et al., 2002). Altered catalytic activity has been shown for variants of UGT1A6, -1A7, -1A8 and -2B15, but the biological significance has yet to be proven (Huang et al., 2002; Miners et al., 2002). A polymorphism in UGT2B7 (268His → Tyr) exhibited similar efficiencies for the glucuronidation of a number of substrates for the wild-type and variant enzymes (Bhasker et al., 2000). Functional significance has only been convincingly demonstrated for a polymorphism in a TA repeat element, $(TA)_{5-8}TAA$, of the UGT1A1 promoter. The length of the TA repeat appears to influence *UGT1A1* transcription, i.e. *UGT1A1* gene expression decreases with increasing number of repeats, and results in impaired glucuronidation of bilirubin in Gilbert syndrome. The *UGT1A1* polymorphism was associated with a marginal effect ($p = 0.06$) on the risk for breast cancer in premenopausal but not in postmenopausal African-American women (Guillemette *et al.*, 2000). No association with risk was observed in a larger study of Caucasian women, and levels of circulating estradiol and estrone were not affected by the polymorphism (Guillemette *et al.*, 2001).

(vi)   *Sulfotransferases*

The SULT superfamily currently consists of 10 distinct enzymes that are classified into three families (SULT1, -2 and -4) based on the identity of amino acid sequence (Falany *et al.*, 2000; Glatt *et al.*, 2000; Adjei & Weinshilboum, 2002). Growing recognition of the carcinogenic potential of catechol estrogens has led to increased interest in the role of SULTs in the intracellular metabolism of estrogen (Raftogianis *et al.*, 2000). These studies were initiated by the hypothesis that SULT-mediated estrogen conjugation reduces catechol estrogen levels and thereby decreases the risk for breast cancer.

The identification of new SULT isoforms during the past few years (Falany *et al.*, 2000) has shown that earlier tissue studies frequently encompassed unrecognized isoforms, which obscured the issue of SULT specificity in estrogen conjugation. In a comprehensive study, Adjei and Weinshilboum (2002) prepared the known 10 recombinant SULT isoforms and determined that seven (1A1, 1A2, 1A3, 1E1, 2A1, 2B1a, 2B1b) catalysed the sulfate conjugation of catechol estrogens, whereas three (1B1, 1C1, 4A1) did not.

Although seven SULT isoforms were shown to conjugate estrogens, they differ significantly in their substrate affinity. There is consensus among investigators that only SULT1E1 can conjugate estradiol, and 2- and 4-hydroxyestradiol at nanomolar concentrations, in contrast to the micromolar concentrations observed for SULT1A1, -1A2, -1A3 and -2A1 (Faucher *et al.*, 2001; Adjei & Weinshilboum, 2002). However, there is disagreement with respect to the sulfation of methoxyestrogens at nanomolar concentrations (Spink *et al.*, 2000; Adjei *et al.*, 2003).

Immunocytochemical studies have shown that SULT1E1 is the principal isoform in normal mammary epithelial cells derived from reduction mammoplasties, the non-tumour-derived cell line 184A1 and epithelial cells in normal breast tissues (Spink *et al.*, 2000; Suzuki *et al.*, 2003). Other isoforms, such as SULT1A1, were not detectable immunohistochemically in normal mammary epithelium, although reverse transcription-PCR revealed SULT1A1 and -1A3 mRNA in 184A1 cells (Spink *et al.*, 2000). The expression pattern of SULT was almost converse in breast cancer cell lines and tissues. Virtually every malignant cell line expresses one or more members of the SULT1A subfamily. For example, SULT1A1 protein and mRNA levels were particularly high in BT-20, MCF-7, T47D and ZR-75 cells. In contrast, SULT1E1 was present in trace amounts or undetectable in most malignant cell lines (Spink *et al.*, 2000; Falany *et al.*, 2002). However, SULT1E1 was detected by immunohistochemistry in 50/113 (44.2%) invasive ductal carcinomas (Suzuki *et al.*, 2003). A subgroup analysis of 35 cases showed a significant correlation ($p < 0.01$) between the immunohistochemical SULT1E1 score and *SULT1E1* mRNA levels that was semiquantified by reverse transcriptase-PCR or with SULT1E1 enzymatic activity. Women who had SULT1E1-positive tumours had a better prognosis (longer disease-free interval [$p = 0.0044$] and overall survival [$p = 0.0026$]) than their SULT1E1-negative counterparts (Suzuki *et al.*, 2003). Both the expression of SULT1E1 in normal mammary epithelium and the poor clinical outcome of SULT1E1-negative breast cancers support the view that SULT1E1-mediated conjugation is important in limiting long-term exposure of the mammary glands to carcinogenic catechol estrogens.

The *SULT1A1* and *-1E1* genes contain polymorphisms that are associated with decreased enzyme activity and thermal stability (Carlini *et al.*, 2001; Adjei *et al.*, 2003). Two *SULT1A1* polymorphisms have been described in codons 213Arg → His and 223Met → Val, which result in three alleles, *SULT1A1*1* (213Arg, 223Met), *SULT1A1*2* (213His, 223Met) and *SULT1A1*3* (213Arg, 223Val). Allele frequencies for *SULT1A1*1*, *-*2* and *-*3* were 65, 33 and 1% for Caucasians and 48, 29 and 23% for African-Americans, respectively (Carlini *et al.*, 2001). A kinetic analysis of 2-methoxyestradiol showed similar K_m values for SULT1A1*1 and SULT1A1*2 (0.90 ± 0.12 and 0.81 ± 0.06 µM, respectively) (Spink *et al.*, 2000). Three *SULT1E1* polymorphisms cause amino acid substitutions in codons 22Asp → Tyr, 32Ala → Val and 253Pro → His (Adjei *et al.*, 2003). Kinetic studies with estradiol and the recombinant *SULT1E1* variant 22Tyr revealed an increase in apparent K_m, which resulted in a 40-fold lower activity compared with the wild-type enzyme (Adjei *et al.*, 2003) and is consistent with the location of residue 22 at the entrance of the substrate-binding pocket (Pedersen *et al.*, 2002). The striking decrease in enzyme activity and concentration observed for 32Ala → Val and 22Asp → Tyr are expected to have considerable impact on the mammary metabolism of estrogen. However, the allele frequency of these *SULT1E1* variants is < 1% (Adjei *et al.*, 2003), which is much lower than the variant *SULT1A1* allele frequency, and raises the question whether they are indeed polymorphisms or mutations. One epidemiological study found an increased risk for breast cancer associated with the *SULT1A1*2* genotype (213Arg → His) (155 cases, 328 controls; odds ratio, 1.8; 95% CI, 1.0–3.2; $p = 0.04$) (Zheng *et al.*, 2001). However, another study reported the lack of an association (444 cases, 227 controls; $p = 0.69$) (Seth *et al.*, 2000).

(vii) *Steroid (estrone) sulfatase*

In contrast to the many SULTs, only one steroid sulfatase hydrolyses several sulfated steroids, including estrone sulfate, estradiol sulfate, dehydroepiandrosterone sulfate and cholesterol sulfate (Burns, 1983). Steroid sulfatase is not expressed in normal endometrium but was observed in 65/76 (86%) endometrial carcinomas (Utusunomiya *et al.*, 2004). In contrast, the enzyme is expressed in both normal and malignant breast tissues (Chapman *et al.*, 1995; Utsumi *et al.*, 1999; Miyoshi *et al.*, 2001). Utsunomiya *et al.* (2004) found a positive correlation ($p < 0.05$) between the steroid sulfatase:estrogen SULT ratio and shorter survival in patients with endometrial carcinomas, and suggested that increased steroid sulfatase and decreased estrogen SULT expression may result in increased availability of biologically active estrogens.

Several studies have shown that progestogens can act as 'selective estrogen enzyme modulators' in hormone-responsive breast cancer cells (reviewed by Pasqualini, 2004). Specifically, several progestogens exert an inhibitory effect on estrone sulfatase, which produces estradiol, in conjunction with a stimulatory effect on SULT, which forms the inactive estrogen sulfate. These data help to explain the antiproliferative effect of progestogens in breast tissue. It was also shown in MCF-7 and T47D cells that estradiol inhibited estrone sulfatase in a dose-dependent manner (IC_{50}: concentration of estradiol that inhibits the activity of the enzyme by 50%, 8.8×10^{-10} M and 1.8×10^{-9} M, respectively) and thereby decreased its own formation by blocking the conversion of estrone sulfate to estradiol (Pasqualini & Chetrite, 2001).

(viii) 17β-Hydroxysteroid dehydrogenase

17β-Hydroxysteroid dehydrogenase (17β-HSD) enzyme is responsible for the interconversion of 17-ketosteroids and their active 17β-hydroxysteroid counterparts, such as estrone, estradiol, androstenedione and testosterone. Six human genes that encode isozymes of 17β-HSD have been cloned (Peltoketo et al., 1999). These isozymes are designated types 1–6 or HSD1–HSD6.

17β-HSD1 is a key enzyme in estrogen metabolism because it catalyses the conversion of estrone into the biologically more active estradiol. It is abundantly expressed in ovarian granulosa cells and placental syncytiotrophoblasts (Peltoketo et al., 1999). 17β-HSD1 is detected in certain peripheral tissues, such as breast and endometrium, in addition to steroidogenic cells in the ovary and placenta. However, the degree of expression reported is quite variable. In breast cancers, for example, the detection of *17β-HSD1* mRNA varies from 16 to 100% (Gunnarsson et al., 2001; Oduwole et al., 2004) and the immunohistochemical staining of 17β-HSD1 ranges from 20 to 61% of cases (Poutanen et al., 1992a,b; Sasano et al., 1996; Suzuki et al., 2000; Oduwole et al., 2004). A positive, inverse or no correlation was observed between 17β-HSD1 expression and estrogen receptor-positive status in breast cancers (Sasano et al., 1996; Suzuki et al., 2000; Oduwole et al., 2004). One study observed significantly higher expression of 17β-HSD1 in postmenopausal cancers while another study found no correlation with menopausal status (Suzuki et al., 2000; Miyoshi et al., 2001). Correlation between 17β-HSD1 expression and prognosis has been inconsistent, and either no association or a shorter overall and disease-free survival have been found in breast cancer patients (Suzuki et al., 2000; Oduwole et al., 2004). One reason for the discrepant data on 17β-HSD1 expression could be the amplification of the *17β-HSD1* gene, which was observed in 14.5% of postmenopausal breast cancers (Gunnarsson et al., 2003). However, 17β-HSD1 is not expressed in normal or malignant endometrium (Utsunomiya et al., 2001, 2003).

The *17β-HSD1* gene contains several polymorphisms, including a common one in exon 6 that results in the amino acid substitution 312Ser → Gly (Normand et al., 1993). Several studies found no association of this polymorphism with either breast or endometrial cancers (Feigelson *et al.*, 2001; Wu *et al.*, 2003; Setiawan *et al.*, 2004). This is consistent with experimental data that show no difference in the catalytic activity of recombinant wild-type and variant 312 alleles (Puranen *et al.*, 1994). Nevertheless, one study observed higher plasma levels of estradiol in lean women with the homozygous 312Gly/Gly genotype ($p = 0.01$) (Setiawan *et al.*, 2004).

17β-HSD2 catalyses the conversion of estradiol into less potent estrone. In contrast to 17β-HSD1, expression studies of 17β-HSD2 yielded more consistent results. 17β-HSD2 is expressed in normal mammary epithelium but is frequently absent in breast cancer cells (Miettinen *et al.*, 1999; Ariga *et al.*, 2000; Suzuki *et al.*, 2000; Gunnarsson *et al.*, 2001; Oduwole *et al.*, 2004). *17β-HSD2* mRNA was found in 10–31% of tumours and 17β-HSD2 protein was absent in all breast cancers (Suzuki *et al.*, 2000; Gunnarsson *et al.*, 2001). In contrast, 17β-HSD2 was regularly expressed in normal endometrium and was detected in 75% of endometrial hyperplasias and 37–50% of endometrial carcinomas (Utsunomiya *et al.*, 2001, 2003). Since 17β-HSD2 preferentially catalyses the oxidation of estradiol to less active estrone, it has been suggested that the expression of 17β-HSD2 in proliferative glandular cells of endometrial disorders may represent an in-situ defence mechanism that modulates unopposed estrogenic effects (Utsunomiya *et al.*, 2003).

17β-HSD5 (also known as aldo-keto reductase, AKR1C3) is expressed in normal breast and prostate (Penning *et al.*, 2000). The level of 17β-HSD5 expression in breast cancer specimens was higher than that in normal breast tissue and 65% of 794 tumours labelled 17β-HSD5-positive (Oduwole *et al.*, 2004). Since 17β-HSD5 recognizes a wide range of substrates, including estrogens, androgens, progestogens and prostaglandins, its role in breast tissue is uncertain.

Progestogens have a complex effect on 17β-HSD activity and can direct the interconversion of estrone to estradiol in both directions (reviewed by Pasqualini, 2004). Studies with the hormone-dependent breast cancer cells MCF-7 and T47D have shown that some progestogens stimulate the reductive activity of estrone to estradiol and thereby enhance cell proliferation (Coldham & James, 1990; Poutanen *et al.*, 1990, 1992b; Peltoketo *et al.*, 1996). Other progestogens favour the oxidation of estradiol to estrone and may thereby inhibit cell growth (Chetrite *et al.*, 1999a,b).

(c)   *Tobacco smoke*

Several compounds in tobacco smoke might affect estrogen metabolism by the induction of CYPs (Zeller & Berger, 1989). An epidemiological study of 27 premenopausal women (14 smokers, 13 nonsmokers) showed a significant increase in urinary excretion of 2-hydroxyestrone that is a result of 2-hydroxylation of reversibly oxidized estradiol (Michnovicz *et al.*, 1986). [The concentration of 4-hydroxylated estrogen metabolites was not assessed by this assay.]

Berstein *et al.* (2000) used GC–MS to measure urinary excretion of catechol estrogens in six smoking and 10 nonsmoking postmenopausal women who received 2 mg/day estradiol valerate for 1 month. Before administration of estradiol valerate, smokers had significantly lower excretion of 16-epiestriol and 4-hydroxyestrone than nonsmokers. After administration of estradiol valerate, much higher excretion of 2-hydroxyestrone and 4-hydroxyestradiol was observed in smokers compared with nonsmokers. These data indicate that only the combination of estradiol valerate and smoking (and not smoking itself) leads to an increase in potentially genotoxic catechol estrogens.

4.1.2   Experimental systems

(a)   Estrogen fatty acid esters

Chronic treatment of ovariectomized rats with 0.5 or 5 nmol/day estradiol stearate for 10 or 23 days had a stronger stimulatory effect on mammary gland cell proliferation than treatment with equimolar doses of estradiol (Mills et al., 2001). Two commonly prescribed hypolipidaemic drugs, clofibrate and gemfibrozil, increase the size and number of hepatic peroxisomes upon administration to rodents. Treatment of rats with clofibrate caused a multifold increase in the hepatic microsomal formation of estradiol fatty acids (Xu et al., 2001a). The stimulatory effect of clofibrate on hepatic fatty acid esterification of estradiol was paralleled by enhanced estradiol-induced increases in the formation of lobules in the mammary gland and by increased incorporation of bromodeoxyuridine, a marker of cell proliferation, into these lobules (Xu et al., 2001b).

(b)   Catechol estrogens

Catechol estrogens are carcinogenic in animal experiments. The experimental evidence was reviewed by Cavalieri et al. (2000) and showed that 4-catechol estrogens are more carcinogenic than the isomers 2-hydroxyestrogens. In addition to the induction of renal cancer in hamsters (Liehr et al., 1986), 4-hydroxyestradiol induces uterine adeno-carcinoma, a hormonally related cancer, in mice. Administration of estradiol, 2-hydroxy-estradiol and 4-hydroxyestradiol induced endometrial carcinomas in 7, 12 and 66%, res-pectively, of neonatally treated CD-1 mice (Newbold & Liehr, 2000). However, in adult ACI rats, administration of estradiol but not that of 2- or 4-hydroxyestradiol or 4-hydroxy-estrone induced mammary tumours (Turan et al., 2004).

4.2   Receptor-mediated effects

As indicated in the monograph on Combined estrogen–progestogen contraceptives, there is evidence that not all of the effects of estrogens and progestogens used in hormonal therapy for the menopause are mediated through nuclear or other receptors. In addition, the effects of these steroids probably involve several molecular pathways and cross-talk between receptor- and/or non-receptor-mediated pathways. During the past decade, exten-sive growth in research on the mechanisms of action of hormones and on hormones and cancer has taken place, and several steroid hormone receptor subtypes and non-genomic mechanisms of action have been determined.

Hormonal therapy with 'estrogens only' is effective in the treatment of many aspects of the menopause, but the increased risk for endometrial cancer renders the prescription of combined estrogen–progestogen products for women with a uterus essential. In this context, an ideal progestogen would prevent endometrial cancer and maintain the protective benefits of estrogens, which means that it should have no significant anti-estrogenicity, except in the endometrium.

The various components of hormonal therapy for the menopause have received increased attention in recent years. Information has become available on the progestogens used and on their hormonal activities and their binding affinities to various receptors and proteins. This information is summarized in Tables 17 and 18, which were compiled on the basis of information gathered by Sitruk-Ware (2002), Schindler *et al.* (2003), Shields-Botella *et al.* (2003), Sitruk-Ware (2004a,b) and Wiegratz and Kuhl (2004).

There has also been tremendous growth in research on the effects of postmenopausal hormonal therapy on a variety of non-cancer end-points related to endometrial function (vaginal bleeding), postmenopausal vasomotor symptoms, treatment of problems with the menstrual cycle, skin, bone and related calcium metabolism, the cardiovascular system and lipid metabolism. Many of these effects are probably at least in part mediated by mechanisms of steroid receptors. This topic is reviewed in Section 4.3.

4.2.1   *Combined estrogen–progestogen therapy*

(*a*)   *Humans*

(i)   *Breast*

No data were available on the effects of exposure to combined estrogen–progestogen therapy on the human breast in the previous evaluation (IARC, 1999). During the past 6 years, several reports have been published that are pertinent to this issue.

Hargreaves *et al.* (1998) obtained archival paraffin-embedded breast tissue samples from women who underwent surgery for benign (*n* = 61) or malignant (*n* = 124) breast disease and stained sections from these for the proliferation marker Ki-67 and the progesterone receptor. The median percentage of normal epithelial cells that stained for Ki-67 [using an unspecified antibody] was 0.19% (range, 0–3.66%) in breast samples of 111 women who did not receive hormonal therapy. This was not significantly different from the percentages in normal epithelial cells from 35 women who took estrogen only (0.22%; range, 0–1.44%) or 39 women who took combined estrogen plus progesterone therapy (0.25%; range, 0–2.80%). However, the median percentage of normal epithelial cells that stained for the nuclear progesterone receptor significantly increased from 4.8% (range, 0–39%) in 100 untreated women to 10.2% (range, 0.2–40%) in 31 women who took estrogen only and 6.7% (range, 0–44%) in 36 women who took combined estrogen plus progesterone therapy. This increased expression of the progesterone receptor is consistent with an effect of estrogen on breast cells.

Hofseth *et al.* (1999) obtained breast biopsies from women who were taking oral estrogen–progestogen therapy that contained conjugated equine estrogens (0.3–2.5 mg/day) or micronized 17β-estradiol (0.5–1.0 mg/day) plus medroxyprogesterone acetate (2.5–5.0 mg/day), from women who were taking these estrogens only or from women who did

Table 17. Overview of the spectrum of hormonal activities of progestogens used in hormonal menopausal therapy

Progestogen	Progesto-genic	Anti-estrogenic	Estrogenic	Androgenic	Anti-androgenic	Glucocorticoid	Antimineralo-corticoid
Chlormadinone acetate	+	+	−	−	+	+	−
Cyproterone acetate	+	+	−	−	+, +	+	−
Desogestrel	+	+	−	+	−	±, −	−
Dienogest	+	+, ±	−, ±	−	+, +	−	−
Drospirenone	+, +	+	−	−	+	?, −	+
Dydrogesterone	+	+	−	−	−, ±	?	±
Etonogestrel [3-keto-desogestrel]	+	+	−	+	−	±, +	−
Gestodene	+	+	−	+	−	±, +	+
Levonorgestrel/norgestrel	+	+	−	+	−	−	−
Medroxyprogesterone (acetate)	+	+	−	±	−	+	−
Norethisterone (acetate)	+, +	+	+	+	−	−	−
Progesterone	+, +	+	−	−	±	+	+
Trimegestone	+	+	−	−	±	−	±

Adapted from Wiegratz and Kuhl (2004); second value, for progestogenic activity only from Sitruk-Ware (2002); second value, except for progestogenic activity from Schindler et al. (2003)

+, effective; ±, weakly effective; −, ineffective; ?, unknown

Data are based mainly on animal experiments. The clinical effects of the progestogens are dependent on their tissue concentrations.

No comparable data were available for ethynodiol diacetate.

Note: This information should be viewed as only an indication of the hormonal activity and its order of magnitude of the various progestogens.

Table 18. Relative binding affinities of progestogens used in hormonal therapy for the menopause to steroid receptors and serum binding globulins[a]

Progestogen	PR	AR	ER	GR	MR	SHBG	CBG
Chlormadinone acetate	134	5	0	8	0	0	0
Cyproterone acetate	180	6	0	6	8	0	0
Desogestrel (as 3-keto-desogestrel)	300	20	0	14	0	15	0
Dienogest	10	10	0	1	0	0	0
Drospirenone	70, 19	65, 2	0, < 0.5	6, 3	230, 500	0	0
Dydrogesterone	150	0	?	?	?	?	?
Etonogestrel (3-keto-desogestrel)	300	20	0	14	0	15	0
Gestodene	180, 864	85, 71	0, < 0.02	27, 28	290, 97	40	0
Levonorgestrel/norgestrel	300, 323	45, 58	0	1, 7.5	75, 17	50	0
Medroxyprogesterone acetate	130, 298	5, 36	0, < 0.02	29, 58	160, 3.1	0	0
Norethisterone acetate	150, 134	15, 55	0, 0.15	0, 1.4	0, 2.7	16	0
Norgestimate/nomegestrol acetate	30	0	0	1	0	0	0
Progesterone	100	0	0	10	100	0	36
Trimegestone	660, 588	1, 2.4	0, < 0.02	9, 13	120, 42	?	?
Reference compounds (100%)	Progesterone	Metribolone (R1881)	17β-Estradiol	Dexamethasone (or cortisol)	Aldosterone	5α-Dihydro-testosterone	Cortisol

Adapted from Wiegrazt and Kuhl (2004a,b); second value from Sitruk-Ware (2004)

?, unknown; AR, androgen receptor; CBG, corticoid-binding globulin; ER, estrogen receptor; GR, glucocorticoid receptor; MR, mineralocorticoid receptor; PR, progesterone receptor; SHBG, sex hormone-binding globulin

[a] Values were compiled by these authors by cross-comparison of the literature. Because the results of the various in-vitro experiments depend largely on the incubation conditions and biological materials used, the published values are inconsistent. These values do not reflect the biological effectiveness, but should be viewed as only an indication of the order of magnitude of the binding affinities of the various progestogens. No comparable data were available for ethynodiol diacetate.

not take hormonal treatment. Compared with untreated women ($n = 16$–19), the percentage of epithelial cells in the inter- and intralobular ducts and the duct-lobular units that stained positive for proliferating cell nuclear antigen were significantly ($p < 0.01$) increased by approximately twofold in women who took estrogen alone ($n = 21$) and those who took estrogen plus progestogen ($n = 15$; ducts only); staining was increased by almost threefold in the duct-lobular unit cells of women who took estrogen plus progestogen ($n = 19$; $p < 0.01$). When another marker of proliferation (Ki-67) was examined, similar differences were found, but only the difference (approximately sixfold) for the duct-lobular unit cells of women who took estrogen plus progestogen was statistically significant ($p < 0.05$). There was a positive correlation between the percentage of epithelial breast cells that stained for markers of proliferation with the duration of both types of hormonal treatment, but this was only statistically significant for the treatment with estrogen plus progestogen when the Ki-67 marker was considered ($p = 0.03$). There was also a significant increase ($p \leq 0.01$) in the percentage of breast tissue occupied by epithelium, i.e. twofold for women who took estrogen only and threefold for women who took estrogen plus progestogen. The percentage of epithelial cells that were positive for the nuclear staining for the progesterone receptor was increased three- to fourfold ($p < 0.01$) in women who took estrogen only and approximately twofold in the lobular units of women who took estrogen plus progestogen ($p < 0.05$); again, the observed increase in the expression of the progesterone receptor is consistent with an effect of estrogen on these cells. No differences were observed in nuclear staining for the estrogen receptor.

Conner et al. (2001) studied 12 women who were treated continuously with 17β-estra-diol (50 µg per day by skin patch) and either oral (5 mg per day) medroxyprogesterone acetate or vaginal (8 mg every 2 days) progesterone on days 15–26 of each cycle. They obtained fine needle aspiration biopsies during the last 2 days of the estrogen part of the cycle and during day 25 or 26 at the end of the estrogen plus progestogen part of the cycle after 6–8 weeks and after 14–16 weeks of treatment. The percentage of epithelial cells that stained for Ki-67 (using the MIB-1 antibody) was 1.4% at the end of the estrogen phase and 2.1% at the end of the estrogen plus progestogen phase of the cycle, but this was not statistically significant. There was no difference in Ki-67 staining between the two proges-togen treatments. In follow-up studies, Conner et al. (2003, 2004a) examined women who received continuous oral 17β-estradiol (2 mg per day) plus norethisterone acetate (1 mg per day) or 17β-estradiol valerate (2 mg per day) plus dienogest (2 mg per day) for 6 months. In the first study, two groups of 13–17 women received estrogen plus either norethisterone acetate or estrogen plus dienogest. For both treatments combined, the mean percentage of epithelial cells that stained for Ki-67 in fine needle aspiration was statistically significantly increased ($p < 0.001$) from 2.2% ($n = 28$; median, 1.4%; range, 0–11.7%) at baseline to 9.1% ($n = 30$; median, 7.6%; range, 0–27.1%) after 3 months and 8.0% ($n = 31$; median, 5.7%; range, 0–25.9%) after 6 months of treatment. One woman who had a high baseline proliferation index showed a decrease in proliferation after treatment. The increases in cell proliferation index were similar for both hormonal treatments (Conner et al., 2003). In the second study of 83 women who were treated with 17β-estradiol (2 mg per day) plus norethisterone acetate (1 mg per day), the mean percentage of epithelial cells that stained for Ki-67 in fine needle aspiration biopsies was significantly ($p < 0.01$) increased from 2.2% (median, 1.9%; range, 0–11.9%) at baseline to 6.4% (median, 5.0%; range, 0–20.4%) after 6 months of treatment. There was a negative correlation between the rate of epithelial proliferation in this study and total and free serum testosterone levels (Conner et al., 2004a).

Valdivia et al. (2004) obtained breast core biopsies from 19 women at baseline and after treatment for 12 months with continuous conjugated equine estrogen (0.625 mg per day) and medroxyprogesterone acetate (5 mg per day). Of these women, 15 responded with an increase in percentage of epithelial cells that stained for Ki-67, one exhibited a decrease and three women had no change in this parameter; the increase from baseline was probably statistically significant, but this was not clear. Expression of the apoptosis marker Bcl-2 was increased in nine women, decreased in five and unchanged in five.

The results of all but one of these studies indicate that combined estrogen–progestogen menopausal therapy increases the rate of cell proliferation in the breast. The addition of progestogens appears to enhance significantly the modest increase in the rate of breast cell proliferation caused by estrogen-only therapy. This is consistent with the notion of an increase in risk for breast cancer associated with combined estrogen–progestogen meno-pausal therapy over that associated with estrogen-only menopausal therapy (see also IARC, 1999). Only the study of archival surgical specimens of women with breast disease by Hargreaves et al. (1998) did not show an increase in breast cell proliferation associated with combined estrogen–progestogen menopausal therapy. The other studies used either fine needle aspirates or core biopsies from women without breast disease, which may explain the discrepancy.

Mammographic density is a strong identifier of risk for sporadic breast cancer that exceeds the risk associated with elevated circulating levels of 17β-estradiol (Santen, 2003). Risk for breast cancer was increased in a number of case–control studies in which mammographic density was not only subjectively evaluated by radiologists but was also assessed by observer bias-free, automated, computer-assisted techniques. The relative risks were in the order of 4–6 for subjective evaluations and 3–4 for computer-assisted evaluations (Byng et al., 1997; Yaffe et al., 1998; Boyd et al., 1999; Li et al., 2005). A number of recent studies have reported on the effects of estrogen–progestogen therapy on mammographic density. Valdivia et al. (2004) (see study details above) observed an increase in mammographic density (BI-RADS method) in 11/19 women (58%) who took conjugated equine estrogen plus medroxyprogesterone acetate for 12 months, while density was decreased in only one woman and was unchanged in seven.

Conner et al. (2004b) randomized women to continuous oral treatment for 6 months with either 17β-estradiol (2 mg per day) plus norethisterone acetate (1 mg per day) (22 women) or 17β-estradiol valerate (2 mg per day) plus dienogest (2 mg per day) (23 women). Both treatments resulted in an increase in mammographic density (Wolfe method) over baseline values in 50–60% of these women; this change was statistically significant.

Christodoulakos *et al.* (2003) randomized 94 women to continuous oral treatment for 12 months with conjugated equine estrogen alone (0.625 mg per day) (25 women), equine estrogen (0.625 mg per day) plus medroxyprogesterone acetate (5 mg per day) (34 women) or 17β-estradiol (2 mg per day) plus norethisterone acetate (1 mg per day) (35 women); 27 untreated control women were also included. Mammographic density (Wolfe classification method) increased in 12% of women who took equine estrogen plus medroxyprogesterone acetate, 31% of women who took 17β-estradiol plus norethisterone acetate and in 8% of women who took estrogen only, whereas density did not increase in any of the control women. Density decreased in 26% of control women but in none of the women who took hormonal treatment. The difference from controls was statistically significant for all three treatment groups.

Georgiev and Manassiev (2002) found that breast density increased in 16% of 19 women who were treated with continuous oral 17β-estradiol (2 mg per day) plus dienogest (2 mg per day) or 17β-estradiol (2 mg per day) plus norethisterone acetate (1 mg per day) and were followed annually by mammography for 4 years using the Wolfe method.

Sendag *et al.* (2001) compared women who received continuous oral treatment with 17β-estradiol (2 mg per day) plus norethisterone acetate (1 mg per day) (44 women), conjugated equine estrogen (0.625 mg per day) plus medroxyprogesterone acetate (5 mg per day) (17 women), equine estrogen only (0.625 mg per day) (20 women) or transdermal 17β-estradiol (3.9 mg per week) (56 women) and 44 women who received a variety of sequential treatments with estrogen and estrogen plus progestogen. The mean follow-up was 20 months (range, 12–96 months) and the Wolfe method was used to assess breast density. Density was increased in 31% of women who took continuous estrogen plus progestogen and in 4% of women who took estrogen only, but did not change in women who received the sequential treatments with estrogen plus progestogen. More women (34%) who took the continuous treatment with 17β-estradiol plus norethisterone acetate had increased breast density than those who took continuous estrogen plus medroxyprogesterone acetate (24%).

Colacurci *et al.* (2001) randomized women to continuous treatment with transdermal 17β-estradiol (0.05 mg per day) plus nomegestrol acetate at one of two doses (5 mg per day, 26 women; or 2.5 mg per day, 25 women), 17β-estradiol only (23 women) or no treatment (controls; 23 women). Mammographic density (Wolfe method) after 12 months of treatment was increased in 35% and 43% of the women who took estrogen plus the high and low dose of nomegestrol acetate, respectively, in 21% of women who took estrogen only and in none of the control women. The differences from the control group were statistically significant.

Erel *et al.* (2001) assigned women to continuous oral treatment with conjugated equine estrogen (0.625 mg per day) plus medroxyprogesterone acetate (2.5 mg per day) (26 women), continuous treatment with estrogen (0.625 mg per day) plus medroxyprogesterone acetate (10 mg/day) for the last 10 days of the 28-day cycle (21 women) or continuous treatment with estrogen only (0.625 mg per day) (23 women). Women were followed by mammography for 4 years using the Wolfe method to assess breast density. Density was increased in 35% of women who took continuous estrogen plus progestogen, in 19% of women who took estrogen plus cyclic progestogen and in 22% of women who took estrogen only. Although the differences between these three groups were not statistically significant, the results suggest that treatment with continuous estrogen plus progestogen is more likely to increase breast density than treatment with continuous estrogen only or estrogen plus sequential progestogen.

Lundström et al. (2001) studied women who took continuous oral conjugated equine estrogen (0.625 mg per day) plus medroxyprogesterone acetate (5 mg per day) (52 women) or estriol (2 mg per day) (51 women) or used a transdermal patch of 17β-estradiol (0.05 mg per day) (55 women) and were followed every 2 years by mammography using the Wolfe method to assess breast density. Density increased over baseline at the first 2-year visit in 40% of women who took continuous estrogen plus progestogen, in 6% of women who took oral estrogen only and in 2% of women who used a transdermal patch of estrogen only.

Collectively, these studies consistently show that approximately one third of women treated with continuous estrogen (by any route) plus oral progestogen respond with increased mammographic breast density. Treatment with continuous estrogen plus sequential progestogen resulted in fewer women developing increased breast density than treatment with continuous estrogen plus progestogen. Estrogen-only treatment appeared to result in increased breast density in fewer women. These findings correspond to the supposition that continuous estrogen plus progestogen therapy results in an increased risk for breast cancer.

(ii)   Uterus

In the previous evaluation (IARC, 1999), it was concluded that the addition of progestogens reduces the increased rate of cell proliferation in the endometrium that is seen with estrogen-only therapy. The effects of estrogen only and their reduction by progestogens were dose-related. Two previous studies from the 1980s on cell proliferation concerned combined treatment with conjugated equine estrogens (Premarin®) and norethisterone. At least nine additional studies have been conducted with norethisterone, all but one of which combined the treatment with 17β-estradiol. In addition, studies have been carried out on six other progestogens combined with estrogen therapy. Many of these studies include histopathological analysis of endometrial biopsies. Although many studies have taken care to standardize this analysis, it should be noted that there is considerable potential for significant inter-observer and inter-study variation (Wright et al., 2002)

Norethisterone (acetate) plus estrogen

Cameron et al. (1997) followed 14 postmenopausal women for 3 months during which they were treated with a dermal patch that released 0.05 mg per day 17β-estradiol for 7 days alternated with a patch that released 0.05 mg per day 17β-estradiol plus 0.25 mg per day norethisterone acetate for 3 days. End-of-study endometrial biopsies were obtained at the end of an estrogen-only period and at the end of an estrogen plus norethisterone acetate period. Staining for the proliferation marker Ki-67 was reduced at the end of the estrogen plus norethisterone acetate period compared with the estrogen-only period, but staining for estrogen (α) and progesterone receptors and histological endometrial thickness did not differ. No endometrial hyperplasia was found.

Johannisson *et al.* (1997) randomized postmenopausal women in an open-label dermal patch study to continuous 0.05 mg per day 17β-estradiol plus doses of norethisterone acetate of 0.17 or 0.35 mg per day either continuously or sequentially on days 14–28. A reference group (not randomized) was treated with a continuous 0.05-mg per day 17β-estradiol patch and orally with either 1 mg per day norethisterone acetate or 20 mg per day dydrogesterone during the last 14 days of each cycle. End-of-study endometrial biopsies were obtained from 107–124 women per group after 13 cycles of 28 days. No significant differences were observed in the percentage of women with atrophic or proliferative endometrial histology and no malignancies occurred; only one case of endometrial hyperplasia developed in the group that received 17β-estradiol plus sequential norethisterone acetate at 0.35 mg per day.

Habiba *et al.* (1998) studied 103 postmenopausal women who were treated orally with 2 mg per day 17β-estradiol valcrate continuously and 1 mg per day norethisterone on days 16–28 of the cycle. The women received a baseline and end-of-study endometrial biopsy after 6 months of therapy. Most women had inactive or non-secretory endometrial histology at baseline whereas over 90% had secretory morphology after 6 months of treatment. No cases of endometrial hyperplasia or carcinoma occurred.

Dahmoun *et al.* (2004) assigned postmenopausal women to continuous treatment with either 2 mg per day 17β-estradiol plus 1 mg per day norethisterone acetate or 0.625 mg per day conjugated equine estrogens plus 5 mg per day medroxyprogesterone acetate. The two treatment groups were analysed in combination after 1 year of treatment. Staining for the proliferation marker Ki-67 was increased in stromal cells, but was not affected in epithelial cells. Staining for estrogen (α) receptor was reduced in the epithelium but was only slightly reduced in stromal cells. Staining for a marker of apoptosis (TUNEL) and the progesterone receptor in stroma and epithelium were not affected by the treatments, nor was endometrial thickness as assessed by ultrasound.

Kurman *et al.* (2000) conducted a double-blind clinical trial in which postmenopausal women were randomized to continuous oral treatment with 1 mg per day 17β-estradiol only or 1 mg per day 17β-estradiol plus 0.10, 0.25 or 0.50 mg per day norethisterone acetate. End-of-study endometrial biopsies were obtained from 241–251 women per group after 12 months of treatment. In the estrogen-only group, 14.6% of women had endometrial hyperplasia, whereas only 0.8% of women who took estrogen plus 0.10 mg norethisterone acetate and 0.4% of women who took the two higher doses of norethisterone acetate had such lesions. In women over 65 years of age, 4/21 (19%) who took estrogen only had endometrial hyperplasia, while none of the women who received estrogen plus either of the doses of norethisterone acetate had this lesion (0/18, 0/18 and 0/19 women).

Iatrakis *et al.* (2004) conducted an open-label prospective study of continuous oral treatment with 1 mg per day 17β-estradiol and 0.5 mg per day norethisterone acetate of 124 postmenopausal women for up to 3 years. A concurrent control group (not randomized) of

130 untreated women was available. Endometrial thickness, as assessed by ultrasound, was virtually unaffected. In end-of-study endometrial biopsies, no differences in the percentage of women with atrophic, secretory or proliferative histology were observed between the treated and control women. No cases of endometrial hyperplasia or carcinoma occurred.

Wells *et al.* (2002) conducted an open-label prospective study of postmenopausal women who were given continuous oral treatment with 2 mg per day 17β-estradiol plus 1 mg per day norethisterone acetate for up to 5 years; the mean follow-up was 4.4 years. Endometrial biopsies were obtained at baseline, between 24 and 36 months and at the end of the study. Inactive or atrophic endometrium was found in 68/164 (41%) women who had had no hormonal treatment at baseline, in 157/465 (34%) women after 24–36 months of treatment and in 185/398 (46%) women at the end of the study. (The entire cohort consisted of a mixture of women who had had no hormonal treatment and women who had already been taking either sequential or estrogen-only hormonal therapy.) At baseline, 14/164 women had a secretory endometrial histology (9%); this increased to 162/465 (35%) and 102/398 (26%) women after 24–36 months of treatment and at the end of the study, respectively. No cases of endometrial hyperplasia or carcinoma occurred. Sturdee *et al.* (2000) reported on 9 months of follow-up in this study. At baseline the prevalence of complex hyperplasia was 5.3% and that of atypical hyperplasia was 0.7% in the entire group of 1196 women who completed 9 months of treatment, many of whom had previously taken hormonal therapy that may have induced these hyperplastic lesions. None of these women had endometrial hyperplasia after 9 months of treatment and no new cases arose.

Neven *et al.* (2004) reported results of the EURALOX (European double-blind clinical trial on raloxifene) in which postmenopausal women were randomized to continuous oral treatment with 2 mg per day 17β-estradiol plus 1 mg per day norethisterone acetate or 60 mg per day raloxifene alone. End-of-study endometrial biopsies were obtained after 12 months of treatment. The conclusion of a detailed histopathological analysis was that more endometrial pathology occurred in 261 women on estrogen plus norethisterone acetate than in 73 women on raloxifene (polyps, 4.3% versus 2.0%; $p < 0.05$; endometrial proliferation/hyperplasia, 8.8% versus 1.2%; $p < 0.001$; cystic atrophy, 5.5% versus 1.2%; $p < 0.001$). Very few cases of malignant or premalignant endometrial histology occurred in either group.

Portman *et al.* (2003) conducted a double-blind placebo-controlled clinical trial in which postmenopausal women were randomized to continuous oral treatment with placebo, ethinylestradiol at 0.005 mg per day without or with 0.25 or 1.0 mg per day norethisterone acetate, or ethinylestradiol at 0.01 mg per day without or with 0.5 or 1.0 mg per day norethisterone acetate. In addition, an open-label comparison group was given 0.625 mg per day conjugated equine estrogens plus 2.5 mg per day medroxyprogesterone acetate. After 12 months of therapy, 114–121 women in each group received an end-of-study endometrial biopsy. Endometrial hyperplasia was found in 23/118 (19%) of the women who took 0.01 mg per day ethinylestradiol only, but only in a maximum of one woman in each of the other groups. In the estrogen-only groups, 80–90% of women had proliferative endometrial morphology, including the 19% of women with hyperplasia in the group who took 0.01 mg per day ethinylestradiol only. The occurrence of this morphology was reduced to 30–45% of women in all groups who were given co-treatment with nore-thisterone acetate, but was found in 70% of women who took estrogens plus medroxypro-gesterone acetate. The differences between the co-treatment with norethisterone acetate and that with estrogen only or estrogen plus medroxyprogesterone acetate were statistically significant.

Other progestogens plus estrogens

Ferenczy and Gelfand (1997) conducted an open-label prospective study of post-menopausal women who were given continuous oral treatment with 2 mg per day 17β-estradiol and 10 mg dydrogesterone on days 15–28. Baseline biopsies from 146 women who completed the 12-month course of treatment showed predominantly atrophic endo-metrium, whereas biopsies taken after 12 months of treatment showed that endometrial histology was predominantly secretory. One endometrial hyperplasia was found, but no endometrial carcinomas.

Hänggi et al. (1997) randomized 35 postmenopausal women per group to oral treatment with either placebo, 2 mg per day of continuous 17β-estradiol plus 10 mg dydrogesterone on days 15–28 or 0.05 mg per day continuous 17β-estradiol by dermal patch plus 10 mg oral dydrogesterone on days 15–28. Ultrasound assessment revealed a 2.5- to threefold increase over baseline of endometrial thickness after 12 and 24 months of hormonal treatment. Biopsies taken at the same time-points showed a shift from a predominantly inactive or atrophic endometrial histology to a predominantly secretory morphology.

Ross et al. (1997) conducted a double-blind clinical trial in which postmenopausal women were randomized to continuous oral treatment with 2 mg per day 17β-estradiol plus 0.1, 0.25 or 0.5 mg per day trimegestone on days 15–28. In each of the three groups, 10–11 women were available for evaluation. After three cycles, biopsies were taken and 90–100% of the women in all groups had a secretory endometrial morphology; no hyper-plasia was found in any of the groups.

Suvanto-Luukkonen et al. (1998) conducted an open-label clinical trial in which post-menopausal women were randomized to continuous treatment with a skin gel that released 0.15 mg per day 17β-estradiol into the circulation plus either an intrauterine device that released 0.02 mg per day levonorgestrel for up to 5 years, 100 mg per day oral micronized progesterone on days 1–25 or 100–200 mg per day vaginal progesterone on days 1–25. After 12 months of treatment, endometrial thickness (assessed by ultrasound) was not significantly changed from baseline. No change in endometrial histology was observed in end-of-study biopsies in the group that received 17β-estradiol plus intrauterine levo-norgestrel but, in the groups that received 17β-estradiol plus oral or vaginal progesterone, morphology changed from predominantly atrophic at baseline (46/50 cases; 92%) to pre-dominantly proliferative (13/18 cases [72%] in the oral progesterone-treated group and 8/14 cases [57%] in the vaginal progesterone-treated group).

Byrjalsen *et al.* (1999) conducted a double-blind clinical trial in which 55–56 post-menopausal women per group were randomized to placebo or continuous oral treatment with 2 mg per day 17β-estradiol plus 0.025 or 0.05 mg per day gestodene sequentially (days 17–28), 1 mg per day 17β-estradiol plus 0.025 mg per day gestodene sequentially (days 17–28) or 1 mg per day 17β-estradiol plus 0.025 mg per day gestodene continuously. After 2 years of follow-up, end-of-study biopsies were obtained and examined histologically. Treatment with continuous estrogen plus gestodene did not change the high percentage of women with atrophic endometrium (83%) compared with placebo (81%) but, in women who received sequential treatments, the majority (54–79%) had a secretory type of endometrial histology. In the latter groups, endometrial thickness, the histo-chemical expression of secretory markers and staining for estrogen and progesterone receptors in the endometrium were increased. One endometrial carcinoma developed in the group who took 1 mg 17β-estradiol and 0.025 mg gestodene sequentially. No cases of endometrial hyperplasia occurred.

van de Weijer *et al.* (1999) randomized 151 women to continuous oral treatment with 1 mg 17β-estradiol plus 5 or 10 mg dydrogesterone on days 15–28. Biopsies at baseline and after 13 cycles revealed that 98% of these women had no endometrial lesions; only one woman in each group developed either proliferative changes or hyperplasia.

Wahab *et al.* (1999) conducted a double-blind clinical trial in which postmenopausal women were randomized to continuous oral treatment with 2 mg per day 17β-estradiol plus 0.05, 0.1, 0.25 or 0.5 mg per day trimegestone on days 15–28. After 6 months of follow-up, biopsies were taken and compared with those of untreated control women who were not randomized. Extensive morphometric analysis of the endometrium was carried out. In the endometrium of treated women compared with that of untreated women, there was evidence of somewhat smaller glands and a clearly significantly reduced area occu-pied by glands, but no change in the number of glands per unit area. Glands with evidence of secretion were less frequent in the high-dose group only. Discriminant analysis revealed a significant relation with dose for the all histomorphometric parameters combined.

Jondet *et al.* (2002) randomized postmenopausal women to treatment with a skin gel that releascd 1.5 mg per day 17β-estradiol on days 1–24 plus oral administration of either 10 mg per day chlormadinone acetate (42 women) or 200 mg per day progesterone (63 women) on days 10–24. Endometrial biopsies were taken at baseline and at the end of the study (18 months). There was a shift in atrophic morphology from 92% of women who were affected at baseline to 20–27% who were affected after 18 months of treatment; at the same point in time, 63–77% of women had a secretory endometrial morphology versus 3% at baseline.

Drospirenone (1, 2 or 3 mg) in combination with 1 mg 17β-estradiol is a continuous combined product used in hormonal therapy. Phase II/III trials of these combinations have demonstrated that, at all three doses of drospirenone, the combination is associated with a highly favourable safety profile, with excellent endometrial protection after 1 and 2 years (no cases of hyperplasia or cancer) (Rubig, 2003).

The combination of 2 mg estradiol valerate with 2 mg dienogest is the first continuous combined hormonal menopausal therapy preparation to contain a progestogen with substantial anti-androgenic activity. This combination was compared with a continuous combination of 2 mg estradiol plus 1 mg norethisterone acetate. In a large-scale study (1501 women) (Von Schoultz, 2003), biopsy and ultrasound assessment demonstrated that estradiol valerate plus dienogest quickly and effectively achieved endometrial atrophy in the vast majority of subjects, which indicates a protective effect on the endometrium.

Fugère *et al.* (2000) conducted a double-blind clinical trial in which postmenopausal women were randomized to continuous treatment with 0.625 mg per day conjugated equine estrogens plus 2.5 mg per day medroxyprogesterone acetate (69 women) or 150 mg per day raloxifene (67 women). Endometrial thickness, as assessed by ultrasound, increased slightly but significantly after 1 and 2 years of follow-up in the group given estrogen plus progestogen but no change was observed in the raloxifene-treated group. In the former group, more women developed benign proliferative endometrial changes (19–24%) when biopsies were taken 1 and 2 years after the start of treatment, whereas in the raloxifene-treated group only 6% of women developed such changes, which did not differ from baseline (4–6%).

Chang *et al.* (2003) conducted a double-blind clinical trial in which postmenopausal women were randomized to 0.625 mg per day conjugated equine estrogens on days 1–25 plus 5 (102 women) or 10 (66 women) mg per day medroxyprogesterone acetate or 20 mg per day dydrogesterone (73 women) sequentially on days 12–25. After 10–12 cycles, no statistically significant changes in endometrial thickness were observed by ultrasound assessment. End-of-study biopsies were taken and flow cytometric analysis was performed on endometrial tissue. No differences in cell-cycle distribution were observed among the three treatment groups, in all of which 61–81% of women had secretory or proliferative endometrial morphology. Endometrial hyperplasia was found in two cases in the group that took 0.625 mg equine estrogens plus 5 mg medroxyprogesterone acetate. No cases of endometrial carcinoma occurred.

Overall, these studies confirm that addition of progestogens to estrogen therapy for the menopause prevents the development of endometrial hyperplasia and reduces the increased rate of endometrial cell proliferation caused by estrogen only. This beneficial effect was found for all progestogens studied, regardless of the route of administration and dose. Norethisterone was the most frequently studied progestogen and, even at the lowest dose examined in randomized studies (in the range of 0.1 mg per day), there was a maximal protective effect for both estrogen-induced hyperplasia and cell proliferation. Treatment with some, but not all, progestogens given sequentially in combination with continuous estrogen treatment resulted in increased endometrial thickness, but this has not been studied in a sufficiently rigorous fashion to draw any conclusion. Most women treated with estrogen only and, to a lesser extent, women who took the combined therapy had a proliferative or secretory type endometrial histology, whereas most untreated postmenopausal women have atrophic or inactive endometrial morphology.

(iii)   *Other effects of hormonal therapy*

Conner *et al.* (2004b) (see above for study details) found statistically significant reductions in free and total serum testosterone and increases in sex hormone-binding globulin (SHBG) caused by the combination of 17β-estradiol and norethisterone, but no change in insulin-like growth factor (IGF)-I levels. However, the combination of 17β-estradiol and norethisterone (acetate) or dienogest did not alter total serum testosterone levels in another study (Conner *et al.*, 2003; see above for details), although it also increased SHBG but did not affect IGF-I. Dören *et al.* (2001) and Hofling *et al.* (2005) reported essentially the same findings in postmenopausal women treated with 17β-estradiol (2 mg per day) and norethisterone acetate (1 mg per day) for 6 or 12 months but found a decrease in the circulating levels of IGF-binding protein-1 and -3, no effects on dehydroepiandrosterone or its sulfate and only minor effects on androstenedione. However, Chatterton *et al.* (2005) found a reduction in the level of dehydroepiandrosterone sulfate in women who took Prempro® (conjugated estrogens plus medroxyprogesterone acetate).

Other studies have investigated the effects of treatment with progestogen plus estrogen on the IGF axis in more detail and have found that a variety of progestogens in combination with 17β-estradiol result in decreases in total and free IGF-I and IGF binding protein-3, increases in IGF-binding protein-1 and no effect on IGF-II (Heald *et al.*, 2000; Campagnoli *et al.*, 2002). The magnitude of these effects appears to depend on the type of progestogens used (Biglia *et al.*, 2003; Campagnoli *et al.*, 2003), but apparently not on the route of administration of the estrogen and progestogens (Raudaskoski *et al.*, 1998). However, in another study, significant differences were found between the effects of transdermal and oral treatment on IGF-I, SHBG and growth hormone-binding protein (Nugent *et al.*, 2003).

Another issue is the possibility that the various regimens used in hormonal therapy for the menopause may affect the metabolism of the hormonal agents used, as suggested by studies of estrogen metabolism (Seeger *et al.*, 2000; Mueck *et al.*, 2001, 2002) (see also Section 4.1).

These studies may suggest reduced androgenic stimulation, e.g. of the breast, and changes in the IGF axis. However, several of the progestogens used, such as norethisterone, have androgenic activity themselves and antigonadotropic effects reported for progestogens such as norethisterone may not be mediated by androgen receptor mechanisms (Couzinet *et al.*, 1996). Furthermore, there is a lack of consistency in many observations, such as the inconsistent effects reported on the IGF axis. Nevertheless, these studies raise the possibility of complex interactions of the agents used in hormonal therapy for the menopause with various hormonal systems.

(*b*)   *Experimental systems*

(i)   *Animal studies*

Three studies of the effects of hormonal therapy regimens in cynomolgus monkeys that had been surgically rendered postmenopausal are summarized in Section 3.1.2 (Cline *et al.*,

1996, 1998; 2002a,b). In these studies, continuous treatment with conjugated equine estrogens slightly increased the rate of cell proliferation in the mammary gland after 2–3 years of exposure, but this increase was not statistically significant. Addition of medroxyprogesterone acetate to the continuous treatment with estrogen increased the rate of cell proliferation in the lobuloalveolar mammary tissue by 50–100% over control values. Staining of mammary tissue for progesterone receptor, an indicator of estrogenic activity, was markedly increased by treatment with estrogen only and this effect was reduced by the addition of progestogen to the treatment. A preliminary study (Isaksson *et al.*, 2003) explored the effect of the same regimens on the immunohistochemical mammary expression of progesterone receptor-A and -B subtypes in cynomolgus monkeys. Treatment with progestogen alone did not significantly affect cell proliferation or expression of the progesterone receptor-A and -B. However, when ethinylestradiol plus norethisterone acetate was used as a regimen for only 1 year, cell proliferation was not increased (Suparto *et al.*, 2003). One study of short duration in mice injected with 17β-estradiol and progesterone also found increased mammary cell proliferation in the combined estrogen plus progestogen group compared with the control groups (Raafat *et al.*, 2001).

[These results are consistent with the observations in breast tissue of women who took conjugated equine estrogen plus medroxyprogesterone acetate as hormonal menopausal therapy but not those who took ethinylestradiol plus norethisterone.]

(ii)   *Cell culture and other studies*

Studies of the effects of estrogen–progestogen combinations on breast cell proliferation *in vitro* were carried out with 17β-estradiol and a variety of progestogens, doses and treatment regimens. Lippert *et al.* (2000, 2001, 2002), Mueck *et al.* (2003) and Seeger *et al.* (2003a,b) determined the in-vitro effects of a range of progestogens on the proliferation of MCF-7 breast cancer cells induced by 10 nM 17β-estradiol, either combined for 5–7 days or sequentially using estrogen only for 4–5 days followed by combined exposure for 3–5 days. Although the results of these studies are not completely identical, they generally showed that norethisterone, medroxyprogesterone acetate, progesterone, chlormadinone acetate, dienogest, 3-keto-desogestrel, gestodene and levonorgestrel counteracted the cell proliferation induced by 17β-estradiol in these estrogen receptor-positive cells. The effects were stronger when exposure to the estrogen and progestogens occurred simultaneously for 5–10 days than when the progestogens were added 4–5 days after the start of estrogen treatment for 3–5 days in some, but not in all studies (Lippert *et al.*, 2000, 2001). Although the consistency across these studies was not perfect, the continuous regimen with progesterone generally produced the strongest counteraction to the 17β-estradiol-induced stimulation of cell proliferation; medroxyprogesterone acetate gave an intermediate and norethisterone gave the weakest counteraction (Seeger *et al.*, 2003a). The inhibitory effect required concentrations of progestogens greater than 1 nM. The equine estrogens, equilin and 17α-dihydroequilin, induced cell proliferation to a lesser extent than 17β-estradiol and progestogens inhibited their activity to a lesser extent than that of 17β-estradiol (Mueck *et al.*,

2003). [These findings suggest a protective effect on breast cancer of combined exposure to estrogen–progestogen but this does not correlate with the epidemiological data.]

Franke and Vermes (2002, 2003) and Franke *et al.* (2003) observed similar effects, but the potencies of progestogens to inhibit 17β-estradiol-induced cell proliferation differed from those found previously (Lippert *et al.*, 2001; Mueck *et al.*, 2003; Seeger *et al.*, 2003a,b), which may be related to the fact that they measured an indicator of cell proliferation, cyclin D, and not proliferation *per se*. They also found that apoptosis (measured by flow cytometry) was induced by 17β-estradiol and enhanced by progestogens, but the actual data were not presented in their reports. However, they used single high doses of both hormones (1 μM) and one time-point — 6 days of continuous treatment. Treatment of T47D human breast cancer cells with 17β-estradiol and medroxyprogesterone acetate resulted in a variety of changes in gene expression patterns (Mrusek *et al.*, 2005). [Although the biological significance of these findings is not clear at present, the changes in gene expression patterns differed between treatments with estrogen only and those with estrogen plus progestogen.]

The endometrial effects of 17β-estradiol (10 nM) with or without medroxyprogesterone acetate (100 nM) were studied by Bläuer *et al.* (2005) in an organotypic culture system of primary human endometrial cells. 17β-Estradiol significantly doubled the percentage of cells that stained for Ki-67 over control values, whereas addition of the progestogen significantly reduced the percentage of Ki-67-positive cells to 50–70% of control values. The apparent effect of 17β-estradiol on cell proliferation required the presence of stromal cells and raised the possibility that the effect is indirect and stroma-mediated. These findings correlate with the supposition that the addition of progestogens to estrogen therapy confers a protective effect for the endometrium. Treatment of primary human endometrial cells with 17β-estradiol in the presence or absence of norethisterone acetate resulted in a variety of changes in gene expression patterns that differed depending on the presence of progestogen (Oehler *et al.*, 2002). [Although the biological significance of these findings is not clear at present, the differences in gene expression patterns between treatment with estrogen only and estrogen plus progestogen may, once confirmed and extended, provide a mechanistic basis for differences in the known biological effects of the two treatments.]

4.2.2   *Individual estrogens and progestogens*

(*a*)   *Humans*

No new data were available to the Working Group.

(*b*)   *Experimental systems*

(i)   *Estrogens*

Only one new study of estrogenic compounds that are used in hormonal therapy for the menopause (conjugated equine estrogens, ethinylestradiol or mestranol) that is relevant to the evaluation of the carcinogenic risk of such therapy via the oral or other routes has been carried out since the previous evaluation (IARC, 1999).

17β-Estradiol has been shown to increase the generation of reactive oxygen species through anchorage- and integrin-dependent signalling to mitochondria. The 17β-estradiol-induced reactive oxygen species increased the phosphorylation of c-Jun and cyclic adenosine monophosphate-response element-binding protein and increased the transcriptional activity of redox-sensitive transcription factors, activator protein 1 and the phosphorylated element-binding protein; these are involved in growth of estrogen-dependent cancer cells (Felty *et al.*, 2005a). Inhibitors of protein synthesis, transcription and replication and function of mitochondria, as well as antioxidants, effectively reduced the estrogen-induced growth of breast cancer cells by blocking the estrogen-induced G_1/S transition of G_0-arrested MCF-7 cells (Felty *et al.*, 2005b). These authors suggested that, in addition to the receptor activity of estrogens, other factors such as reactive oxygen species may be involved in the early growth of cancer cells (Felty *et al.*, 2005b).

(ii)   *Progestogens*

New studies of progestogens, including those most recently introduced, have been conducted that may be relevant to an evaluation of the carcinogenic risk of combined hormonal therapy via the oral or other routes, but no new studies were available on chlormadinone acetate, ethynodiol diacetate or norethynodrel.

Many studies described the influence of substituting active groups on the basic molecule of several progestogens — desogestrel, (3-keto-)desogestrel (etonogestrel), gestodene, levonorgestrel, norethisterone and drospirenone — on receptor binding, receptor transactivation and in-vivo hormonal activities (Deckers *et al.*, 2000; Schoonen *et al.*, 2000a; Garciá-Becerra *et al.*, 2004); these are summarized in Section 4.2.3(*b*) of the monograph on Combined estrogen–progestrogen contraceptives in this volume.

A few studies have examined the role of estrogen and progesterone receptor subtypes on the activities of progestogens and their divergent tissue-specific effects. Estrogen receptor α but not estrogen receptor β appears to be activated by the A-ring 5α-reduced metabolites of both norethisterone and gestodene which have weak estrogenic activity (Larrea *et al.*, 2001). However, Pasapera *et al.* (2002) found that the same metabolites of norethisterone activated both estrogen receptors α and β, and Rabe *et al.* (2000) obtained similar results for norethisterone but not for gestodene. These divergent findings may be related to the fact that the former study used HeLa and Chinese hamster ovary cells, whereas the latter studies used CV-1 monkey kidney cells and T-47D breast cancer cells or COS7 cells. Progesterone, norethisterone, levonorgestrel, desogestrol and gestodene are progestogens that are used in hormonal therapy and contraception. They bind with approximately equal affinity to the progesterone receptor subtypes A and B in MCF-7 cells, in Chinese hamster ovary cells stably transfected with these receptor subtypes and in in-vivo assays (Schoonen *et al.*, 1998). However, after supertransfection of these receptor subtypes in different Chinese hamster ovary cell subclones, differences among the progestogens tested were found in the stimulation of reporter genes for the two receptor subtypes in different clones (Dijkema *et al.*, 1998). These studies illustrate the critical roles of both meta-bolism and receptor-subtype specificity in the various hormonal effects of progestogens, while tissue or cell specificity appears to be another critical determinant of the activities of progestogens on receptor subtypes.

Progestogens may potentially affect not only factors that are related to tumour deve-lopment and tumour cell growth. Some new evidence suggests that they may also affect factors that are related to tumour progression, such as angiogenesis. However, this is an emerging field of research that does not allow any conclusions to be drawn at present. For example, medroxyprogesterone acetate, progesterone, norethisterone, norgestrel and nor-ethynodrel are mediated by the progesterone receptor B and have been shown to induce vascular endothelial growth factor in human breast cancer cells (Wu *et al.*, 2004). Dieno-gest, on the contrary, was shown to inhibit tumour cell-induced angiogenesis (Nakamura *et al.*, 1999) (See also Section 4.2.3(*b*) of the monograph on Combined estrogen–proges-togen contraceptives).

Dydrogesterone inhibits the activity of estrogen sulfatase and 17β-HSD in the human breast cancer cell lines MCF-7 and T-47D and inhibits the conversion of estrone to 17β-estradiol in these cells (Chetrite *et al.*, 2004).

Medroxyprogesterone acetate stimulated proliferation of the progesterone receptor-positive breast cancer cell line T-47D in a time-dependent manner with a biphasic dose–response (Thuneke *et al.*, 2000). Induction of cyclin D1 was found to parallel the stimu-lation of cell proliferation at the same (fairly high) dose of 250 nM. In addition, medroxy-progesterone acetate appears to inhibit the induction of apoptosis by serum depletion of several human breast cancer cell lines at a non-cytotoxic dose of 10 nM. However, this effect was only found in progesterone receptor-positive cell lines and not in the progeste-rone receptor-negative cell line MDA-MB-231, which suggests that this is a progesterone receptor-mediated effect (Ory *et al.*, 2001).

A study of norethisterone by Schoonen *et al.* (2000b) indicates that some of its various 3β- and 5α-reduced metabolites are much stronger estrogens or androgens *in vivo* than the parent compound. Their respective receptor-binding affinities and receptor-transactivation activities correlate with this observation. Rabe *et al.* (2000) found that norethisterone mo-derately transactivated estrogen receptor α in COS7 cells in a manner that was inversely related to dose. It transactivated estrogen receptor β somewhat more strongly; a concentra-tion of 0.1 nM was strongly estrogenic (85% that of ethinylestradiol, which is 100% estro-genic) but higher (1 nM) and lower (0.01 nM) concentrations were far less estrogenic.

Nomegestrol acetate is a strong progestogen that is relatively devoid of other hormonal activities. Its properties have been reviewed by Shields-Botella *et al.* (2003).

Nestorone and trimegestone are newly synthesised progestogens that are less progesto-genic than nomegestrol acetate but have activities that are in the same range as those of pro-gesterone itself and are also relatively devoid of other hormonal activities. The properties and activities of nestorone have been reviewed and described by Kumar *et al.* (2000), Tuba *et al.* (2000) and Sitruk-Ware *et al.* (2003), and those of trimegestone by Zhang *et al.* (2000), Lundeen *et al.* (2001) and Winneker *et al.* (2003).

Progesterone is a natural progestogen that is used in a highly bioavailable, micronized form in hormonal therapy in combination with estrogens (de Lignières, 1999). Differential metabolism occurs in normal and malignant human breast tissue and results in 4-pregnene and 5α-pregnane metabolites that have opposite effects on MCF-7 breast cancer cell proliferation *in vitro* (Wiebe *et al.*, 2000). The 5α-pregnane metabolites stimulate, whereas the 4-pregnene metabolites inhibit cell proliferation. Progesterone and 17β-estradiol affect IGF-I and IGF-binding protein -2 and -3 in a complex but non-synergistic manner, and not all of these effects can be blocked by the anti-estrogen tamoxifen or the anti-progestogen RU486 (mifepristone) (Milewicz *et al.*, 2005a). Similarly, progesterone has been shown to stimulate local production of growth hormone in human breast cancer explants, which cannot be counteracted by RU486 (Milewicz *et al.*, 2005b). Progesterone inhibits the 17β-estradiol-stimulated proliferation of MCF-7 cells more strongly than either medroxy-progesterone acetate or norethisterone (Seeger *et al.*, 2003a); this may have implications for the risk for breast cancer in women who are treated with either progesterone or a synthetic progestogen in combination with estrogen (Fournier *et al.*, 2005).

Medroxyprogesterone acetate or synthetic progestogen R5020 (as surrogate of progesterone) induced distinctly different changes in gene expression in progesterone receptor-negative Ishikawa endometrial cells that had been stably transfected with either progesterone receptor A or B (Smid-Koopman *et al.*, 2005). In both cases, however, the cells responded to medroxyprogesterone acetate or synthetic progestogen R5020 by growth inhibition and induction of apoptosis, which suggests that there is no difference between the two subtypes in the molecular pathways involved in these responses. In a rat endometrial cell line that expresses progesterone receptor, however, progestogen R5020 prevented apoptosis; this was counteracted by RU486 (Pecci *et al.*, 1997). [These results indicate that the progesterone receptor is required for these types of response of endometrial cells to progestogens, but suggest that the responses are highly cell type-specific.]

4.3   Side-effects other than genetic or cancer-related effects

Estrogen–progestogen therapy was designed to provide estrogen to women in order to relieve the vasomotor effects of the menopause and progestogen to modulate the adverse effects of estrogen on the uterus. The actual effects of the combination of these two types of hormone may differ from those of estrogen alone, depending on the target tissue considered. The addition of progestogen may ameliorate the adverse effects of estrogen at some sites, but counteract its possible beneficial effects at other sites. The complexity and interactions of estrogen–progestogen combinations should be borne in mind when considering these therapies.

4.3.1   *Cardiovascular effects*

It is generally believed that women are relatively protected from the development of coronary artery disease until the menopause: the incidence of cardiovascular disease in women lags behinds that in men by approximately 20 years (Colditz *et al.*, 1987; Grundy *et al.*, 1999). Ovarian hormones appear to be involved in the maintenance of these lower rates, since ovariectomized women who do not take hormonal therapy have an incidence of cardiovascular disease similar to that of men of the same age and, at any given age, postmenopausal women have a higher incidence of cardiovascular disease than women who menstruate normally (Wuest *et al.*, 1953; Gordon *et al.*, 1978).

A large body of evidence from observational studies has suggested that postmenopausal hormonal supplementation is associated with a 35–50% reduction in cardiovascular mortality and morbidity (Stampfer & Colditz, 1991). However, the majority of case–control and cohort studies on this subject have been conducted on women who used estrogen-only therapy. These hypothetical benefits have not been confirmed by several recent randomized trials of generally asymptomatic postmenopausal women (Hulley *et al.*, 1998; Herrington *et al.*, 2000; Manson *et al.*, 2003; Anderson *et al.*, 2004). Progestogens that are added to estrogens in combined hormonal therapy to reduce the risk for uterine malignancy have a number of potential adverse effects on the cardiovascular system, which may alter their efficacy in postmenopausal women. [Because combined hormonal therapy is so widely used, it is of pivotal importance to know whether or not it has an effect on cardiovascular disease.] Progestogens can have various effects on the vasomotor system, which are dependent on the agent and the dose regimen, and may also induce vasoconstriction of estrogenized vessels (Horwitz & Horwitz, 1982; Lin *et al.*, 1982).

It should be noted that hormonal therapy is designed to address symptoms that are related to reduced production of female hormones in the peri- and postmenopausal intervals. The menopause may involve changes other than cessation of estrogen and progestogen production, and the use of exogenous hormones may not mimic premenopausal physiology.

(a)   *Biological effects of estrogens on the cardiovascular system*

The putative protective effect of estrogens on the cardiovascular system has for a long time been associated with their beneficial effect on the metabolism and deposition of cholesterol, which contributes to the inhibition of the formation of atherosclerotic plaque in the arterial walls (Bush & Barrett-Connor, 1985; Bush *et al.*, 1987). Although early reports suggested that up to 50% of the protective effect of estrogens on coronary artery disease was attributable to favourable changes in plasma lipids, it is now believed that the changes in lipids induced by estrogens are probably not relevant (Rossouw, 2000; Rossouw *et al.*, 2002).

Estrogen deprivation has been associated with an increased risk for coronary artery disease and poorer vascular functions in women (Wuest *et al.*, 1953; Gordon *et al.*, 1978; Colditz *et al.*, 1987). Acute and chronic administration of estrogens to estrogen-deficient individuals restores the endothelium-dependent vasodilatation of coronary arteries that is lost after the menopause (Herrington *et al.*, 1994; Collins *et al.*, 1995; Volterrani *et al.*, 1995).

In the past decade, it has become clear that ovarian hormones have significant effects on arterial blood flow (Gilligan *et al.*, 1994a; Reis *et al.*, 1994; Collins *et al.*, 1995). The vascular effects of ovarian hormones may differ according to their chemical structure, and it is important not only to differentiate the effects of estrogens from those of progestogens but also to distinguish between the effects of different estrogens. Estrogens induce vaso-dilation while estrogen depletion leads to vasomotor instability, diminished vasodilatory activity and enhanced sensitivity to vasoconstrictor stimuli (Kronenberg *et al.*, 1984; Penotti *et al.*, 1993; Gilligan *et al.*, 1994a; Herrington *et al.*, 1994; Reis *et al.*, 1994; Collins *et al.*, 1995). Ovarian hormones act at all levels of the arterial structure — the endothelium, the vascular smooth muscle and the nerve endings in the adventitia in almost all the arterial systems; they act very rapidly and at both non-genomic and genomic levels (Kronenberg *et al.*, 1984; Jiang *et al.*, 1991, 1992a; Penotti *et al.*, 1993; Gilligan *et al.*, 1994a; Herrington *et al.*, 1994; Reis *et al.*, 1994; Collins *et al.*, 1995).

(i)   *Calcium-antagonistic action of estrogens*

Early in-vitro studies showed that 17β-estradiol has a relaxing effect on isolated rabbit and human coronary artery rings and cardiac myocytes contracted both by activation of receptor-operated and potential-operated calcium channels, due to a calcium-antagonistic effect (Jiang *et al.*, 1991, 1992a,b; Chester *et al.*, 1995). Subsequent in-vitro studies in animals and humans produced further evidence that estrogens have calcium-antagonistic properties, which account for a new non-endothelium-dependent mechanism of relaxation of coronary and peripheral arteries. The calcium-antagonistic property of estrogen was con-firmed in coronary vascular myocytes by measuring cytosolic concentration, contraction and calcium current. Sudhir *et al.* (1995) demonstrated that estrogens cause dilation of coronary conductance and resistance arteries in dogs when administered acutely into the coronary circulation. This in-vivo effect was shown to be endothelium-independent and partially mediated by effects on calcium channels. Calcium-antagonistic properties of estrogen have also been demonstrated in uterine arteries, cardiac myocytes and vascular smooth muscle cells (Stice *et al.*, 1987; Jiang *et al.*, 1991, 1992a; Sudhir *et al.*, 1995). Since it has been proposed that calcium channel blockers may reduce the progression of athero-sclerosis in animals, it has been suggested that estrogens may reduce the progression of coronary artery disease by a similar mechanism in humans (Collins *et al.*, 1993).

(ii)   *Endothelial action of estrogens*

Another important component of the effect of estrogens on the vascular system is mediated through the endothelium. In-vivo studies have demonstrated that estrogens poten-tiate the endothelium-dependent vasodilator response to acetylcholine in the coronary arteries of animals and humans (Gilligan *et al.*, 1994a; Reis *et al.*, 1994; Collins *et al.*, 1995). The effect of estrogens on the restoration of altered endothelial function was demonstrated *in vitro*, and in animals and humans *in vivo* in different vascular beds. Williams *et al.* (1990) reported that a reversal of acetylcholine-induced vasoconstriction was produced by subcutaneous implants of 17β-estradiol in ovariectomized monkeys fed an atherogenic diet for 30 months. Volterrani *et al.* (1995) showed that 17β-estradiol reduces peripheral vascular resistance and increases peripheral blood flow in menopausal women. Collins *et al.* (1995) showed that acute administration of 17β-estradiol reverses the coronary constrictor effect of acetylcholine in postmenopausal women with coronary artery disease and that the effect is gender-dependent. Reis *et al.* (1994) demonstrated an increase in coronary blood flow and epicardial cross-sectional area and decreased resistance in postmenopausal women 15 min after an intravenous infusion of ethinylestradiol. Abnormal coronary vasomotor responses to acetylcholine were also attenuated. Similar results were obtained by Gilligan *et al.* (1994a,b) in women who received continuous infusions of estrogens to achieve physiological concentrations of intracoronary 17β-estradiol. These studies indicated that estrogens influence vascular tone by enhancing the production of an endothelium-derived relaxant factor (nitric oxide). Estrogen receptors have been identified in endothelial cells from human aorta, and coronary and umbilical arteries (Kim-Schulze *et al.*, 1996; Venkov *et al.*, 1996). Caulin-Glaser *et al.* (1997) demonstrated that estradiol induced a rapid (within 30 min) increase in the production of nitric oxide in human umbilical vein endothelial cells grown in cell culture and that this action was inhibited when the estradiol receptor was blocked. Estrogen can induce calcium-dependent nitric oxide synthase activity, which results in an increased release of nitric oxide. Using inhibitors of nitric oxide synthase, Tagawa *et al.* (1997) demonstrated that estrogens considerably improve both nitric oxide-mediated and non nitric oxide-mediated vasodilation in the peripheral vasculature of the forearm in humans.

Since coronary artery tone plays a significant role in the pathogenesis of ischaemic cardiac syndromes, the effect of estrogens on the reactivity of coronary arteries may be important to the cardiovascular effects of these hormones. Rosano *et al.* (2006) showed that intracoronary administration of 17β-estradiol attenuates the vasoconstrictor effect of methylergometrine in women with coronary artery disease, which suggests that 17β-estradiol has a direct effect on the smooth muscle of coronary vessels in humans.

(iii) *Inflammatory effects of estrogens*

C-Reactive protein is a marker of inflammation that has been associated with the risk for coronary heart disease in menopausal women (Ridker *et al.*, 2000; Pradhan *et al.*, 2002). Estrogen administered with or without progestogen rapidly and substantially increases plasma concentrations of C-reactive protein in menopausal women (van Baal *et al.*, 1999; Cushman *et al.*, 1999; Ridker *et al.*, 1999). The effects of hormonal therapy on other markers of inflammation are not consistent with those on C-reactive protein, which suggests that they may be related to metabolic hepatic activation (Silvestri *et al.*, 2003). [The extent to which hormonal therapy affects cardiovascular risk through inflammation is unknown.]

(iv) *Route of administration*

To establish differences in alteration of some risk factors for cardiovascular disease (such as lipoproteins, fibrinogen) according to the route of administration of hormonal menopausal therapy, a study was carried out among women aged 50–65 years who received hormones orally, transdermally or by implantation. Initial therapy consisted of oral or transdermal estrogen alone for 3 months, followed by concomitant cyclical, continuous oral or transdermal administration of norethisterone, as appropriate, for a further 3 months. A separate group of women received an implant of estrogen only followed by an implant of estrogen and testosterone combined. All regimes lowered LDL cholesterol; the oral route was more potent than the parenteral route. Risk factors for cardiovascular disease were significantly reduced in women who used both oral and transdermal estrogen–progestogen therapy compared with untreated menopausal women (controls), although some of the benefit of estrogen alone on fibrinogen and HDL were attenuated (Seed *et al.*, 2002).

(b)   *Biological effects of progestogens on the cardiovascular system*

Progesterone receptors are present in the arterial wall, and the effects of progestogens on arteries are therefore probably mediated by these receptors as well as by down-regulation of the estradiol receptor. Progestogen therapy has various effects on arterial function; it can stabilize arteries that are in a state of vasomotor instability, but may also induce vasoconstriction of estrogenized vessels (Mercuro *et al.*, 1999). Because progestogens have estrogenic effects in some systems and also have progestational mineralo-corticoid and androgenic effects, there has been some concern that combined estrogen–progestogen therapy may modify some of the effects of estrogens on the cardiovascular system (Williams *et al.*, 1994; Adams *et al.*, 1997).

(i)   *Progestogens and lipid profile*

Estrogen-only therapy lowers total serum cholesterol and LDL cholesterol, increases HDL cholesterol and produces an effect upon plasma triglycerides, which is dependent upon the route of administration of the estrogens and the baseline plasma levels of lipids (Walsh *et al.*, 1991). It also stimulates the removal of cholesterol from the systemic circulation, which results in an increase in reverse cholesterol transport (Tikkanen *et al.*, 1982).

In contrast to estrogens, progestogens induce hepatic lipase activity, which increases the degradation of HDL-cholesterol. Accordingly, the addition of a progestogen to estrogens tends to attenuate the increase in serum HDL-cholesterol and the decrease in LDL-cholesterol that are obtained with estrogen only, an effect that may be related to the biochemical structure, dose, androgenic potency and regimen of the progestogen. Progestogens that have pure progestogenic activity do not alter lipid metabolism; 19-nortestosterone derivatives reduce HDL cholesterol, while 17α-hydroxyprogesterone derivatives and non-androgenic progestogens (19-norpregnane derivatives) seem to have little effect and progesterone has no detrimental effect on plasma lipids (Tikkanen *et al.*, 1986; Rijpkema *et al.*, 1990; Walsh *et al.*, 1991; The Writing Group for the PEPI Trial, 1995).

(ii)   *Progestogens and coronary atherosclerosis*

The vasodilatory and anti-atherogenic effects of estrogens on normal and diseased arteries are well known. Estrogens may influence the progression of coronary athero-sclerosis and, when administered either acutely or chronically, may reverse acetylcholine-induced vasoconstriction in both animals and humans. When administered in combination with estrogens, progestogens may interfere with these effects.

Adams *et al.* (1997) evaluated the effect of estrogen-only and estrogen–progestogen therapy in ovariectomized monkeys fed an atherogenic diet and found that estrogens alone or in association with progesterone or medroxyprogesterone acetate significantly reduced (by 50–70%) the degree of coronary atherosclerosis when therapy began soon after oophorectomy, but not when it began later (Williams *et al.*, 1994, 1995; Adams *et al.*, 1997; Clarkson *et al.*, 1998, 2001). Nevertheless, it should be noted that the effect of progestogens on the arteries of non-human primates may be mediated by different metabolic pathways than those present in human arteries. Therefore, the effects of proges-togens on atherosclerosis and vascular function cannot be extrapolated fully from animals to humans.

In a randomized, placebo-controlled trial, Herrington *et al.* (2000) compared the effect of hormonal supplementation with conjugated equine estrogens alone or in combi-nation with medroxyprogesterone acetate on the progression of coronary atherosclerosis in normocholesterolaemic postmenopausal women (aged $\geq$ 55 years) with proven coro-nary artery disease. After a mean follow-up of 3.2 years, no significant difference in mean coronary artery stenosis was found between women allocated to estrogen alone, estrogen plus progestogen or placebo.

The evaluation of intima-media thickening of arteries may help to identify initial stages of atherosclerosis. Several studies have shown that long-term estrogen therapy or combined hormonal therapy are effective in delaying the progression of early stages of atherosclerosis by reducing the intimal thickening in users of hormone compared with non-users (Espeland *et al.*, 1995a; Liang *et al.*, 1997; Hodis *et al.*, 2001).

At present, no role has been established for combined hormonal therapy in the preven-tion of the progression of atherosclerosis in postmenopausal women. From a preventive aspect, the inhibition of plaque formation and progression of small plaques is more impor-tant than a reduction in the size of pre-existing atherosclerotic plaques.

(iii)   *Progestogens and vascular reactivity*

Progestogens have vasoactive properties that are partly mediated by non-nuclear receptors. Since the expression of these receptors on the cell surface is influenced by levels of circulating estrogen, exposure to estrogens may affect the response of the vascular tree to progestogens.

Several studies have evaluated the effect of progesterone and other progestogens on coronary arteries *in vitro* and have demonstrated an endothelium-independent mechanism of relaxation that differs minimally between a variety of substances (Jiang *et al.*, 1992c). Miller and Vanhoutte (1991) assessed relaxation in coronary artery strips from ovariectomized dogs treated with estrogen, progesterone or estrogen plus progesterone. The relaxation response was similar in the coronary arteries of animals that received estrogen and in those that received progesterone, while it was minimally reduced in the group treated with the combined therapy. Therefore, it seems that there is little or no detrimental effect of progesterone on vasomotility, at least *in vitro* (Rosano *et al.*, 2003). However, pure progesterone is not commonly used in combined hormonal therapy.

Studies carried out *in vivo* suggested that synthetic progestogens may antagonize the dilator effect of estrogens in experimental animals. Two studies evaluated the separate and combined effects of conjugated equine estrogens and medroxyprogesterone acetate on the coronary reactivity of atherosclerotic monkeys. Exposure to estrogen increased coronary dilator responses and blood flow reserve, while co-administration of the progestogen resulted in a 50% reduction in dilation (Williams *et al.*, 1994; Adams *et al.*, 1997). Again, the effect of synthetic progestogens cannot be fully translated to women, due to the different metabolic pathways that operate in animals and humans.

Androgenic progestogens have been reported to reduce the beneficial effect of estrogens on vascular reactivity to a greater extent than progesterone and less androgenic progestogens; similar results were found in studies of carotid artery stiffness (Vitale *et al.*, 2001; Rosano et *al.*, 2001; Gambacciani *et al.*, 2002; Rosano *et al.*, 2003).

(c)   Biological effects of hormones on risk for thrombosis

Estrogens have many different effects on the coagulation system. These include increases in the levels of prothrombin fragments 1 + 2 and reductions in those of the anticoagulant factors, protein S and antithrombin, and may also occur after transdermal administration (Teede, *et al.*, 2000; Post *et al.*, 2003). These modifications predict a change towards a more pro-coagulant state (which was confirmed in studies that examined activated protein C resistance or thrombin generation) that is not counterbalanced by an increase in fibrinolytic activity (Teede *et al.*, 2000). It is currently unclear how these effects are induced at the molecular level of the estrogen receptor. At the cellular level, these effects are probably under genetic control, because the haemostatic system of some women appears to be more sensitive to the effect of estrogens than that of others. How estrogens and progestogens interact in their effect on thrombosis is also unclear. It appears that estrogens are pro-thrombotic rather than pro-atherogenic, which explains an increase in risk for thrombosis in former users (Bloemenkamp et *al.*, 1998; Koh *et al.*, 1999); again genetic factors may play an important role (Bloemenkamp *et al.*, 2002).

Selective modulators of the estrogen receptor, such as tamoxifen and raloxifene, have anti-estrogenic effects on breast and endometrial tissue and are used in the treatment and prevention of breast cancer. However, these drugs have estrogenic effects on blood clotting (Peverill, 2003).

(d)   *Effects of the use of estrogen and estrogen plus progestogen on the risk for cardiovascular disease*

(i)   *Coronary heart disease*

The effects of hormonal therapy on coronary heart disease have been evaluated in two randomized trials. The HERS and the WHI have provided critical data on the effect of hormonal therapy on primary and secondary prevention in postmenopausal women with or without coronary artery disease (Hulley *et al.*, 1998; Rossouw *et al.*, 2002). Neither study found a protective effect of fixed-dose hormonal therapy. For continuous combined hormones, the WHI reported a hazard ratio for coronary heart disease of 1.24 (95% CI, 1.00–1.54) over an average of 5.2 years of follow-up; most of the apparent risk occurred during the first year (hazard ratio, 1.81; 95% CI, 1.09–3.01). These effects did not differ by age (Manson *et al.*, 2003). In the HERS secondary prevention trial, the hazard ratio for coronary heart disease for the same combined hormonal therapy over an average of 4.1 years of follow-up was 0.99 (95% CI, 0.80–1.22) with some evidence of an increased risk in the first year (Hulley *et al.*, 1998). The WHI found no significant effects on the risk for coronary heart disease of estrogen alone over an average of 6.8 years of follow-up (hazard ratio, 0.91; 95% CI, 0.75–1.12). The data suggested the possibility that younger women experience a reduction in risk (*p* value for interaction, 0.14; hazard ratio, 0.56; 95% CI, 0.30–1.03) (Anderson *et al.*, 2004).

Few epidemiological studies have investigated the effect of combined hormones, but all have suggested that estrogen plus progestogen therapy may be more effective than estrogen therapy alone in the reduction of cardiovascular events. The majority of the observational studies suggested that the risk for coronary artery disease was reduced in women who received both estrogen only and estrogen–progestogen therapy (Stampfer & Colditz, 1991).

All of the observational studies were conducted in healthy women who used hormonal therapy for reasons other than the menopause and who were generally at low risk for coronary heart disease. The effect of the adjunct of a progestogen to estrogens in women who are at increased risk for cardiovascular disease may differ. The discrepancies with the randomized trials require that the observational studies be viewed cautiously. Biases inherent in cohort and case–control studies and variability of dosing, duration and other time-dependent effects of hormonal therapy must be taken into account in order to present a balanced view of the results. Careful control for confounding and an allowance for an adverse effect during the first 2 years of exposure, with attenuation of this effect in subsequent years, has been shown to align the results from observational studies with those of randomized trials (Prentice *et al.*, 2005). Petitti (1994) argued that compliance bias could account for some of the observed benefits. It has been suggested that the women who were included in the hormonal therapy groups were of higher socioeconomic class, had healthier habits and exercised regularly. Barrett-Connor (1991) demonstrated that a healthy women bias exists at least for the women who were included in the Rancho Bernardo (CA, USA) study population (Barrett-Connor *et al.*, 1989). Not all study populations were restricted to upper class retirement areas, however, and no socioeconomic differences were noted in the Nurses' Health Study (Grodstein *et al.*, 2000) or other studies. Selection bias probably exists in nearly all studies, since women who take hormonal therapy tend to exercise more and have healthier habits. Therefore, estimates of risk reduction in women who take ovarian hormones may be biased towards finding a protective effect that may be due in part to a healthier lifestyle (Nelson *et al.*, 2002a).

(ii)   *Stroke*

The WHI trial reported an increase in risk for stroke from estrogen plus progestogen therapy (hazard ratio, 1.31; 95% CI, 1.02–1.68) that was restricted to ischaemic stroke (hazard ratio, 1.44; 95% CI, 1.09–1.90) (Wassertheil-Smoller *et al.*, 2003). The WHI trial of estrogen alone was interrupted because of the observed increase in risk for stroke (hazard ratio, 1.39; 95% CI, 1.10–1.77) (Anderson *et al.*, 2004). The HERS trial reported a hazard ratio for estrogen plus progestogen of 1.18 (95% CI, 0.83–1.66) for non-fatal stroke and 1.61 (95% CI, 0.73–3.55) for fatal stroke during an average follow-up of 4.1 years (Simon *et al.*, 2001a). The Women's Estrogen for Stroke Trial conducted on 664 postmenopausal women who had had a recent ischaemic stroke or a transient ischaemic attack found no beneficial effect of 17β-estradiol (1 mg per day) for stroke (hazard ratio, 1.1; 95% CI, 0.8–1.6) or mortality (hazard ratio, 1.2; 95% CI, 0.8–1.8) after a mean follow-up of 2.8 years (Viscoli *et al.*, 2001). A meta-analysis of randomized trials found a significant increase in risk for stroke (relative risk, 1.44; 95% CI, 1.10–1.89) with no substantial variation between studies (Gabriel-Sanchéz *et al.*, 2005).

A meta-analysis of nine observational studies suggested that hormonal therapy is associated with a small increase in risk for stroke (relative risk, 1.12; 95% CI, 1.01–1.23) that is primarily confined to thromboembolic stroke (relative risk, 1.20; 95% CI, 1.01–1.40) (Nelson *et al.*, 2002b).

(iii)   *Thrombosis*

The risk for venous thrombotic disease was increased twofold (hazard ratio, 2.06; 95% CI, 1.57–2.70) for estrogen plus progestogen in the WHI trial (Cushman *et al.*, 2004) and almost threefold in the HERS trial (hazard ratio, 2.89; 95% CI, 1.50–5.58) (Hulley *et al.*, 1998). Pulmonary embolism and deep vein thrombosis were similarly affected. The WHI trial reported a smaller increase with estrogen alone (hazard ratio, 1.33; 95% CI, 0.99–1.79) (Anderson *et al.*, 2004).

(e)   *Estrogen–progestogen therapy in postmenopausal women*

The divergent results of observational and randomized studies on cardiovascular endpoints have led many authors to stress the superiority of randomized clinical trials over observational studies, but have not solved the dilemma of the effect of hormonal therapy on the cardiovascular system. The discrepancies in the results of observational and randomized studies are related to methodological issues and to differences between study populations, hormonal regimens and time- and age-dependent biological effects of hormones during different periods of the lives of women. Observational studies typically did not distinguish between the hormonal regimens used, whereas the randomized studies examined a fixed dose of continuous combined conjugated equine estrogens plus medroxyprogesterone acetate. Although the treatment regimens in the two types of study differed, the dose of estrogen and progestogen used probably played an important role. More recent progestogens that have fewer androgenic and mineralo-corticoid effects may influence the risks for cardiovascular disease differently. Several varied opinions on the potential cardiovascular effects — beneficial and adverse — of hormonal therapy for postmenopausal women are still emerging, and the selection of patients, dose regimen and timing of treatment are probably critical (Rosano *et al.*, 2004).

It is possible that factors other than methodological differences may explain the divergent effects of hormonal therapy noted in observational and randomized studies. The randomized clinical studies were conducted exceptionally well and methodological design is not an issue. A key difference between the observational and randomized studies is the women under study: in the observational studies, the exposed women chose to take hormonal therapy for menopausal symptoms and represented long-term compliers while, in the randomized studies, the absence of severe menopausal symptoms was a prerequisite for inclusion in the study. This seemingly small difference may have important implications, since symptomatic women are younger and have clinical symptoms that suggest an effect of a lack of estrogen on several organs or systems. The low prevalence of symptoms may indicate a physiological adaptation to lower levels of ovarian hormone in these women, due to a slow decline in estrogen levels or the long time lapse since menopause, and therefore a new homeostasis. These and other biological explanations for the divergent results of observational and randomized studies should be considered in detail (Rosano *et al.*, 2004).

(i)   *Ageing and cardiovascular response to estrogen–progestogen therapy*

Several studies that evaluated the effect of hormonal therapy on intermediate markers of coronary heart disease in women and in non-human primates indicated substantial benefits, although they also suggested some adverse effects (Scarabin *et al.*, 1999; Walsh *et al.*, 2000; Silvestri *et al.*, 2003). Clinical and experimental evidence suggests that the putative cardio-protective and anti-atherogenic effects of ovarian hormones are receptor-mediated and endothelium-dependent (Caulin-Glaser *et al.*, 1997; Mikkola *et al.*, 1998). Both estrogen receptors and endothelial function are markedly influenced by the time at which estrogen deprivation and progression of the atherosclerotic injury occur. Evidence indicates that expression of the estrogen receptor in the arterial wall is sharply diminished with increasing age, which might be related to an age-related increase in methylation of the promoter region of the estrogen receptor gene in vascular areas with atherosclerosis (Post *et al.*, 1999).

Time since menopause and the presence of atherosclerosis are associated with a reduced cardio-protective effect of estrogens, while the unfavourable effects of hormones on coagulation remain unaltered. Therefore, in early postmenopausal women such as those included in observational studies, hormonal therapy may be cardio-protective because of the responsiveness of the endothelium to estrogens while, in late postmenopausal women, hormonal therapy has either no effect or even a detrimental effect because of the pre-dominance of the pro-coagulant or plaque-destabilizing effects over the vasculo-protective effects. It is possible that hormonal therapy inhibits atherosclerosis in younger women but may not be able to inhibit progression of atherosclerosis and complicated plaques that lead to coronary events in older women. This hypothesis has also been suggested by randomized studies of postmenopausal cynomolgus monkeys in which estrogens had no effect on the extent of coronary artery plaque in those assigned to estrogen alone or to estrogen com-bined with medroxyprogesterone acetate beginning 2 years (approximately 6 human years) after oophorectomy (Williams *et al.*, 1995). When given to younger monkeys soon after oophorectomy, hormonal treatment resulted in a 50% reduction in the extent of plaques (Clarkson *et al.*, 2001; Mikkola & Clarkson, 2002).

The effect of atherosclerosis and ageing on the vascular responsiveness to hormonal menopausal therapy has been also analysed in several clinical studies (Herrington *et al.*, 2001). In the Cardiovascular Health Study, women (over 65 years of age) who had esta-blished cardiovascular disease had a flow-mediated vasodilator response that was equal among women who used hormones (estrogen alone or estrogen combined with pro-gestogen) and those who did not; among women (over 65 years of age) who had no cardio-vascular disease, users of hormones had a 40% better response than non-users (Herrington *et al.*, 2001). In the Estrogen Replacement and Atherosclerosis Trial, a randomized trial that involved women (aged ≥ 55 years) who had documented coronary disease, no effect of estrogen alone or of estrogen combined with progestogen was found on the diameter of coronary arteries (Herrington *et al.*, 2000). In contrast, in the Estrogen in the Prevention of Atherosclerosis Trial, in which younger women (aged ≥ 45 years) who had no cardio-vascular disease were randomly assigned to 17β-estradiol or placebo, the average rate of progression of carotid atherosclerosis was lower in women assigned to estrogen (Hodis *et al.*, 2001).

(ii)   *Characteristics of the study populations*

Women recruited in the randomized studies comprised a broader age range and were representative of individuals for whom prevention interventions would be contemplated. Observational studies recruited women who were exposed to hormonal therapy primarily for short-term relief of menopausal symptoms and longer-term use for the prevention or treatment of osteoporosis. Recently, a new class of progestational agents with anti-aldo-steronic properties has been developed: the prototype of this class is drospirenone, a proges-tational agent that can reduce water retention, body weight and blood pressure (Keam & Wagstaff, 2003). The addition of this newer progestogen to estrogens in hormonal therapy schemes may help to minimize the side-effects of estrogen therapy that are related to water and salt retention and may represent a new strategy for the treatment of postmenopausal women (Pollow *et al.*, 1992; Krattenmacher, 2000).

In a randomized trial of 230 hypertensive postmenopausal women, treatment with dros-pirenone plus 17β-estradiol was not associated with a higher incidence of hyperkalaemia than treatment with placebo in patients with and without type-2 diabetes mellitus and concomitant use of angiotensin-converting enzyme inhibitors, angiotensin receptor anta-gonists or ibuprofen. Drospirenone plus 17β-estradiol was found to reduce both systolic and diastolic blood pressure compared with the placebo group (Preston *et al.*, 2005).

Body mass index is an important marker of endogenous estrogen in postmenopausal women and has been associated with risk for cardiovascular disease especially when it is ≥ 25 kg/m^2 (Wilson *et al.*, 2002). In a very large cohort of 290 827 postmenopausal women, the coronary benefits of hormonal therapy were found exclusively in women with a lower body mass index (< 22 kg/m^2) (Rodriguez *et al.*, 2001). In the WHI, there was no significant interaction with body mass index, which mean was 28.5 (standard deviation [SD], 5.9) (Manson *et al.*, 2003).

Randomized studies of hormones in younger women who seek treatment for meno-pausal symptoms are not informative with regard to hormonal effects on rates of cardio-vascular disease, because of the very low incidence rates in this population.

4.3.2   *Other effects*

(*a*)   *Established benefits*

(i)   *Control of vasomotor symptoms*

The primary indication for use of hormonal therapy during the menopause is vaso-motor symptoms. Numerous studies have documented the beneficial effects of estrogen, either alone or combined with progestogen, for the relief of hot flushes/flashes and night sweats. MacLennan *et al.* (2004b) recently reviewed the randomized, double-blind placebo controlled trials of hormonal therapy and reported a summary measure of the reduction in the frequency of hot flushes of 75% (95% CI, 64.3–82.3%) relative to placebo, accom-panied by similarly important reductions in the severity of symptoms.

(ii)   *Prevention of osteoporosis and fractures*

Hormonal therapy has also been shown to be effective for the prevention or treatment of osteoporosis and bone fractures. In the WHI trial, the risk for hip fractures was reduced by both estrogen alone (hazard ratio, 0.61; 95% CI, 0.41–0.91) and by estrogen plus proges-togen (hazard ratio, 0.67; 95% CI, 0.47–0.96) (Cauley *et al.*, 2003; Anderson *et al.*, 2004). Beneficial effects on bone mineral density have been shown for other hormonal preparations (Recker *et al.*, 1999; Lees & Stevenson, 2001; Arrenbrecht & Boermans, 2002; Civitelli *et al.*, 2002).

(*b*)   *Overview of evidence for other effects*

The efficacy of hormonal therapy for the above indications has typically been esta-blished in randomized trials of up to a few hundred women and a follow-up of a few months for vasomotor symptoms and 3 years for osteoporosis. These trials lack sufficient power to establish rates of disease or rarer side-effects with adequate precision. Further, because of the strong evidence for beneficial effects on vasomotor symptoms, such trials often lack a placebo group, which obscures any inference of hormonal effects on other outcomes. Two large randomized trials, the WHI (Rossouw et al., 2002) and the HERS (Grady et al., 1998) are the primary exceptions. Both of these were randomized, double-blinded, placebo-controlled trials of hormonal therapies that tested chronic disease prevention strategies in the USA. The WHI trial involved separate placebo-controlled comparisons of estrogen plus progestogen (conjugated equine estrogens plus medroxyprogesterone acetate) in 16 608 postmenopausal women aged 50–79 years with an uterus and estrogen alone in 10 739 postmenopausal women in the same age range with prior hysterectomy (Stefanick et al., 2003). The HERS trial tested the same combined hormonal regimen in 2764 postmenopausal women under 80 years of age who had a uterus and documented coronary artery disease. Additional details for both trials are provided in Section 2. Because of the strength of the evidence derived from these two studies, most of the information summarized here on other effects of hormonal therapy relies on data from these trials. For many outcomes, important additional information derives from the Postmenopausal Estrogen/Progestin Interventions (PEPI) study, another randomized, double-blinded, placebo-controlled trial conducted in the USA to evaluate the effects of three combined hormonal regimens and one estrogen-alone therapy on biomarkers of cardiovascular disease in 840 postmenopausal women aged 45–65 years (Espeland et al., 1995b). Data from other randomized trials are described only when they contradict these findings or introduce different inferences. There is also an immense body of data from observational studies that include many features of health that cannot be summarized adequately here. Mention is made of these data only when significant controversy exists between the findings from trials and observational studies.

      (i)   *Quality of life and symptoms associated with menopause or ageing*

Quality of life

Improvement in other symptoms that are commonly associated with ageing or menopause have been reported, occasionally in conjunction with overall quality of life. The reported benefits vary across studies; the differences are probably attributable to the populations studied and the dimensions of symptoms and quality of life used. No clinically significant effects on measures of general quality of life were observed with estrogen plus progestogen therapy in the WHI trial (Hays et al., 2003a) despite significant improvements in vasomotor symptoms and vaginal or genital dryness (Barnabei et al., 2005). In the HERS trial, estrogen plus progestogen decreased hot flushes, vaginal dryness and sleep troubles (Barnebei et al., 2002) and improved depression scores, but was associated with worsening of some health measures (i.e. more rapid decline in physical function scores and in energy/fatigue) (Hlatky et al., 2002). Trials designed specifically to test the effect of hormonal therapy on vasomotor symptoms as their primary objective generally reported an improvement in quality of life, derived primarily from the relief of hot flushes, night sweats and related conditions (e.g. Wiklund et al., 1993).

Vaginal bleeding

Common side-effects of hormonal therapy are vaginal bleeding, breast tenderness, urinary incontinence and headaches. Among women with a uterus, bleeding rates vary by type of hormonal therapy, schedule of progestogen, age and time since initiation of therapy. The prevalence of bleeding with both sequential and continuous formulations has led to numerous attempts to identify hormonal therapy regimens that provide good relief of vasomotor symptoms while minimizing bleeding (e.g. Saure et al., 1996; Al-Azzawi et al., 1999; Cano et al., 1999; Saure et al., 2000; Mendoza et al., 2002). Intermittent and continuous treatment with progestogen has been used to reduce bleeding, especially in older women. In the WHI estrogen plus progestogen trial, 51% of women randomized to continuous combined therapy but less than 5% of women who took placebo reported vaginal bleeding within the first 6 months. The proportion who reported bleeding in the active hormonal therapy group declined thereafter but remained above 11% throughout the study (Barnabei et al., 2005). These estimates do not take into account the non-compliance to the therapy (approximately 42% by year 5) (Rossouw et al., 2002), some of which was a result of bleeding. Most of the bleeding in the active hormonal therapy group was classified as spotting (Barnabei et al., 2005). Bleeding, especially after the first few months of use, causes concern and may lead to significantly increased rates of endometrial biopsy (Anderson et al., 2003). Intermittent treatment provides only a marginal improvement in bleeding rates (Cano et al., 1999), but some studies have found reduced bleeding with higher doses of progestogen (Al-Azzawi et al., 1999). Many smaller randomized trials lacked either a placebo control or a common active treatment control group against which to judge the relative effects. Nevertheless, few significant differences in symptom control or vaginal bleeding were reported.

Breast symptoms

The frequency of breast symptoms, variously reported as breast tenderness, discomfort, pain or mastalgia, is also significantly increased by hormonal therapy. In the WHI trial, 9.3% of asymptomatic women randomized to combined hormones reported breast tenderness at year 1 compared with 2.4% who took placebo, and this proportion remained elevated at year 3 (odds ratio, 2.55; 95% CI, 0.98–6.64) (Barnabei et al., 2005). In the PEPI trial, the risk for greater breast discomfort was doubled by all three combined hormonal regimens relative to placebo (range of odds ratios, 1.92–2.33). Corresponding risks for estrogen alone were not increased over those for placebo (odds ratio, 1.16; 95% CI, 0.70–1.93) (Greendale et al., 1998), which suggests that these breast symptoms may be an effect of protestogen.

Mammographic screening

Use of exogenous hormones interferes with mammographic screening. In the WHI trial, Chlebowski *et al.* (2003) reported that 9.4% of women assigned to combined hormones had an abnormal mammogram during the first year of use compared with 5.4% of placebo-treated women ($p < 0.001$), a period during which there was no excess incidence of breast cancer. This pattern of increased incidence of mammographic abnormalities persisted throughout the follow-up. In a study ancillary to the PEPI trial, Greendale *et al.* (2003) reported increased breast density with all three combined hormonal regimens (change from baseline in adjusted mean mammographic per cent density ranged from 3.1 to 4.8%), which was significantly different from the rate of change in the placebo group (–0.07%; 95% CI, –1.50–1.38%). Use of estrogen alone resulted in a non-significant 1.17% (95% CI, –0.28–2.62%) adjusted mean change, which again suggests that progestogen is the active agent in these breast changes. However, in a randomized, double-blinded, placebo-controlled multi-arm trial of raloxifene and estrogen, the mean breast density in women who took estrogen was significantly greater than that in the other arms (Freedman *et al.*, 2001).

Urinary incontinence

Urinary incontinence is adversely affected by hormonal therapy. Asymptomatic women randomized to estrogen alone in the WHI Trial experienced an increased risk for self-reported urinary incontinence at 1 year, including all subtypes: stress (hazard ratio, 2.15; 95% CI, 1.77–2.62), urge (hazard ratio, 1.32; 95% CI, 1.10–1.58) and mixed urinary incontinence (hazard ratio, 1.79; 95% CI, 1.26–2.53). The addition of medroxyprogesterone acetate did not alter these effects substantially. Among women who reported urinary incontinence at baseline, the risk for worsening the self-reported frequency of incontinence, amount of leakage, limitation in activities and bother associated with the symptoms was significantly elevated by both hormonal regimens at 1 year (Hendrix *et al.*, 2005). In a 3-year randomized, double-blind, placebo-controlled osteoporosis prevention trial (Goldstein *et al.*, 2005), 7% of 158 women randomized to conjugated equine estrogens reported new or worsening urinary incontinence compared with 1.3% of the 152 women randomized to placebo ($p \leq 0.02$). In the HERS trial, Grady *et al.* (2001) found that 39% of women who took estrogen plus progestogen reported worsening symptoms compared with 27% of women who took placebo ($p = 0.001$). Several smaller, short-term, randomized, double-blind, placebo-controlled trials of hormonal therapy have been carried out in incontinent women (Wilson *et al.*, 1987; Fantl *et al.*, 1996; Jackson *et al.*, 1999); some of these used objective measurements of response, but none identified any significant therapeutic response.

Headaches

Frequency and duration of headaches may be affected by hormonal therapy. In the WHI trial, the incidence of headaches or migraines in the placebo-treated group was 4.7% and was modestly increased by estrogen plus progestogen at 1 year to 5.8% (odds ratio,

1.26; 95% CI, 1.08–1.46) (Barnabei *et al.*, 2005). Vestergaard *et al.* (2003) did not find an effect on the occurrence of headache after 5 years in the Danish Osteoporosis Prevention Study. In women who are known to suffer from migraine headaches, however, there is evidence of an increase in the frequency of attacks, the number of days with headache and analgesic consumption over 6 months of observation during continuous combined, continuous sequential or cyclical sequential hormonal therapy (Facchinetti *et al.*, 2002).

(ii)   *Incidence of disease*

In addition to the more common symptoms associated with hormonal therapy, there is increasing evidence of hormonal effects on other clinical outcomes.

Gallbladder disease

Randomized trials have shown a significant increase in the rates of gallbladder disease and biliary tract surgical procedures following hormonal therapy. In the WHI trial, Cirillo *et al.* (2005) reported a hazard ratio for estrogen alone of 1.67 (95% CI, 1.35–2.06) for the incidence of hospitalized gallbladder disease or related surgical procedures over an average of 7.1 years of follow-up and a hazard ratio for estrogen plus progestogen of 1.59 (95% CI, 1.28–1.97) over a mean 5.6 years of follow-up (attributable risk of 31 and 20 cases per 10 000 person–years, respectively). The HERS results on estrogen plus progestogen for the same combined outcome over the initial mean 4.1 years of follow-up were similar (hazard ratio, 1.38; 95% CI, 1.00–1.92) (Simon *et al.*, 2001b) and became significant (hazard ratio, 1.48; 95% CI, 1.12–1.95) during the 6.8-year average open-label extended follow-up period (Hulley *et al.*, 2002). [The Working Group noted that these results suggest that the effect is primarily a function of estrogen alone and may be dependent on duration.] Several observational studies have also found evidence of an adverse effect of hormonal therapy on gallbladder disease (e.g. Mamdani *et al.*, 2000; Boland *et al.*, 2002).

Dementia and cognitive function

Despite preliminary evidence of improved cognitive function following hormonal therapy, randomized trials have not provided evidence of a benefit. On the contrary, data from these trials suggest an increased risk for dementia and a negative impact on cognitive function in women randomized to hormones. The strongest evidence derives from the WHI Memory Study, which is an ancillary study of women over 65 years of age at randomization into one of the WHI hormone trials. In this subset of older participants, the combined hormonal therapy group experienced a significantly increased risk for probable dementia relative to the placebo-treated group (hazard ratio, 2.05; 95% CI, 1.21–3.48) over an average of 4 years of follow-up (Shumaker *et al.*, 2003). A somewhat smaller increase was observed with estrogen alone relative to placebo (hazard ratio, 1.49; 95% CI, 0.83–2.66) over an average of 5 years (Shumaker *et al.*, 2004). The increases in the incidence of probable dementia were not explained by those observed in the incidence of stroke. Rapp *et al.* (2003) and Espeland *et al.* (2004) found an adverse effect of hormonal therapy on global cognitive function for both combined hormones and estrogen alone.

Grady *et al.* (2002b) reported no significant differences between the effects of estrogen plus progestogen and placebo among women at 10 HERS centres from six end-of-study measurements of cognitive function (mean age at time of testing, 71 ± 6 years). One measurement, verbal fluency, was significantly worse ($p = 0.02$) in women who were randomized to estrogen plus progestogen. In the PEPI trial, in which the average age of participants was 56 years (SD, 4.3 years; somewhat younger than those in the WHI or HERS), no significant differences were found between the placebo-treated group and the four hormonal therapy groups at 12 or 36 months for self-reported forgetfulness, concentration or distraction (Reboussin *et al.*, 1998). No randomized trial has been conducted to examine the risk for dementia in younger women. Several very small, short-term randomized trials of hormonal therapy in women with dementia have been conducted (Henderson *et al.*, 2000; Mulnard *et al.*, 2000; Asthana *et al.*, 2001), each of which reported some modest improvements in a subset of the cognitive measurements examined but no consistent pattern of effects.

In contrast, observational studies have mostly reported substantially lower rates of dementia associated with hormonal therapy but with variable relationships between duration and recency of use. In a Cache County Study report, women who had ever used hormonal therapy had a reduced risk for Alzheimer disease compared with non-users (odds ratio, 0.59; 95% CI, 0.35–0.96); the reduction was concentrated in former users or those who had more than 10 years of exposure. The risk for Alzheimer disease in current users of hormonal therapy was not affected (odds ratio, 1.08; 95% CI, 0.59–1.91). According to the authors, this pattern of effects suggests a limited window of time in which a beneficial effect of hormonal therapy on the risk for Alzheimer disease exists (Zandi *et al.*, 2002). Baldereschi *et al.* (1998) reported a reduced risk for Alzheimer disease with ever use of estrogen (odds ratio, 0.28; 95% CI, 0.08–0.98) in the Italian Longitudinal Study on Aging, which was an analysis of data from 1582 postmenopausal women in eight Italian cities. A similar reduction in risk for Alzheimer disease was reported in the Baltimore Longitudinal Study of Aging cohort of 472 peri- or postmenopausal women (mean age at enrollment, 61.5 years). After 16 years of follow-up, the hazard ratio for Alzheimer disease for ever use of oral or transdermal estrogen was 0.46 (95% CI, 0.21–1.00), but no effect of duration was observed (Kawas *et al.*, 1997). Paganini-Hill and Henderson (1994) reported a reduced risk for dementia in users of estrogen (odds ratio, 0.69; 95% CI, 0.46–1.03) and evidence of a stronger effect with higher dose and longer duration of use in a nested case–control study within the Leisure World cohort of southern California.

[Whether hormonal therapy used early in the menopausal period has a beneficial effect on dementia rates or whether these observed reductions arise from subtle patterns of prescription, adherence, survival or other biases remains unanswered.]

Diabetes

The risk for non-insulin-dependent diabetes has been found to be reduced by use of estrogen plus progestogen. In the WHI trial, rates of self-reported diabetes were reduced by 21% (95% CI, 7–33%) (Margolis *et al.*, 2004), and the observed reduction in the HERS trial was 35% (95% CI, 11–52%) (Kanaya *et al.*, 2003), each of which was accompanied by corresponding changes in fasting glucose and insulin levels.

Other diseases or conditions

The potential impact of hormonal therapy on other age-related health conditions (e.g. osteoarthritis, rheumatoid arthritis, lupus, macular degeneration, cataract, Parkinson disease) has been examined in observational studies and in some randomized trials. The evidence for substantial effects on these disease processes is limited at this time, but additional studies would provide much needed clarification (Cooper *et al.*, 2002; d'Elia *et al.*, 2003; Abramov *et al.*, 2004; Currie *et al.*, 2004; Freeman *et al.*, 2004).

Mortality

Randomized trials have not shown a statistically significant effect on mortality during average intervention periods that ranged from 5.2 to 6.8 years (Hulley *et al.*, 2002; Roussouw *et al.*, 2002; Anderson *et al.*, 2004). Additional follow-up of the WHI cohorts will be of particular interest. A recent meta-analysis of 30 trials also found no effect of hormonal therapy on mortality (odds ratio, 0.98; 95% CI, 0.87–1.18). Further analyses suggested a possible reduction in mortality due to factors other than cancer or cardiovascular disease (Salpeter *et al.*, 2004).

4.4   Genetic and related effects

Estrogen may contribute to the promotion of uterine, breast, ovarian and cervix tumours. It is thought to sustain the growth of preneoplastic and malignant cells by acting through estrogen receptor-mediated signalling pathways that regulate the production of growth factors that maintain clonal growth of both cell types. Epidemiological observations and mathematical models derived therefrom have suggested that most malignant cells accumulate several genetic changes in the genes or chromosomes as they evolve into cancer. Since the previous evaluation (IARC, 1999), many studies in experimental systems on the possible direct genetic and genotoxic effects of steroid sex hormones as a factor in carcinogenesis have been published, and these are summarized in Tables 19 and 20. The data that are now available indicate more strongly that some of these hormones and their metabolites can cause DNA damage, which can potentially induce genetic alterations in cells.

As described in detail in Section 4.1 of this monograph, estrogens, i.e. estrone, 17β-estradiol, estriol and 17α-ethinylestradiol, are activated by aromatic hydroxylation at the C-2 and C-4 positions that is catalysed by CYPs. Subsequently, peroxidase enzymes convert them into catechol estrogens, i.e. 2-hydroxyestrogens and 4-hydroxyestrogens (Roy & Liehr, 1999; Cavalieri *et al.*, 2000; Roy & Singh, 2004). Catalytic oxidation of these two catechol estrogens gives rise to the corresponding estrogen-2,3-quinone and estrogen-3,4-quinone, which react with DNA to form adducts (Roy & Liehr, 1999;

Table 19. Genetic and related effects of estrogens in experimental systems

Test system	Results[a] Without exogenous metabolic system	Results[a] With exogenous metabolic system	Dose (LED or HID)[b]	Reference
Estradiol				
Gene mutation, Chinese hamster V79 cells, *Hprt* locus, *in vitro*	+	NT	0.01 nM [0.0027 ng/mL]	Kong et al. (2000)
Gene mutation, Syrian hamster embryo cells, Na$^+$/K$^+$ ATPase, *Hprt* locus, *in vitro*	–	NT	10 µg/mL	Tsutsui et al. (2000a)
Chromosomal aberrations, Syrian hamster embryo cells *in vitro*	–	NT	10 µg/mL	Tsutsui et al. (2000a)
Aneuploidy, Syrian hamster embryo cells *in vitro*	+	NT	1 µg/mL	Tsutsui et al. (2000a)
DNA single-strand breaks, comet assay, human peripheral blood lymphocytes *in vitro*	+	NT	50 µM [13.6 µg/mL]	Anderson et al. (1997)
DNA single-strand breaks, comet assay, human sperm *in vitro*	+	NT	10 µM [2.7 µg/mL]	Anderson et al. (1997)
DNA single-strand breaks, human MCF-7 cells *in vitro*	+	NT	1 nM [0.27 ng/mL]	Yared et al. (2002)
DNA single-strand breaks, human MCF-7 cells *in vitro*	+	NT	10 nM [2.7 ng/mL]	Rajapakse et al. (2005)
Sister chromosome exchange, human peripheral blood lymphocytes *in vitro*	+	+	25 µg	Ahmad et al. (2000)
Micronucleus formation, human MCF-7 cells *in vitro*	–	NT	1 nM [0.27 ng/mL]	Yared et al. (2002)
Chromosomal aberrations, human peripheral blood lymphocytes *in vitro*	–	+	25 µg	Ahmad et al. (2000)
Chromosomal aberrations, human peripheral blood lymphocytes *in vitro*	–	+	10 µg	Ahmad et al. (2000)
Aneuploidy, human MCF-7 cells *in vitro*	–	NT	3.6 µM [1 µg/mL]	Fernandez et al. (2005)
Micronucleus formation, mouse bone-marrow cells *in vivo*	–		150 mg/kg bw ip	Ashby et al. (1997)
Micronucleus formation, rat and mouse bone-marrow cells *in vivo*	–		1250 mg/kg bw ip	Shelby et al. (1997)
2-Hydroxyestradiol				
Gene mutation, Syrian hamster embryo cells, Na$^+$/K$^+$ ATPase, *Hprt* locus, *in vitro*	–	NT	3 µg/mL	Tsutsui et al. (2000a)
Chromosomal aberrations, Syrian hamster embryo cells *in vitro*	+	NT	3 µg/mL	Tsutsui et al. (2000a)
Aneuploidy, Syrian hamster embryo cells *in vitro*	+	NT	1 µg/mL	Tsutsui et al. (2000a)

Table 19 (contd)

Test system	Results[a]		Dose (LED or HID)[b]	Reference
	Without exogenous metabolic system	With exogenous metabolic system		
DNA single-strand breaks, human MCF-7 cells *in vitro*	+	NT	100 nM [30 ng/mL]	Rajapakse *et al.* (2005)
Aneuploidy, human MCF-7 cells *in vitro*	–	NT	3.6 μM [1 μg/mL]	Fernandez *et al.* (2005)
4-Hydroxyestradiol				
Gene mutation, Syrian hamster embryo cells, Na$^+$/K$^+$ ATPase, *Hprt* locus, *in vitro*	+	NT	1 μg/mL	Tsutsui *et al.* (2000a)
Chromosomal aberrations, Syrian hamster embryo cells *in vitro*	+	NT	3 μg/mL	Tsutsui *et al.* (2000a)
Aneuploidy, Syrian hamster embryo cells *in vitro*	+	NT	1 μg/mL	Tsutsui *et al.* (2000a)
DNA single-strand breaks, human MCF-7 cells *in vitro*	+	NT	100 nM [30 ng/mL]	Rajapakse *et al.* (2005)
Aneuploidy, human MCF-7 cells *in vitro*	–	NT	3.6 μM [1 μg/mL]	Fernandez *et al.* (2005)
2-Methoxyestradiol				
Gene mutation, Syrian hamster embryo cells, Na$^+$/K$^+$ ATPase, *in vitro*	+	NT	0.1 μg/mL	Tsutsui *et al.* (2000b)
Gene mutation, Syrian hamster embryo cells, *Hprt* locus, *in vitro*	+	NT	0.3 μg/mL	Tsutsui *et al.* (2000b)
Chromosomal aberrations, Syrian hamster embryo cells *in vitro*	+	NT	0.3 μg/mL	Tsutsui *et al.* (2000b)
Aneuploidy, Syrian hamster embryo cells *in vitro*	+	NT	0.3 μg/mL	Tsutsui *et al.* (2000b)
Estrone				
Gene mutation, Syrian hamster embryo cells, Na$^+$/K$^+$ ATPase, *Hprt* locus, *in vitro*	–	NT	10 μg/mL	Tsutsui *et al.* (2000a)
Chromosomal aberrations, Syrian hamster embryo cells *in vitro*	+	NT	10 μg/mL	Tsutsui *et al.* (2000a)
Aneuploidy, Syrian hamster embryo cells *in vitro*	+	NT	30 μg/mL	Tsutsui *et al.* (2000a)
DNA single-strand breaks, comet assay human MCF-7 cells *in vitro*	+	NT	0.1 nM [0.03 ng/mL]	Yared *et al.* (2002)

Table 19 (contd)

Test system	Results[a]		Dose (LED or HID)[b]	Reference
	Without exogenous metabolic system	With exogenous metabolic system		
Micronucleus formation, human MCF-7 cells *in vitro*	+	NT	0.1 nM [0.03 ng/mL]	Yared *et al.* (2002)
2-Hydroxyestrone				
Gene mutation, Syrian hamster embryo cells, Na^+/K^+ ATPase, *Hprt* locus, *in vitro*	−	NT	10 µg/mL	Tsutsui *et al.* (2000a)
Chromosomal aberrations, Syrian hamster embryo cells *in vitro*	+	NT	3 µg/mL	Tsutsui *et al.* (2000a)
Aneuploidy, Syrian hamster embryo cells *in vitro*	+	NT	0.3 µg/mL	Tsutsui *et al.* (2000a)
4-Hydroxyestrone				
Gene mutation, Syrian hamster embryo cells, Na^+/K^+ ATPase, *in vitro*	+	NT	3 µg/mL	Tsutsui *et al.* (2000a)
Gene mutation, Syrian hamster embryo cells, *Hprt* locus, *in vitro*	+	NT	1 µg/mL	Tsutsui *et al.* (2000a)
Chromosomal aberrations, Syrian hamster embryo cells *in vitro*	+	NT	3 µg/mL	Tsutsui *et al.* (2000a)
Aneuploidy, Syrian hamster embryo cells *in vitro*	+	NT	3 µg/mL	Tsutsui *et al.* (2000a)
2-Methoxyestrone				
Gene mutation, Syrian hamster embryo cells, Na^+/K^+ ATPase, *Hprt* locus, *in vitro*	−	NT	10 µg/mL	Tsutsui *et al.* (2000a)
Chromosomal aberrations, Syrian hamster embryo cells *in vitro*	−	NT	10 µg/mL	Tsutsui *et al.* (2000a)
Aneuploidy, Syrian hamster embryo cells *in vitro*	+	NT	10 µg/mL	Tsutsui *et al.* (2000a)
16α-Hydroxyestrone				
Gene mutation, Syrian hamster embryo cells, Na^+/K^+ ATPase, *Hprt* locus, *in vitro*	−	NT	10 µg/mL	Tsutsui *et al.* (2000a)
Chromosomal aberrations, Syrian hamster embryo cells *in vitro*	−	NT	10 µg/mL	Tsutsui *et al.* (2000a)
Aneuploidy, Syrian hamster embryo cells *in vitro*	+	NT	10 µg/mL	Tsutsui *et al.* (2000a)

COMBINED ESTROGEN–PROTESTOGEN MENOPAUSAL THERAPY   321

Table 19 (contd)

Test system	Results[a] Without exogenous metabolic system	Results[a] With exogenous metabolic system	Dose (LED or HID)[b]	Reference
Estriol				
Gene mutation, Syrian hamster embryo cells, Na$^+$/K$^+$ ATPase, Hprt locus, in vitro	–	NT	10 µg/mL	Tsutsui et al. (2000a)
Chromosomal aberrations, Syrian hamster embryo cells in vitro	–	NT	10 µg/mL	Tsutsui et al. (2000a)
Aneuploidy, Syrian hamster embryo cells in vitro	–	NT	10 µg/mL	Tsutsui et al. (2000a)
DNA single-strand breaks, human MCF-7 cells in vitro	+	NT	10 nM [3 ng/mL]	Yared et al. (2002)
Micronucleus formation, human MCF-7 cells in vitro	–	NT	0.1 mM [28.9 µg/mL]	Yared et al. (2002)
Ethinylestradiol				
Salmonella typhimurium TA100, TA1535, TA98, TA97a, reverse mutation	–	–	10 mg/plate	Hundel et al. (1997)
Unscheduled DNA synthesis, rat hepatocytes in vitro	+	NT	1 µM [0.3 µg/mL]	Martelli et al. (2003)
Unscheduled DNA synthesis, human hepatocytes in vitro	–	NT	50 µM [15 µg/mL]	Martelli et al. (2003)
Sister chromosome exchange, human peripheral blood lymphocytes in vitro	+	+	1 µg/mL	Hundal et al. (1997)
Chromosomal aberrations, human peripheral blood lymphocytes in vitro	+	NT	1 µg/mL[c] 48 h	Hundal et al. (1997)
Chromosomal aberrations, human peripheral blood lymphocytes in vitro	–	+	10 µg/mL[d] 6 h	Hundal et al. (1997)
Sister chromosome exchange, mouse bone-marrow cells in vivo	+		1 mg/kg bw ip	Hundal et al. (1997)
Micronucleus formation, mouse bone-marrow cells in vivo	+		1 mg/kg bw ip	Hundal et al. (1997)

[a] +, positive; –, negative; NT, not tested
[b] LED, lowest effective dose; HID, highest ineffective dose; ip, intraperitoneal
[c] Tested for 48 h without exogenous metabolic system only
[d] Tested with exogenous metabolic system only for 6 h. The result was negative without exogenous metabolic system after an exposure of 6 h.

Table 20. Genetic and related effects of progestogens in experimental animals

Test system	Results[a]		Dose (LED or HID)[b]	Reference
	Without exogenous metabolic system	With exogenous metabolic system		
Progesterone				
Unscheduled DNA synthesis, rat hepatocytes *in vitro*	–	NT	50 μM [15.7 μg/mL]	Martelli *et al.* (2003)
Unscheduled DNA synthesis, human hepatocytes *in vitro*	–	NT	50 μM [15.7 μg/mL]	Martelli *et al.* (2003)
Micronucleus formation, rat liver *in vivo*	+		100 mg/kg bw po	Martelli *et al.* (1998)
Medroxyprogesterone				
Unscheduled DNA synthesis, rat hepatocytes *in vitro*	–	NT	50 μM [17.2 μg/mL]	Martelli *et al.* (2003)
Unscheduled DNA synthesis, human hepatocytes *in vitro*	–	NT	50 μM [17.2 μg/mL]	Martelli *et al.* (2003)
Norethisterone				
Unscheduled DNA synthesis, rat hepatocytes *in vitro*	±	NT	10 μM [3 μg/mL]	Martelli *et al.* (2003)
Unscheduled DNA synthesis, human hepatocytes *in vitro*	–	NT	50 μM [15 μg/mL]	Martelli *et al.* (2003)
Sister chromosome exchange, human peripheral blood lymphocytes *in vitro*	–	–	75 μg/mL	Ahmad *et al.* (2001)
Chromosomal aberrations, human peripheral blood lymphocytes *in vitro*	–	–	75 μg /mL	Ahmad *et al.* (2001)
Micronucleus formation, rat liver *in vivo*	–		100 mg/kg bw po	Martelli *et al.* (1998)
Norgestrel				
Sister chromosome exchange, human peripheral blood lymphocytes *in vitro*	+	+	25 μg/mL	Ahmad *et al.* (2001)
Chromosomal aberrations, human peripheral blood lymphocytes *in vitro*	+	+	25 μg/mL	Ahmad *et al.* (2001)
Chromosomal aberrations, human peripheral blood lymphocytes *in vitro*	–	+	10 μg/mL	Ahmad *et al.* (2001)

Table 20 (contd)

Test system	Results[a]		Dose (LED or HID)[b]	Reference
	Without exogenous metabolic system	With exogenous metabolic system		
Cyproterone acetate				
DNA single-strand breaks, comet assay, rat hepatocytes *in vitro*	+	NT	10 μM [4 μg/mL]	Mattioli *et al.* (2004)
Unscheduled DNA synthesis, male rat hepatocytes *in vitro*	–	NT	10 μM [4 μg/mL]	Mattioli *et al.* (2004)
Unscheduled DNA synthesis, female rat hepatocytes *in vitro*	+	NT	10 μM [4 μg/mL]	Mattioli *et al.* (2004)
Gene mutation, Big Blue™ transgenic Fischer 344 rats, *LacI* gene, *in vivo*	+		75 mg/kg bw × 1 po	Krebs *et al.* (1998)
Levonorgestrel				
Gene mutation, mouse lymphoma L5178Y cells *in vitro*	–	NT	NG	Jordan (2002)
Chromosomal aberrations, Chinese hamster ovary fibroblasts *in vitro*	–	NT	NG	Jordan (2002)
Desogestrel				
Salmonella typhimurium [strains NG], reverse mutation	–	–	NG	Jordan (2002)
Micronucleus formation, female rat liver *in vivo*	–		NG	Jordan (2002)
Potassium canrenoate				
DNA single-strand breaks, rat hepatocytes *in vitro*	+	NT	10 μM [3.7 μg/mL]	Martelli *et al.* (1999)
Unscheduled DNA synthesis, rat liver *in vitro*	+	NT	30 μM [11 μg/mL]	Martelli *et al.* (1999)
Micronucleus formation, rat hepatocytes *in vitro*	+	NT	30 μM [11 μg/mL]	Martelli *et al.* (1999)
DNA single-strand breaks, human hepatocytes *in vitro*	+	NT	30 μM [11 μg/mL]	Martelli *et al.* (1999)
DNA single-strand breaks, human peripheral blood lymphocytes *in vitro*	–	NT	90 μM [33 μg/mL]	Martelli *et al.* (1999)
Unscheduled DNA synthesis, human liver *in vitro*	–	NT	90 μM [33 μg/mL]	Martelli *et al.* (1999)
Micronucleus formation, human hepatocytes *in vitro*	–	NT	90 μM [33 μg/mL]	Martelli *et al.* (1999)
Micronucleus formation, human peripheral blood lymphocytes *in vitro*	–	NT	90 μM [33 μg/mL]	Martelli *et al.* (1999)

Table 20 (contd)

Test system	Results[a]		Dose (LED or HID)[b]	Reference
	Without exogenous metabolic system	With exogenous metabolic system		
DNA single-strand breaks, male rat liver *in vivo*	+		325 mg/kg bw po	Martelli *et al.* (2002)
DNA single-strand breaks, female rat thyroid and bone marrow *in vivo*	+		325 mg/kg bw po	Martelli *et al.* (2002)
DNA single-strand breaks, rat testes and ovary *in vivo*	+		81 mg/kg bw po	Martelli *et al.* (2002)
Micronucleus formation, rat liver *in vivo*	–		325 mg/kg bw po	Martelli *et al.* (2002)
Micronucleus formation, rat bone marrow polychromatic erythrocytes *in vivo*	–		325 mg/kg bw po	Martelli *et al.* (2002)
Drospirenone				
Unscheduled DNA synthesis, rat hepatocytes *in vitro*	+	NT	1 µM [0.36 µg/mL]	Martelli *et al.* (2003)
Unscheduled DNA synthesis, human hepatocytes *in vitro*	–	NT	50 µM [18.3 µg/mL]	Martelli *et al.* (2003)

[a] +, positive; –, negative; ±, equivocal; NT, not tested
[b] LED, lowest effective dose; HID, highest ineffective dose; NG, not given; po, oral

Cavalieri *et al.*, 2000). These adducts can form stable modifications that remain in the DNA unless they are removed by repair. Alternatively, the modified bases can be released from DNA by destabilization of the glycosydic bond and result in the formation of depurinated or depyrimidinated sites (Cavalieri *et al.*, 2000).

4.4.1 *Humans*

At present, only two studies have reported the presence of catechol estrogen adducts in human breast tissue. Embrechts *et al.* (2003) analysed estrogen adducts in the DNA from 18 human samples: five malignant breast tumour samples, five samples of tissues adjacent to the tumour and eight alcohol-fixed and paraffin-embedded malignant breast tumour samples. Almost every DNA sample showed the presence of deoxyguanosine adducts of 4-hydroxyestradiol and 4-hydroxyestrone. In four patients who had used conjugated equine estrogens, 4-hydroxyequilenin–DNA adducts, derived from conjugated equine estrogen metabolites, were detected. In seven patients, deoxyadenosine adducts of 4-hydroxy-17α-ethinylestradiol were observed. The formation of catechol estrogen quinone-derived DNA adducts has also been reported in two breast samples that were collected from one woman with and one woman without breast cancer (Markushin *et al.*, 2003). The catechol quinone-derived adducts identified were 4-hydroxyestradiol-1-N3-adenosine, 4-hydroxyestrone-1-N3-adenosine and 4-hydroxyestradiol-1-N7-guanine.

4.4.2 *Experimental systems* (Tables 19 and 20)

Liquid chromatographic–tandem MS analysis of mammary fat pads of rats injected with 4-hydroxyequilenin showed a dose-dependent increase in DNA single-strand breaks and formation of alkylated guanine adducts that are prone to depurination; stable cyclic deoxyguanosine and deoxyadenosine adducts and other oxidized bases were also observed (Zhang *et al.*, 2001). Injection of 4-hydroxyestradiol or estradiol-3,4-quinone into the mammary glands of female ACI rats resulted in formation of the depurinating adducts 4-hydroxyestradiol-1-N3-adenosine and 4-hydroxyestradiol-1-N7-guanosine (Li *et al.*, 2004). 4-Hydroxyestradiol-GSH conjugates were also detected. Recently, 4-hydroxy catechol estrogen conjugates with GSH or its hydrolytic products (cysteine and *N*-acetylcysteine) were detected in picomole amounts both in tumours and hyperplastic mammary tissues from ERKO/Wnt-1 mice and demonstrated the formation of estrogen-3,4-quinones (Devanesan *et al.*, 2001). DNA adducts derived from 2-hydroxyestrogen-quinone have been shown to be mutagenic, and primarily produced G→T and A→T mutations in simian kidney (COS-7) cells (Terashima *et al.*, 2001). Estradiol-3,4-quinone reacted rapidly to form 4-hydroxyestradiol-1-N3-adenosine adducts that are depurinating adducts. Numerous A→G mutations in H-*ras* DNA were observed in SENCAR mouse skin treated with estradiol-3,4-quinone (Chakravarti *et al.*, 2001). [These studies indicate that certain estrogen metabolites can react with DNA to form adducts. Such adducts or the apurinic sites they generate in DNA can give rise to mutations and these, in turn, could contribute to the development of tumours.]

Recently, it was reported that estrogen-induced mammary gland tumours in female ACI rats show losses and gains in chromosomes. Cells with an increased copy number of the *c-myc* gene (7q33), one on each of the three homologues of a trisomy of chromosome 7, were observed. A frequency of aneuploidy of 61% in sporadic invasive human ductal breast cancers and 71% in ductal carcinoma *in situ* was also observed. The authors asserted that the estrogen-induced mammary tumours in female ACI rats resembled human ductal carcinoma *in situ* and invasive ductal breast cancer because they are aneuploid and exhibit a high frequency of *c-myc* amplification (Li *et al.*, 2002).

Mitochondria are significant targets of estrogen (reviewed by Roy *et al.*, 2004; Felty & Roy, 2005a,b). Recently Felty *et al.* (2005a) reported that physiological concentrations of 17β-estradiol stimulate a rapid production of intracellular reactive oxygen species which, in epithelial cells, depends on cell adhesion, the cytoskeleton and integrins. Induction of the production of reactive oxygen species by estradiol occurs much more rapidly than the estrogen receptor-mediated interaction with the genome. Furthermore, estradiol-stimulated production of reactive oxygen species does not depend on the presence of the estrogen receptor in breast cancer cells because it was equal in both estrogen receptor-positive cell lines MCF7, T47D and ZR75.1 and the estrogen receptor-negative cell line MDA-MB 468. Exposure of human mammary epithelial cells to 2- or 4-hydroxyestradiol has been shown to produce reactive oxygen species and a subsequent increase in the formation of 8-OHdG (Hurh *et al.*, 2004; Chen *et al.*, 2005). This finding shows that formation of reactive oxygen species following exposure to estradiol could explain oxidative damage in hormone-dependent tumours and subsequent genetic alterations reported earlier (Malins & Haimanot, 1991; Musarrat *et al.*, 1996; Yamamoto *et al.*, 1996; Malins *et al.*, 2001). Mutations have recently been reported to occur following exposures to physiological and pharmacological concentrations of estrogens (Kong *et al.*, 2000; Singh *et al.*, 2005).

It has been shown that catechol estrogens can induce aldehydic DNA lesions in calf thymus DNA (Lin *et al.*, 2003). Equilin and equilenin are major constituents of Premarin®, a widely prescribed drug used in estrogen therapy for the menopause. These equine estrogens are metabolized, respectively, to 4-hydroxyequilin and 4-hydroxyequilenin, which, in turn, are oxidized to products that react with DNA. Mutations induced by 4-hydroxyequilin have been identified in supF plasmid shuttle vectors that were transfected in human fibroblast cells (Yasui *et al.*, 2003).

5. Summary of Data Reported and Evaluation

5.1   Exposure data

Combined estrogen–progestogen menopausal therapy involves the co-administration of an estrogen and a progestogen to peri- or postmenopausal women. These hormones may be given as individual compounds administered simultaneously or as combination preparations. Early treatment regimens included estrogen only. After a substantial increase in the 1960s and early 1970s, the use of these regimens declined after 1975 when a strong association with endometrial cancer was found. When the addition of a progestogen was introduced as a strategy to reduce this risk, the use of hormonal menopausal therapy again increased steadily in the 1980s, particularly in developed countries. Combined estrogen–progestogen menopausal therapy is now administered to women who have not undergone a hysterectomy, whereas estrogen-only menopausal treatment tends to be prescribed to hysterectomized women. Although combined hormonal therapy was initially indicated for the control of menopausal symptoms, its application was expanded in the 1990s to include the treatment or prevention of a range of conditions related to ageing. However, since 2002, dramatic declines in use followed the report of a broad range of adverse effects in the Women's Health Initiative Estrogen Plus Progestin Trial in the USA. Reflecting this new evidence, practices are returning to a narrower set of indications directed at the short-term treatment of menopausal symptoms.

Combined estrogen–progestogen formulations are frequently used in hormonal menopausal therapy, although separate administration of each hormonal component is still prevalent. Commercial preparations are available for oral, vaginal and transdermal administration. Currently, continuous exposure to both hormones (both estrogen and progestogen at fixed daily doses) is common, particularly in the USA, whereas cyclical dosing, in which progestogen is added periodically to daily estrogen, is prevalent in other countries. Other scheduling strategies are also used occasionally. Some formulations and doses that are currently available for combined hormonal therapy are new and their possible long-term adverse effects have not been evaluated.

Combined hormonal therapy is much more commonly used in developed than in developing countries. At the peak of use in 1999, approximately 20 million women in developed countries used combined hormonal therapy, including 50% of women aged 50–65 years in the USA. Use has fallen by more than 50% since 2002, particularly for continuous combined hormonal therapy. Use in some developing countries also has declined modestly, although the data are more limited. Among peri- and postmenopausal women in developed countries, current users of combined hormonal therapy tend to be younger and more highly educated, to have a lower body mass and to use health care more regularly than non-users. The characteristics of users are known to vary between countries and to change over time.

5.2   Human carcinogenicity data

Breast cancer

Two large randomized trials, 10 cohort studies and seven case–control studies reported on the relationship between the use of combined estrogen–progestogen menopausal therapy and breast cancer in postmenopausal women. The studies consistently reported an increased risk for breast cancer in users of combined estrogen–progestogen therapy compared with non-users. The increased risk was greater than that in users of estrogen alone. The available evidence was inadequate to evaluate whether or not the risk for breast cancer varies according to the progestogenic content of the therapy or its dose, or according to the number of days each month that the progestogens are added to the estrogen therapy. Observational studies showed that the relative risk was greater for lobular than for ductal cancers. The increase in the risk for breast cancer was largely confined to current or recent users, and the risk increased with increasing duration of use of the combined hormonal therapy.

Endometrial cancer

One randomized trial, four cohort studies and eight case–control studies reported on the relationship between use of combined estrogen–progestogen menopausal therapy and the risk for endometrial cancer in postmenopausal women. The risk for endometrial cancer was inversely associated with the number of days per month that progestogens were added to the regimen. The addition of progestogens to estrogen therapy for less than 10 days per month was associated with a significantly higher risk for endometrial cancer than never use of hormonal therapy, and the risk increased with increasing duration of use of that regimen. Estrogen therapy with daily progestogens was associated with a risk for endometrial cancer similar to, and possibly lower than, that found in women who had never used hormonal therapy. In contrast, the use of estrogens alone was associated with a considerably higher risk than that of any combined estrogen–progestogen regimen. Use of combined estrogen–progestogen menopausal therapy began relatively recently and, as yet, there is little information on its effects on the risk for endometrial cancer many years after cessation of use. The available evidence was inadequate to evaluate whether or not the risk for endometrial cancer varies according to the type or daily dose of progestogen.

Cervical cancer

The data from two randomized trials were inadequate to suggest that combined estrogen–progestogen hormonal therapy alters the risk for human papillomavirus infection or cervical cancer, and are of limited statistical power.

Ovarian cancer

Data from one randomized trial and two cohort and four case–control studies were inadequate to evaluate an association between ovarian cancer and combined estrogen–progestogen hormonal therapy.

Colorectal cancer

Two randomized trials and four cohort and three case–control studies provided information on the use of combined estrogen–progestogen hormonal therapy and the risk for colorectal cancer. None showed significantly elevated risks in women who had used these preparations for any length of time. Seven studies showed relative risks below 1.0 and the risk was significantly reduced in two, which suggests a potential protective effect. The reduced risk tended to be observed among recent users and did not appear to be related to duration of use.

Other cancers

Large randomized trials provided the only substantial data on risk for lung cancer, which was slightly but not significantly elevated in users of combined estrogen–progestogen hormonal therapy. Observational data on lung cancer include both slightly increased and slightly reduced rates in users of such combined hormonal therapy. Data on cancer at other sites, including the liver, were too limited for evaluation.

5.3   Animal carcinogenicity data

Relatively few studies have been carried out to examine the tumorigenic effects of combined hormonal therapy in animals.

Oral administration of combined hormonal therapy in mice that are prone to develop mammary tumours resulted in similar incidences of mammary tumours in controls and in animals treated with conjugated equine estrogens alone and with conjugated equine estrogens plus medroxyprogesterone acetate. However, tumour latency was reduced in animals treated with conjugated equine estrogens plus medroxyprogesterone acetate. Conjugated equine estrogens plus medroxyprogesterone acetate suppressed the development of uterine adenomyosis.

Oral administration of conjugated equine estrogens alone or with medroxyprogesterone acetate to ovariectomized rats pretreated with the carcinogen 7,12-dimethylbenz[*a*]-anthracene increased the incidence of mammary tumours with equal frequency and to a level equal to that in non-ovariectomized controls.

5.4   Other relevant data

Absorption, distribution, metabolism and excretion

Various combinations of estrogens and progestogens are used for hormonal menopausal therapy. Since steroids penetrate normal skin easily, a variety of systems have been developed that deliver estrogens and progestogens parenterally (e.g. transdermal patches), thus by-passing the liver.

While the mechanisms of absorption and distribution of estrogens and progestogens have been known for a number of years, only recently has an understanding of the genes that encode the enzymes which control the enzymatic steps involved in steroid metabolism been acquired. This applies especially to the oxidative metabolism of estrogen. The phase I enzymes cytochrome P450 1A1 and 1B1 catalyse the production of catechol estrogen and metabolites of estrogen quinone that can induce the formation of DNA adducts. This is counteracted by the phase II enzymes, catechol-*O*-methyltransferase and glutathione

S-transferase P1, which reduce the levels of catechol and quinones by forming methoxy-estrogens and glutathione conjugates. Polymorphic variants of these and other enzymes occur frequently in the population and several are associated with altered enzyme function. A large body of epidemiological data has failed to identify a consistent association between exposure to hormones and risk for cancer with any single enzyme variant. However, possible interactions between these genes need to be examined.

Progestogens are discussed in the monograph on Combined estrogen–progestogen contraceptives.

Receptor-mediated effects

The use of combined estrogen–progestogen menopausal therapy increases the rate of cell proliferation in the postmenopausal human breast, and appears to enhance significantly the modest increase in breast-cell proliferation induced by estrogen alone. Oral administration of conjugated equine estrogens alone or in combination with medroxyprogesterone acetate to ovariectomized monkeys resulted in an increase in epithelial cell proliferation and epithelial density in the mammary gland, as determined histologically, whereas the combination of conjugated equine estrogens and norethisterone acetate did not. The effects were greater with conjugated equine estrogens plus medroxyprogesterone acetate than with conjugated equine estrogens or medroxyprogesterone alone. Subcutaneous implantation of 17β-estradiol alone or in combination with progesterone for 3 days into ovariectomized monkeys resulted in a slight increase in epithelial cell proliferation in the mammary gland as did intraperitoneal administration of 17β-estradiol alone or in combination with progesterone to ovariectomized mice; the effect in mice was greater with 17β-estradiol plus progesterone than with 17β-estradiol alone. Approximately one-third of women treated with daily estrogen (by any route) plus daily oral progestogen develop increased mammographic breast density. In contrast, following treatments with estrogen daily plus progestogen less frequently than daily, a smaller proportion of women develop increased breast density. The addition of progestogens to estrogen therapy for the menopause prevents the development of endometrial hyperplasia and reduces the increased rate of endometrial cell proliferation induced by treatment with estrogen only. This effect has been found for all progestogens studied, regardless of the route of administration or dose. Inadequate data were available to the Working Group on duration of treatment or time since cessation of treatment.

Cardiovascular effects of estrogen and progestogen

Randomized trials that studied combined hormonal menopausal therapy did not show a protective effect of a fixed single dose of conjugated equine estrogens with or without medroxyprogesterone acetate on the incidence of coronary heart disease, although a large body of literature from observational studies suggests that such treatment confers benefits for this disease. These discrepancies have not been fully resolved but may arise from methodological limitations in some observational studies. Randomized trials have consistently reported a small adverse effect of combined hormonal therapy on the incidence of stroke, which is generally supported by observational studies. Evidence of an increase in the incidence of venous thromboembolism from hormonal therapy, particularly with estrogen plus progestogen, has been found in both randomized trials and observational studies, and is supported by mechanistic studies. The overall evidence relies heavily on studies of conjugated equine estrogens and medroxyprogesterone acetate, the data from which suggest a small increase in risk for broadly defined cardiovascular disease as a whole. The extent to which these results apply to other estrogens and progestogens, doses or routes of administration is not known.

Other effects

The beneficial effects of combined hormonal menopausal therapy have been established unambiguously for vasomotor symptoms, osteoporosis and fractures, with moderate evidence for a reduced risk for non-insulin-dependent diabetes. The evidence for an increase in breast density and an increase in the prevalence of breast tenderness and vaginal bleeding is also unambiguous. There is strongly suggestive evidence of interference in mammographic screening associated with breast density and an increase in problems of urinary incontinence. There is consistent evidence for an increase in the risk for gallbladder disease. Results for cognitive function and dementia are less clear. In women who initiate therapy later in life (≥ 65 years of age), randomized trials have provided evidence of a small deleterious effect on cognitive function and an increased risk for dementia. The cognitive effects in women who initiate therapy at younger ages are still uncertain. Randomized trials did not show substantial effects on mortality or on the quality of life, other than the relief of symptoms related to the menopause.

Genetic and related effects

Data on the genetic effects of estrogens and their derivatives indicate that these compounds give rise to reactive metabolites and reactive oxygen species that can induce DNA damage. The evidence reported since the previous evaluation further substantiates the premise that these mechanisms could contribute to the induction of cancer by estrogens. New evidence demonstrates that DNA adducts that are expected to result from the metabolites of catechol estrogen are found in humans, experimental animals and in-vitro systems and that exposure to estrogens generates reactive oxygen species. While these new findings increase the plausibility of these pathways as mechanisms of estrogen-related carcinogenesis, they do not prove that these are the major pathways to estrogen-related cancers. The way in which progestogens might influence the genotoxicity of estrogens is not known.

Receptor-mediated responses to hormones are a plausible and probably necessary mechanism for hormonal carcinogenesis. The results of research over the past few years add considerable support for a direct genotoxic effect of hormones or their associated by-products such as reactive oxygen species. Current knowledge does not allow a conclusion as to whether either of these mechanisms is the major determinant of hormonally induced cancer. It is entirely possible that both mechanisms contribute to and are necessary for carcinogenesis. Cessation of hormonal treatment may reduce the receptor-mediated effects while gene damage may be more persistent.

5.5 Evaluation

There is *sufficient evidence* in humans for the carcinogenicity of combined estrogen–progestogen menopausal therapy in the breast.

There is *evidence suggesting lack of carcinogenicity* in humans for combined estrogen–progestogen menopausal therapy in the colorectum.

There is *sufficient evidence* in humans for the carcinogenicity of combined estrogen–progestogen menopausal therapy in the endometrium when progestogens are taken for fewer than 10 days per month, and there is *evidence suggesting lack of carcinogenicity* in the endometrium when progestogens are taken daily. The risk for endometrial cancer is inversely associated with the number of days per month that progestogens are added to the regimen.

There is *limited evidence* in experimental animals for the carcinogenicity of conjugated equine estrogens plus medroxyprogesterone acetate.

Overall evaluation

Combined estrogen–progestogen menopausal therapy is *carcinogenic to humans (Group 1).*

6. References

Abramov, Y., Borik, S., Yahalom, C., Fatum, M., Avgil, G., Brzezinski, A. & Banin, E. (2004) The effect of hormone therapy on the risk for age-related maculopathy in postmenopausal women. *Menopause*, **11**, 62–68

Adams, M.R., Register, T.C., Golden, D.L., Wagner, JD. & Williams, J.K. (1997) Medroxyprogesterone acetate antagonizes inhibitory effects of conjugated equine estrogens on coronary artery atherosclerosis. *Arterioscler. Thromb. vasc. Biol.*, **17**, 217–221

Adjei, A.A. & Weinshilboum, R.M. (2002) Catecholestrogen sulfation: Possible role in carcinogenesis. *Biochem. biophys. Res. Commun.*, **292**, 402–408

Adjei, A.A., Thomae, B.A., Prondzinski, J.L., Eckloff, B.W., Wieben, E.D. & Weinshilboum, R.M. (2003) Human estrogen sulfotransferase (SULT1E1) pharmacogenomics: Gene resequencing and functional genomics. *Br. J. Pharmacol.*, **139**, 1373–1382

Ahmad, M.E., Shadab, G.G.H.A., Hoda, A. & Afzal, M. (2000) Genotoxic effects of estradiol-17β on human lymphocyte chromosomes. *Mutat. Res.*, **466**, 109–115

Ahmad, M.E., Shadab, G.G.H.A., Azfer, M.A. & Afzal, M. (2001) Evaluation of genotoxic potential of synthetic progestins-norethindrone and norgestrel in human lymphocytes in vitro. *Mutat. Res.*, **494**, 13–20

Aitken, J.M., Hart, D.M. & Lindsay, R. (1973) Oestrogen replacement therapy for prevention of osteoporosis after oophorectomy. *Br. med. J.*, **3**, 515–518

Al-Azzawi, F., Wahab, M., Thompson, J., Whitehead, M. & Thompson, W. (1999) Acceptability and patterns of uterine bleeding in sequential trimegestone-based hormone replacement therapy: A dose-ranging study. *Hum. Reprod.*, **14**, 636–641

Albert, C., Vallée, M., Beaudry, G., Belanger, A. & Hum, D.W. (1999) The monkey and human uridine diphosphate-glucuronosyltransferase UGT1A9, expressed in steroid target tissues, are estrogen-conjugating enzymes. *Endocrinology*, **140**, 3292–3302

Alpert, L.C., Schecter, R.L., Berry, D.A., Melnychuk, D., Peters, W.P., Caruso, J.A., Townsend, A.J. & Batist, G. (1997) Relation of glutathione S-transferase alpha and mu isoforms to response to therapy in human breast cancer. *Clin. Cancer Res.*, **3**, 661–667

American College of Physicians (1992) Guidelines for counseling postmenopausal women about preventive hormone therapy. *Ann. intern. Med.*, **117**, 1038–1041

Anderson, D., Dobrzynska, M.M. & Basaran, N. (1997) Effect of various genotoxins and reproductive toxins in human lymphocytes and sperm in the Comet assay. *Teratog. Carcinog. Mutag.*, **17**, 29–43

Anderson, G.L., Judd, H.L., Kaunitz, A.M., Barad, D.H., Beresford, S.A.A., Pettinger, M., Liu, J., McNeeley, G. & Lopez, A.M. for the Women's Health Initiative Investigators (2003) Effects of estrogen plus progestin on gynecologic cancers and associated diagnostic procedures. *J. Am. med. Assoc.*, **290**, 1739–1748

Anderson, G.L., Limacher, M., Assaf, A.R., Bassford, T., Beresford, S.A.A., Black, H., Bonds, D., Brunner, R., Brzyski, R., Caan, B., Chlebowski, R., Curb, D., Gass, M., Hays, J., Heiss, G., Hendrix, S., Howard, B.V., Hsia, J., Hubbell, A., Jackson, R., Johnson, K.C., Judd, H., Kotchen, J.M., Kuller, L., LaCroix, A.Z., Lanc, D., Langer, R.D., Lasser, N., Lewis, C.E., Manson, J., Margolis, K., Ockene, J., O'Sullivan, M.J., Phillips, L., Prentice, R.L., Ritenbaugh, C., Robbins, J., Rossouw, J.E., Sarto, G., Stefanick, M.L., Van Horn, L., Wactawski-Wende, J., Wallace, R. & Wassertheil-Smoller, S. for the Women's Health Initiative Steering Committee (2004) Effects of conjugated equine estrogen in postmenopausal women with hysterectomy: The Women's Health Initiative randomized controlled trial. *J. Am. med. Assoc.*, **291**, 1701–1712

Ariga, N., Moriya, T., Suzuki, T., Kimura, M., Ohuchi, N., Satomi, S. & Sasano, H. (2000) 17β-Hydroxysteroid dehydrogenase type 1 and type 2 in ductal carcinoma in situ and intraductal proliferative lesions of the human breast. *Anticancer Res.*, **20**, 1101–1108

Arrenbrecht, S. & Boermans, A.J.M. (2002) Effects of transdermal estradiol delivered by a matrix patch on bone density in hysterectomized, postmenopausal women: A 2-year placebo-controlled trial. *Osteoporos. int.*, **13**, 176–183

Ashby, J., Fletcher, K., Williams, C., Odum, J. & Tinwell, H. (1997) Lack of activity of estradiol in rodent bone marrow micronucleus assays. *Mutat. Res.*, **395**, 83–88

Asthana, S., Baker, L.D., Craft, S., Stanczyk, F.Z., Veith, R.C., Raskind, M.A. & Plymate, S.R. (2001) High-dose estradiol improves cognition for women with AD. Results of a randomized study. *Neurology*, **57**, 605–612 van Baal, W.M., Kenemans, P., van der Mooren, M.J., Kessel, H., Emeis, J.J. & Stehouwer, C.D.A. (1999) Increased C-reactive protein levels during short-term hormone replacement therapy in healthy postmenopausal women. *Thromb. Haemost.*, **81**, 925–928

Badawi, A.F., Cavalieri, E.L. & Rogan, E.G. (2001) Role of human cytochrome P450 1A1, 1A2, 1B1, and 3A4 in the 2-, 4-, and 16α-hydroxylation of 17β-estradiol. *Metabolism*, **50**, 1001–1003

Bailey, L.R., Roodi, N., Dupont, W.D. & Parl, F.F. (1998) Association of cytochrome P450 *1B1* (*CYP1B1*) polymorphism with steroid receptor status in breast cancer. *Cancer Res.*, **58**, 5038–5041

Bakken, K., Alsaker, E., Eggen, A.E. & Lund, E. (2004) Hormone replacement therapy and incidence of hormone-dependent cancers in the Norwegian Women and Cancer Study. *Int. J. Cancer*, **112**, 130–134

Baldereschi, M., Di Carlo, A., Lepore, V., Bracco, L., Maggi, S., Grigoletto, F., Scarlato, G. & Amaducci, L. for the ILSA Working Group (1998) Estrogen-replacement therapy and Alzheimer's disease in the Italian Longitudinal Study on Aging. *Neurology*, **50**, 996–1002

Banks, E., Beral, V., Cameron, R., Hogg, A., Langley, N., Barnes, I., Bull, D., Elliman, J. & Harris, C.L. (2001) Agreement between general practice prescription data and self-reported use of hormone replacement therapy and treatment for various illnesses. *J. Epidemiol. Biostat.*, **6**, 357–363

Banks, E., Barnes, I., Baker, K. & Key, T.J. for the EPIC Working Group on Reproductive and Hormonal Factors (2002) Use of hormonal therapy for menopause in nine European countries. In: Riboli, E & Lambert, R., eds, *Nutrition and Lifestyle: Opportunities for Cancer Prevention* (IARC Scientific Publications No. 156), Lyon, pp. 301–303

Banks, E., Reeves, G., Beral, V., Bull, D., Crossley, B., Simmonds, M., Hilton, E., Bailey, S., Barrett, N., Briers, P., English, R., Jackson, A., Kutt, E., Lavelle, J., Rockall, L., Wallis, M.G., Wilson, M. & Patnick, J. (2004) Influence of personal characteristics of individual women on sensitivity and specificity of mammography in the Million Women Study: Cohort study. *Br. med. J.*, **329**, 477

Barnabei, V.M., Grady, D., Stovall, D.W., Cauley, J.A., Lin, F., Stuenkel, C.A., Stefanick, M.L. & Pickar, J.H. (2002) Menopausal symptoms in older women and the effects of treatment with hormone therapy. *Obstet. Gynecol.*, **100**, 1209–1218

Barnabei, V.M., Cochrane, B.B., Aragaki, A.K., Nygaard, I., Williams, R.S., McGovern, P.G., Young, R.L., Wells, E.C., O'Sullivan, M.J., Chen, B., Schenken, R. & Johnson, S.R. for the Women's Health Initiative Investigators (2005) Menopausal symptoms and treatment-related effects of estrogen and progestin in the Women's Health Initiative. *Obstet. Gynecol.*, **105**, 1063–1073

Barrett-Connor, E. (1991) Postmenopausal estrogen and prevention bias. *Ann. intern. Med.*, **115**, 455–456

Barrett-Connor, E., Wingard, D.L. & Criqui, M.H. (1989) Postmenopausal estrogen use and heart disease risk factors in the 1980s. Rancho Bernardo, Calif, revisited. *J. Am. med. Assoc.*, **261**, 2095–2100

Benet-Rodriguez, M., Carvajal García-Pando, A., Garcia del Pozo, J., Alvarez Requejo, A. & Vega Alonso, T. (2002) [Hormonal replacement therapy in Spain]. *Med. clin.*, **119**, 4–8 (in Spanish)

Beral, V., Banks, E., Reeves, G. & Appleby, P. (1999) Use of HRT and the subsequent risk of cancer. *J. Epidemiol. Biostat.*, **4**, 191–210

Beral, V. and the Million Women Study Collaborators (2003) Breast cancer and hormone-replacement therapy in the Million Women Study. *Lancet*, **362**, 419–427

Beral, V., Bull, D., Reeves, G. & Million Women Study Collaborators (2005) Endometrial cancer and hormone-replacement therapy in the Million Women Study. *Lancet*, **365**, 1543–1551

Beresford, S.A., Weiss, N.S., Voigt, L.F. & McKnight, B. (1997) Risk of endometrial cancer in relation to use of oestrogen combined with cyclic progestagen therapy in postmenopausal women. *Lancet*, **349**, 458–461

Bernstein, L.M., Tsyrlina, E.V., Kolesnik, O.S., Gamajunova, V.B. & Adlercreutz, H. (2000) Catecholestrogens excretion in smoking and non-smoking postmenopausal women receiving estrogen replacement therapy. *Steroid Biochem. mol. Biol.*, **72**, 143–147

Bhasker, C.R., McKinnon, W., Stone, A., Lo, A.C., Kubota, T., Ishizaki, T. & Miners, J.O. (2000) Genetic polymorphism of UDP-glucuronosyltransferase 2B7 (UGT2B7) at amino acid 268: Ethnic diversity of alleles and potential clinical significance. *Pharmacogenetics*, **10**, 679–685

Biglia, N., Ambroggio, S., Ponzone, R., Sgro, L., Ujcic, E., Dato, F.A. & Sismondi, P. (2003) Modification of serum IGF-I, IGFBPs and SHBG levels by different HRT regimens. *Maturitas*, **45**, 283–291

Bilgrami, I., Blower, K., Feng, J., Stefanko, G. & Tan, E. (2004) Changes in the use of hormone replacement therapy in New Zealand following the publication of the Women's Health Initiative Trial. *N.Z. med. J.*, **117**, U1175

Bläuer, M., Heinonen, P.K., Martikainen, P.M., Tomas, E. & Ylikomi, T. (2005) A novel organotypic culture model for normal human endometrium: Regulation of epithelial cell proliferation by estradiol and medroxyprogesterone acetate. *Hum. Reprod.*, **20**, 864–871

Bloemenkamp, K.W.M., Rosendaal, F.R., Helmerhorst, F.M., Koster, T., Bertina, R.M. & Vandenbroucke, J.P. (1998) Hemostatic effects of oral contraceptives in women who developed deep-vein thrombosis while using oral contraceptives. *Thromb. Haemost.*, **80**, 382–387

Bloemenkamp, K.W.M., de Maat, M.P.M., Dersjant-Roorda, M.C., Helmerhorst, F.M. & Kluft, C. (2002) Genetic polymorphisms modify the response of factor VII to oral contraceptive use: An example of gene–environment interaction. *Vasc. Pharmacol.*, **39**, 131–136

Boland, L.L., Folsom, A.R., Rosamond, W.D & Atherosclerosis Risk in Communities (ARIC) Study Investigators (2002) Hyperinsulinemia, dyslipidemia, and obesity as risk factors for hospitalized gallbladder disease. A prospective study. *Ann. Epidemiol.*, **12**, 131–140

Bolton, J.L., Trush, M.A., Penning, T.M., Dryhurst, G. & Monks, T.J. (2000) Role of quinones in toxicology. *Chem. Res. Toxicol.*, **13**, 135–160

Bosetti, C., Negri, E., Franceschi, S., Trichopoulos, D., Beral, V. & La Vecchia, C. (2001) Relationship between postmenopausal hormone replacement therapy and ovarian cancer. *J. Am. med. Assoc.*, **285**, 3089

Boyd, N.F., Lockwood, G.A., Martin, L.J., Knight, J.A., Jong, R.A., Fishell, E., Byng, J.W., Yaffe, M.J. & Tritchler, D.L. (1999) Mammographic densities and risk of breast cancer among subjects with a family history of this disease. *J. natl Cancer Inst.*, **91**, 1404–1408

Bradlow, H.L., Telang, N.T., Sepkovic, D.W. & Osborne, M.P. (1996) 2-Hydroxyestrone: The 'good' estrogen. *J. Endocrinol.*, **150** (Suppl.), S259–S265

Brinton, L.A. & Hoover, R.N. for the Endometrial Cancer Collaborative Group (1993) Estrogen replacement therapy and endometrial cancer risk: Unresolved issues. *Obstet. Gynecol.*, **81**, 265–271

Bromley, S.E., de Vries, C.S. & Farmer, R.D.T. (2004) Utilisation of hormone replacement therapy in the United Kingdom. A descriptive study using the general practice research database. *Br. J. Obstet. Gynaecol.*, **111**, 369–376

Brueggemeier, R.W., Bhat, A.S., Lovely, C.J., Coughenour, H.D., Joomprabutra, S., Weitzel, D.H., Vandre, D.D., Yusuf, F. & Burak, W.E., Jr (2001) 2-Methoxymethylestradiol: A new 2-methoxy estrogen analog that exhibits antiproliferative activity and alters tubulin dynamics. *J. steroid Biochem. mol. Biol.*, **78**, 145–156

Buist, D.S.M., LaCroix, A.Z., Newton, K.M. & Keenan, N.L. (1999) Are long-term hormone replacement therapy users different from short-term and never users? *Am. J. Epidemiol.*, **149**, 275–281

Buist, D.S.M., Newton, K.M., Miglioretti, D.L., Beverly, K., Connelly, M.T., Andrade, S., Hartsfield, C.L., Wei, F., Chan, K.A. & Kessler, L. (2004) Hormone therapy prescribing patterns in the United States. *Obstet. Gynecol.*, **104**, 1042–1050

Burns, G.R.J. (1983) Purification and partial characterization of arylsulphatase C from human placental microsomes. *Biochim. biophys. Acta*, **759**, 199–204

Bush, T.L. & Barrett-Connor, E. (1985) Noncontraceptive estrogen use and cardiovascular disease. *Epidemiol. Rev.*, **7**, 89–104

Bush, T.L., Barrett-Connor, E., Cowan, L.D., Criqui, M.H., Wallace, R.B., Suchindran, C.M., Tyroler, H.A. & Rifkind, B.M. (1987) Cardiovascular mortality and noncontraceptive use of estrogen in women: Results from the Lipid Research Clinics Program Follow-up Study. *Circulation*, **75**, 1102–1109

Byng, J.W., Yaffe, M.J., Lockwood, G.A., Little, L.E., Tritchler, D.L. & Boyd, N.F. (1997) Automated analysis of mammographic densities and breast carcinoma risk. *Cancer*, **80**, 66–74

Byrjalsen, I., Bjarnason, N.H. & Christiansen, C. (1999) Progestational effects of combinations of gestodene on the postmenopausal endometrium during hormone replacement therapy. *Am. J. Obstet. Gynecol.*, **180**, 539–549

Cameron, S.T., Critchley, H.O.D., Glasier, A.F., Williams, A.R. & Baird, D.T. (1997) Continuous transdermal oestrogen and interrupted progestogen as a novel bleed-free regimen of hormone replacement therapy for postmenopausal women. *Br. J. Obstet. Gynaecol.*, **104**, 1184–1190

Campagnoli, C., Colombo, P., De Aloysio, D., Gambacciani, M., Grazioli, I., Nappi, C., Serra, G.B. & Genazzani, A.R. (2002) Positive effects on cardiovascular and breast metabolic markers of oral estradiol and dydrogesterone in comparison with transdermal estradiol and norethisterone acetate. *Maturitas*, **41**, 299–311

Campagnoli, C., Abba, C., Ambroggio, S. & Peris, C. (2003) Differential effects of progestins on the circulating IGF-I system. *Maturitas.*, **46** (Suppl. 1), S39–S44

Campbell, S. & Whitehead, M. (1977) Oestrogen therapy and the menopausal syndrome. *Clin. Obstet. Gynaecol.*, **4**, 31–47

Cano, A., Tarin, J.J. & Duenas, J.L. (1999) Two-year prospective, randomized trial comparing an innovative twice-a-week progestin regimen with a continuous combined regimen as postmenopausal hormone therapy. *Fertil. Steril.*, **71**, 129–136

Cao, K., Stack, D.E., Ramanathan, R., Gross, M.L., Rogan, E.G. & Cavalieri, E.L. (1998) Synthesis and structure elucidation of estrogen quinones conjugated with cysteine, *N*-acetylcysteine, and glutathione. *Chem. Res. Toxicol.*, **11**, 909–916

Carlini, E.J., Raftogianis, R.B., Wood, T.C., Jin, F., Zheng, W., Rebbeck, T.R. & Weinshilboum, R.M. (2001) Sulfation pharmacogenetics: *SULT1A1* and *SULT1A2* allele frequencies in Caucasian, Chinese and African-American subjects. *Pharmacogenetics*, **11**, 57–68

Carney, P.A., Tosteson, A.N.A., Titus-Ernstoff, L., Weiss, J.E., Goodrich, M.E., Manganiello, P. & Kasales, C.J. (2006) Hormone therapies in women aged 40 and older: Prevalence and correlates of use. *Maturitas*, **53**, 65–76

Castagnetta, L.A.M., Granata, O.M., Traina, A., Ravazzolo, B., Amoroso, M., Miele, M., Bellavia, V., Agostara, B. & Carruba, G. (2002) Tissue content of hydroxyestrogens in relation to survival of breast cancer patients. *Clin. Cancer Res.*, **8**, 3146–3155

Cauley, J.A., Robbins, J., Chen, Z., Cummings, S.R., Jackson, R.D., LaCroix, A.Z., LeBoff, M., Lewis, C.E., McGowan, J., Neuner, J., Pettinger, M., Stefanick, M.L., Wactawski-Wende, J. & Watts, N.B. for the Women's Health Initiative Investigators (2003) Effects of estrogen plus progestin on risk of fracture and bone mineral density: The Women's Health Initiative Randomized Trial. *J. Am. med. Assoc.*, **290**, 1729–1738

Caulin-Glaser, T., Garcia-Cardena, G., Sarrel, P., Sessa, W.C. & Bender, J.R. (1997) 17β-Estradiol regulation of human endothelial cell basal nitric oxide release, independent of cytosolic Ca^{2+} mobilization. *Circ. Res.*, **81**, 885–892

Cavalieri, E., Frenkel, K., Liehr, J.G., Rogan, E. & Roy, D. (2000) Estrogens as endogenous genotoxic agents — DNA adducts and mutations. *J. natl Cancer Inst. Monogr.*, **27**, 75–93

Chakravarti, D., Mailander, P.C., Li, K.M., Higginbotham, S., Zhang, H.L., Gross, M.L., Meza, J.L., Cavalieri, E.L. & Rogan, E.G. (2001) Evidence that a burst of DNA depurination in SENCAR mouse skin induces error-prone repair and forms mutations in the H-ras gene. *Oncogene*, **20**, 7945–7953

Chang, T.-C., Chen, M., Lien, Y.-R., Chen, R.-J. & Chow, S.-N. (2003) Comparison of the difference in histopathology and cell cycle kinetics among the postmenopausal endometrium treated with different progestins in sequential-combined hormone replacement therapy. *Menopause*, **10**, 172–178

Chapman, O., Purohit, A., Wang, D.Y., Ghilchik, M.W. & Reed, M.J. (1995) Oestrone sulphatase activity in normal and malignant breast tissues: Relationship with tumour location. *Anticancer Res.*, **15**, 1467–1472

Chatterton, R.T., Jr, Geiger, A.S., Mateo, E.T., Helenowski, I.B. & Gann, P.H. (2005) Comparison of hormone levels in nipple aspirate fluid of pre- and postmenopausal women: Effect of oral contraceptives and hormone replacement. *J. clin. Endocrinol. Metab.*, **90**, 1686–1691

Chen, Z.-H., Na, H.-K., Hurh, Y.-J. & Surh, Y.-J. (2005) 4-Hydroxyestradiol induces oxidative stress and apoptosis in human mammary epithelial cells: Possible protection by NF-κB and ERK/MAPK. *Toxicol. appl. Pharmacol.*, **208**, 46–56

Cheng, Z., Rios, G.R., King, C.D., Coffman, B.L., Green, M.D., Mojarrabi, B., Mackenzie, P.I. & Tephly, T.R. (1998) Glucuronidation of catechol estrogens by expressed human UDP-glucuronosyltransferases (UGTs) 1A1, 1A3, and 2B7. *Toxicol. Sci.*, **45**, 52–57

Chester, H., Jiang, C., Borland, J.A., Yacoub, M.H. & Collins, P. (1995) Oestrogen relaxes human epicardial coronary arteries through non-endothelium-dependent mechanisms. *Coron. Artery Dis.*, **6**, 417–422

Chetrite, G.S., Kloosterboer, H.J., Philippe, J.C. & Pasqualini, J.R. (1999a) Effects of Org OD14 (Livial®) and its metabolites on 17β-hydroxysteroid dehydrogenase activity in hormone-dependent MCF-7 and T-47D breast cancer cells. *Anticancer Res.*, **19**, 261–267

Chetrite, G.S., Ebert, C., Wright, F., Philippe, J.-C. & Pasqualini, J.R. (1999b) Effect of Medrogestone on 17β-hydroxysteroid dehydrogenase activity in the hormone-dependent MCF-7 and T-47D human breast cancer cell lines. *J. steroid Biochem. mol. Biol.*, **68**, 51–56

Chetrite, G.S., Thole, H.H., Philippe, J.-C. & Pasqualini, J.R. (2004) Dydrogesterone (Duphaston) and its 20-dihydro-derivative as selective estrogen enzyme modulators in human breast cancer cell lines. Effect on sulfatase and on 17β-hydroxysteroid dehydrogenase (17β-HSD) activity. *Anticancer Res.*, **24**, 1433–1438

Chlebowski, R.T., Hendrix, S.L., Langer, R.D., Stefanick, M.L., Gass, M., Lane, D., Rodabough, R.J., Gilligan, M.A., Cyr, M.G., Thomson, C.A., Khandekar, J., Petrovich, H. & McTiernan, A. for the WHI Investigators (2003) Influence of estrogen plus progestin on breast cancer and mammography in healthy postmenopausal women: The Women's Health Initiative Randomized Trial. *J. Am. med. Assoc.*, **289**, 3243–3253

Chlebowski, R.T., Wactawski-Wende, J., Ritenbaugh, C., Hubbell, F.A., Ascensao, J., Rodabough, R.J., Rosenberg, C.A., Taylor, V.M., Harris, R., Chen, C., Adams-Campbell, L.L. & White, E. for the Women's Health Initiative Investigators (2004) Estrogen plus progestin and colorectal cancer in postmenopausal women. *New Engl. J. Med.*, **350**, 991–1004

Christodoulakos, G.E., Lambrinoudaki, I.V., Panoulis, K.P.C., Vourtsi, A.D., Vlachos, L., Georgiou, E. & Creatsas, G.C. (2003) The effect of various regimens of hormone replacement therapy on mammographic breast density. *Maturitas*, **45**, 109–118

Cirillo, D.J., Wallace, R.B., Rodabough, R.J., Greenland, P., LaCroix, A.Z., Limacher, M.C. & Larson, J.C. (2005) Effect of estrogen therapy on gallbladder disease. *J. Am. med. Assoc.*, **293**, 330–339

Civitelli, R., Pilgram, T.K., Dotson, M., Muckerman, J., Lewandowski, N., Armamento-Villareal, R., Yokoyama-Crothers, N., Kardaris, E.E., Hauser J., Cohen, S. & Hildebolt, C.F. (2002) Alveolar and postcranial bone density in postmenopausal women receiving hormone/estrogen replacement therapy. A randomized, double-blind, placebo-controlled trial. *Arch. intern. Med.*, **162**, 1409–1415

Clarkson, T.B., Anthony, M.S. & Jerome, C.P. (1998) Lack of effect of raloxifene on coronary artery atherosclerosis of postmenopausal monkeys. *J. clin. Endocrinol. Metab.*, **83**, 721–726

Clarkson, T.B., Anthony, M.S. & Morgan, T.M. (2001) Inhibition of postmenopausal atherosclerosis progression: A comparison of the effects of conjugated equine estrogens and soy phyto-estrogens. *J. clin. Endocrinol. Metab.*, **86**, 41–47

Cline, J.M., Soderqvist, G., von Schoultz, E., Skoog, L. & von Schoultz, B. (1996) Effects of hormone replacement therapy on the mammary gland of surgically postmenopausal cyno-molgus macaques. *Am. J. Obstet. Gynecol.*, **174**, 93–100

Cline, J.M., Soderqvist, G., von Schoultz, E., Skoog, L. & von Schoultz, B. (1998) Effects of conju-gated estrogens, medroxyprogesterone acetate, and tamoxifen on the mammary glands of macaques. *Breast Cancer Res. Treat.*, **48**, 221–229

Cline, J.M., Register, T.C. & Clarkson, T.B. (2002a) Effects of tibolone and hormone replacement therapy on the breast of cynomolgus monkeys. *Menopause*, **9**, 422–429

Cline, J.M., Register, T.C., & Clarkson, T.B. (2002b) Comparative effects of tibolone and conju-gated equine estrogens with and without medroxyprogesterone acetate on the reproductive tract of female cynomulgus monkeys. *Menopause*, **9**, 242–252

Colacurci, N., Fornaro, F., de Franciscis, P., Palermo, M. & del Vecchio, W. (2001) Effects of diffe-rent types of hormone replacement therapy on mammographic density. *Maturitas*, **40**, 159–164

Coldham, N.G. & James, V.H.T. (1990) A possible mechanism for increased breast cell prolifera-tion by progestins through increased reductive 17β-hydroxysteroid dehydrogenase activity. *Int. J. Cancer*, **45**, 174–178

Colditz, G.A., Willett, W.C., Stampfer, M.J., Rosner, B., Speizer, F.E. & Hennekens, C.H. (1987) Menopause and the risk of coronary heart disease in women. *New Engl. J. Med.*, **316**, 1105–1110

Colditz, G.A., Egan, K.M. & Stampfer, M.J. (1993) Hormone replacement therapy and risk of breast cancer: Results from epidemiologic studies. *Am. J. Obstet. Gynecol.*, **168**, 1473–1480

Collaborative Group on Hormonal Factors in Breast Cancer (1997) Breast cancer and hormone replacement therapy: Collaborative reanalysis of data from 51 epidemiological studies of 52,705 women with breast cancer and 108,411 women without breast cancer. *Lancet*, **350**, 1047–1059

Collins, P., Rosano, G.M., Jiang, C., Lindsay, D., Sarrel, P.M. & Poole-Wilson, P.A. (1993) Cardio-vascular protection by oestrogen — A calcium antagonist effect? *Lancet*, **341**, 1264–1265

Collins, P., Rosano, G.M., Sarrel, P.M., Ulrich, L., Adamopoulos, S., Beale, C.M., McNeill, J.G. & Poole-Wilson, P.A. (1995) 17β-Estradiol attenuates acetylcholine-induced coronary arterial constriction in women but not men with coronary heart disease. *Circulation*, **92**, 24–30

Conner, P., Skoog, L. & Söderqvist, G. (2001) Breast epithelial proliferation in postmenopausal women evaluated through fine-needle-aspiration cytology. *Climacteric*, **4**, 7–12

Conner, P., Söderqvist, G., Skoog, L., Gräser, T., Walter, F., Tani, E., Carlström, K. & von Schoultz, B. (2003) Breast cell proliferation in postmenopausal women during HRT evaluated through fine needle aspiration cytology. *Breast Cancer Res. Treat.*, **78**, 159–165

Conner, P., Christow, A., Kersemaekers, W., Söderqvist, G., Skoog, L., Carlström, K., Tani, E., Mol-Arts, M. & von Schoultz, B. (2004a) A comparative study of breast cell proliferation during hormone replacement therapy: Effects of tibolon and continuous combined estrogen–progestogen treatment. *Climacteric*, **7**, 50–58

Conner, P., Svane, G., Azavedo, E., Söderqvist, G., Carlström, K., Gräser, T., Walter, F. & von Schoultz, B. (2004b) Mammographic breast density, hormones and growth factors during continuous combined hormone therapy. *Fertil. Steril.*, **81**, 1617–1623

Cooper, G.S., Dooley, M.A., Treadwell, E.L., St Clair, E.W. & Gilkeson, G.S. (2002) Hormonal and reproductive risk factors for development of systemic lupus erythematosus. *Arthrit. Rheum.*, **7**, 1830–1839

Coughlin, S.S., Giustozzi, A., Smith, S.J. & Lee, N.C. (2000) A meta-analysis of estrogen replacement therapy and risk of epithelial ovarian cancer. *J. clin. Epidemiol.*, **53**, 367–375

Couzinet, B., Young, J., Brailly, S., Chanson, P., Thomas, J.L. & Schaison, G. (1996) The antigonadotropic activity of progestins (19-nortestosterone and 19-norprogesterone derivatives) is not mediated through the androgen receptor. *J. clin Endocrinol. Metab.*, **81**, 4218–4223

Csizmadi, I., Collet, J.-P., Benedetti, A., Boivin, J.-F. & Hanley, J.A. (2004) The effects of transdermal and oral oestrogen replacement therapy on colorectal cancer risk in postmenopausal women. *Br. J. Cancer*, **90**, 76–81

Currie, L.J., Harrison, M.B., Trugman, J.M., Bennett, J.P. & Wooten, F. (2004) Postmenopausal estrogen use affects risk for Parkinson disease. *Arch. Neurol.*, **61**, 886–888

Cushman, M., Legault, C., Barrett-Connor, E., Stefanick, M.L., Kessler, C., Judd, H.L., Sakkinen, P.A. & Tracy, R.P. (1999) Effect of postmenopausal hormones on inflammation-sensitive proteins: The Postmenopausal Estrogen/Progestin Interventions (PEPI) Study. *Circulation*, **100**, 717–722

Cushman, M., Kuller, L.H., Prentice, R., Rodabough, R.J., Psaty, B.M., Stafford, R.S., Sidney, S. & Rosendaal, F.R. (2004) Estrogen plus progestin and risk of venous thrombosis. *J. Am. med. Assoc.*, **292**, 1573–1580

Dahmoun, M., Ödmark, I.-S., Risberg, B., Karlsson, M.G., Pavlenko, T. & Backstrom, T. (2004) Apoptosis, proliferation, and sex steroid receptors in postmenopausal endometrium before and during HRT. *Maturitas*, **49**, 114–123

Daling, J.R., Malone, K.E., Doody, D.R., Voigt, L.F., Bernstein, L., Coates, R.J., Marchbanks, P.A., Norman, S.A., Weiss, L.K., Ursin, G., Berlin, J.A., Burkman, R.T., Deapen, D., Folger, S.G., McDonald, J.A., Simon, M.S., Strom, B.L., Wingo, P.A. & Spirtas, R. (2002) Relation of regimens of combined hormone replacement therapy to lobular, ductal, and other histologic types of breast carcinoma. *Cancer*, **95**, 2455–2464

Davis, S.R., Dinatale, I., Rivera-Woll, L. & Davison, S. (2005) Postmenopausal hormone therapy: From monkey glands to transdermal patches. *J. Endocrinol.*, **185**, 207–222

Dawling, S., Roodi, N., Mernaugh, R.L., Wang, X. & Parl, F.F. (2001) Catechol-*O*-methyltransferase (COMT)-mediated metabolism of catechol estrogens: Comparison of wild-type and variant COMT isoforms. *Cancer Res.*, **61**, 6716–6722

Dawling, S., Roodi, N. & Parl, F.F. (2003) Methoxyestrogens exert feedback inhibition on cytochrome P450 1A1 and 1B1. *Cancer Res.*, **63**, 3127–3132

Dawling, S., Hachey, D.L., Roodi, N. & Parl, F.F. (2004) In vitro model of mammary estrogen metabolism: Structural and kinetic differences between catechol estrogens 2- and 4-hydroxyestradiol. *Chem. Res. Toxicol.*, **17**, 1258–1264

Deckers, G.H., Schoonen, W.G.E.J. & Kloosterboer, H.J. (2000) Influence of the substitution of 11-methylene, delta[15], and/or 18-methyl groups in norethisterone on receptor binding, transactivation assays and biological activities in animals. *J. steroid Biochem. mol. Biol.*, **74**, 83–92

Devanesan, P., Santen, R.J., Bocchinfuso, W.P., Korach, K.S., Rogan, E.G. & Cavalieri, E. (2001) Catechol estrogen metabolites and conjugates in mammary tumors and hyperplastic tissue from estrogen receptor-α knock-out (ERKO)/Wnt-1 mice: Implications for initiation of mammary tumors. *Carcinogenesis*, **22**, 1573–1576

De Vivo, I, Hankinson, S.E., Li, L., Colditz, G.A. & Hunter, D.J. (2002) Association of *CYP1B1* polymorphisms and breast cancer risk. *Cancer Epidemiol. Biomarkers Prev.*, **11**, 489–492

Dijkema, R., Schoonen, W.G.E.J., Teuwen, R., van der Struik, S.E., de Ries, R.J.H., van der Kar, B.A.T. & Olijve, W. (1998) Human progesterone receptor A and B isoforms in CHO cells. I. Stable transfection of receptor and receptor-responsive reporter genes: Transcription modulation by (anti)progestagens. *J. steroid Biochem. mol. Biol.*, **64**, 147–156

Donker, G.A., Spreeuwenberg, P., Bartelds, A.I.M., van der Velden, K. & Foets, M. (2000) Hormone replacement therapy: Changes in frequency and type of prescription by Dutch GPs during the last decade of the millennium. *Fam. Pract.*, **17**, 508–513

Dören, M., Rübig, A., Coelingh Bennink, H.J.T. & Holzgreve, W. (2001) Differential effects on the androgen status of postmenopausal women treated with tibolone and continuous combined estradiol and norethindrone acetate replacement therapy. *Fertil. Steril.*, **75**, 554–559

Ekström, H., Esseveld, J. & Hovelius, B. (2003) Associations between attitudes toward hormone therapy and current use of it in middle-aged women. *Maturitas*, **46**, 45–57

d'Elia, H.F., Larsen, A., Mattsson, L.-A., Waltbrand, E., Kvist, G., Mellström, D., Saxne, T., Ohlsson, C., Nordborg, E. & Carlsten, H. (2003) Influence of hormone replacement therapy on disease progression and bone mineral density in rheumatoid arthritis. *J. Rheumatol.* **30**, 1456–1463

El-Rayes, B.F., Ali, S., Heilbrun, L.K., Lababidi, S., Bouwman, D., Visscher, D. & Philip, P.A. (2003) Cytochrome P450 and glutathione transferase expression in human breast cancer. *Clin. Cancer Res.*, **9**, 1705–1709

Embrechts, J., Lemiere, F., Van Dongen, W., Esmans, E.L., Buytaert, P., Van Marck, E., Kockx, M. & Makar, A. (2003) Detection of estrogen DNA-adducts in human breast tumor tissue and healthy tissue by combined nano LC–nano ES tandem mass spectrometry. *J. Am. Soc. mass Spectrom.*, **14**, 482–491

Erel, C.T., Esen, G., Seyisoglu, H., Elter, K., Uras, C., Ertungealp, E. & Aksu, M.F. (2001) Mammographic density increase in women receiving different hormone replacement regimens. *Maturitas*, **40**, 151–157

Espeland, M.A., Applegate, W., Furberg, C.D., Lefkowitz, D., Rice, L. & Hunninghake, D. for the ACAPS Investigators (1995a) Estrogen replacement therapy and progression of intimal-medial thickness in the carotid arteries of postmenopausal women. *Am. J. Epidemiol.*, **142**, 1011–1019

Espeland, M.A., Bush, T.L., Mebane-Sims, I., Stefanick, M.L., Johnson, S., Sherwin, R. & Waclawiw, M. for the PEPI Trial Investigators (1995b) Rationale, design, and conduct of the PEPI Trial. *Control. clin. Trials*, **16**, 3S–19S

Espeland, M.A., Rapp. S.R., Shumaker, S.A., Brunner, R., Manson, J.E., Sherwin, B.B., Hsia, J., Margolis, K.L., Hogan, P.E., Wallace, R., Dailey, M., Freeman, R. & Hays, J. for the Women's Health Initiative Memory Study Investigators (2004) Conjugated equine estrogens and global cognitive function in postmenopausal women. Women's Health Initiative Memory Study. *J. Am. med. Assoc.*, **291**, 2959–2968

Ewertz, M., Mellemkjaer, L., Poulsen, A.H., Friis, S., Sorensen, H.T., Pedersen, L., McLaughlin, J.K. & Olsen, J.H. (2005) Hormone use for menopausal symptoms and risk of breast cancer. A Danish cohort study. *Br. J. Cancer*, **92**, 1293–1297

Facchinetti, F., Nappi, R.E., Tirelli, A., Polatti, F. & Nappi, G. (2002) Hormone supplementation differently affects migraine in postmenopausal women. *Headache*, **42**, 924–929

Falany, C.N., Xie, X., Wang, J., Ferrer, J. & Falany, J.L. (2000) Molecular cloning and expression of novel sulphotransferase-like cDNAs from human and rat brain. *Biochem. J.*, **346**, 857–864

Falany, J.L., Macrina, N. & Falany, C.N. (2002) Regulation of MCF-7 breast cancer cell growth by β-estradiol sulfation. *Breast Cancer Res. Treat.*, **74**, 167–176

Falk, R.T., Rossi, S.C., Fears, T.R., Sepkovic, D.W., Migella, A., Adlercreutz, H., Donaldson, J., Bradlow, H.L. & Ziegler, R.G. (2000) A new ELISA kit for measuring urinary 2-hydroxy-estrone, 16α-hydroxyestrone, and their ratio: Reproducibility, validity, and assay performance after freeze-thaw cycling and preservation by boric acid. *Cancer Epidemiol. Biomarkers Prev.*, **9**, 81–87

Fantl, J.A., Bump, R.C., Robinson, D., McClish, D.K., Wyman, J.R. & the Continence Program for Women Research Group (1996) Efficacy of estrogen supplementation in the treatment of urinary incontinence. *Obstet. Gynecol.*, **88**, 745–749

Faucher, F., Lacoste, L., Dufort, I. & Luu-The, V. (2001) High metabolization of catecholestrogens by type 1 estrogen sulfotransferase (hEST1). *J. steroid Biochem. mol. Biol.*, **77**, 83–86

Feigelson, H.S., McKean-Cowdin, R., Coetzee, G.A., Stram, D.O., Kolonel, L.N. & Henderson, B.E. (2001) Building a multigenic model of breast cancer susceptibility: *CYP17* and *HSD17B1* are two important candidates. *Cancer Res.*, **61**, 785–789

Felty, Q. & Roy, D. (2005a) Mitochondrial signals to nucleus regulate estrogen-induced cell growth. *Med. Hypotheses*, **64**, 133–141

Felty, Q. & Roy, D. (2005b) Estrogen, mitochondria, and growth of cancer and non-cancer cells. *J. Carcinog.*, **4**, 1

Felty, Q., Singh, K.P. & Roy, D. (2005a) Estrogen-induced G_1/S transition of G_0-arrested estrogen-dependent breast cancer cells is regulated by mitochondrial oxidant signaling. *Oncogene*, **24**, 4883–4893

Felty, Q., Xiong, W.-C., Sun, D., Sarkar, S., Singh, K.P., Parkash, J. & Roy, D. (2005b) Estrogen-induced mitochondrial reactive oxygen species as signal-transducing messengers. *Biochemistry*, **44**, 6900–6909

Ferenczy, A. & Gelfand, M.M. (1997) Endometrial histology and bleeding patterns in post-menopausal women taking sequential, combined estradiol and dydrogesterone. *Maturitas*, **26**, 219–226

Fernandez, S.V., Russo, I.H., Lareef, M., Balsara, B. & Russo, J. (2005) Comparative genomic hybridization of human breast epithelial cells transformed by estrogen and its metabolites. *Int. J. Oncol.*, **26**, 691–695

Fournier, A., Berrino, F., Riboli, E., Avenel, V. & Clavel-Chapelon, F. (2005) Breast cancer risk in relation to different types of hormone replacement therapy in the E3N-EPIC cohort. *Int. J. Cancer*, **114**, 448–454

Franke, H.R. & Vermes, I. (2002) The effect of continuous combined 17β-oestradiol and dihydro-dydrogesterone on apoptotic cell death and proliferation of human breast cancer cells in vitro. *Eur. J. Cancer*, **38** (Suppl.), S69–S70

Franke, H.R. & Vermes, I. (2003) Differential effects of progestogens on breast cancer cell lines. *Maturitas*, **46** (Suppl. 1), S55–S58

Franke, H.R., Kole, S., Ciftci, Z., Haanen, C. & Vermes, I. (2003) In vitro effects of estradiol, dydrogesterone, tamoxifen and cyclophosphamide on proliferation vs. death in human breast cancer cells. *Cancer Lett.*, **190**, 113–118

Freedman, M., San Martin, J., O'Gorman, J., Eckert, S., Lippman, M.E., Lo, S.-C.B., Walls, E.L. & Zeng, J. (2001) Digitized mammography: A clinical trial of postmenopausal women randomly assigned to receive raloxifene, estrogen, or placebo. *J. natl Cancer Inst.*, **93**, 51–56

Freeman, E.E., Munoz, B., Schein, O.D. & West, S.K. (2004) Incidence and progression of lens opacities. Effect of hormone replacement therapy and reproductive factors. *Epidemiology*, **15**, 451–457

Fugère, P., Scheele, W.H., Shah, A., Strack, T.R., Glant, M.D. & Jolly, E. (2000) Uterine effects of raloxifene in comparison with continuous–combined hormone replacement therapy in post-menopausal women. *Am. J. Obstet. Gynecol.*, **182**, 568–574

Gabriel-Sánchez, R., Carmona, L., Roque, M., Sánchez-Gómez. L.M. & Bonfill, X. (2005) Hormone replacement therapy for preventing cardiovascular disease in post-menopausal women. *Cochrane Database. Syst. Rev.*, CD002229

Gall, W.E., Zawada, G., Mojarrabi, B., Tephly, T.R., Green, M.D., Coffman, B.L., Mackenzie, P.I. & Radominska-Pandya, A. (1999) Differential glucuronidation of bile acids, androgens and estrogens by human UGT1A3 and 2B7. *J. steroid Biochem. mol. Biol.*, **70**, 101–108

Gambacciani, M., Monteleone, P., Vitale, C., Silvestri, A., Fini, M., Genazzani, A.R. & Rosano, G.M.C. (2002) Dydrogesterone does not reverse the effects of estradiol on endothelium-dependant vasodilation in postmenopausal women: A randomized clinical trial. *Maturitas*, **43**, 117–123

Gambrell, R.D. (1986) Prevention of endometrial cancer with progestogens. *Maturitas*, **8**, 159–168

Garciá-Becerra, R., Cooney, A.J., Borja-Cacho, E., Lemus, A.E., Pérez-Palacios, G. & Larrea, F. (2004) Comparative evaluation of androgen and progesterone receptor transcription selectivity indices of 19-nortestosterone-derived progestins. *J. steroid Biochem. mol. Biol.*, **91**, 21–27

Garg, P.P., Kerlikowske, K., Subak, L. & Grady, D. (1998) Hormone replacement therapy and the risk of epithelial ovarian carcinoma: A meta-analysis. *Obstet. Gynecol.*, **92**, 472–479

Garte, S., Gaspari, L., Alexandrie, A.K., Ambrosone, C., Autrup, H., Autrup, J.L., Baranova, H., Bathum, L., Benhamou, S., Boffetta, P., Bouchardy, C., Breskvar, K., Brockmoller, J., Cascorbi, I., Clapper, M.L., Coutelle, C., Daly, A., Dell'Omo, M., Dolzan, V., Dresler, C.M., Fryer, A., Haugen, A., Hein, D.W., Hildesheim, A., Hirvonen, A., Hsieh, L.-L., Ingelman-Sundberg, M., Kalina, I., Kang, D., Kihara, M., Kiyohara, C., Kremers, P., Lazarus, P., Le Marchand, L., Lechner, M.C., van Lieshout, E.M.M., London, S., Manni, J.J., Maugard, C.M., Morita, S., Nazar-Stewart, V., Noda, K., Oda, Y., Parl, F.F., Pastorelli, R., Persson, I., Peters, W.H.M., Rannug, A., Rebbeck, T., Risch, A., Roelandt, L., Romkes, M., Ryberg, D., Salagovic, J., Schoket, B., Seidegard, J., Shields, P.G., Sim, E., Sinnet, D., Strange, R.C., Stücker, I., Sugimura, H., To-Figueras, J., Vineis, P., Yu, M.C. & Taioli, E. (2001) Metabolic gene polymorphism frequencies in control populations. *Cancer Epidemiol. Biomarkers Prev.*, **10**, 1239–1248

Georgiev, D.B. & Manassiev, N.A. (2002) Effect of long-term continuous combined hormone replacement therapy with estradiol valerate and either dienogest or norethisterone acetate on mammographic density in postmenopausal women. *Medscape Womens Health*, **7**, 1

Gestl, S.A., Green, M.D., Shearer, D.A., Frauenhoffer, E., Tephly, T.R. & Weisz, J. (2002) Expression of UGT2B7, a UDP-glucuronosyltransferase implicated in the metabolism of 4-hydroxyestrone and all-*trans* retinoic acid, in normal human breast parenchyma and in invasive and *in situ* breast cancers. *Am. J. Pathol.*, **160**, 1467–1479

Gilligan, D.M., Quyyumi, A.A. & Cannon, R.O., III (1994a) Effects of physiological levels of estrogen on coronary vasomotor function in postmenopausal women. *Circulation*, **89**, 2545–2551

Gilligan, D.M., Badar, D.M., Panza, J.A., Quyyumi, A.A. & Cannon, R.O., III (1994b) Acute vascular effects of estrogen in postmenopausal women. *Circulation*, **90**, 786–791

Glatt, H., Engelke, C.E., Pabel, U., Teubner, W., Jones, A.L., Coughtrie, M.W., Andrae, U., Falany, C.N. & Meinl, W. (2000) Sulfotransferases: Genetics and role in toxicology. *Toxicol. Lett.*, **112–113**, 341–348

Glud, E., Kjaer, S.K., Thomsen, B.L., Hogdall, C., Christensen, L., Hogdall, E., Bock, J.E. & Blaakaer, J. (2004) Hormone therapy and the impact of estrogen intake on the risk of ovarian cancer. *Arch. intern. Med.*, **164**, 2253–2259

Goldstein, S.R., Johnson, S., Watts, N.B., Ciaccia, A.V., Elmerick, D. & Muram, D. (2005) Incidence of urinary incontinence in postmenopausal women treated with raloxifene or estrogen. *Menopause*, **12**, 160–164

Goodman, M.T., McDuffie, K., Kolonel, L.N., Terada, K., Donlon, T.A., Wilkens, L.R., Guo, C. & Le Marchand, L. (2001) Case–control study of ovarian cancer and polymorphisms in genes involved in catecholestrogen formation and metabolism. *Cancer Epidemiol. Biomarkers Prev.*, **10**, 209–216

Goodman, J.E., Lavigne, J.A., Wu, K., Helzlsouer, K.J., Strickland, P.T., Selhub, J. & Yager, J.D. (2001) *COMT* genotype, micronutrients in the folate metabolic pathway and breast cancer risk. *Carcinogenesis*, **22**, 1661–1665

Goodman, J.E., Jensen, L.T., He, P. & Yager, J.D. (2002) Characterization of human soluble high and low activity catechol-*O*-methyltransferase catalyzed catechol estrogen methylation. *Pharmacogenetics*, **12**, 517–528

Gordon, T., Kannel, W.B., Hjortland, M.C. & McNamara, P.M. (1978) Menopause and coronary heart disease. The Framingham Study. *Ann. intern. Med.*, **89**, 157–161

Goth-Goldstein, R., Stampfer, M.R., Erdmann, C.A. & Russell, M. (2000) Interindividual variation in *CYP1A1* expression in breast tissue and the role of genetic polymorphism. *Carcinogenesis*, **21**, 2119–2122

Grady, D., Rubin, S.M., Petitti, D.B., Fox, C.S., Black, D., Ettinger, B., Ernster, V.L. & Cummings, S.R. (1992) Hormone therapy to prevent disease and prolong life in postmenopausal women. *Ann. intern. Med.*, **117**, 1016–1037

Grady, D., Applegate, W., Bush, T., Furberg, C., Riggs, B. & Hulley, S.B., for the HERS Research Group (1998) Heart and Estrogen/Progestin Replacement Study (HERS): Design, methods, and baseline characteristics. *Control. clin. Trials,* **19**, 314–335

Grady, D., Brown, J.S., Vittinghoff, E., Applegate, W., Varner, E. & Snyder, T. for the HERS Research Group (2001) Postmenopausal hormones and incontinence: The Heart and Estrogen/Progestin Replacement Study. *Obstet. Gynecol.*, **97**, 116–120

Grady, D., Herrington, D., Bittner, V., Blumenthal, R., Davidson, M., Hlatky, M., Hsia, J., Hulley, S., Herd, A., Khan, S., Newby, L.K., Waters, D., Vittinghoff, E. & Wenger, N. for the HERS Research Group (2002a) Cardiovascular disease outcomes during 6.8 years of hormone therapy: Heart and Estrogen/Progestin Replacement Study follow-up (HERS II). *J. Am. med. Assoc.*, **288**, 49–57

Grady, D., Yaffe, K., Kristof, M., Lin, F., Richards, C. & Barrett-Connor, E. (2002b) Effect of post-menopausal hormone therapy on cognitive function: The Heart and Estrogen/progestin Replacement Study. *Am. J. Med.*, **113**, 543–548

Greendale, G.A., Reboussin, B.A., Hogan, P., Barnabei, V.M., Shumaker, S., Johnson, S. & Barrett-Connor, E. for the Postmenopausal Estrogen/Progestin Interventions Trial Investigators (1998) Symptom relief and side effects of postmenopausal hormones: Results from the Postmenopausal Estrogen/Progestin Interventions Trial. *Obstet. Gynecol.*, **92**, 982–988

Greendale, G.A., Lee, N.P. & Arriola, E.R. (1999) The menopause. *Lancet*, **353**, 571–580

Greendale, G.A., Reboussin, B.A., Slone, S., Wasilauskas, C., Pike, M.C. & Ursin, G. (2003) Post-menopausal hormone therapy and change in mammographic density. *J. natl Cancer Inst.*, **95**, 30–37

Grodstein, F., Manson, J.E., Colditz, G.A., Willett, W.C., Speizer, F.E. & Stampfer, M.J. (2000) A prospective, observational study of postmenopausal hormone therapy and primary prevention of cardiovascular disease. *Ann. intern. Med.*, **133**, 933–941

Grundy, S.M., Pasternak, R., Greenland, P., Smith, S. & Fuster, V. (1999) Assessment of cardio-vascular risk by use of multiple-risk-factor assessment equations: A statement for healthcare professionals from the American Heart Association and the American College of Cardiology. *J. Am. Coll. Cardiol.*, **34**, 1348–1359

Guillemette, C., Millikan, R.C., Newman, B. & Housman, D.E. (2000) Genetic polymorphisms in uridine diphospho-glucuronosyltransferase 1A1 and association with breast cancer among African Americans. *Cancer Res.*, **60**, 950–956

Guillemette, C., De Vivo, I., Hankinson, S.E., Haiman, C.A., Spiegelman, D., Housman, D.E. & Hunter, D.J. (2001) Association of genetic polymorphisms in UGT1A1 with breast cancer and plasma hormone levels. *Cancer Epidemiol. Biomarkers Prev.*, **10**, 711–714

Gunnarsson, C., Olsson, B.M. & Stål, O. (2001) Abnormal expression of 17β-hydroxysteroid dehydrogenases in breast cancer predicts late recurrence. *Cancer Res.*, **61**, 8448–8451

Gunnarsson, C., Ahnström, M., Kirschner, K., Olsson, B., Nordenskjöld, B., Rutqvist, L.E., Skoog, L. & Stål, O. (2003) Amplification of *HSD17B1* and *ERBB2* in primary breast cancer. *Oncogene*, **22**, 34–40

Haas, J.S., Kaplan, C.P., Gerstenberger, E.P. & Kerlikowske, K. (2004) Changes in the use of postmenopausal hormone therapy after the publication of clinical trial results. *Ann. intern. Med.*, **140**, 184–188

Habiba, M.A., Bell, S.C. & Al-Azzawi, F. (1998) Endometrial responses to hormone replacement therapy: Histological features compared with those of late luteal phase endometrium. *Hum. Reprod.*, **13**, 1674–1682

Hachey, D.L., Dawling, S., Roodi, N. & Parl, F.F. (2003) Sequential action of phase I and II enzymes cytochrome P450 1B1 and glutathione S-transferase P1 in mammary estrogen metabolism. *Cancer Res.*, **63**, 8492–8499

Hammond, C.B., Jelovsek, F.R., Lee, K.L., Creasman, W.T. & Parker, R.T. (1979) Effects of long-term estrogen replacement therapy. II. Neoplasia. *Am. J. Obstet. Gynecol.*, **133**, 537–547

Hänggi, W., Bersinger, N., Altermatt, H.J. & Birkhäuser, M.H. (1997) Comparison of transvaginal ultrasonography and endometrial biopsy in endometrial surveillance in postmenopausal HRT users. *Maturitas*, **27**, 133–143

Hanna, I.H., Dawling, S., Roodi, N., Guengerich, F.P. & Parl, F.F. (2000) Cytochrome P450 *1B1* (*CYP1B1*) pharmacogenetics: Association of polymorphisms with functional differences in estrogen hydroxylation activity. *Cancer Res.*, **60**, 3440–3444

Hannaford, P. & Elliot, A. (2005) Use of exogenous hormones by women and colorectal cancer: Evidence from the Royal College of General Practitioners' Oral Contraception Study. *Contraception*, **71**, 95–98

Hargreaves, D.F., Knox, F., Swindell, R., Potten, C.S. & Bundred, N.J. (1998) Epithelial proliferation and hormone receptor status in the normal post-menopausal breast and the effects of hormone replacement therapy. *Br. J. Cancer*, **78**, 945–949

Hays, J., Ockene, J.K., Brunner, R.L., Kotchen, J.M., Manson, J.E., Patterson, R.E., Aragaki, A.K., Shumaker, S.A., Brzyski, R.G., LaCroix, A.Z., Granek, I.A. & Valanis, B.G. for the Women's Health Initiative Investigators (2003a) Effects of estrogen plus progestin on health-related quality of life. *New Engl. J. Med.*, **348**, 1839–1854

Hays, J., Hunt, J.R., Hubbell, F.A., Anderson, G.L., Limacher, M., Allen, C. & Rossouw, J.E. (2003b) The Women's Health Initiative recruitment methods and results. *Ann. Epidemiol.*, **13**, S18–S77

Heald, A., Selby, P.L., White, A. & Gibson, J.M. (2000) Progestins abrogate estrogen-induced changes in the insulin-like growth factor axis. *Am. J. Obstet. Gynecol.*, **183**, 593–600

Henderson, V.W., Paganini-Hill, A., Miller, B.L., Elble, R.J., Reyes, P.F., Shoupe, D., McCleary, C.A., Klein, R.A., Hake, A.M. & Farlow, M.R. (2000) Estrogen for Alzheimer's disease in women: Randomized, double-blind, placebo-controlled trial. *Neurology*, **54**, 295–301

Hendrix, S.L., Cochrane, B.B., Nygaard, I.E., Handa, V.L., Barnabei, V.M., Iglesia, C., Aragaki, A., Naughton, M.J., Wallace, R.B. & McNeeley, S.G. (2005) Effects of estrogen with and without progestin on urinary incontinence. *J. Am. med. Assoc.*, **293**, 935–948

Heng, D., Gao, F., Jong, R., Fishell, E., Yaffe, M., Martin, L., Li, T., Stone, J., Sun, L., & Hopper, J. (2004) Risk factors for breast cancer associated with mammographic features in Singaporean chinese women. *Cancer Epidemiol. Biomarkers Prev.*, **13**, 1751–1758

Herrington, D.M., Braden, G.A., Williams, J.K. & Morgan, T.M. (1994) Endothelial-dependent coronary vasomotor responsiveness in postmenopausal women with and without estrogen replacement therapy. *Am. J. Cardiol.*, **73**, 951–952

Herrington, D.M., Reboussin, D.M., Brosnihan, K.B., Sharp, P.C., Shumaker, S.A., Snyder, T.E., Furberg, C.D., Kowalchuk, G.J., Stuckey, T.D., Rogers, W.J., Givens, D.H. & Waters, D. (2000) Effects of estrogen replacement on the progression of coronary–artery atherosclerosis. *New Engl. J. Med.*, **343**, 522–529

Herrington, D.M., Espeland, M.A., Crouse, J.R., III, Robertson, J., Riley, W.A., McBurnie, M.A. & Burke, G.L. (2001) Estrogen replacement and brachial artery flow-mediated vasodilation in older women. *Arterioscler. Thromb. vasc. Biol.*, **21**, 1955–1961

Hersh, A.L., Stefanick, M.L. & Stafford, R.S. (2004) National use of postmenopausal hormone therapy: Annual trends and response to recent evidence. *J. Am. med. Assoc.*, **291**, 47–53

Hill, D.A., Weiss, N.S., Beresford, S.A., Voigt, L.F., Daling, J.R., Stanford, J.L. & Self, S. (2000) Continuous combined hormone replacement therapy and risk of endometrial cancer. *Am. J. Obstet. Gynecol.*, **183**, 1456–1461

Hirvonen, E. (1996) Progestins. *Maturitas*, **23** (Suppl.), S13–S18

Hlatky, M.A., Boothroyd, D., Vittinghoff, E., Sharp, P. & Whooley, M.A. for the HERS Research Group (2002) Quality-of-life and depressive symptoms in postmenopausal women after receiving hormone therapy. Results from the Heart and Estrogen/Progestin Replacement Study (HERS) Trial. *J. Am. med. Assoc.*, **287**, 591–597

Ho, G.H., Luo, X.W., Ji, C.Y., Foo, S.C. & Ng E.H. (1998) Urinary 2/16α-hydroxyestrone ratio: Correlation with serum insulin-like growth factor binding protein-3 and a potential biomarker of breast cancer risk. *Ann. Acad. Med. Singapore*, **27**, 294–299

Hochberg, R.B. (1998) Biological esterification of steroids. *Endocr. Rev.*, **19**, 331–348

Hodis, H.N., Mack, W.J., Lobo, R.A., Shoupe, D., Sevanian, A., Mahrer, P.R., Selzer, R.H., Liu, C.-R., Liu, C.-H. & Azen, S.P. (2001) Estrogen in the prevention of atherosclerosis. A randomized, double-blind, placebo-controlled trial. *Ann. intern. Med.*, **135**, 939–953

Hoffmann, H., Hillesheim, H.G., Güttner, J., Stade, K., Merbt, E.-M., Holle, K., Oettel, M., Strecke, J., Hesse, G., Horn, U., Valentin, U., Lemke, H., Chemnitius, K.H., Schimmel, I., Deufrains, J., Hesse, V., Keil, E., Klinger, G., Klinger, G., Stelzner, A., Furcht, R., Gaida, P., Anke, M., Dettmann, R., Kramp, B. & Robiller, F. (1983) Long term toxicological studies on the progestin STS 557. *Exp. clin. Endocrinol.*, **81**, 179–196

Hofling, M., Carlström, K., Svane, G., Azavedo, E., Kloosterboer, H. & von Schoultz, B. (2005) Different effects of tibolone and continuous combined estrogen plus progestogen hormone therapy on sex hormone binding globulin and free testosterone levels—An association with mammographic density. *Gynecol. Endocrinol.*, **20**, 110–115

Hofseth, L.J., Raafat, A.M., Osuch, J.R., Pathak, D.R., Slomski, C.A. & Haslam, S.Z. (1999) Hormone replacement therapy with estrogen or estrogen plus medroxyprogesterone acetate is associated with increased epithelial proliferation in the normal postmenopausal breast. *J. clin. Endocrinol. Metab.*, **84**, 4559–4565

Hong, C.-C., Thompson, H.J., Jiang, C., Hammond, G.L., Tritchler, D., Yaffe, M. & Boyd, N.F. (2003) Val158Met polymorphism in *catechol-O-methyltransferase* gene associated with risk factors for breast cancer. *Cancer Epidemiol. Biomarkers Prev.*, **12**, 838–847

Hoover, R., Gray, L.A., Sr, Cole, P. & MacMahon, B. (1976) Menopausal estrogens and breast cancer. *New Engl. J. Med.*, **295**, 401–405

Horwitz, K.B. & Horwitz, L.D. (1982) Canine vascular tissues are targets for androgens, estrogens, progestins, and glucocorticoids. *J. clin. Invest.*, **69**, 750–758

Hu, X., Xia, H., Srivastava, S.K., Herzog, C., Awasthi, Y.C., Ji, X., Zimniak, P. & Singh, S.V. (1997) Activity of four allelic forms of glutathione S-transferase hGSTP1-1 for diol epoxides of polycyclic aromatic hydrocarbons. *Biochem. biophys. Res. Commun.*, **238**, 397–402

Huang, C.-S., Shen, C.-Y., Chang, K.-J., Hsu, S.-M. & Chern, H.-D. (1999) Cytochrome P4501A1 polymorphism as a susceptibility factor for breast cancer in postmenopausal Chinese women in Taiwan. *Br. J. Cancer*, **80**, 1838–1843

Huang, P., Feng, L., Oldham, E.A., Keating, M.J. & Plunkett, W. (2000) Superoxide dismutase as a target for the selective killing of cancer cells. *Nature*, **407**, 390–395

Huang, Y.H., Galijatovic, A., Nguyen, N., Geske, D., Beaton, D., Green, J., Green, M., Peters, W.H. & Tukey, R.H. (2002) Identification and functional characterization of UDP-glucurono-syltransferases UGT1A8*1, UGT1A8*2 and UGT1A8*3. *Pharmacogenetics*, **12**, 287–297

Hulley, S., Furberg, C., Barrett-Connor, E., Cauley, J., Grady, D., Haskell, W., Knopp, R., Lowery, M., Satterfield, S., Schrott, H., Vittinghoff, E. & Hunninghake, D. for the HERS Research Group (2002) Noncardiovascular disease outcomes during 6.8 years of hormone therapy: Heart and Estrogen/Progestin Replacement Study follow-up (HERS II). *J. Am. med. Assoc.*, **288**, 58–66

Hulley, S., Grady, D., Bush, T., Furberg, C., Herrington, D., Riggs, B. & Vittinghoff, E. (1998) Randomized trial of estrogen plus progestin for secondary prevention of coronary heart disease in postmenopausal women. Heart and Estrogen/Progestin Replacement Study (HERS) Research Group. *J. Am. med. Assoc.*, **280**, 605–613

Hundal, B.S., Dhillon, V.S. & Sidhu, I.S. (1997) Genotoxic potential of estrogens. *Mutat. Res.*, **389**, 173–181

Hurh, Y.-J., Chen, Z.-H., Na, H.-K., Han, S.-Y. & Surh, Y.-J. (2004) 2-Hydroxyestradiol induces oxidative DNA damage and apoptosis in human mammary epithelial cells. *J. Toxicol. environ Health*, **A67**, 1939–1953

IARC (1979) *IARC Monographs on the Evaluation of the Carcinogenic Risks of Chemicals to Humans*, Vol. 21, *Sex Hormones (II)*, Lyon

IARC (1999) *IARC Monographs on the Evaluation of Carcinogenic Risks to Humans*, Vol. 72, *Hormonal Contraception and Post-menopausal Hormonal Therapy*, Lyon

IARC (2007) *IARC Monographs on the Evaluation of Carcinogenic Risks to Humans*, Vol. 90, *Human Papillomaviruses*, Lyon

Iatrakis, G., Tsionis, C., Antoniadis, S. & Kourounis, G. (2004) Effect on endometrium of combined oestrogen–progestogen replacement therapy of 1 mg 17β-estradiol and 0.5 mg norethisterone acetate. *Clin. exp. Obstet. Gynecol.*, **31**, 50–52

IMS Health (2005) *IMS Health MIDAS*, June

Isaksson, E., Wang, H., Sahlin, L., von Schoultz, B., Cline, J.M. & von Schoultz, E. (2003) Effects of long-term HRT and tamoxifen on the expression of progesterone receptors A and B in breast tissue from surgically postmenopausal cynomolgus macaques. *Breast Cancer Res. Treat.*, **79**, 233–239

Jackson, S., Shepherd, A., Brookes, S. & Abrams, P. (1999) The effect of oestrogen supplementation on post-menopausal urinary stress incontinence: A double-blind placebo-controlled trial. *Br. J. Obstet. Gynaecol.*, **106**, 711–718

Jacobs, E.J., White, E., Weiss, N.S., Heckbert, S.R., LaCroix, A. & Barlow, W.E. (1999) Hormone replacement therapy and colon cancer among members of a health maintenance organization. *Epidemiology*, **10**, 445–451

Jain, M.G., Rohan, T.E. & Howe, G.R. (2000) Hormone replacement therapy and endometrial cancer in Ontario, Canada. *J. clin. Epidemiol.*, **53**, 385–391

Jefcoate, C.R., Liehr, J.G., Santen, R.J., Sutter, T.R., Yager, J.D., Yue, W., Santner, S.J., Tekmal, R., Demers, L., Pauley, R., Naftolin, F., Mor, G. & Berstein, L. (2000) Tissue-specific synthesis and oxidative metabolism of estrogens. *J. natl Cancer Inst. Monogr.*, **27**, 95–112

Jernström, H., Bendahl, P.O., Lidfeldt, J., Nerbrand, C., Agardh, C.D. & Samsioe, G. (2003a) A prospective study of different types of hormone replacement therapy use and the risk of subsequent breast cancer: The Women's Health in the Lund Area (WHILA) study (Sweden). *Cancer Causes Control*, **14**, 673–680

Jernström, H., Klug, T.L., Sepkovic, D.W., Bradlow, H.L. & Narod, S.A. (2003b) Predictors of the plasma ratio of 2-hydroxyestrone to 16α-hydroxyestrone among pre-menopausal, nulliparous women from four ethnic groups. *Carcinogenesis*, **24**, 991–1005

Ji, X., Blaszczyk, J., Xiao, B., O'Donnell, R., Hu, X., Herzog, C., Singh, S.V. & Zimniak, P. (1999) Structure and function of residue 104 and water molecules in the xenobiotic substrate-binding site in human glutathione *S*-transferase P1-1. *Biochemistry*, **38**, 10231–10238

Jiang, C., Sarrel, P.M., Lindsay, D.C., Poole-Wilson, P.A. & Collins, P. (1991) Endothelium-independent relaxation of rabbit coronary artery by 17 β-oestradiol *in vitro*. *Br J Pharmacol.*, **104**, 1033–1037

Jiang, C., Poole-Wilson, P.A., Sarrel, P.M., Mochizuki, S., Collins, P. & MacLeod, K.T. (1992a) Effect of 17β-oestradiol on contraction, Ca^{2+} current and intracellular free Ca^{2+} in guinea-pig isolated cardiac myocytes. *Br. J. Pharmacol.*, **106**, 739–745

Jiang, C., Sarrel, P.M., Poole-Wilson, P.A., & Collins, P. (1992b) Acute effect of 17β-estradiol on rabbit coronary artery contractile responses to endothelin-1. *Am. J. Physiol.*, **263**, H271–H275

Jiang, C., Sarrel, P.M., Lindsay, D.C., Poole-Wilson, P.A. & Collins, P. (1992c) Progesterone induces endothelium-independent relaxation of rabbit coronary artery in vitro. *Eur. J. Pharmacol.*, **211**, 163–167

Jick, S.S., Walker, A.M. & Jick, H. (1993) Estrogens, progesterone, and endometrial cancer. *Epidemiology*, **4**, 20–24

Johannisson, E., Holinka, C.F. & Arrenbrecht, S. (1997) Transdermal sequential and continuous hormone replacement regimens with estradiol and norethisterone acetate in postmenopausal women: Effects on the endometrium. *Int. J. Fertil. Womens Med.*, **42** (Suppl. 2), 388–398

Jolleys, J.V. & Olesen, F. (1996) A comparative study of prescribing of hormone replacement therapy in USA and Europe. *Maturitas*, **23**, 47–53

Jondet, M., Maroni, M., Yaneva, H., Brin, S., Peltier-Pujol, F. & Pelissier, C. (2002) Comparative endometrial histology in postmenopausal women with sequential hormone replacement therapy of estradiol and either chlormadinone acetate or micronized progesterone. *Maturitas*, **41**, 115–121

Jordan, A. (2002) Toxicology of progestogens of implantable contraceptives for women. *Contraception*, **65**, 3–8

Kanaya, A.M., Herrington, D., Vittinghoff, E., Lin, F., Grady, D., Bittner, V., Cauley, J.A. & Barrett-Connor, E. for the Heart and Estrogen/Progestin Replacement Study (2003) Glycemic effects of postmenopausal hormone therapy: The Heart and Estrogen/Progestin Replacement Study. A randomized, double-blind, placebo-controlled trial. *Ann. intern. Med.*, **138**, 1–9

Karolinska Institutet (2007) [http://www.imm.ki.se/CYPalleles/cyp1A1.htm], accessed 20 December 2007

Kawas, C., Resnick, S., Morrison, A., Brookmeyer, R., Corrada, M., Zonderman, A., Bacal, C., Lingle, D.D. & Metter, E. (1997) A prospective study of estrogen replacement therapy and the risk of developing Alzheimer's disease: The Baltimore Longitudinal Study of Aging. *Neurology*, **48**, 1517–1521

Keam, S.J. & Wagstaff, A.J. (2003) Ethinylestradiol/drospirenone: A review of its use as an oral contraceptive. *Treat. Endocrinol.*, **2**, 49–70

Kelley, K., Engqvist-Goldstein, A., Montali, J.A., Wheatley, J.B., Schmidt, D.E., Jr & Kauvar, L.M. (1994) Variability of glutathione *S*-transferase isoenzyme patterns in matched normal and cancer human breast tissue. *Biochem. J.*, **304**, 843–848

Kennedy, D.L., Baum, C. & Forbes, M.B. (1985) Noncontraceptive estrogens and progestins: Use patterns over time. *Obstet. Gynecol.*, **65**, 441–446

Kim-Schulze, S., McGowen, K.A., Hubchak, S.C., Cid, M.C., Martin, M.B., Kleinman, H.K., Greene, G.L. & Schnaper, H.W. (1996) Expression of an estrogen receptor by human coronary artery and umbilical vein endothelial cells. *Circulation*, **94**, 1402–1407

King, C.D., Rios, G.R., Green, M.D. & Tephly, T.R. (2000) UDP-glucuronosyltransferases. *Curr. Drug Metab.*, **1**, 143–161

Kirsh, V. & Kreigcr, N. (2002) Estrogen and estrogen–progestin replacement therapy and risk of postmenopausal breast cancer in Canada. *Cancer Causes Control*, **13**, 583–590

Kisselev, P., Schunck, W.-H., Roots, I. & Schwarz, D. (2005) Association of CYP1A1 polymorphisms with differential metabolic activation of 17β-estradiol and estrone. *Cancer Res.*, **65**, 2972–2978

Klauber, N., Parangi, S., Flynn, E., Hamel, E. & D'Amato, R.J. (1997) Inhibition of angiogenesis and breast cancer in mice by the microtubule inhibitors 2-methoxyestradiol and taxol. *Cancer Res.*, **57**, 81–86

Koh, K.K., Horne, M.K., III & Cannon, R.O., III (1999) Effects of hormone replacement therapy on coagulation, fibrinolysis, and thrombosis risk in postmenopausal women. *Thromb. Haemost.*, **82**, 626–633

Kong, L.-Y., Szaniszlo, P., Albrecht, T. & Liehr, J.G. (2000) Frequency and molecular analysis of *Hprt* mutations induced by estradiol in Chinese hamster V79 cells. *Int. J. Oncol.*, **17**, 1141–1149

Krajinovic, M., Ghadirian, P., Richer, C., Sinnett, H., Gandini, S., Perret, C., LaCroix, A., Labuda, D. & Sinnett, D. (2001) Genetic susceptibility to breast cancer in French-Canadians: Role of carcinogen-metabolizing enzymes and gene–environment interactions. *Int. J. Cancer*, **92**, 220–225

Krattenmacher, R. (2000) Drospirenone: Pharmacology and pharmacokinetics of a unique progestogen. *Contraception*, **62**, 29–38

Krebs, O., Schafer, B., Wolff, T., Oesterle, D., Deml, E., Sund, M. & Favor, J. (1998) The DNA damaging drug cyproterone acetate causes gene mutations and induces glutathione-S-transferase P in the liver of female Big Blue™ transgenic F344 rats. *Carcinogenesis*, **19**, 241–245

Kronenberg, F., Cote, L.J., Linkie, D.M., Dyrenfurth, I. & Downey, J.A. (1984) Menopausal hot flashes: Thermoregulatory, cardiovascular, and circulating catecholamine and LH changes. *Maturitas*, **6**, 31–43

Kumar, N., Koide, S.S., Tsong, Y.-Y. & Sundaram, K. (2000) Nestorone: A progestin with a unique pharmacological profile. *Steroids*, **65**, 629–636

Kurman, R.J., Félix, J.C., Archer, D.F., Nanavati, N., Arce, J.-C. & Moyer, D.L. (2000) Norethindrone acetate and estradiol-induced endometrial hyperplasia. *Obstet. Gynecol.*, **96**, 373–379

Lacey, J.V., Jr, Mink, P.J., Lubin, J.H., Sherman, M.E., Troisi, R., Hartge, P., Schatzkin, A. & Schairer, C. (2002) Menopausal hormone replacement therapy and risk of ovarian cancer. *J. Am. med. Assoc.*, **288**, 334–341

Lachman, H.M., Papolos, D.F., Saito, T., Yu, Y.M., Szumlanski, C.L. & Weinshilboum, R.M. (1996) Human catechol-*O*-methyltransferase pharmacogenetics: Description of a functional polymorphism and its potential application to neuropsychiatric disorders. *Pharmacogenetics*, **6**, 243–250

Larrea, F., Garcia-Beccera, R., Lemus, A.E., Garcia, G.A., Pérez-Palacios, Jackson, K.J., Coleman, K.M., Dace, R., Smith, C.L. & Cooney, A.J. (2001) A-ring reduced metabolites of 19-nor synthetic progestins as subtype selective agonists for ERα. *Endocrinology*, 3791–3799

Larsen, M.C., Angus, W.G.R., Brake, P.B., Eltom, S.E., Sukow, K.A. & Jefcoate, C.R. (1998) Characterization of CYP1B1 and CYP1A1 expression in human mammary epithelial cells: Role of the aryl hydrocarbon receptor in polycyclic aromatic hydrocarbon metabolism. *Cancer Res.*, **58**, 2366–2374

Lautala, P., Ulmanen, I. & Taskinen, J. (2001) Molecular mechanisms controlling the rate and specificity of catechol O-methylation by human soluble catechol O-methyltransferase. *Mol. Pharmacol.*, **59**, 393–402

LaVallee, T.M., Zhan, X.H., Johnson, M.S., Herbstritt, C.J., Swartz, G., Williams, M.S., Hembrough, W.A., Green, S.J. & Pribluda, V.S. (2003) 2-Methoxyestradiol up-regulates death receptor 5 and induces apoptosis through activation of the extrinsic pathway. *Cancer Res.*, **63**, 468–475

Lavigne, J.A., Goodman, J.E., Fonong, T., Odwin, S., He, P., Roberts, D.W. & Yager, J.D. (2001) The effects of catechol-*O*-methyltransferase inhibition on estrogen metabolite and oxidative DNA damage levels in estradiol-treated MCF-7 cells. *Cancer Res.*, **61**, 7488–7494

Lee, A.J., Kosh, J.W., Conney, A.H. & Zhu, B.T. (2001) Characterization of the NADPH-dependent metabolism of 17β-estradiol to multiple metabolites by human liver microsomes and selectively expressed human cytochrome P450 3A4 and 3A5. *J. Pharmacol. exp. Ther.*, **298**, 420–432

Lee, A.J., Mills, L.H., Kosh, J.W., Conney, A.H. & Zhu, B.T. (2002) NADPH-dependent metabolism of estrone by human liver microsomes. *J. Pharmacol. exp. Ther.*, **300**, 838–849

Lee, A.J., Cai, M.X., Thomas, P.E., Conney, A.H. & Zhu, B.T. (2003a) Characterization of the oxidative metabolites of 17β-estradiol and estrone formed by 15 selectively expressed human cytochrome P450 isoforms. *Endocrinology*, **144**, 3382–3398

Lee, A.J., Conney, A.H. & Zhu, B.T. (2003b) Human cytochrome P450 3A7 has a distinct high catalytic activity for the 16α-hydroxylation of estrone but not 17β-estradiol. *Cancer Res.*, **63**, 6532–6536

Lees, B. & Stevenson, J.C. (2001) The prevention of osteoporosis using sequential low-dose hormone replacement therapy with estradiol-17β and dydrogesterone. *Osteoporos. int.*, **12**, 251–258

Lévesque, E., Beaulieu, M., Hum, D.W. & Bélanger, A. (1999) Characterization and substrate specificity of UGT2B4 (E⁴⁵⁸): A UDP-glucuronosyltransferase encoded by a polymorphic gene. *Pharmacogenetics*, **9**, 207–216

Lewis, D.F.V., Gillam, E.M.J., Everett, S.A. & Shimada, T. (2003) Molecular modelling of human CYP1B1 substrate interactions and investigation of allelic variant effects on metabolism. *Chem.-biol. Interact.*, **145**, 281–295

Li, C.I., Weiss, N.S., Stanford, J.L. & Daling, J.R. (2000) Hormone replacement therapy in relation to risk of lobular and ductal breast carcinoma in middle-aged women. *Cancer*, **88**, 2570–2577

Li, D.N., Seidel, A., Pritchard, M.P., Wolf, C.R. & Friedberg, T. (2000) Polymorphisms in P450 *CYP1B1* affect the conversion of estradiol to the potentially carcinogenic metabolite 4-hydroxyestradiol. *Pharmacogenetics*, **10**, 343–353

Li, J.J., Papa, D., Davis, M.F., Weroha, S.J., Aldaz, C.M., El Bayoumy, K., Ballenger, J., Tawfik, O. & Li, S.A. (2002) Ploidy differences between hormone- and chemical carcinogen-induced rat mammary neoplasms: Comparison to invasive human ductal breast cancer. *Mol. Carcinog.*, **33**, 56–65

Li, C.I., Malone, K.E., Porter, P.L., Weiss, N.S., Tang, M.T., Cushing-Haugen, K.L. & Daling, J.R. (2003) Relationship between long durations and different regimens of hormone therapy and risk of breast cancer. *J. Am. med. Assoc.*, **289**, 3254–3263

Li, K.-M., Todorovic, R., Devanesan, P., Higginbotham, S., Köfeler, H., Ramanathan, R., Gross, M.L., Rogen, E.G. & Cavalieri, E.L. (2004) Metabolism and DNA binding studies of 4-hydroxyestradiol and estradiol-3,4-quinone *in vitro* and in female ACI rat mammary gland *in vivo*. *Carcinogenesis*, **25**, 289–297

Li, T., Sun, L., Miller, N., Nicklee, T., Woo, J., Hulse-Smith, L., Tsao, M.-S., Khokha, R., Martin, L. & Boyd, N. (2005) The association of measured breast tissue characteristics with mammographic density and other risk factors for breast cancer. *Cancer Epidemiol. Biomarkers Prev.*, **14**, 343–349

Liang, Y.-L., Teede, H., Shiel, L.M., Thomas, A., Craven, R., Sachithanandan, N., McNeil, J.J., Cameron, J.D., Dart, A. & McGrath, B.P. (1997) Effects of oestrogen and progesterone on age-related changes in arteries of postmenopausal women. *Clin. exp. Pharmacol. Physiol.*, **24**, 457–459

Liehr, J.G. & Ricci, M.J. (1996) 4-Hydroxylation of estrogens as marker of human mammary tumors. *Proc. natl Acad. Sci. USA*, **93**, 3294–3296

Liehr, J.G., Fang, W.-F., Sirbasku, D.A. & Ari-Ulubelen, A. (1986) Carcinogenicity of catechol estrogens in Syrian hamsters. *J. steroid Biochem.*, **24**, 353–356

de Lignières, B. (1999) Oral micronized progesterone. *Clin. Ther.*, **21**, 41–60

Lin, A.L., McGill, H.C., Jr & Shain, S.A. (1982) Hormone receptors of the baboon cardiovascular system. Biochemical characterization of aortic and myocardial cytoplasmic progesterone receptors. *Circ. Res.*, **50**, 610–616

Lin, P.-H., Nakamura, J., Yamaguchi, S., Asakura, S. & Swenberg, J.A. (2003) Aldehydic DNA lesions induced by catechol estrogens in calf thymus DNA. *Carcinogenesis*, **24**, 1133–1141

Lindsay, R., Hart, D.M., Forrest, C. & Baird, C. (1980) Prevention of spinal osteoporosis in oophorectomised women. *Lancet*, **ii**, 1151–1154

Lippert, C., Seeger, H., Wallwiener, D. & Mueck, A.O. (2000) Comparison of the effects of continuous combined and sequential combined medroxyprogesterone acetate–estradiol treatment on the proliferation of MCF-7 cells. *Climacteric*, **3**, 271–277

Lippert, C., Seeger, H., Wallwiener, D. & Mueck, A.O. (2001) The effect of medroxyprogesterone acetate and norethisterone on the estradiol stimulated proliferation in MCF-7 cells: Comparison of continuous combined versus sequential combined estradiol/progestin treatment. *Eur. J. Gynaecol. Oncol.*, **22**, 331–335

Lippert, C., Seeger, H., Wallwiener, D. & Mueck, A.O. (2002) Tibolone versus 17β-estradiol/norethisterone: Effects on the proliferation of human breast cancer cells. *Eur. J. Gynaec. Oncol.*, **23**, 127–130

Lundberg, V., Tolonen, H., Stegmayr, B., Kuulasmaa, K. & Asplund, K. (2004) Use of oral contraceptives and hormone replacement therapy in the WHO MONICA project. *Maturitas*, **48**, 39–49

Lundeen, S.G., Zhang, Z., Zhu, Y., Carver, J.M. & Winneker, R.C. (2001) Rat uterine complement C3 expression as a model for progesterone receptor modulators: Characterization of the new progestin trimegestone. *J. steroid Biochem. mol. Biol.*, **78**, 137–143

Lundström, E., Wilczek, B., von Palffy, Z., Soderqvist, G. & von Schoultz, B. (2001) Mammographic breast density during hormone replacement therapy: Effects of continuous combination, unopposed transdermal and low-potency estrogen regimens. *Climacteric*, **4**, 42–48

MacLaren, A. & Woods, N.F. (2001) Midlife women making hormone therapy decisions. *Womens Health Issues*, **11**, 216–230

MacLennan, A.H., Taylor, A.W. & Wilson, D.H. (2004a) Hormone therapy use after the Women's Health Initiative. *Climacteric*, **7**, 138–142

MacLennan, A.H., Broadbent, J.L., Lester, S. & Moore V. (2004b) Oral oestrogen and combined oestrogen/progestogen therapy versus placebo for hot flushes. *The Cochrane Database Syst. Rev.*, **4**

Magnusson, C., Baron, J.A., Correia, N., Bergstrom, R., Adami, H.O. & Persson, I. (1999) Breast-cancer risk following long-term oestrogen– and oestrogen–progestin-replacement therapy. *Int. J. Cancer*, **81**, 339–344

Majumdar, S.R., Almasi, E.A. & Stafford, R.S. (2004) Promotion and prescribing of hormone therapy after report of harm by the Women's Health Initiative. *J. Am. med. Assoc.*, **292**, 1983–1988

Malins, D.C. & Haimanot, R. (1991) Major alterations in the nucleotide structure of DNA in cancer of the female breast. *Cancer Res.*, **51**, 5430–5432

Malins, D.C., Johnson, P.M., Wheeler, T.M., Barker, E.A., Polissar, N.L. & Vinson, M.A. (2001) Age-related radical-induced DNA damage is linked to prostate cancer. *Cancer Res.*, **61**, 6025–6028

Mamdani, M.M., Tu, K., van Walraven, C., Austin, P.C. & Naylor, C.D. (2000) Postmenopausal estrogen replacement therapy and increased rates of cholecystectomy and appendectomy. *Can. med. Assoc. J.*, **162**, 1421–1424

Manson, J.E., Hsia, J., Johnson, K.C., Rossouw, J.E., Assaf, A.R., Lasser, N.L., Trevisan, M., Black, H.R., Heckbert, S.R., Detrano, R., Strickland, O.L., Wong, N.D., Crouse, J.R., Stein, E. & Cushman, M. for the Women's Health Initiative Investigators (2003) Estrogen plus progestin and the risk of coronary heart disease. *New Engl. J. Med.*, **349**, 523–534

Manzoli, L., Di Giovanni, P., Del Duca, L., De Aloysio, D., Festi, D., Capodicasa, S., Monastra, G., Romano, F. & Staniscia, T. (2004) Use of hormone replacement therapy in Italian women aged 50–70 years. *Maturitas*, **49**, 241–251

Margolis, K.L., Bonds, D.F., Rodabough, R.J., Tinker, L., Phillips, L.S., Allen, C., Bassford, T., Burke, G., Torrens, J. & Howard, B.V. (2004) Effect of oestrogen plus progestin on the incidence of diabetes in postmenopausal women: Results from the Women's Health Initiative Hormone Trial. *Diabetologia*, **47**, 1175–1187

Markushin, Y., Zhong, W., Cavalieri, E.L., Rogan, E.G., Small, G.J., Yeung, E.S. & Jankowiak, R. (2003) Spectral characterization of catechol estrogen quinone (CEQ)-derived DNA adducts and their identification in human breast tissue extract. *Chem. Res. Toxicol.*, **16**, 1107–1117

Martelli, A., Mereto, E., Ghia, M., Orsi, P., Allavena, A., De Pascalis, C.R. & Brambilla, G. (1998) Induction of micronuclei and of enzyme-altered foci in the liver of female rats exposed to progesterone and three synthetic progestins. *Mutat. Res.*, **419**, 33–41

Martelli, A., Mattioli, F., Carrozzino, R., Ferraris, E., Marchese, M., Angiola, M. & Brambilla, G. (1999) Genotoxicity testing of potassium canrenoate in cultured rat and human cells. *Mutagenesis*, **14**, 463–472

Martelli, A., Carrozzino, R., Mattioli, F., Bucci, G., Lamarino, G. & Brambilla, G. (2002) DNA damage in tissues of rat treated with potassium canrenoate. *Toxicology*, **171**, 95–103

Martelli, A., Mattioli, F., Angiola, M., Reimann, R. & Brambilla, G. (2003) Species, sex and interindividual differences in DNA repair induced by nine sex steroids in primary cultures of rat and human hepatocytes. *Mutat. Res.*, **536**, 69–78

Mattioli, F., Garbero, C., Gosmar, M., Manfredi, V., Carrozzino, R., Martelli, A. & Brambilla, G. (2004) DNA fragmentation, DNA repair and apoptosis induced in primary rat hepatocytes by dienogest, dydrogesterone and 1,4,6-androstatriene-17β-ol-3-one acetate. *Mutat. Res.*, **564**, 21–29

Maugard, C.M., Charrier, J., Pitard, A., Campion, L., Akande, O., Pleasants, L. & Ali-Osman, F. (2001) Genetic polymorphism at the glutathione S-transferase (GST) P1 locus is a breast cancer risk modifier. *Int. J. Cancer*, **91**, 334–339

McFadyen, M.C.E., Breeman, S., Payne, S., Stirk, C., Miller, I.D., Melvin, W.T. & Murray, G.I. (1999) Immunohistochemical localization of cytochrome P450 CYP1B1 in breast cancer with monoclonal antibodies specific for CYP1B1. *J. Histochem. Cytochem.*, **47**, 1457–1464

McGrath, M., Hankinson, S.E., Arbeitman, L., Colditz, G.A., Hunter, D.J. & De Vivo, I. (2004) Cytochrome P450 1B1 and catechol-*O*-methyltransferase polymorphisms and endometrial cancer susceptibility. *Carcinogenesis*, **25**, 559–565

McKnight, B., Voigt, L.F., Beresford, S.A. & Weiss, N.S. (1998) Re: Estrogen–progestin replacement therapy and endometrial cancer. *J. natl Cancer Inst.*, **90**, 164–166

McLellan, R.A., Oscarson, M., Hidestrand, M., Leidvik, B., Jonsson, E., Otter, C. & Ingelman-Sundberg, M. (2000) Characterization and functional analysis of two common human cytochrome P450 1B1 variants. *Arch. Biochem. Biophys.*, **378**, 175–181

Meilahn, E.N., De Stavola, B., Allen, D.S., Fentiman, I., Bradlow, H.L., Sepkovic, D.W. & Kuller, L.H. (1998) Do urinary oestrogen metabolites predict breast cancer? Guernsey III cohort follow-up. *Br. J. Cancer*, **78**, 1250–1255

Mendoza, N., Pisón, J.A., Fernandez, M., Sánchez, M.C., Malde, J. & Miranda, J.A. (2002) Prospective, randomised study with three HRT regimens in postmenopausal women with an intact uterus. *Maturitas*, **41**, 289–298

Mercuro, G., Pitzalis, L., Podda, A., Zoncu, S., Pilia, I., Melis, G.B. & Cherchi, A. (1999) Effects of acute administration of natural progesterone on peripheral vascular responsiveness in healthy postmenopausal women. *Am. J. Cardiol.*, **84**, 214–218

Merom, D., Ifrah, A., Cohen-Manheim, I., Chinich, A. & Green, M.S. (2002) Factors predicting current use of hormone replacement therapy among menopausal Jewish women in Israel. The National Women's Health Interview Survey, 1998. *Israeli med. Assoc. J.*, **4**, 671–676

Metcalfe, S. (2004) *HT Use in New Zealand: A Patient-level Analysis of Pharmhouse Data*, unpublished report released under the Official Information Act, October 2004

Michnovicz, J.J., Hershcopf, R.J., Naganuma, H., Bradlow, H.L. & Fishman, J. (1986) Increased 2-hydroxylation of estradiol as a possible mechanism for the anti-estrogenic effect of cigarette smoking. *New Engl. J. Med.*, **315**, 1305–1309

Miettinen, M., Mustonen, M., Poutanen, M., Isomaa, V., Wickman, M., Soderqvist, G., Vihko, R. & Vihko, P. (1999) 17β-Hydroxysteroid dehydrogenases in normal human mammary epithelial cells and breast tissue. *Breast Cancer Res. Treat.*, **57**, 175–182

Mikkola, T.S. & Clarkson, T.B. (2002) Estrogen replacement therapy, atherosclerosis, and vascular function. *Cardiovasc. Res.*, **53**, 605–619

Mikkola, T., Viinikka, L. & Ylikorkala, O. (1998) Estrogen and postmenopausal estrogen/progestin therapy: Effect on endothelium-dependent prostacyclin, nitric oxide and endothelin-1 production. *Eur. J. Obstet. Gynecol.*, **79**, 75–82

Milewicz, T., Gregoraszczuk, E.L., Sztefko, K., Augustowska, K., Krzysiek, J. & Rys, J. (2005a) Lack of synergy between estrogen and progesterone on local IGF-I, IGFBP-3 and IGFBP-2 secretion by both hormone-dependent and hormone-independent breast cancer explants in vitro. Effect of tamoxifen and mifepristone (RU 486). *Growth Horm. IGF Res.*, **15**, 140–147

Milewicz, T., Gregoraszczuk, E.L., Augustowska, K., Krzysiek, J., Sztefko, K. & Rys, J. (2005b) Progesterone but not estradiol-17β potentiates local GH secretions by hormone-dependent breast cancer explants. An *in vitro* study. *Exp. clin. Endocrinol. Diabetes*, **113**, 127–132

Miller, V.M. & Vanhoutte, P.M. (1991) Progesterone and modulation of endothelium-dependent responses in canine coronary arteries. *Am. J. Physiol.*, **261**, R1022–R1027

Million Women Study Collaborators (2002) Patterns of use of hormone replacement therapy in one million women in Britain, 1996–2000. *Br. J. Obstet. Gynaecol.*, **109**, 1319–1330

Million Women Study Collaborators (2005) Endometrial cancer and hormone-replacement therapy in the Million Women Study. *Lancet*, **365**, 1543–1551

Mills, L.H., Lee, A.J., Parlow, A.F. & Zhu, B.T. (2001) Preferential growth stimulation of mammary glands over uterine endometrium in female rats by a naturally occurring estradiol-17β-fatty acid ester. *Cancer Res.*, **61**, 5764–5770

Miners, J.O., McKinnon, R.A. & Mackenzie, P.I. (2002) Genetic polymorphisms of UDP-glucuronosyltransferases and their functional significance. *Toxicology*, **181–182**, 453–456

Mitrunen, K. & Hirvonen, A. (2003) Molecular epidemiology of sporadic breast cancer. The role of polymorphic genes involved in oestrogen biosynthesis and metabolism. *Mutat. Res.*, **544**, 9–41

Miyairi, S., Maeda, K., Oe, T., Kato, T. & Naganuma, A. (1999) Effect of metal ions on the stable adduct formation of 16α-hydroxyestrone with a primary amine via the Heyns rearrangement. *Steroids*, **64**, 252–258

Miyoshi, Y., Ando, A., Shiba, E., Taguchi, T., Tamaki, Y. & Noguchi, S. (2001) Involvement of up-regulation of 17β-hydroxysteroid dehydrogenase type 1 in maintenance of intratumoral high estradiol levels in postmenopausal breast cancers. *Int. J. Cancer*, **94**, 685–689

Mizunuma, H., Honjo, H., Aso, T., Urabe, M., Ohta, H., Kobayashi, S., Sagara, Y., Sanada, M., Tanaka, K., Dobashi, K., Hayashi, K. & Ohama, K. (2001) Postmenopausal hormone replacement therapy use and risk of endometrial cancer in Japanese women. *Climacteric*, **4**, 293–298

Mrusek. S., Classen-Linke, I., Vloet, A., Beier, H.M. & Krusche, C.A. (2005) Estradiol and medroxyprogesterone acetate regulated genes in T47D breast cancer cells. *Mol. cell. Endocrinol.*, **235**, 39–50

Mueck, A.O., Seeger, H., Gräser, T., Oettel, M. & Lippert, T.H. (2001) The effects of postmenopausal hormone replacement therapy and oral contraceptives on the endogenous estradiol metabolism. *Horm. Metab. Res.*, **33**, 744–747

Mueck, A.O., Seeger, H. & Wallwiener, D. (2002) Impact of hormone replacement therapy on endogenous estradiol metabolism in postmenopausal women. *Maturitas*, **43**, 87–93

Mueck, A.O., Seeger, H. & Wallwiener, D. (2003) Comparison of the proliferative effects of estradiol and conjugated equine estrogens on human breast cancer cells and impact of continuous combined progestogen addition. *Climacteric*, **6**, 221–227

Mueller, J.E., Döring, A., Heier, M. & Löwel, H. (2002) Prevalence and determinants of hormone replacement therapy in German women 1984–1995. *Maturitas*, **43**, 95–104

Mulnard, R.A., Cotman, C.W., Kawas, C., van Dyck, C.H., Sano, M., Doody, R., Koss, E., Pfeiffer, E., Jin, S., Gamst, A., Grundman, M., Thomas, R. & Thal, L.J. for the Alzheimer's Disease Cooperative Study (2000) Estrogen replacement therapy for treatment of mild to moderate Alzheimer disease. A randomized controlled trial. *J. Am. med. Assoc.*, **283**, 1007–1015

Murray, G.I., Taylor, M.C., McFadyen, M.C.E., McKay, J.A., Greenlee, W.F., Burke, M.D. & Melvin, W.T. (1997) Tumor-specific expression of cytochrome P450 CYP1B1. *Cancer Res.*, **57**, 3026–3031

Murray, G.I., Melvin, W.T., Greenlee, W.F. & Burke, M.D. (2001) Regulation, function, and tissue-specific expression of cytochrome P450 CYP1B1. *Ann. Rev. Pharmacol. Toxicol.*, **41**, 297–316

Musarrat, J., Arezina-Wilson, J. & Wani, A.A. (1996) Prognostic and aetiological relevance of 8-hydroxyguanosine in human breast carcinogenesis. *Eur. J. Cancer*, **32A**, 1209–1214

Muti, P., Bradlow, H.L., Micheli, A., Krogh, V., Freudenheim, J.L., Schünemann, H.J., Stanulla, M., Yang, J., Sepkovic, D.W., Trevisan, M. &. Berrino, F. (2000) Estrogen metabolism and risk of breast cancer: A prospective study of the 2:16α-hydroxyestrone ratio in premenopausal and postmenopausal women. *Epidemiology*, **11**, 635–640

Nachtigall, L.E., Nachtigall, R.H., Nachtigall, R.D. & Beckman, E.M. (1979) Estrogen replacement therapy. I: A 10 year prospective study in the relationship to osteoporosis. *Obstet. Gynecol.*, **53**, 277–281

Nakamura, M., Katsuki, Y., Shibutani, Y. & Oikawa, T. (1999) Dienogest, a synthetic steroid, suppresses both embryonic and tumor-cell-induced angiogenesis. *Eur. J. Pharmacol.*, **386**, 33–40

Negri, E., Tzonou, A., Beral, V., Lagiou, P., Trichopoulos, D., Parazzini, F., Franceschi, S., Booth, M. & La Vecchia, C. (1999) Hormonal therapy for menopause and ovarian cancer in a collaborative re-analysis of European studies. *Int. J. Cancer*, **80**, 848–851

Nelson, H.D., Humphrey, L.L., LeBlanc, E., Miller, J., Takano, L., Chan, B.K.S., Nygren, P., Allan, J.D. & Teutsch, S.M, (2002a) *Postmenopausal Hormone Replacement Therapy for the Primary Prevention of Chronic Conditions: A Summary of the Evidence for the U.S. Preventive Services Task Force.* [https://www.preventiveservices.ahrg.gov]

Nelson, H.D., Humphrey, L.L., Nygren, P., Teutsch, S.M. & Allan, J.D. (2002b) Postmenopausal hormone replacement therapy. *J. Am. med. Assoc.*, **288**, 872–881

Neven, P., Quail, D., Levrier, M., Aguas, F., Thé, H.S., De Geyter, C., Glant, M.D., Beck, H., Bosio-LeGoux, B., Schmitt, H., Hottgenroth, A. & Nickelsen, T. (2004) Uterine effects of estrogen plus progestin therapy and raloxifene: Adjudicated results from the EURALOX study. *Obstet. Gynecol.*, **103**, 881–891

Newbold, R.R. & Liehr, J.G. (2000) Induction of uterine adenocarcinoma in CD-1 mice by catechol estrogens. *Cancer Res.*, **60**, 235–237

Newcomb, P.A. & Storer, B.E. (1995) Postmenopausal hormone use and risk of large-bowel cancer. *J. natl Cancer Inst.*, **87**, 1067–71

Newcomb, P. A. & Trentham-Dietz, A. (2003) Patterns of postmenopausal progestin use with estrogen in relation to endometrial cancer (United States). *Cancer Causes Control*, **14**, 195–201

Newcomb, P.A., Titus-Ernstoff, L., Egan, K.M., Trentham-Dietz, A., Baron, J.A., Storer, B.E., Willett, W.C. & Stampfer, M.J. (2002) Postmenopausal estrogen and progestin use in relation to breast cancer risk. *Cancer Epidemiol. Biomarkers Prev.*, **11**, 593–600

Nichols, H.B., Trentham-Dietz, A., Hampton, J.M. & Newcomb, P.A. (2005) Oral contraceptives use, reproductive factors, and colorectal cancer risk: Findings from Wisconsin. *Cancer Epidemiol. Biomarkers Prev.*, **14**, 1212–1218

Normand, T., Narod, S., Labrie, F. & Simard, J. (1993) Detection of polymorphisms in the estradiol 17α-hydroxysteroid dehydrogenase II gene at the EDH17B2 locus on 17q11-q21. *Hum. mol. Genet.*, **2**, 479–483

North American Menopause Society (2004) Recommendations for estrogen and progestogen use in peri- and postmenopausal women: October 2004 position statement of The North American Menopause Society. *Menopause*, **11**, 589–600

Nugent, A.G., Leung, K.-C., Sullivan, D., Reutens, A.T. & Ho, K.K.Y. (2003) Modulation by progestogens of the effects of oestrogen on hepatic endocrine function in postmenopausal women. *Clin. Endocrinol.*, **59**, 690–698

Oduwole, O.O., Li, Y., Isomaa, V.V., Mäntyniemi, A., Pulkka, A.E., Soini, Y. & Vihko, P.T. (2004) 17β-Hydroxysteroid dehydrogenase type 1 is an independent prognostic marker in breast cancer. *Cancer Res.*, **64**, 7604–7609

Oehler, M.K., MacKenzie, I.Z., Wallwiener, D., Bicknell, R. & Rees, M.C.P. (2002) Wnt-7a is upregulated by norethisterone in human endometrial epithelial cells: A possible mechanism by which progestogens reduce the risk of estrogen-induced endometrial neoplasia. *Cancer Lett.*, **186**, 75–81

Olsson, H.L., Ingvar, C. & Bladstrom, A. (2003) Hormone replacement therapy containing progestins and given continuously increases breast carcinoma risk in Sweden. *Cancer*, **97**, 1387–1392

Ory, K., Lebeau, J., Levalois, C., Bishay, K., Fouchet, P., Allemand, I., Therwath, A. & Chevillard, S. (2001) Apoptosis inhibition mediated by medroxyprogesterone acetate treatment of breast cancer cell lines. *Breast Cancer Res. Treat.*, **68**, 187–198

Paganini-Hill, A. (1999) Estrogen replacement therapy and colorectal cancer risk in elderly women. *Dis. Colon Rectum*, **42**, 1300–1305

Paganini-Hill, A. & Henderson, V.W. (1994) Estrogen deficiency and risk of Alzheimer's disease in women. *Am. J. Epidemiol.*, **140**, 256–261

Pahuja, S.L., Zielinski, J.E., Giordano, G., McMurray, W.J. & Hochberg, R.B. (1991) The biosynthesis of D-ring fatty acid esters of estriol. *J. biol. Chem.*, **266**, 7410–7416

Palmlund, I. (1997) The social construction of menopause as risk. *J. psychosom. Obstet. Gynaecol.*, **18**, 87–94

Paria, B.C., Lim, H., Wang, X.-N., Liehr, J., Das, S.K. & Dey, S.K. (1998) Coordination of differential effects of primary estrogen and catecholestrogen on two distinct targets mediates embryo implantation in the mouse. *Endocrinology*, **139**, 5235–5246

Paria, B.C., Lim, H., Das, S.K., Reese, J. & Dey, S.K. (2000) Molecular signaling in uterine receptivity for implantation. *Semin. Cell dev. Biol.*, **11**, 67–76

Pasapera, A.M., Gutierrez-Sagal, R., Herrera, J., Galicia-Canales, N., Garcia de la More, M. & Ulloa-Aguirre, A. (2002) Norethisterone is bioconverted to oestrogenic compounds that activate both the oestrogen receptor α and oestrogen receptor β in vitro. *Eur. J. Pharmacol.*, **452**, 347–355

Pasley, B.H., Standfast, S.J. & Katz, S.H. (1984) Prescribing estrogen during menopause: Physician survey of practices in 1974 and 1981. *Public Health Rep.*, **99**, 424–429

Pasqualini, J.R. (2003) Differential effects of progestins on breast tissue enzymes. *Maturitas*, **46** (Suppl. 1), S45–S54

Pasqualini, J.R. (2004) The selective estrogen enzyme modulators in breast cancer: A review. *Biochim. biophys. Acta*, **1654**, 123–143

Pasqualini, J.R. & Chetrite, G. (2001) Paradoxical effect of estradiol: It can block its own bioformation in human breast cancer cells. *J. steroid Biochem. mol. Biol.*, **78**, 21–24

Pasqualini, J.R., Chetrite, G., Blacker, C., Feinstein, M.-C., Delalonde, L., Talbi, M. & Maloche, C. (1996) Concentrations of estrone, estradiol, and estrone sulfate and evaluation of sulfatase and aromatase activities in pre- and postmenopausal breast cancer patients. *J. clin. Endocrinol. Metab.*, **81**, 1460–1464

Pecci, A., Scholz, A., Pelster, D. & Beato, M. (1997) Progestins prevent apoptosis in a rat endometrial cell line and increase the ratio of $bcl-X_L$ to $bcl-X_s$. *J. biol. Chem.* **272**, 11791–11798

Pedersen, L.C., Petrotchenko, E., Shevtsov, S. & Negishi, M. (2002) Crystal structure of the human estrogen sulfotransferase-PAPS complex: Evidence for catalytic role of Ser[137] in the sulfuryl transfer reaction. *J. biol. Chem.*, **277**, 17928–17932

Peltoketo, H., Isomaa, V., Poutanen, M. & Vihko, R. (1996) Expression and regulation of 17β-hydroxysteroid dehydrogenase type 1. *J. Endocrinol.*, **150** (Suppl.), 21–30

Peltoketo, H., Vihko, P. & Vihko, R. (1999) Regulation of estrogen action: Role of 17β-hydroxysteroid dehydrogenases. *Vitam. Horm.*, **55**, 353–398

Penning, T.M., Burczynski, M.E., Jez, J.M., Hung, C.-F., Lin, H.-K., Ma, H., Moore, M., Palackal, N. & Ratnam, K. (2000) Human 3α-hydroxysteroid dehydrogenase isoforms (AKR1C1-AKR1C4) of the aldo-keto reductase superfamily: Functional plasticity and tissue distribution reveals roles in the inactivation and formation of male and female sex hormones. *Biochem. J.*, **351**, 67–77

Penotti, M., Nencioni, T., Gabrielli, L., Farina, M., Castiglioni, E. & Polvani, F. (1993) Blood flow variations in internal carotid and middle cerebral arteries induced by postmenopausal hormone replacement therapy. *Am. J. Obstet. Gynecol.*, **169**, 1226–1232

Persson, I., Adami, H.-O., Bergkvist, L., Lindgren, A., Pettersson, B., Hoover, R. & Schairer, C. (1989) Risk of endometrial cancer after treatment with oestrogens alone or in conjunction with progestogens: Results of a prospective study. *Br. med. J.*, **298**, 147–151

Persson, I., Yuen, J., Bergkvist, L. & Schairer, C. (1996) Cancer incidence and mortality in women receiving estrogen and estrogen-progestin replacement therapy — Long-term follow-up of a Swedish cohort. *Int. J. Cancer*, **67**, 327–332

Persson, I., Weiderpass, E., Bergkvist, L., Bergstrom, R. & Schairer, C. (1999) Risks of breast and endometrial cancer after estrogen and estrogen–progestin replacement. *Cancer Causes Control*, **10**, 253–260

Petitti, D.B. (1994) Coronary heart disease and estrogen replacement therapy. Can compliance bias explain the results of observational studies? *Ann. Epidemiol.*, **4**, 115–118

Peverill, R.E. (2003) Hormone therapy and venous thromboembolism. *Best Pract. and Res. clin. Endocrin. Metab.*, **17**, 149–164

Pike, M.C., Peters, R.K., Cozen, W., Probst-Hensch, N.M., Felix, J.C., Wan, P.C. & Mack, T.M. (1997) Estrogen–progestin replacement therapy and endometrial cancer. *J. natl Cancer Inst.*, **89**, 1110–1116

Pike, M.C., Pearce, C.L., Peters, R., Cozen, W., Wan, P. & Wu, A.H. (2004) Hormonal factors and the risk of invasive ovarian cancer: A population-based case–control study. *Fertil. Steril.*, **82**, 186–195

Pollow, K., Juchem, M., Elger, W., Jacobi, N., Hoffmann, G. & Mobus, V. (1992) Dihydrospirorenone (ZK30595): A novel synthetic progestagen — Characterization of binding to different receptor proteins. *Contraception*, **46**, 561–574

Portman, D.J., Symons, J.P., Wilborn, W. & Kempfert, N.J. (2003) A randomized, double-blind, placebo-controlled, multicenter study that assessed the endometrial effects of norethindrone acetate plus ethinyl estradiol versus ethinyl estradiol alone. *Am. J. Obstet. Gynecol.*, **188**, 334–342

Post, W.S., Goldschmidt-Clermont, P.J., Wilhide, C.C., Heldman, A.W., Sussman, M.S., Ouyang, P., Milliken, E.E. & Issa, J.P. (1999) Methylation of the estrogen receptor gene is associated with aging and atherosclerosis in the cardiovascular system. *Cardiovasc. Res.*, **43**, 985–991

Post, M.S., Christella, M., Thomassen, L.G.D., van der Mooren, M.J., van Baal, W.M., Rosing, J., Kenemans, P. & Stehouwer, C.D.A. (2003) Effect of oral and transdermal estrogen replacement therapy on hemostatic variables associated with venous thrombosis. A randomized, placebo-controlled study in postmenopausal women. *Arterioscler. Thromb. vasc. Biol.*, **23**, 1116–1121

Poutanen, M., Isomaa, V., Kainulainen, K. & Vihko, R. (1990) Progestin induction of 17β-hydroxysteroid dehydrogenase enzyme protein in the T-47D human breast-cancer cell line. *Int. J. Cancer*, **46**, 897–901

Poutanen, M., Isomaa, V., Lehto, V.-P. & Vihko, R. (1992a) Immunological analysis of 17β-hydroxysteroid dehydrogenase in benign and malignant human breast tissue. *Int. J. Cancer*, **50**, 386–390

Poutanen, M., Moncharmont, B. & Vihko, R. (1992b) 17β-Hydroxysteroid dehydrogenase gene expression in human breast cancer cells: Regulation of expression by a progestin. *Cancer Res.*, **52**, 290–294

Pradhan, A.D., Manson, J.E., Rossouw, J.E., Siscovick, D.S., Mouton, C.P., Rifai, N., Wallace, R.B., Jackson, R.D., Pettinger, M.B. & Ridker, P.M. (2002) Inflammatory biomarkers, hormone replacement therapy, and incident coronary heart disease: Prospective analysis from the Women's Health Initiative Observational Study. *J. Am. med. Assoc.*, **288**, 980–987

Prentice, R.L., Langer, R., Stefanick, M.L., Howard, B.V., Pettinger, M., Anderson, G., Barad, D., Curb, J.D., Kotchen, J., Kuller, L., Limacher, M. & Wactawski-Wende, J. for the Women's Health Initiative Investigators. (2005) Combined postmenopausal hormone therapy and cardiovascular disease: Toward resolving the discrepancy between observational studies and the Women's Health Initiative Clinical Trial. *Am. J. Epidemiol.*, **162**, 404–414

Preston, R.A., White, W.B., Pitt, B., Bakris, G., Norris, P.M. & Hanes, V. (2005) Effects of drospi-renone/17β-estradiol on blood pressure and potassium balance in hypertensive postmeno-pausal women. *Am. J. Hypertens.*, **18**, 797–804

Pribluda, V.S., Gubish, E.R., Jr, LaVallee, T.M., Treston, A., Swartz, G.M. & Green, S.J. (2000) 2-Methoxyestradiol: An endogenous antiangiogenic and antiproliferative drug candidate. *Cancer Metast. Rev.*, **19**, 173–179

Prihartono, N., Palmer, J.R., Louik, C., Shapiro, S. & Rosenberg, L. (2000) A case–control study of use of postmenopausal female hormone supplements in relation to the risk of large bowel cancer. *Cancer Epidemiol. Biomarkers Prev.*, **9**, 443–447

Progetto Menopausa Italia Study Group (2001) General and medical factors associated with hormone replacement therapy among women attending menopause clinics in Italy. *Meno-pause*, **8**, 290–295

Pukkala, E., Tulenheimo-Silfvast, A. & Leminen, A. (2001) Incidence of cancer among women using long versus monthly cycle hormonal replacement therapy, Finland 1994–1997. *Cancer Causes Control*, **12**, 111–115

Puranen, T.J., Poutanen, M.H., Peltoketo, H.E., Vihko, P.T. & Vihko, R.K. (1994) Site-directed mutagenesis of the putative active site of human 17β-hydroxysteroid dehydrogenase type 1. *Biochem. J.*, **304**, 289–293

Purdie, D.M., Bain, C.J., Siskind, V., Russell, P., Hacker, N.F., Ward, B.G., Quinn, M.A. & Green, A.C. (1999) Hormone replacement therapy and risk of epithelial ovarian cancer. *Br. J. Cancer*, **81**, 559–563

Raafat, A.M., Hofseth, L.J., Li, S., Bennett, J.M. & Haslam, S.Z. (1999) A mouse model to study the effects of hormone replacement therapy on normal mammary gland during menopause: Enhanced proliferative response to estrogen in late postmenopausal mice. *Endocrinology*, **140**, 2570–2580

Raafat, A.M., Hofseth, L.J. & Haslam, S.Z. (2001) Proliferative effects of combination estrogen and progesterone replacement therapy on the normal postmenopausal mammary gland in a murine model. *Am. J. Obstet. Gynecol.*, **184**, 340–349

Rabe, T., Bohlmann, M.K., Rehberger-Schneider, S. & Prifti, S. (2000) Induction of estrogen receptor-α and -β activities by synthetic progestins. *Gynecol. Endocrinol.*, **14**, 118–126

Rachon, D., Zdrojewski, T., Suchecka-Rachon, K., Szpakowski, P., Bandosz, P., Manikowski, A. & Wyrzykowski, B. (2004) Knowledge and use of hormone replacement therapy among Polish women: Estimates from a nationally representative study HORTPOL 2002. *Maturitas*, **47**, 31–37

Raftogianis, R., Creveling, C., Weinshilboum, R. & Weisz, J. (2000) Estrogen metabolism by conjugation. *J. natl Cancer Inst. Monogr.*, **27**, 113–124

Rajapakse, N., Butterworth, M. & Kortenkamp, A. (2005) Detection of DNA strand breaks and oxidized DNA bases at the single-cell level resulting from exposure to estradiol and hydroxylated metabolites. *Environ. mol. Mutag.*, **45**, 397–404

Ramanathan, R., Cao, K., Cavalieri, E. & Gross, M.L. (1998) Mass spectrometric methods for distinguishing structural isomers of glutathione conjugates of estrone and estradiol. *J. Am. Soc. mass Spectrom.*, **9**, 612–619

Rapp, S.R., Espeland, M.A., Shumaker, S.A., Henderson, V.W., Brunner, R.L., Manson, J.E., Gass, M.L.S., Stefanick, M.L., Lane, D.S., Hays, J., Johnson, K.C., Coker, L.H., Dailey, M. & Bowen, D. for the WHIMS Investigators (2003) Effect of estrogen plus progestin on global cognitive function in postmenopausal women: The Women's Health Initiative Memory Study: A randomized controlled trial. *J. Am. med. Assoc.*, **289**, 2663–2672

Raudaskoski, T., Knip, M. & Laatikainen, T. (1998) Plasma insulin-like growth factor-I and its binding proteins 1 and 3 during continuous nonoral and oral combined hormone replacement therapy. *Menopause*, **5**, 217–222

Reboussin, B.A., Greendale, G.A. & Espeland, M.A. (1998) Effect of hormone replacement therapy on self-reported cognitive symptoms: Results from the Postmenopausal Estrogen/Progestin Interventions (PEPI) Trial. *Climacteric*, **1**, 172–179

Recker, R.R., Davies, M., Dowd, R.M. & Heaney, R.P. (1999) The effect of low-dose continuous estrogen and progesterone therapy with calcium and vitamin D on bone in elderly women. A randomized, controlled trial. *Ann. intern. Med.*, **130**, 897–904

Reis, S.E., Gloth, S.T., Blumenthal, R.S., Resar, J.R., Zacur, H.A., Gerstenblith, G. & Brinker, J.A. (1994) Ethinyl estradiol acutely attenuates abnormal coronary vasomotor responses to acetylcholine in postmenopausal women. *Circulation*, **89**, 52–60

Ridker, P.M., Hennekens, C.H., Rifai, N., Buring, J.E. & Manson, J.E. (1999) Hormone replacement therapy and increased plasma concentration of C-reactive protein. *Circulation*, **100**, 713–716

Ridker, P.M., Hennekens, C.H., Buring, J.E. & Rifai, N. (2000) C-Reactive protein and other markers of inflammation in the prediction of cardiovascular disease in women. *New Engl. J. Med.*, **342**, 836–843

Rijpkema, A.H.M., van der Sanden, A.A. & Ruijs, A.H.C. (1990) Effects of post-menopausal oestrogen–progestogen replacement therapy on serum lipids and lipoproteins: A review. *Maturitas*, **12**, 259–285

Riman, T., Dickman, P.W., Nilsson, S., Correia, N., Nordlinder, H., Magnusson, C.M. & Persson, I.R. (2001) Risk factors for epithelial borderline ovarian tumors: Results of a Swedish case–control study. *Gynecol. Oncol.*, **83**, 575–585

Riman, T., Dickman, P.W., Nilsson, S., Correia, N., Nordlinder, H., Magnusson, C.M., Weiderpass, E. & Persson, I.R. (2002) Hormone replacement therapy and the risk of invasive epithelial ovarian cancer in Swedish women. *J. natl Cancer Inst.*, **94**, 497–504

Risch, H.A. & Howe, G.R. (1995) Menopausal hormone use and colorectal cancer in Saskatchewan: A record linkage cohort study. *Cancer Epidemiol. Biomarkers Prev.*, **4**, 21–28

Rodriguez, C., Calle, E.E., Patel, A.V., Tatham, L.M., Jacobs, E.J. & Thun, M.J. (2001) Effect of body mass on the association between estrogen replacement therapy and mortality among elderly US women. *Am. J. Epidemiol.*, **153**, 145–152

Rogan, E.G., Badawi, A.F., Devanesan, P.D., Meza, J.L., Edney, J.A., West, W.W., Higginbotham, S.M. & Cavalieri, E.L. (2003) Relative imbalances in estrogen metabolism and conjugation in breast tissue of women with carcinoma: Potential biomarkers of susceptibility to cancer. *Carcinogenesis,* **24**, 697–702

Rosano, G.M.C., Mercuro, G., Vitale, C., Rossini, P., Galetta, P. & Fini, M. (2001) How progestins influence the cardiovascular effect of hormone replacement therapy. *Gynecol. Endocrinol.,* **15** (Suppl. 6), 9–17

Rosano, G.M.C., Vitale, C., Silvestri, A. & Fini, M. (2003) Metabolic and vascular effect of progestins in post-menopausal women. Implications for cardioprotection. *Maturitas,* **46** (Suppl. 1), S17–S29

Rosano, G.M.C., Vitale, C. & Lello, S. (2004) Postmenopausal hormone therapy: Lessons from observational and randomized studies. *Endocrine,* **24**, 251–254

Rosano, G.M.C., Collins, P., Gerbara, O., Sheiban, I., Silvestri, A., Wajngarten, M., Ramires, J.A., Fini, M. & Mercuro, G. (2006) Effect of estradiol 17β upon coronary artery vasoconstrictor response to methylergometrine maleate in female menopausal patients. *Int. J. Cardiol.,* **107**, 254–259

Ross, R.K., Paganini-Hill, A., Mack, T.M., Arthur, M. & Henderson, B.E. (1981) Menopausal oestrogen therapy and protection from death from ischaemic heart disease. *Lancet,* **i**, 858–860

Ross, D., Godfree, V., Cooper, A., Pryse-Davies, J. & Whitehead, M.I. (1997) Endometrial effects of three doses of trimegestone, a new orally active progestogen, on the postmenopausal endometrium. *Maturitas,* **28**, 83–88

Ross, R.K., Paganini-Hill, A., Wan, P.C. & Pike, M.C. (2000) Effect of hormone replacement therapy on breast cancer risk: Estrogen versus estrogen plus progestin. *J. natl Cancer Inst.,* **92**, 328–332

Rossouw, J.E. (2000) Debate: The potential role of estrogen in the prevention of heart disease in women after menopause. *Curr. Control Trials cardiovasc. Med.,* **1**, 135–138

Rossouw, J.E., Anderson, G.L., Prentice, R.L., LaCroix, A.Z., Kooperberg, C., Stefanick, M.L., Jackson, R.D., Beresford, S.A.A., Howard, B.V., Johnson, K.C., Kotchen, J.M. & Ockene, J. for the Writing Group for the Women's Health Initiative Investigators (2002) Risks and benefits of estrogen plus progestin in healthy postmenopausal women: Principal results from the Women's Health Initiative Randomized Controlled Trial. *J. Am. med. Assoc.,* **288**, 321–333

Roy, D. & Liehr, G. (1999) Estrogen, DNA damage and mutations. *Mutat. Res,* **424**, 107–115

Roy, D. & Singh, K.P. (2004) Estrogen-induced genetic alterations and their role in carcinogenicity. *Curr. Genom.,* **5**, 245–257

Roy, D., Parkash, J. & Narayan, S. (2004) Genetics and bioenergetics of mitochondria influencing the etiology and pharmacology of steroidal hormones. *Curr. Pharmacogenom.,* **2**, 379–390

Rubig, A. (2003) Drospirenone: A new cardiovascular-active progestin with antialdosterone and antiandrogenic properties. *Climacteric,* **6** (Suppl. 3), 49–54

Rylander-Rudqvist, T., Wedrén, S., Jonasdottir, G., Ahlberg, S., Weiderpass, E., Persson, I. & Ingelman-Sundberg, M. (2004) Cytochrome P450 1B1 gene polymorphisms and postmenopausal endometrial cancer risk. *Cancer Epidemiol. Biomarkers Prev.,* **13**, 1515–1520

Sakamoto, S., Kudo, H., Suzuki, S., Mitamura, T., Sassa, S., Kuwa, K., Chun, Z., Yoshimura, S., Maemura, M., Nakayama, T. & Shinoda, H. (1997a) Additional effects of medroxyprogesterone acetate on mammary tumors in oophorectomized, estrogenized, DMBA-treated rats. *Anticancer Res.,* **17**, 4583–4588

Sakamoto, S., Mori, T., Shinoda, H., Sassa, S. & Koyama, T. (1997b) Effects of conjugated estro-gens with or without medroxyprogesterone acetate on mammary carcinogenesis, uterine adenomyosis and femur in mice. *Acta anat.*, **159**, 204–208

Salpeter, S.R., Walsh, J.M.E., Greyber, E., Ormiston, T.M. & Salpeter, E.E. (2004) Mortality asso-ciated with hormone replacement therapy in younger and older women. *J. gen. intern. Med.*, **19**, 791–804

Santen, R.J. (2003) Risk of breast cancer with progestins: Critical assessment of current data. *Steroids*, **68**, 953–964

Sasaki, M., Tanaka, Y., Kaneuchi, M., Sakuragi, N. & Dahiya, R. (2003) CYP1B1 gene polymor-phisms have higher risk for endometrial cancer, and positive correlations with estrogen receptor α and estrogen receptor β expressions. *Cancer Res.*, **63**, 3913–3918

Sasano, H., Frost, A.R., Saitoh, R., Harada, N., Poutanen, M., Vihko, R., Bulun, S.E., Silverberg, S.G. & Nagura, H. (1996) Aromatase and 17β-hydroxysteroid dehydrogenase type 1 in human breast carcinoma. *J. clin. Endocrinol. Metab.*, **81**, 4042–4046

Saure, A., Hirvonen, E., Milsom, I., Christensen, A. & Damber, M.-G. (1996) A randomized, double-blind, multicentre study comparing the clinical effects of two sequential estra-diol–progestin combinations containing either desogestrel or norethisterone acetate in climac-teric women with estrogen deficiency symptoms. *Maturitas*, **24**, 111–118

Saure, A., Planellas, J., Poulsen, H.K. & Jaszczak, P. (2000) A double-blind, randomized, compa-rative study evaluating clinical effects of two sequential estradiol–progestogen combinations containing either desogestrel or medroxyprogesterone acetate in climacteric women. *Matu-ritas*, **34**, 133–142

Scarabin, P.-Y., Alhenc-Gelas, M., Oger, E. & Plu-Bureau, G. (1999) Hormone replacement therapy and circulating ICAM-1 in postmenopausal women — A randomised controlled trial. *Thromb. Haemost.*, **81**, 673–675

Schabath, M.B., Wu, X., Vassilopoulou-Sellin, R., Vaporciyan, A.A. & Spitz, M.R. (2004) Hormone replacement therapy and lung cancer risk: A case–control analysis. *Clin. Cancer Res.*, **10**, 113–123

Schairer, C., Lubin, J., Troisi, R., Sturgeon, S., Brinton, L. & Hoover, R. (2000) Menopausal estrogen and estrogen–progestin replacement therapy and breast cancer risk. *J. Am. med. Assoc.*, **283**, 485–491

Schindler, A.E., Campagnoli, C., Druckmann, R., Huber, J., Pasqualini, J.R., Schweppe, K.W. & Thijssen, J.H.H. (2003) Classification and pharmacology of progestins. *Maturitas*, **46** (Suppl. 1), 7–16

Schoonen, W.G.E.J., Dijkema, R., de Ries, R.J.H., Wagenaars, J.L., Joosten, J.W.H., de Gooyer, M.E., Deckers, G.H. & Kloosterboer, H.J. (1998) Human progesterone receptor A and B iso-forms in CHO cells. II. Comparison of binding, transactivation and ED_{50} values of several synthetic (anti)progestagens *in vitro* in CHO and MCF-7 cells and *in vivo* in rabbits and rats. *J. steroid Biochem. mol. Biol.*, **64**, 157–170

Schoonen, W.G.E.J., Deckers, G., de Gooijer, M.E., de Ries, R., Mathijssen-Mommers, G., Hamersma, H. & Kloosterboer, H.J. (2000a) Contraceptive progestins. Various 11-substituents combined with four 17-substituents: 17α-Ethynyl, five- and six-membered spiromethylene ethers or six-membered spiromethylene lactones. *J. steroid Biochem. mol. Biol.*, **74**, 109–123

Schoonen, W.G.E.J., Deckers, G.H., de Gooijer, M.E., de Ries, R. & Kloosterboer, H.J. (2000b) Hormonal properties of norethisterone, 7α-methyl-norethisterone and their derivatives. *J. steroid Biochem. mol. Biol.*, **74**, 213–222

Schumacher, G. & Neuhaus, P. (2001) The physiological estrogen metabolite 2-methoxyestradiol reduces tumor growth and induces apoptosis in human solid tumors. *J. Cancer Res. clin. Oncol.*, **127**, 405–410

Schumacher, G., Kataoka, M., Roth, J.A. & Mukhopadhyay, T. (1999) Potent antitumor activity of 2-methoxyestradiol in human pancreatic cancer cell lines. *Clin. Cancer Res.*, **5**, 493–499

Schütze, N., Vollmer, G., Tiemann, I., Geiger, M. & Knuppen, R. (1993) Catecholestrogens are MCF-7 cell estrogen receptor agonists. *J. steroid Biochem. mol. Biol.*, **46**, 781–789

Schütze, N., Vollmer, G. & Knuppen, R. (1994) Catecholestrogens are agonists of estrogen receptor dependent gene expression in MCF-7 cells. *J. steroid Biochem. mol. Biol.*, **48**, 453–461

Seed, M., Sands, R.H., McLaren, M., Kirk, G. & Darko, D. (2000) The effect of hormone replacement therapy and route of administration on selected cardiovascular risk factors in post-menopausal women. *Fam. Pract.*, **17**, 479–507

Seeger, H., Mueck, A.O. & Lippert, T.H. (2000) Effect of norethisterone acetate on estrogen metabolism in postmenopausal women. *Horm. Metab. Res.*, **32**, 436–439

Seeger, H., Wallwiener, D. & Mueck, A.O. (2003a) Comparison of the effect of progesterone, medroxyprogesterone acetate and norethisterone on the proliferation of human breast cancer cells. *J. Br. Menopause Soc.*, **9**, 36–38

Seeger, H., Wallwiener, D. & Mueck, A.O. (2003b) The effect of progesterone and synthetic progestins on serum- and estradiol-stimulated proliferation of human breast cancer cells. *Horm. Metab. Res.*, **35**, 76–80

Sendag, F., Terek, M.C., Ozsener, S., Oztekin, K., Bilgin, O., Bilgen, I. & Memis, A. (2001) Mammographic density changes during different postmenopausal hormone replacement therapies. *Fertil. Steril.*, **76**, 445–450

Seth, P., Lunetta, K.L., Bell, D.W., Gray, H., Nasser, S.M., Rhei, E., Kaelin, C.M., Iglehart, D.J., Marks, J.R., Garber, J.E., Haber, D.A. & Polyak, K. (2000) Phenol sulfotransferases: Hormonal regulation, polymorphism, and age of onset of breast cancer. *Cancer Res.*, **60**, 6859–6863

Setiawan, V.W., Hankinson, S.E., Colditz, G.A., Hunter, D.J. & De Vivo, I. (2004) *HSD17B1* gene polymorphisms and risk of endometrial and breast cancer. *Cancer Epidemiol. Biomarkers Prev.*, **13**, 213–219

Shapiro, S. (2003) Risks of estrogen plus progestin therapy: A sensitivity analysis of findings in the Women's Health Initiative Randomized Controlled Trial. *Climacteric*, **6**, 302–310

Shelby, M.D., Tice, R.R. & Witt, K.L. (1997) 17-β-Estradiol fails to induce micronuclei in the bone marrow cells of rodents. *Mutat. Res.*, **395**, 89–90

Shields-Botella, J., Duc, I., Duranti, E., Puccio, F., Bonnet, P., Delansorne, R. & Paris, J. (2003) An overview of nomegestrol acetate selective receptor binding and lack of estrogenic action on hormone-dependent cancer cells. *J. steroid Biochem. mol. Biol.*, **87**, 111–122

Shimada, T., Watanabe, J., Kawajiri, K., Sutter, T.R., Guengerich, F.P., Gillam, E.M. & Inoue, K. (1999) Catalytic properties of polymorphic human cytochrome P450 1B1 variants. *Carcinogenesis*, **20**, 1607–1613

Shumaker, S.A., Legault, C., Rapp, S.R., Thal, L., Wallace, R.B., Ockene, J.K., Hendrix, S.L., Jones, B.N., III, Assaf, A.R., Jackson, R.D., Kotchen, J.M., Wassertheil-Smoller, S. & Wactawski-Wende, J. for the WHIMS Investigators (2003) Estrogen plus progestin and the incidence of dementia and mild cognitive impairment in postmenopausal women. The Women's Health Initiative Memory Study: A randomized controlled trial. *J. Am. med. Assoc.*, **289**, 2651–2662

Shumaker, S.A., Legault, C., Kuller, L., Rapp, S.R., Thal, L., Lane, D.S., Fillit, H., Stefanick, M.L., Hendrix, S.L., Lewis, C.E., Masaki, K. & Coker, L.H. for the Women's Health Initiative Memory Study Investigators (2004) Conjugated equine estrogens and incidence of probable dementia and mild cognitive impairment in postmenopausal women. Women's Health Initiative Memory Study. *J. Am. med. Assoc.*, **291**, 2947–2958

Silvestri, A., Gebara, O., Vitale, C., Wajngarten, M., Leonardo, F., Ramires, J.A.F., Fini, M., Mercuro, G. & Rosano, G.M. (2003) Increased levels of C-reactive protein after oral hormone replacement therapy may not be related to an increased inflammatory response. *Circulation*, **107**, 3165–3169

Simon, J.A., Hsia, J., Cauley, J.A., Richards, C., Harris, F., Fong, J., Barrett-Connor, E. & Hulley, S.B. (2001a) Postmenopausal hormone therapy and risk of stroke: The Heart and Estrogen–Progestin Replacement Study (HERS). *Circulation*, **103**, 638–642

Simon, J.A., Hunninghake, D.B., Agarwal, S.K., Lin, F., Cauley, J.A., Ireland, C.C. & Pickar, J.H. for the Heart and Estrogen/Progestin Replacement Study (HERS) Research Group (2001b) Effect of estrogen plus progestin on risk for biliary tract surgery in postmenopausal women with coronary artery disease. *Ann. intern. Med.*, **135**, 493–501

Singh, K., López-Guerrero, J.A., Llombart-Bosch, A. & Roy, D. (2005) Estrogen-induced mutations and its role in the development of tumorigenesis. In: Li, J.J., Li, S.A. & Llombarts-Bosch, A., eds, *Hormonal Carcinogenesis IV*, New York, Springer-Verlag, pp. 475–479

Sit, A.S., Modugno, F., Weissfeld, J.L., Berga, S.L.& Ness, R.B. (2002) Hormone replacement therapy formulations and risk of epithelial ovarian carcinoma. *Gynecol. Oncol.*, **86**, 118–123

Sitruk-Ware, R. (2002) Progestogens in hormonal replacement therapy: New molecules, risks, and benefits. *Menopause*, **9**, 6–15

Sitruk-Ware, R. (2004a) Pharmacological profile of progestins. *Maturitas*, **47**, 277–283

Sitruk-Ware, R. (2004b) New progestogens: A review of their effects in perimenopausal and post-menopausal women. *Drugs Aging*, **21**, 865–883

Sitruk-Ware, R., Small, M., Kumar, N., Tsong, Y.Y., Sundaram, K. & Jackanicz, T. (2003) Nesto-rone: Clinical applications for contraception and HRT. *Steroids*, **68**, 907–913

Smart, J. & Daly, A.K. (2000) Variation in induced CYP1A1 levels: Relationship to CYP1A1, Ah receptor and *GSTM1* polymorphisms. *Pharmacogenetics*, **10**, 11–24

Smid-Koopman, E., Kuhne, L.C.M., Hanekamp, E.E., Gielen, S.C.J.P., De Ruiter, P.E., Grootegoed, J.A., Helmerhorst, T.J.M., Burger, C.W., Brinkmann, A.O., Huikeshoven, F.J. & Blok, L.J. (2005) Progesterone-induced inhibition of growth and differential regulation of gene expression in PRA- and/or PRB-expressing endometrial cancer cell lines. *J. Soc. gynecol. Invest.*, **12**, 285–292

Smith, D.C., Prentice, R., Thompson, D.J. & Herrmann, W.L. (1975) Association of exogenous estrogen and endometrial carcinoma. *New Engl. J. Med.*, **293**, 1164–1167

Smith, E.M., Johnson, S.R., Figuerres, E.J., Mendoza, M., Fedderson, D., Haugen, T.H. & Turek, L.P. (1997) The frequency of human papillomavirus detection in postmenopausal women on hormone replacement therapy. *Gynecol. Oncol.*, **65**, 441–446

Spink, B.C., Katz, B.H., Hussain, M.M., Pang, S., Connor, S.P., Aldous, K.M., Gierthy, J.F. & Spink, D.C. (2000) SULT1A1 catalyzes 2-methoxyestradiol sulfonation in MCF-7 breast cancer cells. *Carcinogenesis*, **21**, 1947–1957

Stafford, R.S., Saglam, D., Causino, N. & Blumenthal, D. (1998) The declining impact of race and insurance status on hormone replacement therapy. *Menopause*, **5**, 140–144

Stahlberg, C., Pedersen, A.T., Lynge, E., Andersen, Z.J., Keiding, N., Hundrup, Y.A., Obel, E.B. & Ottesen, B. (2004) Increased risk of breast cancer following different regimens of hormone replacement therapy frequently used in Europe. *Int. J. Cancer*, **109**, 721–727

Stampfer, M.J. & Colditz, G.A. (1991) Estrogen replacement therapy and coronary heart disease: A quantitative assessment of the epidemiologic evidence. *Prev. Med.*, **20**, 47–63

Stefanick, M.L., Cochrane, B.B., Hsia, J., Barad, D.H., Liu, J.H. & Johnson, S.R. (2003) The Women's Health Initiative postmenopausal hormone trials: Overview and baseline characteristics of participants. *Ann. Epidemiol.*, **13**, S78–S86

Stice, S.L., Ford, S.P., Rosazza, J.P. & Van Orden, D.E. (1987) Role of 4-hydroxylated estradiol in reducing Ca^{2+} uptake of uterine arterial smooth muscle cells through potential-sensitive channels. *Biol. Reprod.*, **36**, 361–368

Stoilov, I., Akarsu, A.N., Alozie, I., Child, A., Barsoum-Homsy, M., Turacli, M.E., Or, M., Lewis, R.A., Ozdemir, N., Brice, G., Aktan, S.G., Chevrette, L., Coca-Prados, M. & Sarfarazi, M. (1998) Sequence analysis and homology modeling suggest that primary congenital glaucoma on 2p21 results from mutations disrupting either the hinge region or the conserved core structures of cytochrome P4501B1. *Am. J. hum. Genet.* **62**, 573–584

Strickler, R.C. (2003) Women's Health Initiative results: A glass more empty than full. *Fertil. Steril.*, **80**, 488–490

Strothmann, A. & Schneider, H.P.G. (2003) Hormone therapy: The European women's perspective. *Climacteric*, **6**, 337–346

Sturdee, D.W., Ulrich, L.G., Barlow, D.H., Wells, M., Campbell, M.J., Vessey, M.P., Nielsen, B., Anderson, M.C. & Bragg, A.J. (2000) The endometrial response to sequential and continuous combined oestrogen–progestogen replacement therapy. *Br. J. Obstet. Gynaecol.*, **107**, 1392–1400

Sudhir, K., Chou, T.M., Mullen, W.L., Hausmann, D., Collins, P., Yock, P.G. & Chatterjee, K. (1995) Mechanisms of estrogen-induced vasodilation: In vivo studies in canine coronary conductance and resistance arteries. *J. Am. Coll. Cardiol.*, **26**, 807–814

Suparto, I.H., Williams, J.K., Cline, J.M., Anthony, M.S. & Fox, J.L. (2003) Contrasting effects of two hormone replacement therapies on the cardiovascular and mammary gland outcomes in surgically postmenopausal monkeys. *Am. J. Obstet. Gynecol.*, **188**, 1132–1140

Suvanto-Luukkonen, E., Malinen, H., Sundström, H., Penttinen, J. & Kauppila, A. (1998) Endometrial morphology during hormone replacement therapy with estradiol gel combined to levo-norgestrel-releasing intrauterine device or natural progesterone. *Acta obstet. gynecol. scand.*, **77**, 758–763

Suzuki, T., Moriya, T., Ariga, N., Kaneko, C., Kanazawa, M. & Sasano, H. (2000) 17β-Hydroxy-steroid dehydrogenase type 1 and type 2 in human breast carcinoma: A correlation to clinico-pathological parameters. *Br. J. Cancer*, **82**, 518–523

Suzuki, T., Nakata, T., Miki, Y., Kaneko, C., Moriya, T., Ishida, T., Akinaga, S., Hirakawa, H., Kimura, M. & Sasano, H. (2003) Estrogen sulfotransferase and steroid sulfatase in human breast carcinoma. *Cancer Res.*, **63**, 2762–2770

Syvänen, A.-C., Tilgmann, C., Rinne, J. & Ulmanen, I. (1997) Genetic polymorphism of catechol-O-methyltransferase (COMT): Correlation of genotype with individual variation of S-COMT activity and comparison of the allele frequencies in the normal population and Parkinsonian patients in Finland. *Pharmacogenetics*, **7**, 65–71

Tagawa, H., Shimokawa, H., Tagawa, T., Kuroiwa-Matsumoto, M., Hirooka, Y. & Takeshita, A. (1997) Short-term estrogen augments both nitric oxide-mediated and non-nitric oxide-mediated endothelium-dependent forearm vasodilation in postmenopausal women. *J. cardiovasc. Pharmacol.*, **30**, 481–488

Tang, Y.M., Green, B.L., Chen, G.F., Thompson, P.A., Lang, N.P., Shinde, A., Lin, D.X., Tan, W., Lyn-Cook, B.D., Hammons, G.J. & Kadlubar, F.F. (2000) Human *CYP1B1 Leu^{432}Val* gene polymorphism: Ethnic distribution in African-Americans, Caucasians and Chinese; oestradiol hydroxylase activity; and distribution in prostate cancer cases and controls. *Pharmacogenetics*, **10**, 761–766

Teede, H.J., McGrath, B.P., Smolich, J.J., Malan, E., Kotsopoulos, D., Liang, Y.-L. & Peverill, R.E. (2000) Postmenopausal hormone replacement therapy increases coagulation activity and fibrinolysis. *Arterioscler. Thromb. vasc. Biol.*, **20**, 1404–1409

Terashima, I., Suzuki, N. & Shibutani, S. (2001) Mutagenic properties of estrogen quinone-derived DNA adducts in simian kidney cells. *Biochemistry*, **40**, 166–172

Thom, M.H., White, P.J., Williams, R.M., Sturdee, D.W., Paterson, M.E.L., Wade-Evans, T. & Studd, J.W.W. (1979) Prevention and treatment of endometrial disease in climacteric women receiving oestrogen therapy. *Lancet*, **ii**, 455–457

Thuneke, I., Schulte, H.M. & Bamberger, A.-M. (2000) Biphasic effect of medroxyprogesterone-acetate (MPA) treatment on proliferation and cyclin D1 gene transcription in T47D breast cancer cells. *Breast Cancer Res. Treat.*, **63**, 243–248

Tikkanen, M.J., Nikkilä, E.A., Kuusi, T. & Sipinen, S.U. (1982) High density lipoprotein-2 and hepatic lipase: Reciprocal changes produced by estrogen and norgestrel. *J. clin. Endocrinol. Metab.*, **54**, 1113–1117

Tikkanen, M.J., Kuusi, T., Nikkilä, E.A. & Sipinen, S. (1986) Post-menopausal hormone replacement therapy: Effects of progestogens on serum lipids and lipoproteins. A review. *Maturitas*, **8**, 7–17

Tinley, T.L., Leal, R.M., Randall-Hlubek, D.A., Cessac, J.W., Wilkens, L.R., Rao, P.N. & Mooberry, S.L. (2003) Novel 2-methoxyestradiol analogues with antitumor activity. *Cancer Res.*, **63**, 1538–1549

Tjønneland, A., Christensen, J., Thomsen, B.L., Olsen, A., Overvad, K., Ewertz, M. & Mellemkjaer, L. (2004) Hormone replacement therapy in relation to breast carcinoma incidence rate ratios: A prospective Danish cohort study. *Cancer*, **100**, 2328–2337

Todorovic, R., Devanesan, P., Higginbotham, S., Zhao, J., Gross, M.L., Rogan, E.G. & Cavalieri, E.L. (2001) Analysis of potential biomarkers of estrogen-initiated cancer in the urine of Syrian golden hamsters treated with 4-hydroxyestradiol. *Carcinogenesis*, **22**, 905–911

Townsend, J. (1998) Hormone replacement therapy: Assessment of present use, costs, and trends. *Br. J. gen. Pract.*, **48**, 955–958

Troisi, R.J., Schairer, C., Chow, W.-H., Schatzkin, A., Brinton, L.A. & Fraumeni, J.F., Jr (1997) A prospective study of menopausal hormones and risk of colorectal cancer (United States). *Cancer Causes Control*, **8**, 130–138

Tsutsui, T., Tamura, Y., Hagiwara, M., Miyachi, T., Hikiba, H., Kubo, C. & Barrett, J.C. (2000) Induction of mammalian cell transformation and genotoxicity by 2-methoxyestradiol, an endogenous metabolite of estrogen. *Carcinogenesis*, **21**, 735–740

Tsutsui, T., Tamura, Y., Yagi, E. & Barrett, J.C. (2000a) Involvement of genotoxic effects in the initiation of estrogen-induced cellular transformation: Studies using Syrian hamster embryo cells treated with 17β-estradiol and eight of its metabolites. *Int. J. Cancer*, **86**, 8–14

Tsutsui, T., Tamura, Y., Hagiwara, M., Miyachi, T., Hikiba, H., Kubo, C. & Barrett, J.C. (2000b) Induction of mammalian cell transformation and genotoxicity by 2-methoxyestradiol, an endogenous metabolite of estrogen. *Carcinogenesis*, **21**, 735–740

Tuba, Z., Bardin, C.W., Dancsi, A., Francsics-Czinege, E., Molnar, C., Csorgei, J., Falkay, G., Koide, S.S., Kumar, N., Sundaram, K., Dukat-Abrok, V. & Balogh, G. (2000) Synthesis and biological activity of a new progestogen, 16-methylene-17α-hydroxy-18-methyl-19-nor-pregn-4-ene-3,20-dione acetate. *Steroids*, **65**, 266–274

Tukey, R.H. & Strassburg, C.P. (2000) Human UDP-glucuronosyltransferases: Metabolism, expression, and disease. *Ann. Rev. Pharmacol. Toxicol.*, **40**, 581–616

Turan, V.K., Sanchez, R.I., Li, J.J., Li, S.A., Reuhl, K.R., Thomas, P.E., Conney, A.H., Gallo, M.A., Kauffman, F.C. & Mesia-Vela, S. (2004) The effects of steroidal estrogens in ACI rat mammary carcinogenesis: 17β-Estradiol, 2-hydroxyestradiol, 4-hydroxyestradiol, 16α-hydroxyestradiol, and 4-hydroxyestrone. *J. Endocrinol.*, **183**, 91–99

Turgeon, D., Carrier, J.-S., Lévesque, E., Hum, D.W. & Bélanger, A. (2001) Relative enzymatic activity, protein stability, and tissue distribution of human steroid-metabolizing UGT2B subfamily members. *Endocrinology*, **142**, 778–787

Tworoger, S.S., Chubak, J., Aiello, E.J., Ulrich, C.M., Atkinson, C., Potter, J.D., Yasui, Y., Stapleton, P.L., Lampe, J.W., Farin, F.M., Stanczyk, F.Z. & McTiernan, A. (2004) Association of *CYP17*, *CYP19*, *CYP1B1*, and *COMT* polymorphisms with serum and urinary sex hormone concentrations in postmenopausal women. *Cancer Epidemiol. Biomarkers Prev.*, **13**, 94–101

Ursin, G., London, S., Stanczyk, F.Z., Gentzschein, E., Paganini-Hill, A., Ross, R.K. & Pike, M.C. (1999) Urinary 2-hydroxyestrone/16α-hydroxyestrone ratio and risk of breast cancer in postmenopausal women. *J. natl Cancer Inst.*, **91**, 1067–1072

Ursin, G., Wilson, M., Henderson, B.E., Kolonel, L.N., Monroe, K., Lee, H.-P., Seow, A., Yu, M.C., Stanczyk, F.Z. & Gentzschein, E. (2001) Do urinary estrogen metabolites reflect the differences in breast cancer risk between Singapore Chinese and United States African-American and white women? *Cancer Res.*, **61**, 3326–3329

Ursin, G., London, S., Yang, D., Tseng, C.-C., Pike, M.C., Bernstein, L., Stanczyk, F.Z. & Gentzschein, E. (2002) Urinary 2-hydroxyestrone/16α-hydroxyestrone ratio and family history of breast cancer in premenopausal women. *Breast Cancer Res. Treat.*, **72**, 139–143

US Preventive Service Task Force (2002) Postmenopausal hormone replacement therapy for primary prevention of chronic conditions: Recommendations and rationale. *Ann. intern. Med.*, **137**, 834–839

Utsumi, T., Yoshimura, N., Takeuchi, S., Ando, J., Maruta, M., Maeda, K. & Harada, N. (1999) Steroid sulfatase expression is an independent predictor of recurrence in human breast cancer. *Cancer Res.*, **59**, 377–381

Utsunomiya, H., Suzuki, T., Kaneko, C., Takeyama, J., Nakamura, J., Kimura, K., Yoshihama, M., Harada, N., Ito, K., Konno, R., Sato, S., Okamura, K. & Sasano, H. (2001) The analyses of

17β-hydroxysteroid dehydrogenase isozymes in human endometrial hyperplasia and carcinoma. *J. clin. Endocrinol. Metab.*, **86**, 3436–3443

Utsunomiya, H., Suzuki, T., Ito, K., Moriya, T., Konno, R., Sato, S., Yaegashi, N., Okamura, K. & Sasano, H. (2003) The correlation between the response to progestogen treatment and the expression of progesterone receptor β and 17β-hydroxysteroid dehydrogenase type 2 in human endometrial carcinoma. *Clin. Endocrinol.*, **58**, 696–703

Utsunomiya, H., Ito, K., Suzuki, T., Kitamura, T., Kaneko, C., Nakata, T., Niikura, H., Okamura, K., Yaegashi, N. & Sasano, H. (2004) Steroid sulfatase and estrogen sulfotransferase in human endometrial carcinoma. *Clin. Cancer Res.*, **10**, 5850–5856

Valdivia, I., Campodonico, I., Tapia, A., Capetillo, M., Espinoza, A. & Lavin, P. (2004) Effects of tibolone and continuous combined hormone therapy on mammographic breast density and breast histochemical markers in postmenopausal women. *Fertil. Steril.*, **81**, 617–623

Vallée, M., Albert, C., Beaudry, G., Hum, D.W. & Bélanger, A. (2001) Isolation and characterization of the monkey UDP-glucuronosyltransferase cDNA clone monUGT1A01 active on bilirubin and estrogens. *J. steroid Biochem. mol. Biol.*, **77**, 239–249

Venkov, C.D., Rankin, A.B. & Vaughan, D.E. (1996) Identification of authentic estrogen receptor in cultured endothelial cells. *Circulation*, **94**, 727–733

Vestergaard, P., Hermann, A.P., Stilgren, L., Tofteng, C.L., Sorensen, O.H., Eiken, P., Nielsen, S.P. & Mosekilde, L. (2003) Effects of 5 years of hormonal replacement therapy on menopausal symptoms and blood pressure — A randomised controlled study. *Maturitas*, **46**, 123–132

Vihma, V., Adlercreutz, H., Tiitinen, A., Kiuru, P., Wähälä, K. & Tikkanen, M.J. (2001) Quantitative determination of estradiol fatty acid esters in human pregnancy serum and ovarian follicular fluid. *Clin. Chem.*, **47**, 1256–1262

Vihma, V., Tiitinen, A., Ylikorkala, O. & Tikkanen, M.J. (2003a) Quantitative determination of estradiol fatty acid esters in lipoprotein fractions in human blood. *J. clin. Endocrinol. Metab.*, **88**, 2552–2555

Vihma, V., Vehkavaara, S., Yki-Järvinen, H., Hohtari, H. & Tikkanen, M.J. (2003b) Differential effects of oral and transdermal estradiol treatment on circulating estradiol fatty acid ester concentrations in postmenopausal women. *J. clin. Endocrinol. Metab.*, **88**, 588–593

Viscoli, C.M., Brass, L.M., Kernan, W.N., Sarrel, P.M., Suissa, S. & Horwitz, R.I. (2001) A clinical trial of estrogen-replacement therapy after ischemic stroke. *New Engl. J. Med.*, **345**, 1243–1249

Vitale, C., Fini, M., Leonardo, F., Rossini, P., Cerquetani, E., Onorati, D. & Rosano, G.M.C. (2001) Effect of estradiol valerate alone or in association with cyproterone acetate upon vascular function of postmenopausal women at increased risk for cardiovascular disease. *Maturitas*, **40**, 239–245

Voigt, L.F., Weiss, N.S., Chu, J., Daling, J.R., McKnight, B. & van Belle, G. (1991) Progestagen supplementation of exogenous oestrogens and risk of endometrial cancer. *Lancet*, **338**, 274–277

Volterrani, M., Rosano, G., Coats, A., Beale, C. & Collins, P. (1995) Estrogen acutely increases peripheral blood flow in postmenopausal women. *Am. J. Med.*, **99**, 119–122

Von Schoultz, B. (2003) Clinical efficacy and safety of combined estradiol valerate and dienogest: A new no-bleed treatment. *Climacteric*, **6** (Suppl. 2), 24–32

Wahab, M., Thompson, J., Hamid, B., Deen, S. & Al-Azzawi, F. (1999) Endometrial histomorphometry of trimegestone-based sequential hormone replacement therapy: A weighted comparison with the endometrium of the natural cycle. *Hum. Reprod.*, **14**, 2609–2618

Walsh, B.W., Schiff, I., Rosner, B., Greenberg, L., Ravnikar, V. & Sacks, F.M. (1991) Effects of postmenopausal estrogen replacement on the concentrations and metabolism of plasma lipoproteins. *New Engl. J. Med.*, **325**, 1196–1204

Walsh, B.W., Paul, S., Wild, R.A., Dean, R.A., Tracy, R.P., Cox, D.A. & Anderson, P.W. (2000) The effects of hormone replacement therapy and raloxifene on C-reactive protein and homocysteine in healthy postmenopausal women: A randomized, controlled trial. *J. clin. Endocrinol. Metab.*, **85**, 214–218

Wang, Z., Yang, D., Mohanakrishnan, A.K., Fanwick, P.E., Nampoothiri, P., Hamel, E. & Cushman, M. (2000) Synthesis of B-ring homologated estradiol analogues that modulate tubulin polymerization and microtubule stability. *J. med. Chem.*, **43**, 2419–2429

Wassertheil-Smoller, S., Hendrix, S.L., Limacher, M., Heiss, G., Kooperberg, C., Baird, A., Kotchen, T., Curb, J.D., Black, H., Rossouw, J.E., Aragaki, A., Safford, M., Stein, E., Laowattana, S. & Mysiw, W.J. for the WHI Investigators (2003) Effect of estrogen plus progestin on stroke in postmenopausal women: The Women's Health Initiative: A randomized trial. *J. Am. med. Assoc.*, **289**, 2673–2684

Watanabe, J., Shimada, T., Gillam, E.M., Ikuta, T., Suemasu, K., Higashi, Y., Gotoh, O. & Kawajiri, K. (2000) Association of CYP1B1 genetic polymorphism with incidence to breast and lung cancer. *Pharmacogenetics*, **10**, 25–33

Wathen, C.N., Feig, D.S., Feightner, J.W., Abramson, B.L., Cheung, A.M. & the Canadian Task Force on Preventive Health Care (2004) Hormone replacement therapy for the primary prevention of chronic diseases: Recommendation statement from the Canadian Task Force on Preventive Health Care. *Can. med. Assoc. J.*, **170**, 1535–1537

Weiderpass, E., Adami, H.-O., Baron, J.A., Magnusson, C., Bergstrom, R., Lindgren, A., Correia, N. & Persson, I. (1999) Risk of endometrial cancer following estrogen replacement with and without progestins. *J. natl Cancer Inst.*, **91**, 1131–1137

van de Weijer, P.H.M., Scholten, P.C., van der Mooren, M.J., Barentsen, R. & Kenemans, P. (1999) Bleeding patterns and endometrial histology during administration of low-dose estradiol sequentially combined with dydrogesterone. *Climacteric*, **2**, 101–109

Weiss, L.K., Burkman, R.T., Cushing-Haugen, K.L., Voigt, L.F., Simon, M.S., Daling, J.R., Norman, S.A., Bernstein, L., Ursin, G., Marchbanks, P.A., Strom, B.L., Berlin, J.A., Weber, A.L., Doody, D.R., Wingo, P.A., McDonald, J.A., Malone, K.E., Folger, S.G. & Spirtas, R. (2002) Hormone replacement therapy regimens and breast cancer risk. *Obstet. Gynecol.*, **100**, 1148–1158

Weisz, J., Fritz-Wolz, G., Gestl, S., Clawson, G.A., Creveling, C.R., Liehr, J.G. & Dabbs, D. (2000) Nuclear localization of catechol-*O*-methyltransferase in neoplastic and nonneoplastic mammary epithelial cells. *Am. J. Pathol.*, **156**, 1841–1848

Wells, M., Sturdee, D.W., Barlow, D.H., Ulrich, L.G., O'Brien, K., Campbell, M.J., Vessey, M.P. & Bragg, A.J. (2002) Effect on endometrium of long term treatment with continuous combined oestrogen–progestogen replacement therapy: Follow up study. *Br. med. J.*, **325**, 239–242

Wen, W., Cai, Q., Shu, X.O., Cheng, J.R., Parl, F., Pierce, L., Gao, Y.-T. & Zheng, W. (2005) Cytochrome P450 1B1 and catechol-*O*-methyltransferase genetic polymorphisms and breast cancer risk in Chinese women: Results from the Shanghai Breast Cancer Study and a meta-analysis. *Cancer Epidemiol. Biomarkers Prev.*, **14**, 329–335

Whitehead, M.I., Townsend, P.T., Pryse-Davies, J., Ryder, T.A. & King, R.J.B. (1981) Effects of estrogens and progestins on the biochemistry and morphology of the postmenopausal endometrium. *New Engl. J. Med.*, **305**, 1599–1605

Wiebe, J.P., Muzia, D., Hu, J., Szwajcer, D., Hill, S.A. & Seachrist, J.L. (2000) The 4-pregnene and 5α-pregnane progesterone metabolites formed in nontumorous and tumorous breast tissue have opposite effects on breast cell proliferation and adhesion. *Cancer Res.*, **60**, 936–943

Wiegratz, I. & Kuhl, H. (2004) Progestogen therapies: Differences in clinical effects? *Trends Endocrinol. Metab.*, **15**, 277–285

Wiklund, I., Karlberg, J. & Mattsson, L.-A. (1993) Quality of life of postmenopausal women on a regimen of transdermal estradiol therapy: A double-blind placebo-controlled study. *Am. J. Obstet. Gynecol.*, **168**, 824–830

Williams, J.K., Adams, M.R. & Klopfenstein, H.S. (1990) Estrogen modulates responses of atherosclerotic coronary arteries. *Circulation*, **81**, 1680–1687

Williams, J.K., Honoré, E.K., Washburn, S.A. & Clarkson, T.B. (1994) Effects of hormone replacement therapy on reactivity of atherosclerotic coronary arteries in cynomolgus monkeys. *J. Am. Coll. Cardiol.*, **24**, 1757–1761

Williams, J.K., Anthony, M.S., Honore, E.K., Herrington, D.M., Morgan, T.M., Register, T.C. & Clarkson, T.B. (1995) Regression of atherosclerosis in female monkeys. *Arterioscler. Thromb. vasc. Biol.*, **15**, 827–836

Wilson, P.D., Faragher, B., Butler, B., Bu'lock, D., Robinson, E.L. & Brown, A.D.G. (1987) Treatment with oral piperazine oestrone sulphate for genuine stress incontinence in postmenopausal women. *Br. J. Obstet. Gynaecol.*, **94**, 568–574

Wilson, P.W.F., D'Agostino, R.B., Sullivan, L., Parise, H. & Kannel, W.B. (2002) Overweight and obesity as determinants of cardiovascular risk: The Framingham experience. *Arch. intern. Med.*, **162**, 1867–1872

Winneker, R.C., Bitran, D. & Zhang, Z. (2003) The preclinical biology of a new potent and selective progestin: Trimegestone. *Steroids*, **68**, 915–920

Women's Health Initiative Steering Committee (2004) Effects of conjugated equine estrogen in postmenopausal women with hysterectomy: The Women's Health Initiative Randomized Controlled Trial. *J. Am. med. Assoc.*, **291**, 1701–1712

Women's Health Initiative Study Group (1998) Design of the Women's Health Initiative clinical trial and observational study. *Control clin. Trials.*, **19**, 61–109

Wright, T.C., Holinka, C.F., Ferenczy, A., Gatsonis, C.A., Mutter, G.L., Nicosia, S. & Richart, R.M. (2002) Estradiol-induced hyperplasia in endometrial biopsies from women on hormone replacement therapy. *Am. J. surg. Pathol.*, **26**, 1269–1275

Writing Group for the PEPI Trial (1995) Effects of estrogen or estrogen/progestin regimens on heart disease risk factors in postmenopausal women. The Postmenopausal Estrogen/Progestin Interventions (PEPI) Trial. *J. Am. med. Assoc.*, **273**, 199–208

Writing Group for the Women's Health Initiative Investigators (2002) Risks and benefits of estrogen plus progestin in healthy premenopausal women. Principal results from the Women's Health Initiative Randomized Controlled Trial. *J. Am. med. Assoc.*, **288**, 321–333

Wu, A.H., Seow, A., Arakawa, K., Van Den Berg, D., Lee, H.-P. & Yu, M.C. (2003) HSD17B1 and CYP17 polymorphisms and breast cancer risk among Chinese women in Singapore. *Int. J. Cancer*, **104**, 450–457

Wu, J., Richer, J., Horwitz, K.B. & Hyder, S.M. (2004) Progestin-dependent induction of vascular endothelial growth factor in human breast cancer cells: Preferential regulation by progesterone receptor B. *Cancer Res.*, **64**, 2238–2244

Wuest, J.H., Jr, Dry, T.J. & Edwards, J.E. (1953) The degree of coronary atherosclerosis in bilaterally oophorectomized women. *Circulation*, **7**, 801–809

Xu, S., Zhu, B.T. & Conney, A.H. (2001a) Stimulatory effect of clofibrate and gemfibrozil administration on the formation of fatty acid esters of estradiol by rat liver microsomes. *J. Pharmacol. exp. Ther.*, **296**, 188–197

Xu, S., Zhu, B.T., Cai, M.X. & Conney, A.H. (2001b) Stimulatory effect of clofibrate on the action of estradiol in the mammary gland but not in the uterus of rats. *J. Pharmacol. exp. Ther.*, **297**, 50–56

Yaffe, M.J., Boyd, N.F., Byng, J.W., Jong, R.A., Fishell, E., Lockwood, G.A., Little, L.E. & Tritchler, D.L. (1998) Breast cancer risk and measured mammographic density. *Eur. J. Cancer Prev.*, **7**, S47–S55

Yager, J.D. & Liehr, J.G. (1996) Molecular mechanisms of estrogen carcinogenesis. *Ann. Rev. Pharmacol. Toxicol.*, **36**, 203–232

Yamamoto, R., Tatsuta, M., Yamamoto, T. & Terada, N. (1996) The later administration of progesterone more rapidly activates dormant mouse mammary tumor cells initiated by 3′-methyl-4-dimethylaminoazobenzene. *Cancer Lett.*, **100**, 41–45

Yao, J., Chang, M., Li, Y., Pisha, E., Liu, X., Yao, D., Elguindi, E.C., Blond, S.Y. & Bolton, J.L. (2002) Inhibition of cellular enzymes by equine catechol estrogens in human breast cancer cells: Specificity for glutathione S-transferase P1-1. *Chem. Res. Toxicol.*, **15**, 935–942

Yao, J., Li, Y., Chang, M., Wu, H., Yang, X., Goodman, J.E., Liu, X., Liu, H., Mesecar, A.D., van Breemen, R.B., Yager, D.J. &. Bolton, J.L. (2003) Catechol estrogen 4-hydroxyequilenin is a substrate and an inhibitor of catechol-O-methyltransferase. *Chem. Res. Toxicol.*, **16**, 668–675

Yared, E., McMillan, T.J. & Martin, F.L. (2002) Genotoxic effects of oestrogens in breast cells detected by the micronucleus assay and the Comet assay. *Mutagenesis*, **17**, 345–352

Yasui, M., Matsui, S., Laxmi, Y.R.S., Suzuki, N., Kim, S.Y., Shibutani, S. & Matsuda, T. (2003) Mutagenic events induced by 4-hydroxyequilin in *sup*F shuttle vector plasmid propagated in human cells. *Carcinogenesis*, **24**, 911–917

Yue, T.-L., Wang, X., Louden, C.S., Gupta, S., Pillarisetti, K., Gu, J.-L., Hart, T.K., Lysko, P.G. & Feuerstein, G.Z. (1997) 2-Methoxyestradiol, an endogenous estrogen metabolite, induces apoptosis in endothelial cells and inhibits angiogenesis: Possible role for stress-activated protein kinase signaling pathway and Fas expression. *Mol. Pharmacol.*, **51**, 951–962

Zandi, P.P., Carlson, M.C., Plassman, B.L., Welsh-Bohmer, K.A., Mayer, L.S., Steffens, D.C. & Breitner, J.C.S. for the Cache County Memory Study Investigators (2002) Hormone replacement therapy and incidence of Alzheimer disease in older women. The Cache County Study. *J. Am. med. Assoc.*, **288**, 2123–2129

Zeller, W.J. & Berger, M.R. (1989) Nicotine and estrogen metabolism — Possible implications of smoking for growth and outcome of treatment of hormone-dependent cancer? Discussion of experimental results. *J. Cancer Res. Oncol.*, **115**, 601–603

Zhang, Z., Lundeen, S.G., Zhu, Y., Carver, J.M. & Winneker, R.C. (2000) In vitro characterization of trimegestone: A new potent and selective progestin. *Steroids*, **65**, 637–643

Zhang, F., Swanson, S.M., van Breemen, R.B., Liu, X., Yang, Y., Gu, C. & Bolton, J.L. (2001) Equine estrogen metabolite 4-hydroxyequilenin induces DNA damage in the rat mammary tissues: Formation of single-strand breaks, apurinic sites, stable adducts, and oxidized bases. *Chem. Res. Toxicol.*, **14**, 1654–1659

Zheng, W., Dunning, L., Jin, F. & Holtzman, J. (1998) Correspondence re: G.C. Kabat *et al.*, Urinary estrogen metabolites and breast cancer: A case–control study. Cancer Epidemiol. Biomarkers Prev., *6*, 505–509, 1997. *Cancer Epidemiol. Biomark. Prev.*, **7**, 85–86

Zheng, W., Xie, D.-W., Jin, F., Cheng, J.-R., Dai, Q., Wen, W.-Q., Shu, X.-O. & Gao, Y.-T. (2000) Genetic polymorphism of cytochrome P450-1B1 and risk of breast cancer. *Cancer Epidemiol. Biomarkers Prev.*, **9**, 147–150

Zheng, W., Xie, D., Cerhan, J.R., Sellers, T.A., Wen, W. & Folsom, A.R. (2001) Sulfotransferase 1A1 polymorphism, endogenous estrogen exposure, well-done meat intake, and breast cancer risk. *Cancer Epidemiol. Biomarkers Prev.*, **10**, 89–94

Ziel, H.K. & Finkle, W.D. (1975) Increased risk of endometrial carcinoma among users of conjugated estrogens. *New Engl. J. Med.*, **293**, 1167–1170

Ziel, H.K., Finkle, W.D. & Greenland, S. (1998) Decline in incidence of endometrial cancer following increase in prescriptions for opposed conjugated estrogens in a prepaid health plan. *Gynecol. Oncol.*, **68**, 253–255

ANNEXES

ANNEX 1
CHEMICAL AND PHYSICAL DATA ON COMPOUNDS USED IN COMBINED ESTROGEN–PROGESTOGEN CONTRACEPTIVES AND HORMONAL MENOPAUSAL THERAPY

Annex 1 describes the chemical and physical data, technical products, trends in production by region and uses of estrogens and progestogens in combined estrogen–progestogen contraceptives and hormonal menopausal therapy. Estrogens and progestogens are listed separately in alphabetical order. Trade names for these compounds alone and in combination are given in Annexes 2–4.

Sales are listed according to the regions designated by WHO. These are:

Africa: Algeria, Angola, Benin, Botswana, Burkina Faso, Burundi, Cameroon, Cape Verde, Central African Republic, Chad, Comoros, Congo, Côte d'Ivoire, Democratic Republic of the Congo, Equatorial Guinea, Eritrea, Ethiopia, Gabon, Gambia, Ghana, Guinea, Guinea-Bissau, Kenya, Lesotho, Liberia, Madagascar, Malawi, Mali, Mauritania, Mauritius, Mozambique, Namibia, Niger, Nigeria, Rwanda, Sao Tome and Principe, Senegal, Seychelles, Sierra Leone, South Africa, Swaziland, Togo, Uganda, United Republic of Tanzania, Zambia and Zimbabwe

America (North): Canada, Central America (Antigua and Barbuda, Bahamas, Barbados, Belize, Costa Rica, Cuba, Dominica, El Salvador, Grenada, Guatemala, Haiti, Honduras, Jamaica, Mexico, Nicaragua, Panama, Puerto Rico, Saint Kitts and Nevis, Saint Lucia, Saint Vincent and the Grenadines, Suriname, Trinidad and Tobago), United States of America

America (South): Argentina, Bolivia, Brazil, Chile, Colombia, Dominican Republic, Ecuador, Guyana, Paraguay, Peru, Uruguay, Venezuela

Eastern Mediterranean: Afghanistan, Bahrain, Djibouti, Egypt, Iran (Islamic Republic of), Iraq, Jordan, Kuwait, Lebanon, Libyan Arab Jamahiriya, Morocco, Oman, Pakistan, Qatar, Saudi Arabia, Somalia, Sudan, Syrian Arab Republic, Tunisia, United Arab Emirates, Yemen

Europe: Albania, Andorra, Armenia, Austria, Azerbaijan, Belarus, Belgium, Bosnia and Herzegovina, Bulgaria, Croatia, Cyprus, Czech Republic, Denmark, Estonia, Finland, France, Georgia, Germany, Greece, Hungary, Iceland, Ireland, Israel, Italy, Kazakhstan, Kyrgyzstan, Latvia, Lithuania, Luxembourg, Malta, Monaco, Netherlands, Norway, Poland, Portugal, Republic of Moldova, Romania, Russian Federation, San Marino,

Serbia and Montenegro, Slovakia, Slovenia, Spain, Sweden, Switzerland, Tajikistan, The Former Yugoslav Republic of Macedonia, Turkey, Turkmenistan, Ukraine, United Kingdom of Great Britain and Northern Ireland, Uzbekistan

South-East Asia: Bangladesh, Bhutan, Democratic People's Republic of Korea, Democratic Republic of Timor-Leste, India, Indonesia, Maldives, Myanmar, Nepal, Sri Lanka, Thailand

Western Pacific: Australia, Brunei Darussalam, Cambodia, China, Cook Islands, Fiji, Japan, Kiribati, Lao People's Democratic Republic, Malaysia, Marshall Islands, Micronesia (Federated States of), Mongolia, Nauru, New Zealand, Niue, Palau, Papua New Guinea, Philippines, Republic of Korea, Samoa, Singapore, Solomon Islands, Tokelau, Tonga, Tuvalu, Vanuatu, Viet Nam

1. Estrogens

1.1   Conjugated estrogens

The term 'conjugated estrogens' refers to mixtures of at least eight compounds, including sodium estrone sulfate and sodium equilin sulfate, that are derived wholly or in part from equine urine, are plant-based or are manufactured synthetically from estrone and equilin. Conjugated estrogens contain as concomitant components the sodium sulfate conjugates of 17α-dihydroequilin, 17β-dihydroequilin and 17α-estradiol (Pharmacopeial Convention, 2004).

1.1.1   Nomenclature

Sodium estrone sulfate

Chem. Abstr. Serv. Reg. No.: 438-67-5
Chem. Abstr. Name: 3-(Sulfooxy)-estra-1,3,5(10)-trien-17-one, sodium salt
IUPAC Systematic Name: Estrone, hydrogen sulfate sodium salt
Synonyms: Estrone sodium sulfate; estrone sulfate sodium; estrone sulfate sodium salt; oestrone sodium sulfate; oestrone sulfate sodium; oestrone sulfate sodium salt; sodium estrone sulfate; sodium estrone-3-sulfate; sodium oestrone sulfate; sodium oestrone-3-sulfate; 3-sulfatoxyestra-1,3,5(10)-trien-17-one, sodium salt

Sodium equilin sulfate

Chem. Abstr. Serv. Reg. No.: 16680-47-0
Chem. Abstr. Name: 3-(Sulfooxy)-estra-1,3,5(10),7-tetraen-17-one, sodium salt
IUPAC Systematic Name: 3-Hydroxyestra-1,3,5(10),7-tetraen-17-one, hydrogen sulfate, sodium salt
Synonyms: Equilin, sulfate, sodium salt; equilin sodium sulfate; sodium equilin 3-monosulfate; sodium equilin sulfate

1.1.2   *Structural and molecular formulae and relative molecular mass*

Sodium estrone sulfate

CH$_3$ O

H

H   H

NaO$_3$SO

C$_{18}$H$_{21}$O$_5$S.Na   Relative molecular mass: 372.4

Sodium equilin sulfate

CH$_3$ O

H   H

NaO$_3$SO

C$_{18}$H$_{19}$O$_5$S.Na   Relative molecular mass: 370.4

1.1.3   *Chemical and physical properties*

From Gennaro (2000) and American Hospital Formulary Service (2005)
(*a*)   *Description*: Buff-coloured, odourless or with a slight characteristic odour, amorphous powder (from natural sources); white to light buff, odourless or with a slight odour, crystalline or amorphous powder (synthetic)
(*b*)   *Solubility*: Soluble in water

1.1.4   *Technical products and impurities*

Conjugated estrogens contain 52.5% min. and 61.5% max. sodium estrone sulfate and 22.5% min. and 30.5% max. sodium equilin sulfate; the total of sodium estrone sulfate and sodium equilin sulfate is 79.5% min. and 88.0% max. of the labelled content of conjugated estrogens. Conjugated estrogens contain as concomitant components (as sodium sulfate conjugates) 13.5% min. and 19.5% max. 17α-dihydroequilin, 0.5% min. and 4.0% max. 17β-dihydroequilin and 2.5% min. and 9.5% max. 17α-estradiol of the labelled content of conjugated estrogens (Pharmacopeial Convention, 2004).

Conjugated estrogens are available as tablets for oral administration, as a liquid for parenteral injection and as a 0.0625% vaginal cream (American Hospital Formulary Service, 2005).

Conjugated estrogens (natural) are a mixture that contains the sodium salts of the water-soluble sulfate esters of estrone and equilin derived wholly or in part from equine urine or prepared synthetically from estrone and equilin. Conjugated estrogens (natural) also contain conjugated estrogenic substances of types that are excreted by pregnant mares and include δ8,9-dehydroestrone, 17α-dihydroequilenin, 17β-dihydroequilenin, 17α-dihydroequilin, 17β-dihydroequilin, equilenin, 17α-estradiol and 17β-estradiol (American Hospital Formulary Service, 2005).

Conjugated estrogens (synthetic) are a mixture of conjugated estrogens that are prepared synthetically from plant sources (i.e. soya and yams). Conjugated estrogens (synthetic) are commercially available as preparations that contain a mixture of nine of the 10 known conjugated estrogenic substances that are present in currently available commercial preparations of conjugated estrogens (natural). However, in contrast to currently available preparations of conjugated estrogens (natural), the conjugated estrogenic substances present in conjugated estrogens (synthetic) are prepared entirely synthetically (American Hospital Formulary Service, 2005).

1.1.5   Use

Conjugated estrogens are used mainly in the treatment of menopausal disorders (e.g. vasomotor symptoms, vulvar and vaginal atrophy) and for the prevention and treatment of osteoporosis. Conjugated estrogens are usually administered orally at a dose of 0.3–1.25 mg/day (American Hospital Formulary Service, 2005).

Table 1 presents comparative global data on sales of conjugated estrogens in 1994, 1999 and 2004 (IMS Health, 2005). The regions are broadly as those defined by WHO.

Table 1. Conjugated estrogens used in combined estrogen–progestogen menopausal therapy (thousands of standard units[a])

Region	1994	1999	2004
Africa	7 980	10 814	9 780
Eastern Mediterranean	51	3 102	1 683
Europe	448 555	508 776	192 332
North America	9 250	1 039 067	217 181
South America	15 330	103 701	32 713
South-East Asia	1 162	1 992	9 555
Western Pacific	17 521	70 675	27 576
Total	499 848	1 738 126	490 820

From IMS Health (2005)
[a] Standard units are sales in terms of standard dose units; the standard dose unit for oral products is one tablet or capsule.

1.2   Ethinylestradiol

1.2.1   *Nomenclature*

Chem. Abstr. Serv. Reg. No.: 57-63-6
Deleted CAS Reg. No.: 77538-56-8; 406932-93-2
Chem. Abstr. Name: (17α)-19-Norpregna-1,3,5(10)-trien-20-yne-3,17-diol
IUPAC Systematic Name: 19-Nor-17α-pregna-1,3,5(10)-trien-20-yne-3,17-diol
Synonyms: Ethinylestradiol; 17-ethinylestradiol; 17-ethinyl-3,17-estradiol; 17α-ethi-
nyl-3,17-dihydroxy-Δ1,3,5-estratriene; 17α-ethinylestradiol; 17α-ethinyl-17β-estra-
diol; 17α-ethinylestra-1,3,5(10)-triene-3,17β-diol; 17α-ethinyl-1,3,5(10)-estratriene-
3,17-diol; ethinyloestradiol; 17-ethynyl-3,17-dihydroxy-1,3,5-oestratrione; ethynylestradiol; 17-ethynylestradiol; 17α-ethynylestradiol; 17-ethynylestra-1,3,5(10)-triene-
3,17β-diol; ethynyloestradiol; 19-Nor-17α-pregna-1,3,5(10)-trien-20-yne-3,17β-diol

1.2.2   *Structural and molecular formulae and relative molecular mass*

$C_{20}H_{24}O_2$ Relative molecular mass: 296.4

1.2.3   *Chemical and physical properties of the pure substance*

From O'Neil (2001) and Sweetman (2005), unless otherwise specified
(a)   *Description:* White to creamy or slightly yellowish white, odourless, crystalline
      powder
(b)   *Melting-point:* 182–184 °C
(c)   *Solubility:* Practically insoluble in water; soluble in acetone (1 part in 5), ethanol
      (1 part in 6), chloroform (1 part in 20), dioxane (1 part in 4), diethyl ether (1 part
      in 4) and vegetable oils
(d)   *Optical rotation:* $[\alpha]_D^{20}$, less than –27° to –30° (Pharmacopeial Convention,
      2004; Council of Europe, 2005)

1.2.4   *Technical products and impurities*

Ethinylestradiol is commercially available as tablets either alone or in combination
with progestogens, as described in the monograph on Combined estrogen–progestogen
contraceptives.

Reported impurities include: estradiol, 3-hydroxyestra-1,3,5(10)-trien-17-one (estrone), 19-nor-17α-pregna-1,3,5(10),9(11)-tetraen-20-yne-3,17-diol and 19-norpregna-1,3,5(10)-trien-20-yne-3,17-diol (17β-ethinylestradiol) (British Pharmacopoeial Commission, 2004).

1.2.5   Use

Ethinylestradiol is a synthetic estrogen that acts similarly to estradiol. It is frequently used as the estrogenic component of combined oral contraceptive preparations; a typical daily dose is 20–50 µg. Ethinylestradiol is also used as an emergency contraceptive combined with levonorgestrel or norgestrel. A combined preparation of ethinylestradiol with the anti-androgen cyproterone is used for the hormonal treatment of acne and hirsutism, particularly when contraception is also required. Ethinylestradiol has also been used for hormonal menopausal therapy; doses of 10–20 µg daily were given (in conjunction with a progestogen in women with a uterus). For the treatment of female hypogonadism, 50 µg has been given up to three times daily for 14 consecutive days in every 4 weeks, followed by a progestogen for the next 14 days (Sweetman, 2005).

Table 2 presents comparative global data on sales of ethinylestradiol in 1994, 1999 and 2004 (IMS Health, 2005). The regions are broadly as those defined by WHO.

Table 2. Ethinylestradiol used in combined estrogen–progestogen contraceptives and combined estrogen–progestogen menopausal therapy (thousands of standard units[a])

Region	1994	1999	2004
Combined estrogen–progestogen contraceptives			
Monophasic preparations (< 50 µg estrogen)			
Africa	2 564	2 955	3 881
Eastern Mediterranean	6 353	8 728	7 494
Europe	159 180	197 014	266 090
North America	55 356	67 909	101 390
South America	52 552	69 183	83 406
South-East Asia	11 807	29 288	58 282
Western Pacific	10 414	14 467	25 673
Subtotal	298 225	389 543	546 215
Monophasic preparations (≥ 50 µg estrogen)			
Africa	2 060	1 611	1 364
Eastern Mediterranean	1 942	827	126
Europe	15 319	9 577	4 932
North America	4 343	2 371	1 788
South America	23 611	19 761	14 395
South-East Asia	3 463	12 619	7 794
Western Pacific	2 125	2 000	1 371
Subtotal	52 863	48 765	31 770

Table 2 (contd)

Regions	1994	1999	2004
Biphasic preparations			
Africa	439	429	473
Eastern Mediterranean	70	59	217
Europe	25 126	22 918	18 833
North America	455	1 979	5 634
South America	41	732	1 297
South-East Asia	0	1	2
Western Pacific	312	211	95
Subtotal	26 442	26 330	26 551
Triphasic preparations			
Africa	4 447	5 360	4 477
Eastern Mediterranean	1 586	965	1 860
Europe	62 951	69 133	55 880
North America	39 551	48 081	51 048
South America	13 612	12 400	10 871
South-East Asia	352	2 232	3 389
Western Pacific	8 613	7 829	7 251
Subtotal	131 111	146 000	134 776
Total	508 641	610 638	739 312
Hormonal menopausal therapy			
Africa	226	0	0
Eastern Mediterranean	267	0	0
Europe	34 581	13 016	5 783
North America	1 187	333	81 863
South America	20 039	15 072	19 291
South-East Asia	5 714	5 041	5 297
Western Pacific	52 461	45 300	30 246
Total	114 475	78 761	142 480

From IMS Health (2005)
[a] Standard units are sales in terms of standard dose units; the standard dose unit for oral products is one tablet or capsule.

1.3 Mestranol

1.3.1 *Nomenclature*

Chem. Abstr. Serv. Reg. No.: 72-33-3
Deleted CAS Reg. No.: 43085-54-7; 53445-46-8
Chem. Abstr. Name: (17α)-3-Methoxy-19-norpregna-1,3,5(10)-trien-20-yn-17-ol
IUPAC Systematic Name: 3-Methoxy-19-nor-17α-pregna-1,3,5(10)-trien-20-yn-17-ol

Synonyms: Ethinylestradiol 3-methyl ether; 17α-ethinylestradiol 3-methyl ether; ethinyloestradiol 3-methyl ether; 17α-ethinyloestradiol 3-methyl ether; ethynylestradiol methyl ether; ethynylestradiol 3-methyl ether; 17-ethynylestradiol 3-methyl ether; 17α-ethynylestradiol 3-methyl ether; 17α-ethynylestradiol methyl ether; ethynyloestradiol methyl ether; ethynyloestradiol 3-methyl ether; 17-ethynyloestradiol 3-methyl ether; 17α-ethynyloestradiol 3-methyl ether; 17α-ethynyloestradiol methyl ether; 3-methoxy-17α-ethinylestradiol; 3-methoxy-17α-ethinyloestradiol; 3-methoxy-17α-ethynylestradiol; 3-methoxyethynylestradiol; 3-methoxy-17α-ethynyloestradiol; 3-methoxyethynyloestradiol; 3-methylethynylestradiol; 3-*O*-methylethynylestradiol; 3-methylethynyloestradiol; 3-*O*-methylethynyloestradiol; Δ-MVE

1.3.2   *Structural and molecular formulae and relative molecular mass*

$C_{21}H_{26}O_2$ Relative molecular mass: 310.4

1.3.3   *Chemical and physical properties of the pure substance*

From O'Neil (2001) and Sweetman (2005)
(a) *Description*: White to creamy white, odourless, crystalline powder
(b) *Melting-point*: 150–154 °C
(c) *Solubility*: Practically insoluble in water; sparingly soluble in ethanol; slightly soluble in methanol; soluble in acetone, dioxane and diethyl ether; freely soluble in chloroform
(d) *Optical rotation*: $[\alpha]_D^{20}$, –20° to –24° (British Pharmacopoeial Commission, 2004; Council of Europe, 2005); +2° to +8° (Society of Japanese Pharmacopoeia, 2001; Pharmacopeial Convention, 2004)

1.3.4   *Technical products and impurities*

Mestranol is commercially available as a component of combination tablets with chlormadinone acetate, ethynodiol diacetate, levonorgestrel, lynoestrenol or norethisterone and formerly with norethynodrel (IPPF, 2002; Sweetman, 2005; see the monograph on Combined estrogen–progestogen contraceptives and Annex 2).

1.3.5   *Use*

Mestranol is a synthetic estrogen pro-drug that is rapidly metabolized to ethinylestra-diol; it therefore acts similarly to estradiol. It is used as the estrogen component of combined oral contraceptive preparations at a usual daily dose of 50 µg. The progestogen component is frequently norethisterone. Mestranol has also been used as the estrogen component of some preparations for hormonal menopausal therapy. Administration has usually been in a sequential regimen with doses ranging from 12.5 to 50 µg daily, in combination with a cyclical progestogen (Sweetman, 2005).

Table 3 presents comparative global data on sales of mestranol in 1994, 1999 and 2004 (IMS Health, 2005). The regions are broadly as those defined by WHO.

Table 3. Mestranol used in combined estrogen–progestogen contraceptives and combined estrogen-progestogen menopausal therapy (thousands of standard units)

Region	1994	1999	2000
Combined hormonal contraceptives			
Monophasic preparations (≥ 50 µg estrogen)			
Africa	11	35	42
Europe	1 436	589	45
North America	2 983	1 587	928
South America	1 144	1 253	588
South-East Asia	1 381	882	645
Western Pacific	188	164	181
Subtotal	7 142	4 510	2 430
Biphasic preparations			
Europe	48	0	0
North America	624	479	220
South America	175	78	0
Subtotal	848	557	220
Total	7 990	5 067	2 650
Combined hormonal menopausal therapy			
Europe	2 794	939	0
North America	12 006	10 476	7 930
South-East Asia	299	17	0
Western Pacific	18 287	13 811	9 312
Total	33 386	25 243	17 242

From IMS Health (2005)

[a] Standard units are sales in terms of standard dose units; the standard dose unit for oral products is one tablet or capsule.

1.4 Estradiols

1.4.1 Estradiol

(a) Nomenclature

Chem. Abstr. Serv. Reg. No.: 50-28-2
Chem. Abstr. Name: (17β)-Estra-1,3,5(10)-triene-3,17-diol
IUPAC Systematic Name: Estra-1,3,5(10)-triene-3,17β-diol
Synonyms: Dihydrofollicular hormone; dihydrofolliculin; dihydromenformon; dihydro-theelin; dihydroxyestrin; 3,17β-dihydroxyestra-1,3,5(10)-triene; 3,17-epidihydroxyes-tratriene; β-estradiol; 17β-estradiol; 3,17β-estradiol; (D)-3,17β-estradiol; oestradiol-17β; 17β-oestradiol

(b) Structural and molecular formulae and relative molecular mass

CH₃ OH
H
H
H H
HO

$C_{18}H_{24}O_2$ Relative molecular mass: 272.4

(c) Chemical and physical properties of the pure substance

From O'Neil (2001) and Sweetman (2005)

  (i)   Description: White or creamy white, odourless, crystalline powder
  (ii) Melting-point: 173–179 °C
  (iii) Solubility: Practically insoluble in water; soluble in ethanol (1 part in 28), chloroform (1 part in 435), diethyl ether (1 part in 150), ace-tone, dioxane, and other organic solvents
  (iv) Optical rotation: $[\alpha]_D^{25}$, +76° to +83° (in dioxane)

Estradiol hemihydrate is a white, or almost white, crystalline powder or colourless crystal; it is practically insoluble in water, sparingly soluble in ethanol, slightly soluble in dichloromethane and diethyl ether and soluble in acetone. Approximately 1.03 g estradiol hemihydrate are equivalent to 1 g of the anhydrous substance (Reynolds, 1996).

(d) Technical products and impurities

Estradiol is available commercially as oral and vaginal tablets, as a metered topical gel, as topical transdermal patches, as a vaginal cream and as an extended-release vaginal insert (ring) (American Hospital Formulary Service, 2005; Food and Drug Administra-tion, 2005).

Reported impurities (for estradiol hemihydrate) include: estra-1,3,5(10),9(11)-tetraene-3,17β-diol, estra-1,3,5(10)-triene-3,17α-diol (17α-estradiol), 3-hydroxyestra-1,3,5(10)-trien-17-one (estrone) and 4-methylestra-1,3,5(10)-triene-3,17β-diol (British Pharmacopoeial Commission, 2004).

1.4.2   *Estradiol benzoate*

(*a*)   *Nomenclature*

Chem. Abstr. Serv. Reg. No.: 50-50-0
Chem. Abstr. Name: (17β)-Estra-1,3,5(10)-triene-3,17-diol, 3-benzoate
IUPAC Systematic Name: Estradiol, 3-benzoate
Synonyms: Estradiol benzoate; β-estradiol benzoate, β-estradiol 3-benzoate; 17β-estradiol benzoate; 17β-estradiol 3-benzoate; estradiol monobenzoate; 1,3,5(10)-estratriene-3,17β-diol 3-benzoate; β-oestradiol benzoate; β-oestradiol 3-benzoate; 17β-oestradiol benzoate; 17β-oestradiol 3-benzoate; oestradiol monobenzoate; 1,3,5(10)-oestratriene-3, 17β-diol 3-benzoate

(*b*)   *Structural and molecular formulae and relative molecular mass*

$C_{25}H_{28}O_3$ Relative molecular mass: 376.5

(*c*)   *Chemical and physical properties of the pure substance*

From O'Neil (2001) and Sweetman (2005)
   (i)   *Description*: Almost white crystalline powder or colourless crystals that exhibit polymorphism
   (ii)   *Melting-point*: 191–196 °C
   (iii) *Solubility*: Practically insoluble in water; slightly soluble in ethanol and diethyl ether; sparingly soluble in acetone and vegetable oils; and soluble in dioxane and dichloromethane
   (iv)   *Optical rotation*: $[\alpha]_D^{25}$, +58° to +63° (in dioxane)

(d)   *Technical products and impurities*

Estradiol benzoate is commercially available for injection (oily or aqueous suspension) and implant (Society of Japanese Pharmacopoeia, 2001; British Pharmacopoeial Commission, 2004).

Reported impurities include: estradiol, estra-1,3,5(10)-triene-3,17β-diyl dibenzoate, 17β-hydroxyestra-1,3,5(10),9(11)-tetraen-3-yl benzoate, 3-hydroxyestra-1,3,5(10)-trien-17β-yl benzoate, 17α-hydroxyestra-1,3,5(10)-trien-3-yl benzoate and 17β-hydroxy-4-methylestra-1,3,5(10)-trien-3-yl benzoate (British Pharmacopoeial Commission, 2004).

1.4.3   *Estradiol cypionate*

(a)   *Nomenclature*

Chem. Abstr. Serv. Reg. No.: 313-06-4
Chem. Abstr. Name: (17β)-Estra-1,3,5(10)-triene-3,17-diol, 17-cyclopentanepropanoate
IUPAC Systematic Name: Oestradiol, 17-cyclopentanepropionate
Synonyms: Cyclopentanepropionic acid, 17-ester with oestradiol; cyclopentanepropionic acid, 3-hydroxyestra-1,3,5(10)-trien-17β-yl ester; depo-estradiol cyclopentylpropionate; depoestradiol cypionate; estradiol 17β-cyclopentanepropionate; estradiol cyclopentylpropionate; estradiol 17-cyclopentylpropionate; estradiol 17β-cyclopentylpropionate; 17β-estradiol 17-cyclopentylpropionate; estradiol cypionate; estradiol 17-cypionate; estradiol 17β-cypionate

(b)   *Structural and molecular formulae and relative molecular mass*

C$_{26}$H$_{36}$O$_{3}$ Relative molecular mass: 396.6

(c)   *Chemical and physical properties of the pure substance*

From O'Neil (2001) and Sweetman (2005)

    (i)   *Description*: White, odourless crystalline powder
    (ii)   *Melting-point*: 151–152 °C
    (iii)   *Solubility*: Practically insoluble in water; soluble in ethanol (1 part in 40), chloroform (1 in 7), diethyl ether (1 in 2800), acetone and dioxane
    (iv)   *Optical rotation*: $[\alpha]_D^{25}$, +45° (in chloroform)

(d)   Technical products and impurities

Estradiol cypionate is available commercially as injectable suspensions in oil for parenteral administration (American Hospital Formulary Service, 2005; Food and Drug Administration, 2005).

1.4.4   *Estradiol valerate*

(a)   Nomenclature

Chem. Abstr. Serv. Reg. No.: 979-32-8
Deleted CAS Nos.: 907-12-0; 69557-95-5
Chem. Abstr. Name: (17β)-Estra-1,3,5(10)-triene-3,17-diol, 17-pentanoate
IUPAC Systematic Name: Estradiol 17-valerate
Synonyms: Estradiol 17β-valerate; estradiol valerianate; estra-1,3,5(10)-triene-3,17β-diol 17-valerate; 3-hydroxy-17β-valeroyloxyestra-1,3,5(10)-triene; oestradiol valerate

(b)   Structural and molecular formulae and relative molecular mass

$C_{23}H_{32}O_3$ Relative molecular mass: 356.5

(c)   Chemical and physical properties of the pure substance

From O'Neil (2001) and Sweetman (2005)
    (i)   *Description*: White, odourless, crystalline powder
    (ii)   *Melting-point*: 144–145 °C
    (iii)   *Solubility*: Practically insoluble in water; soluble in benzyl benzoate, dioxane, methanol and castor oil; sparingly soluble in arachis oil and sesame oil

(d)   Technical products and impurities

Estradiol valerate is available commercially as injectable suspensions in oil for parenteral administration; it is also available commercially as tablets alone or in combination with progestogens (IPPF, 2002; American Hospital Formulary Service, 2005; Editions du Vidal, 2005; Sweetman, 2005).

Reported impurities include: estradiol, estra-1,3,5(10)-trien-3,17β-diyl dipentanoate, 3-hydroxyestra-1,3,5(10),9(11)-tetraen-17β-yl pentanoate, 3-hydroxyestra-1,3,5(10)-trien-

17β-yl butanoate (estradiol butyrate), 17β-hydroxyestra-1,3,5(10)-trien-3-yl pentanoate and 3-hydroxy-4-methylestra-1,3,5(10)-trien-17β-yl pentanoate (British Pharmacopoeial Commission, 2004).

Other esters of estradiol that have been reported and that may have been used as pharmaceuticals include: estradiol 17β-acetate 3-benzoate, estradiol 3,17β-dipropionate, estradiol 3,17β-diundecylenate, estradiol 17β-enanthate, estradiol 17β-hexahydrobenzoate, estradiol 17β-phenylpropionate, estradiol 17β-stearate, estradiol 17β-undecylate and polyestradiol phosphate.

1.4.5   Use of estradiols

Estradiol is the most active of the naturally occurring estrogens. Estradiol and its semi-synthetic esters and other natural estrogens are primarily used in hormonal menopausal therapy, whereas synthetic derivatives such as ethinylestradiol and mestranol have a major role as components of combined oral contraceptives. Estradiol may also be used in hormonal therapy for female hypogonadism or primary ovarian failure (Sweetman, 2005).

For hormonal menopausal therapy, oral preparations of estradiol are commonly used, as are transdermal patches. Transdermal gels, subcutaneous implants and a nasal spray are also available. Intramuscular injections were used formerly. In women with a uterus, a progestogen is also required, given cyclically or continuously, and is usually taken orally, although some transdermal preparations are available. Vaginal estradiol preparations are used specifically for the treatment of menopausal atrophic vaginitis; these are generally recommended for short-term use only, if given without a progestogen in women with a uterus, although specific recommendations vary between products (Sweetman, 2005).

For oral use, estradiol or estradiol valerate are normally given; doses are 1–2 mg daily cyclically or, more usually, continuously (Sweetman, 2005).

Estradiol may be used topically as transdermal skin patches to provide a systemic effect; a variety of patches are available that release between 25 and 100 µg estradiol every 24 h. Depending on the preparation, patches are replaced once or twice weekly. Topical gel preparations are also applied for systemic effect: the usual dose is 0.5–1.5 mg estradiol daily. A nasal spray is available that delivers 150 µg estradiol hemihydrate per spray. The usual initial dose is 300 µg daily; maintenance doses are 150–600 µg daily (Sweetman, 2005).

In order to prolong the duration of action, subcutaneous implants of estradiol may be used. The dose of estradiol is generally 25–100 mg and a new implant is given after about 4–8 months according to the concentrations of estrogen (Sweetman, 2005).

Estradiol may be used locally as vaginal tablets, as a 0.01% vaginal cream or as a 3-month vaginal ring (Sweetman, 2005).

Intramuscular injections of estradiol benzoate or valerate esters have been used as oily depot solutions, usually given once every 3–4 weeks. The cypionate, dipropionate, enanthate, hexahydrobenzoate, phenylpropionate and undecylate esters of estradiol have been used similarly. The enanthate and cypionate esters are used as the estrogen component of combined injectable contraceptives (Sweetman, 2005).

Tables 4 and 5 present comparative global data on sales of estradiol and methylestradiol, respectively, in 1994, 1999 and 2004 (IMS Health, 2005). The regions are broadly as those defined by WHO.

Table 4. Estradiol used in combined estrogen–progestogen contraceptives and combined estrogen–progestogen menopausal therapy (thousands of standard units[a])

Region	1994	1999	2004
Combined hormonal contraceptives			
Monophasic preparations (< 50 µg estrogen)			
Eastern Mediterranean	0	0	3 075
South America	0	192	298
Subtotal	0	192	3 372
Biphasic preparations			
Europe	114	222	245
North America	0	0	2
Subtotal	114	222	248
Total	114	414	3 620
Combined hormonal menopausal therapy			
Africa	12 079	18 307	17 130
Eastern Mediterranean	7 849	15 895	23 611
Europe	698 456	1 254 408	854 592
North America	17 233	39 571	114 851
South America	62 451	163 521	136 594
South-East Asia	7 954	21 790	44 194
Western Pacific	12 558	84 200	38 764
Total	818 581	1 597 690	1 229 735

From IMS Health (2005)
[a] Standard units are sales in terms of standard dose units; the standard dose unit for oral products is one tablet or capsule.

Table 5. Methylestradiol used in combined estrogen–progestogen menopausal therapy (thousands of standard units[a])

Region	1994	1999	2004
Eastern Mediterranean	10	0	0
South America	2023	2019	1767
South-East Asia	1694	2857	1839
Total	3727	4876	3606

From IMS Health (2005)
[a] Standard units are sales in terms of standard dose units; the standard dose unit for oral products is one tablet or capsule.

1.5   Estriol

1.5.1   *Nomenclature*

Chem. Abstr. Serv. Reg. No.: 50-27-1
Chem. Abstr. Name: (16α,17β)-Estra-1,3,5(10)-triene-3,16,17-triol
IUPAC Systematic Name: Estriol
Synonyms: Estra-1,3,5(10)-triene-3,16α,17β-triol; estratriol; 16α-estriol; 16α,17β-estriol; 3,16α,17β-estriol; follicular hormone hydrate; 16α-hydroxyestradiol; 3,16α,17β-trihydroxyestra-1,3,5(10)-triene; trihydroxyestrin

1.5.2   *Structural and molecular formulae and relative molecular mass*

$C_{18}H_{24}O_3$ Relative molecular mass: 288.4

1.5.3   *Chemical and physical properties of the pure substance*

From O'Neil (2001) and Sweetman (2005)
(*a*)   *Description*: White, odourless, crystalline powder
(*b*)   *Melting-point*: 282 °C
(*c*)   *Solubility*: Practically insoluble in water; sparingly soluble in ethanol; soluble in acetone, chloroform, dioxane, diethyl ether and vegetable oils; freely soluble in pyridine
(*d*)   *Specific rotation*: $[\alpha]_D^{25}$, +58° (in dioxane)

1.5.4   *Technical products and impurities*

Estriol is commercially available as tablets, pessaries and a cream. Sodium succinate and succinate salts of estriol are also available (Sweetman, 2005).

Reported impurities include: estradiol, estra-1,3,5(10),9(11)-tetraene-3,16α,17β-triol (9,11-didehydroestriol), estra-1,3,5(10)-triene-3,16α,17α-triol (17-epi-estriol), estra-1,3,5(10)-triene-3,16β,17β-triol (16-epi-estriol), estra-1,3,5(10)-triene-3,16β,17α-triol (16,17-epi-estriol), 3-hydroxyestra-1,3,5(10)-trien-17-one (estrone); 3,16α-dihydroxy-estra-1,3,5(10)-trien-17-one, 3-hydroxy-17-oxa-D-homoestra-1,3,5(10)-trien-17a-one and 3-methoxyestra-1,3,5(10)-triene-16α,17β-diol (estriol 3-methyl ether) (British Pharmaco-poeial Commission, 2004).

1.5.5   Use

Estriol is a naturally occurring estrogen that has actions and uses similar to those described for estradiol. It is used for hormonal menopausal therapy. For short-term treatment, oral doses of estriol have been 0.5–3 mg daily given for 1 month, followed by 0.5–1 mg daily. Estriol has also been given in combination with other natural estrogens, such as estradiol and estrone; usual doses of estriol have ranged from about 250 µg to 2 mg daily. It is also administered intravaginally for the short-term treatment of meno-pausal atrophic vaginitis as a 0.01% or 0.1% cream or as pessaries containing 500 µg (Sweetman, 2005).

Table 6 presents comparative global data on sales of estriol in 1994, 1999 and 2004 (IMS Health, 2005). The regions are broadly as those defined by WHO.

Table 6. Estriol used in combined estrogen–progestogen menopausal therapy (thousands of standard units[a])

Region	1994	1999	2004
Europe	85 372	83 465	28 058
South-East Asia	3 151	5 249	6 577
Western Pacific	0	10	71
Total	88 523	88 724	34 706

From IMS Health (2005)
[a] Standard units are sales in terms of standard dose units; the standard dose unit for oral products is one tablet or capsule.

1.6   Estrone

1.6.1   Nomenclature

Chem. Abstr. Serv. Reg. No.: 53-16-7
Deleted CAS Reg. No.: 37242-41-4
Chem. Abstr. Name: 3-Hydroxyestra-1,3,5(10)-trien-17-one
IUPAC Systematic Name: 3-Hydroxyestra-1,2,5(10)-triene-17-one
Synonyms: d-Estrone; d-oestrone

1.6.2   *Structural and molecular formulae and relative molecular mass*

$C_{18}H_{22}O_2$ Relative molecular mass: 270.4

1.6.3   *Chemical and physical properties of the pure substance*

From O'Neil (2001) and Sweetman (2005)

(*a*)   *Description*: White to creamy white, odourless, crystalline powder (exists in three crystalline phases: one monoclinic, the other two orthorhombic)

(*b*)   *Melting-point*: 254.5–256 °C

(*c*)   *Solubility*: Practically insoluble in water (0.003 g/100 mL at 25 °C); soluble in ethanol (1 in 250), chloroform (1 in 110 at 15 °C), acetone (1 in 50 at 50 °C), dioxane and vegetable oils; slightly soluble in diethyl ether and solutions of alkali hydroxides

(*d*)   *Specific rotation*: $[\alpha]_D^{22}$, +152° (in chloroform)

1.6.4   *Technical products and impurities*

Estrone is available commercially as pessaries and as a sterile suspension in water or 0.9% sodium chloride for injection. It is also available as a multicomponent tablet, cream and injectable solution (American Hospital Formulary Service, 2005; APPCo, 2005; Editions du Vidal, 2005).

1.6.5   *Use*

Estrone is a naturally occurring estrogen that has actions and uses similar to those described for estradiol. For hormonal menopausal therapy, estrone has been given orally at a dose of 1.4–2.8 mg daily, in a cyclical or continuous regimen, as a combination product with estradiol and estriol. Estrone has also been administered by intramuscular injection in oily solutions and aqueous suspensions. When used specifically for menopausal atrophic vaginitis, estrone has been administered vaginally (Sweetman, 2005).

Table 7 presents comparative global data on sales of estrone in 1994, 1999 and 2004 (IMS Health, 2005). The regions are broadly as those defined by WHO.

Table 7. Estrone used in combined estrogen–progestogen menopausal therapy (thousands of standard units[a])

Region	1994	1999	2004
Africa	765	754	812
Europe	499	69	48
North America	6	1	0
South America	34	6	0
Total	1305	829	860

From IMS Health (2005)
[a] Standard units are sales in terms of standard dose units; the standard dose unit for oral products is one tablet or capsule.

1.7   Estropipate

1.7.1   *Nomenclature*

Chem. Abstr. Serv. Reg. No.: 7280-37-7
Deleted CAS No.: 29080-16-8
Chem. Abstr. Name: 3-(Sulfooxy)-estra-1,3,5(10)-trien-17-one, compd. with piperazine (1:1)
IUPAC Systematic Name: Estrone, hydrogen sulfate, compd. with piperazine (1:1)
Synonyms: Piperazine estrone sulfate; piperazine oestrone sulfate; 3-sulfatoxyestra-1,3,5(10)-trien-17-one piperazine salt; 3-sulfatoxyoestra-1,3,5(10)-trien-17-one piperazine salt

1.7.2   *Structural and molecular formulae and relative molecular mass*

$C_{22}H_{32}N_2O_5S$ Relative molecular mass: 436.6

1.7.3   *Chemical and physical properties of the pure substance*

From O'Neil (2001) and Sweetman (2005)
(*a*)   *Description*: White to yellowish white, odourless, fine crystalline powder
(*b*)   *Melting-point*: 190 °C; solidifies on further heating and decomposes at 245 °C

(c)   *Solubility*: Very slightly soluble in water, ethanol, chloroform and diethyl ether; soluble in warm water and warm ethanol (1 part in 500)

(d)   *Optical rotation*: $[\alpha]_D^{25}$, +87.8° (in sodium hydroxide)

1.7.4   Technical products and impurities

Estropipate is available as tablets and as a vaginal cream (American Hospital Formulary Service, 2005).

Reported impurities include: estrone (British Pharmacopoeial Commission, 2004).

1.7.5   Use

Estropipate is a semi-synthetic conjugate of estrone with piperazine that is used for hormonal menopausal therapy. Its action is due to estrone to which it is hydrolysed in the body. Estropipate is given orally for the short-term treatment of menopausal symptoms; suggested doses have ranged from 0.75 to 6 mg daily, given cyclically or continuously. When used for longer periods for the prevention of postmenopausal osteoporosis, a daily dose of 0.75 or 1.5 mg is given cyclically or continuously. In women with a uterus, estropipate should be used in conjunction with a progestogen. Estropipate has also been used in the short-term treatment of menopausal atrophic vaginitis as a vaginal cream that contains 0.15%; 2–4 g of cream is applied daily (Sweetman, 2005).

Table 8 presents comparative global data on sales of estropipate in 1994, 1999 and 2004 (IMS Health, 2005). The regions are broadly as those defined by WHO.

Table 8. Estropipate used in combined estrogen–progestogen menopausal therapy (thousands of standard units[a])

Region	1994	1999	2004
Europe	0	121	0
Total	0	121	0

From IMS Health (2005)
[a] Standard units are sales in terms of standard dose units; the standard dose unit for oral products is one tablet or capsule.

1.8   Regulations and guidelines

Guidelines for the use of estrogens are found in national and international pharmacopoeias (Secretaría de Salud, 1994, 1995; Society of Japanese Pharmacopoeia, 2001; Pharmacopeial Convention, 2004; Swiss Pharmaceutical Society, 2004; Council of Europe, 2005; Sweetman, 2005).

2.   Progestogens

2.1   Chlormadinone acetate

2.1.1   *Nomenclature*

Chem. Abstr. Serv. Reg. No.: 302-22-7
Chem. Abstr. Name: 17-(Acetyloxy)-6-chloropregna-4,6-diene-3,20-dione
IUPAC Systematic Name: 6-Chloro-17-hydroxypregna-4,6-diene-3,20-dione, acetate
Synonyms: 17α-Acetoxy-6-chloro-4,6-pregnadiene-3,20-dione; 6-chloro-Δ^6-17-acetoxyprogesterone; 6-chloro-Δ^6-[17α]acetoxyprogesterone

2.1.2   *Structural and molecular formulae and relative molecular mass*

$C_{23}H_{29}ClO_4$ Relative molecular mass: 404.9

2.1.3   *Chemical and physical properties of the pure substance*

From O'Neil (2001) and Society of Japanese Pharmacopoeia (2001)
(*a*)   *Description*: White to light-yellow, odourless crystals
(*b*)   *Melting-point*: 212–214 °C
(*c*)   *Solubility*: Practically insoluble in water; very soluble in chloroform; soluble in acetonitrile; slightly soluble in ethanol and diethyl ether
(*d*)   *Optical rotation*: $[\alpha]_D^{20}$, −10.0° to −14.0° (in acetonitrile) (Society of Japanese Pharmacopoeia, 2001); $[\alpha]_D$, +6° (in chloroform) (O'Neil, 2001)

2.1.4   *Technical products and impurities*

Chlormadinone acetate is available commercially as tablets, either alone or in combination with ethinylestradiol or mestranol (IPPF, 2002).

2.1.5   *Use*

Chlormadinone acetate is a progestogen that is structurally related to progesterone and that may have some anti-androgenic activity. It is given orally either alone or in combination with an estrogen in the treatment of menstrual disorders such as menorrhagia and endometriosis at doses of 2–10 mg daily either cyclically or continuously. It may also be used as the progestogen component of combined oral contraceptives at a dose of 1–2 mg daily, particularly in women with androgen-dependent conditions such as acne and hirsutism (Sweetman, 2005).

Table 9 presents comparative global data on sales of chlormadinone acetate in 1994, 1999 and 2004 (IMS Health, 2005). The regions are broadly as those defined by WHO.

Table 9. Chlormadinone acetate used in combined estrogen–progestogen contraceptives and combined estrogen–progestogen menopausal therapy (thousands of standard units[a])

Region	1994	1999	2004
Combined hormonal contraceptives			
Monophasic preparations (< 50 µg estrogen)			
Eastern Mediterranean	0	0	40
Europe	0	1 768	5 937
North America	0	0	72
South America	0	0	238
Subtotal	0	1 768	6 288
Monophasic preparations (≥ 50 µg estrogen)			
Europe	858	547	0
Subtotal	858	547	0
Biphasic preparations			
Europe	2 312	2 769	1 797
North America	506	329	167
Subtotal	2 818	3 098	1 964
Total	3 676	5 413	8 252
Combined hormonal menopausal therapy			
Africa	226	0	0
Eastern Mediterranean	267	0	0
Europe	860	0	0
North America	12 006	10 476	7 930
Western Pacific	509	365	299
Total	13 868	10 841	8 230

From IMS Health (2005)
[a] Standard units are sales in terms of standard dose units; the standard dose unit for oral products is one tablet or capsule.

2.2   Cyproterone acetate

2.2.1   *Nomenclature*

Chem. Abstr. Serv. Reg. No.: 427-51-0
Chem. Abstr. Name: (1β,2β)-17-(Acetyloxy)-6-chloro-1,2-dihydro-3'H-cyclopropa-[1,2]pregna-1,4,6-triene-3,20-dione
IUPAC Systematic Name: 6-Chloro-1β,2β-dihydro-17-hydroxy-3'H-cyclopropa[1,2]-pregna-1,4,6-triene-3,20-dione acetate
Synonyms: Cyproterone 17-O-acetate; cyproterone 17α-acetate; 1,2α-methylene-6-chloro-17α-acetoxy-4,6-pregnadiene-3,20-dione; 1,2α-methylene-6-chloro-Δ^{4,6}-pregnadien-17α-ol-3,20-dione acetate; 1,2α-methylene-6-chloro-pregna-4,6-diene-3,20-dione 17α-acetate; methylene-6-chloro-17-hydroxy-1α,2α-pregna-4,6-diene-3,20-dione acetate

2.2.2   *Structural and molecular formulae and relative molecular mass*

$C_{24}H_{29}ClO_4$ Relative molecular mass: 416.9

2.2.3   *Chemical and physical properties of the pure substance*

From O'Neil (2001) and Council of Europe (2005)
(*a*)   *Description:* White, crystalline powder
(*b*)   *Melting-point:* 200–201 °C
(*c*)   *Solubility*: Practically insoluble in water; very soluble in dichloromethane and acetone; soluble in methanol; sparingly soluble in ethanol
(*d*)   *Specific rotation:* $[\alpha]_D^{20}$, +152° to +157°

2.2.4   *Technical products and impurities*

Cyproterone acetate is commercially available as tablets and an injectable solution (IPPF, 2002; British Medical Association/Royal Pharmaceutical Society of Great Britain, 2004; APPCo, 2005).

Reported impurities include: 3,20-dioxo-1β,2β-dihydro-3'*H*-cyclopropa[1,2]pregna-1,4,6-trien-17-yl acetate and 6-methoxy-3,20-dioxo-1β,2β-dihydro-3'*H*-cyclopropa[1,2]-pregna-1,4,6-trien-17-yl acetate (British Pharmacopoeial Commission, 2004).

2.2.5   *Use*

Cyproterone acetate is a progestogen that has anti-androgenic properties. It is typically used in conjunction with ethinylestradiol for the control of acne and hirsutism in women, and also provides contraception in these women. The usual oral doses are 2 mg cyproterone acetate with 35 μg ethinylestradiol given daily for 21 days of each menstrual cycle (Sweetman, 2005).

Table 10 presents comparative global data on sales of cyproterone acetate in 1994, 1999 and 2004 (IMS Health, 2005). The regions are broadly as those defined by WHO.

Table 10. Cyproterone acetate used in combined estrogen–progestogen contraceptives, combined estrogen–progestogen menopausal therapy and other uses (thousands of standard units[a])

Region	1994	1999	2004
Combined hormonal contraceptives			
Biphasic preparations			
Europe	114	222	245
Total	114	222	245
Combined hormonal menopausal therapy			
Africa	0	2 064	1 503
Eastern Mediterranean	0	139	1 125
Europe	15 170	84 098	42 379
North America	0	6 322	5 324
South America	323	42 043	25 999
South-East Asia	0	3 461	10 455
Western Pacific	0	1 625	2 577
Total	15 493	139 751	89 363
Oral anti-acne preparations			
Africa	10 015	12 875	15 901
Eastern Mediterranean	3 684	7 312	11 576
Europe	447 961	495 803	627 266
North America	5 995	15 219	36 054
South America	80 570	129 686	254 244
South-East Asia	28 711	31 593	63 107
Western Pacific	17 838	41 116	87 877
Total	594 773	733 603	1 096 026

From IMS Health (2005)

[a] Standard units are sales in terms of standard dose units; the standard dose unit for oral products is one tablet or capsule.

2.3   Desogestrel

2.3.1   *Nomenclature*

Chem. Abstr. Serv. Reg. No.: 54024-22-5
Chem. Abstr. Name: (17α)-13-Ethyl-11-methylene-18,19-dinorpregn-4-en-20-yn-17-ol
IUPAC Systematic Name: 13-Ethyl-11-methylene-18,19-dinor-17α-pregn-4-en-20-yn-17-ol
Synonyms: 13-Ethyl-11-methylene-18,19-dinor-17α-4-pregnen-20-yn-17-ol; 17α-ethynyl-18-methyl-11-methylene-Δ⁴-oestren-17β-ol

2.3.2   *Structural and molecular formulae and relative molecular mass*

$C_{22}H_{30}O$ Relative molecular mass: 310.5

2.3.3   *Chemical and physical properties of the pure substance*

From O'Neil (2001) and Sweetman (2005)
(*a*)   *Description*: White, crystalline powder
(*b*)   *Melting-point*: 109–110 °C
(*c*)   *Solubility*: Practically insoluble in water; slightly soluble in ethanol and ethyl acetate; sparingly soluble in *n*-hexane
(*d*)   *Optical rotation*: $[\alpha]_D^{20}$, +53° to +57° (in chloroform)

2.3.4   *Technical products and impurities*

Desogestrel is available commercially only in combination with ethinylestradiol in tablets for monophasic and triphasic regimens (IPPF, 2002; British Medical Association/ Royal Pharmaceutical Society of Great Britain, 2004; American Hospital Formulary Service, 2005; Editions du Vidal, 2005; Sweetman, 2005).

Reported impurities include: 13-ethyl-16-[13-ethyl-17β-hydroxy-11-methylene-18,19-dinor-17α-pregn-4-en-20-yn-16-ylidene]-11-methylene-18,19-dinor-17α-pregn-4-en-20-yn-17β-ol, 13-ethyl-11-methylene-18,19-dinor-5α,17α-pregn-3-en-20-yn-17-ol (desogestrel D³-isomer) and 11-methylene-19-nor-17α-pregn-4-en-20-yn-17-ol; 13-ethyl-11-methylenegon-4-en-17-one (British Pharmacopoeial Commission, 2004).

2.3.5   *Use*

Desogestrel is a synthetic progestene that is structurally related to levonorgestrel, has actions and uses similar to those of progestogens in general and has little or no androgenic activity. It is used as the progestogenic component of combined mono- and multiphasic oral contraceptive preparations and as a subdermal implantable 'progestogen-only' contraceptive. A typical daily oral dose of 150 µg is used as the progestogenic component of combined oral contraceptive preparations. An oral dose of 75 µg daily is used as a progestogen-only contraceptive (Editions du Vidal, 2005; Sweetman, 2005).

Table 11 presents comparative global data on sales of desogestrel in 1994, 1999 and 2004 (IMS Health, 2005). The regions are broadly as those defined by WHO.

2.4   Drospirenone

2.4.1   *Nomenclature*

Chem. Abst. Services Reg. No.: 67392-87-4

Chem. Abstr. Name: (2′S,6R,7R,8R,9S,10R,13S,14S,15S,16S)-1,3′,4′,6,7,8,9,10,11,12, 13,14,15,16,20,21-Hexadecahydro-10,13-dimethyl-spiro[17H-dicyclopropa-[6,7:15,16]cyclopenta[a]phenanthrene-17,2′ (5′H)-furan]-3,5′ (2H)-dione

Synonyms: Dihydrospirorenone; 1,2-dihydrospirorenone; drospirenona; spiro[17H-dicyclopropa[6,7:15,16]cyclopenta[a]phenanthrene-17,2′ (5′H)-furan]-3,5′ (2H)-dione, 1,3′,4′,6,7,8,9,10,11,12,13,14,15,16,20,21-hexadecahydro-10,13-dimethyl-, [6R-(6α, 7α,8β,9α,10β,13β,14α,15α,16α,17β)]-

2.4.2   *Structural and molecular formulae and relative molecular mass*

C$_{24}$H$_{30}$O$_3$ Relative molecular mass: 366.5

2.4.3   *Chemical and physical properties*

From O'Neil (2001)

(*a*)   *Melting-point*: 201.3 °C

(*b*)   *Optical rotation*: [α]$_D^{22}$, –182° (in chloroform)

Table 11. Desogestrel used in combined estrogen–progestogen contraceptives and combined estrogen–progestogen menopausal therapy (thousands of standard units[a])

Region	1994	1999	2004
Combined hormonal contraceptives			
Monophasic preparations (< 50 μg estrogen)			
Africa	287	231	223
Eastern Mediterranean	495	841	1 129
Europe	65 347	51 877	53 550
North America	9 875	11 326	15 764
South America	7 675	9 952	8 295
South-East Asia	1 618	4 078	5 933
Western Pacific	2 320	2 122	2 237
Subtotal	87 617	80 426	87 131
Monophasic preparations (≥ 50 μg estrogen)			
North America	0	0	19
South America	1	0	0
Subtotal	1	0	19
Biphasic preparations			
Eastern Mediterranean	0	0	148
Europe	3 430	3 893	4 774
North America	0	1 879	5 620
South America	0	732	1 298
South-East Asia	0	1	2
Western Pacific	0	3	46
Subtotal	3 430	6 508	11 888
Triphasic preparations			
Europe	0	120	1 690
North America	0	0	880
Subtotal	0	120	2 571
Total	91 048	87 054	101 609
Combined hormonal menopausal therapy			
Europe	10 563	3 992	2 532
Total	10 563	3 992	2 532

From IMS Health (2005)
[a] Standard units are sales in terms of standard dose units; the standard dose unit for oral products is one tablet or capsule.

2.4.4   *Technical products and impurities*

Drospirenone is available as capsules that contain 3.0 mg drospirenone and 0.030 mg ethinylestradiol as part of an oral contraceptive regimen (IPPF, 2002).

2.4.5   *Use*

Drospirenone is a progestogen with anti-mineralo-corticoid and anti-androgenic acti-vities; it is used as the progestogenic component of a combined oral contraceptive at doses of 3 mg daily (Sweetman, 2005). Its use in hormonal menopausal therapy has also been reported very recently (IMS Health, 2005).

Table 12 presents comparative global data on sales of drospirenone in 1994, 1999 and 2004 (IMS Health, 2005). The regions are broadly as those defined by WHO.

Table 12. Drospirenone used in combined estrogen–progestogen contraceptives and combined estrogen–progestogen menopausal therapy (thousands of standard units[a])

Region	1994	1999	2004
Combined hormonal contraceptives			
Monophasic preparations (< 50 µg estrogen)			
Africa	0	0	293
Eastern Mediterranean	0	0	601
Europe	0	0	25 422
North America	0	0	11 996
South America	0	0	4 129
South East Asia	0	0	92
Western Pacific	0	0	1 087
Total	0	0	43 620
Combined hormonal menopausal therapy			
Africa	0	0	209
Europe	0	0	3 191
Total	0	0	3 400

From IMS Health (2005)
[a] Standard units are sales in terms of standard dose units; the standard dose unit for oral products is one tablet or capsule.

2.5   Dydrogesterone

2.5.1   *Nomenclature*

Chem. Abstr. Serv. Reg. No.: 152-62-5
Chem. Abstr. Name: (9β,10α)-Pregna-4,6-diene-3,20-dione
IUPAC Systematic Name: 10α-Pregna-4,6-diene-3,20-dione
Synonyms: 10α-Isopregnenone; dehydro-retroprogesterone; dehydroprogesterone

2.5.2 *Structural and molecular formulae and relative molecular mass*

$C_{21}H_{28}O_2$ Relative molecular mass: 312.5

2.5.3 *Chemical and physical properties of the pure substance*

From O'Neil (2001) and Sweetman (2005)

(*a*) *Description*: White to pale yellow, odourless, crystalline powder

(*b*) *Melting-point*: 169–170 °C

(*c*) *Solubility*: Practically insoluble in water; soluble in acetone, chloroform (1 in 2), ethanol (1 in 40) and diethyl ether (1 in 200); slightly soluble in fixed oils; sparingly soluble in methanol

(*d*) *Specific rotation*: $[\alpha]_D^{25}$, –484.5° (in chloroform)

2.5.4 *Technical products and impurities*

Dydrogesterone is available commercially as tablets and capsules, either alone or in combination with estradiol (British National Formulary, 2004; APPCo, 2005; Editions du Vidal, 2005).

2.5.5 *Use*

Dydrogesterone is a progestogen that is structurally related to progesterone, but does not have estrogenic or androgenic properties. Together with cyclic or continuous estrogen, dydrogesterone is also given cyclically in oral doses of 10 mg once or twice daily, or continuously in doses of 5 mg daily, for endometrial protection during hormonal menopausal therapy. It is also given orally in the treatment of menstrual disorders such as menorrhagia, usually in a dose of 10 mg twice daily in a cyclical regimen, and for the treatment of endometriosis at a dose of 10 mg two or three times daily cyclically or continuously (British Medical Association, 2004; Sweetman, 2005).

Table 13 presents comparative global data on sales of dydrogesterone in 1994, 1999 and 2004 (IMS Health, 2005). The regions are broadly as those defined by WHO.

Table 13. Dydrogesterone used in a combined estro-gen–progestogen menopausal therapy (thousands of standard units[a])

Region	1994	1999	2004
Africa	0	0	87
Eastern Mediterranean	0	1 226	2 283
Europe	0	51 054	115 892
South America	0	0	2 429
South-East Asia	0	104	3 352
Western Pacific	0	368	570
Total	0	52 752	124 613

From IMS Health (2005)
[a] Standard units are sales in terms of standard dose units; the standard dose unit for oral products is one tablet or capsule.

2.6 Ethynodiol diacetate

2.6.1 *Nomenclature*

Chem. Abstr. Serv. Reg. No.: 297-76-7
Chem. Abstr. Name: (3β,17α)-19-Norpregn-4-en-20-yne-3,17-diol, diacetate
IUPAC Systematic Name: 19-Nor-17α-pregn-4-en-20-yne-3β,17β-diol, diacetate
Synonyms: Ethinodiol diacetate; ethynodiol acetate; β-ethynodiol diacetate

2.6.2 *Structural and molecular formulae and relative molecular mass*

$C_{24}H_{32}O_4$ Relative molecular mass: 384.5

2.6.3 *Chemical and physical properties of the pure substance*

From O'Neil (2001) and Sweetman (2005), unless otherwise noted
(a) *Description:* White, odourless, crystalline powder
(b) *Melting-point:* ~126–127 °C

(c)   *Solubility*: Very slightly soluble to practically insoluble in water; soluble in ethanol; freely to very soluble in chloroform; freely soluble in diethyl ether

(d)   *Optical rotation*: $[\alpha]_D^{20}$, −70° to −76° (in chloroform) (Pharmacopeial Commission, 2004)

2.6.4   *Technical products and impurities*

Ethynodiol diacetate is available commercially alone or as a component of a combination tablet that contains ethynodiol diacetate plus ethinylestradiol or mestranol (Sweetman, 2005).

2.6.5   *Use*

Ethynodiol diacetate is a progestogen that is used as the progestogenic component of combined oral contraceptives and also alone as an oral progestogen-only contraceptive. Typical daily doses are 1–2 mg in combination products and 500 μg for progestogen-only contraceptives (Sweetman, 2005).

Table 14 presents comparative global data on sales of ethynodiol diacetate in 1994, 1999 and 2004 (IMS Health, 2005). The regions are broadly as those defined by WHO.

2.7   Gestodene

2.7.1   *Nomenclature*

Chem. Abstr. Serv. Reg. No.: 60282-87-3
Deleted CAS Reg. No.: 110541-55-4
Chem. Abstr. Name: (17α)-13-Ethyl-17-hydroxy-18,19-dinorpregna-4,15-dien-20-yn-3-one
IUPAC Systematic Name: 13-Ethyl-17-hydroxy-18,19-dinor-17α-pregna-4,15-dien-20-yn-3-one

2.7.2   *Structural and molecular formulae and relative molecular mass*

$C_{21}H_{26}O_2$ Relative molecular mass: 310.4

Table 14. Ethynodiol diacetate used in combined estrogen–progestogen contraceptives and combined estrogen–progestogen menopausal therapy (thousands of standard units[a])

Region	1994	1999	2004
Combined hormonal contraceptives			
Monophasic preparations (< 50 µg estrogen)			
Europe	65	28	0
North America	3 904	4 363	3 239
Western Pacific	32	0	26
Subtotal	4 000	4 390	3 265
Monophasic preparations (≥ 50 µg estrogen)			
Africa	26	0	0
Europe	127	0	0
North America	533	232	40
South America	299	176	62
South-East Asia	778	655	448
Western Pacific	69	6	2
Subtotal	1 832	1 069	551
Biphasic preparations			
South America	9	7	0
Subtotal	9	7	0
Total	5 841	5 466	3 816
Combined hormonal menopausal therapy			
Europe	0	49	0
Western Pacific	2 427	1 283	598
Total	2 427	1 332	598

From IMS Health (2005)
[a] Standard units are sales in terms of standard dose units; the standard dose unit for oral products is one tablet or capsule.

2.7.3   *Chemical and physical properties of the pure substance*

From O'Neil (2001)
(*a*) *Description*: Crystals
(*b*) *Melting-point*: 197.9 °C

2.7.4   *Technical products and impurities*

Gestodene is available commercially as a component of combination tablets with ethinylestradiol (IPPF, 2002; Editions du Vidal, 2005).

2.7.5   *Use*

Gestodene is used as the progestogenic component of combined oral contraceptives; a typical daily dose is 75 µg in monophasic preparations and 50–100 µg in triphasic preparations (Sweetman, 2005).

Table 15 presents comparative global data on sales of gestodene in 1994, 1999 and 2004 (IMS Health, 2005). The regions are broadly as those defined by WHO.

Table 15. Gestodene used in combined estrogen–progestogen contraceptives and combined estrogen–progestogen menopausal therapy (thousands of standard units[a])

Region	1994	1999	2004
Combined hormonal contraceptive			
Monophasic preparations (< 50 µg estrogen)			
Africa	416	580	778
Eastern Mediterranean	305	1 118	2 103
Europe	42 138	49 100	59 460
North America	1 232	1 873	1 864
South America	9 939	16 905	22 829
South-East Asia	1 932	1 661	2 686
Western Pacific	1 111	1 359	1 633
Subtotal	57 072	72 595	91 352
Biphasic preparations			
Europe	1	0	0
Subtotal	1	0	0
Triphasic preparations			
Africa	155	136	84
Europe	11 958	15 204	9 695
South America	0	121	69
Western Pacific	0	53	1
Subtotal	12 113	15 514	9 849
Total	69 186	88 109	101 201
Combined hormonal menopausal therapy			
Europe	0	0	4 980
South America	0	0	1 412
North America	0	0	428
Total	0	0	6 821

From IMS Health (2005)

[a] Standard units are sales in terms of standard dose units; the standard dose unit for oral products is one tablet or capsule.

2.8   Levonorgestrel

2.8.1   *Nomenclature*

Chem. Abstr. Serv. Reg. No.: 797-63-7
Deleted CAS Reg. No.: 797-62-6; 4222-79-1; 121714-72-5
Chem. Abstr. Name: (17α)-13-Ethyl-17-hydroxy-18,19-dinorpregn-4-en-20-yn-3-one
IUPAC Systematic Name: 13-Ethyl-17-hydroxy-18,19-dinor-17α-pregn-4-en-20-yn-3-one
Synonyms: 13-Ethyl-17-ethynyl-17β-hydroxy-4-gonen-3-one; 13-ethyl-17α-ethynyl-17-hydroxygon-4-en-3-one; 13-ethyl-17α-ethynylgon-4-en-17β-ol-3-one; 13β-ethyl-17α-ethynyl-17β-hydroxygon-4-en-3-one; 13-ethyl-17-hydroxy-18,19-dinor-17α-pregn-4-en-20-yn-3-one; 17-ethynyl-18-methyl-19-nortestosterone; 18-methylnorethindrone; l-norgestrel; D-l-norgestrel; D-norgestrel

2.8.2   *Structural and molecular formulae and relative molecular mass*

$C_{21}H_{28}O_2$ Relative molecular mass: 312.5

2.8.3   *Chemical and physical properties of the pure substance*

From O'Neil (2001) and Sweetman (2005)
(a)   *Description*: White or almost white, odourless, crystalline powder
(b)   *Melting-point*: 235–237 °C
(c)   *Solubility*: Practically insoluble in water; slightly soluble in ethanol; sparingly soluble in dichloromethane; soluble in chloroform
(d)   *Specific rotation*: $[\alpha]_D^{20}$, –32.4° (in chloroform)

2.8.4   *Technical products and impurities*

Levonorgestrel is available commercially as a single-ingredient tablet and in combined tablets with estradiol, estradiol valerate, estriol and ethinylestradiol for hormonal therapy (British Pharmacopaeial Commission, 2004). It is also available as an intrauterine system and as a flexible, closed-capsule implant made of silicone rubber tubing (Sweetman, 2005).

Reported impurities include: 13-ethyl-3,4-diethynyl-18,19-dinor-17α-pregn-5-en-20-yn-3β,4α,17-triol, 13-ethyl-3,4-diethynyl-18,19-dinor-17α-pregn-5-en-20-yn-3α,4α,17-triol 13-ethyl-18,19-dinor-17α-pregn-4-en-20-yn-17-ol, 13-ethyl-3-ethynyl-18,19-dinor-

17α-pregna-3,5-dien-20-yn-17-ol, 13-ethyl-17-hydroxy-18,19-dinor-17α-pregna-4,8(14)-dien-20-yn-3-one and 13-ethyl-17-hydroxy-18,19-dinor-17α-pregn-5(10)-en-20-yn-3-one (British Pharmacopoeial Commission, 2004).

2.8.5   *Use*

Levonorgestrel is D-(–)-norgestrel, the active levorotatory form of norgestrel.

Levonorgestrel is more commonly used as a hormonal contraceptive than norgestrel (and is twice as potent) and has androgenic activity. The typical daily dose of levonorgestrel is 30 or 37.5 µg when used as an oral progestogen-only contraceptive, 150–250 µg when used as a combined oral contraceptive in monophasic preparations, and 50–125 µg when used as a combined oral contraceptive in triphasic preparations. Levonorgestrel is also used as a long-acting (up to 5 years) progestogen-only contraceptive administered by subcutaneous implantation. A long-acting intrauterine device is also available for contraception or menorrhagia (Sweetman, 2005).

Levonorgestrel is used as the progestogenic component of hormonal menopausal therapy. A typical oral regimen is 75–250 µg levonorgestrel for 10–12 days of a 28-day cycle. Levonorgestrel may also be given via a combined transdermal patch, applied once weekly for 2 weeks of a 4-week cycle, that releases 10 µg per 24 h together with an estrogen. Alternatively, a patch that releases 7 µg per 24 h together with an estrogen is applied once weekly for continuous hormonal therapy (Sweetman, 2005).

Table 16 presents comparative global data on sales of levonorgestrel in 1994, 1999 and 2004 (IMS Health, 2005). The regions are broadly as those defined by WHO.

2.9   Lynestrenol

2.9.1   *Nomenclature*

Chem. Abstr. Serv. Reg. No.: 52-76-6
Deleted CAS Reg. No.: 60416-16-2
Chem. Abstr. Name: (17α)-19-Norpregn-4-en-20-yn-17-ol
IUPAC Systematic Name: 19-Nor-17α-pregn-4-en-20-yn-17-ol
Synonyms: 3-Desoxynorlutin; Δ^4-17α-ethinylestren-17β-ol; Δ^4-17α-ethinyloestren-17β-ol; ethynylestrenol; ethynyloestrenol; 17α-ethynylestrenol; 17α-ethynyloestrenol; 17α-ethynyl-17β-hydroxy-Δ^4-estrene; 17α-ethynyl-17β-hydroxy-Δ^4-oestrene

Table 16. Levonorgestrel used in combined estrogen–progestogen contraceptives and combined estrogen–progestogen menopausal therapy (thousands of standard units[a])

Region	1994	1999	2001
Combined hormonal contraceptives			
Monophasic preparations (< 50 µg estrogen)			
Africa	1 854	2 142	2 584
Eastern Mediterranean	5 501	6 636	3 364
Europe	31 996	61 292	79 164
North America	10 928	16 583	22 538
South America	34 863	42 064	46 906
South-East Asia	3 640	19 803	42 426
Western Pacific	5 858	9 167	18 916
Subtotal	94 638	157 686	215 897
Monophasic preparations (≥ 50 µg estrogen)			
Africa	30	15	5
Eastern Mediterranean	318	286	66
Europe	7 637	4 679	2 706
North America	1 132	671	537
South America	15 709	15 387	13 050
South-East Asia	238	8 734	3 962
Western Pacific	1 439	1 304	753
Subtotal	26 502	31 077	21 079
Biphasic preparations			
Africa	313	336	400
Eastern Mediterranean	70	59	69
Europe	14 814	13 302	10 835
Western Pacific	312	200	49
Subtotal	15 508	13 896	11 352
Triphasic preparations			
Africa	4 181	5 150	4 353
Eastern Mediterranean	1 586	965	1 860
Europe	43 499	47 396	39 636
North America	21 673	18 226	11 415
South America	13 418	11 908	10 607
South-East Asia	352	2 232	3 389
Western Pacific	8 329	7 545	6 718
Subtotal	93 037	93 421	77 977
Total	229 685	296 080	326 305
Combined hormonal menopausal therapy			
Europe	187 978	231 661	85 112
North America	0	0	790
South America	20 543	20 553	10 889
South-East Asia	0	428	2 054
Western Pacific	354	300	95
Total	208 875	252 942	98 941

From IMS Health (2005)

[a] Standard units are sales in terms of standard dose units; the standard dose unit for oral products is one tablet or capsule.

2.9.2   *Structural and molecular formulae and relative molecular mass*

$C_{20}H_{28}O$ Relative molecular mass: 284.4

2.9.3   *Chemical and physical properties of the pure substance*

From O'Neil (2001) and Sweetman (2005)
(*a*)   *Description*: White, crystalline powder
(*b*)   *Melting-point*: 158–160 °C
(*c*)   *Solubility*: Practically insoluble in water; soluble in ethanol, acetone and diethyl ether; freely soluble in chloroform
(*d*)   *Specific rotation*: $[\alpha]_D$, –13° (in chloroform)

2.9.4   *Technical products and impurities*

Lynestrenol is available commercially as a single-ingredient tablet and as a component of combination tablets that contain ethinylestradiol or mestranol (Reynolds, 1996; IPPF, 2002; Editions du Vidal, 2005).

2.9.5   *Use*

Lynestrenol is used alone or as the progestogenic component of oral contraceptives. Typical oral daily doses for contraception are 0.5 mg when used as a progestogen-only preparation and 0.75–2.5 mg when combined with an estrogen. When used alone for menstrual disorders, doses of 5 to 10 mg daily are given, frequently as cyclical regimens (Sweetman, 2005).

Table 17 presents comparative global data on sales of lynestrenol in 1994, 1999 and 2004 (IMS Health, 2005). The regions are broadly as those defined by WHO.

2.10   *Medroxyprogesterone acetate*

2.10.1   *Nomenclature*

Chem. Abstr. Serv. Reg. No.: 71-58-9
Chem. Abstr. Name: (6α)-17-(Acetyloxy)-6-methylpregn-4-ene-3,20-dione
IUPAC Systematic Name: 17-Hydroxy-6α-methylpregn-4-ene-3,20-dione, acetate

Table 17. Lynoestrenol used in combined estrogen–progestogen contraceptives and combined estrogen–progestogen menopausal therapy (thousands of standard units[a])

Region	1994	1999	2004
Combined hormonal contraceptives			
Monophasic preparations (< 50 µg estrogen)			
Europe	1197	658	538
South America	0	0	13
South-East Asia	23	0	0
Subtotal	1220	658	551
Monophasic preparations (≥ 50 µg estrogen)			
Africa	8	0	0
Eastern Mediterranean	10	0	0
Europe	1619	842	0
North America	114	0	0
South America	1644	1570	581
South-East Asia	1684	2156	2374
Western Pacific	82	76	0
Subtotal	5162	4643	2956
Biphasic preparations			
Africa	7	7	0
Europe	1839	1088	310
South America	41	0	0
Subtotal	1887	1095	310
Total	8269	6396	3817
Combined hormonal menopausal therapy			
Europe	986	407	0
Western Pacific	6676	4373	2344
Total	7662	4780	2344

From IMS Health (2005)
[a] Standard units are sales in terms of standard dose units; the standard dose unit for oral products is one tablet or capsule.

Synonyms: 17α-Acetoxy-6α-methylprogesterone; depomedroxyprogesterone acetate; depo-progestin; depot-medroxyprogesterone acetate; DMPA; 17-hydroxy-6α-methyl-progesterone, acetate; 17α-hydroxy-6α-methylprogesterone acetate; MAP; medroxy-progesterone 17-acetate; 6α-methyl-17-acetoxyprogesterone; 6α-methyl-17α-hydroxyprogesterone acetate

2.10.2   *Structural and molecular formulae and relative molecular mass*

C$_{24}$H$_{34}$O$_4$ Relative molecular mass: 386.5

2.10.3   *Chemical and physical properties of the pure substance*

From O'Neil (2001) and Sweetman (2005)
(*a*)   *Description*: White to off-white, odourless, crystalline powder
(*b*)   *Melting-point*: 207–209 °C
(*c*)   *Solubility*: Practically insoluble in water; slightly soluble in diethyl ether; sparingly soluble in ethanol and methanol; soluble in acetone and dioxane; freely soluble in chloroform and dichloromethane
(*d*)   *Specific rotation*: [α]$_D^{25}$, +61° (in chloroform)

2.10.4   *Technical products and impurities*

Medroxyprogesterone acetate is available commercially as single-ingredient tablets, as combination tablets with conjugated estrogens, estradiol or estradiol cypionate and as sterile suspensions (IPPF, 2002; American Hospital Formulary Service, 2005; Editions du Vidal, 2005).

Reported impurities include: 6α,17a-dimethyl-3,17-dioxo-*D*-homoandrost-4-en-17aα-yl acetate, 6β-hydroxy-6-methyl-3,20-dioxopregn-4-en-17-yl acetate (6β-hydroxymedroxyprogesterone acetate), 17-hydroxy-6α-methylpregn-4-ene-3,20-dione (medroxyprogesterone), 6-methyl-3,20-dioxopregna-4,6-dien-17-yl acetate, 6α-methyl-3,20-dioxo-5β-pregnan-17-yl acetate (4,5β-dihydromedroxyprogesterone acetate), 6β-methyl-3,20-dioxopregn-4-en-17-yl acetate (6-epimedroxyprogesterone acetate) and 6-methylene-3,20-dioxopregn-4-en-17-yl acetate (6-methylenehydroxyprogesterone acetate) (British Pharmacopoeial Commission, 2004).

2.10.5   *Use*

Medroxyprogesterone acetate is given by intramuscular injection as a contraceptive. A combined contraceptive injection that contains 25 mg medroxyprogesterone acetate with 5 mg estradiol cypionate is given monthly. As a progestogen-only contraceptive, a dose of 150 mg is given every 12 weeks.

When used as the progestogen component of hormonal menopausal therapy, medroxyprogesterone acetate is administered orally in a variety of regimens that include 2.5 or 5 mg daily continuously, 5 or 10 mg daily for 12–14 days of a 28-day cycle and 20 mg daily for 14 days of a 91-day cycle (Sweetman, 2005).

It is also used for the treatment of menorrhagia and secondary amenorrhoea and in the palliative treatment of some hormone-dependent malignant neoplasms (Sweetman, 2005).

Table 18 presents comparative global data on sales of medroxyprogesterone acetate in 1994, 1999 and 2004 (IMS Health, 2005). The regions are broadly as those defined by WHO.

Table 18. Medroxyprogesterone acetate used in combined estrogen–progestogen menopausal therapy (thousands of standard units[a])

Region	1994	1999	2004
Africa	0	1 068	2 669
Eastern Mediterranean	0	514	511
Europe	54 980	298 081	167 948
North America	0	1 031 863	219 035
South America	23 322	131 139	41 098
South-East Asia	4 782	6 691	13 091
Western Pacific	6 364	101 908	31 230
Total	89 447	1 571 264	475 583

From IMS Health (2005)
[a] Standard units are sales in terms of standard dose units; the standard dose unit for oral products is one tablet or capsule.

2.11   Megestrol acetate

2.11.1   *Nomenclature*

Chem. Abstr. Serv. Reg. No.: 595-33-5
Chem. Abstr. Name: 17-(Acetyloxy)-6-methylpregna-4,6-diene-3,20-dione
IUPAC Systematic Name: 17-Hydroxy-6-methylpregna-4,6-diene-3,20-dione, acetate
Synonyms: DMAP; megestryl acetate; MGA

2.11.2   *Structural and molecular formulae and relative molecular mass*

C$_{24}$H$_{32}$O$_4$ Relative molecular mass: 384.5

2.11.3   *Chemical and physical properties of the pure substance*

From O'Neil (2001) and Sweetman (2005)
(*a*)   *Description*: White to creamy white, odourless, crystalline powder
(*b*)   *Melting-point*: 214–216 °C
(*c*)   *Solubility*: Practically insoluble in water (2 µg/mL at 37 °C); very soluble in chloroform; soluble in acetone; slightly soluble in diethyl ether and fixed oils; sparingly soluble in ethanol
(*d*)   *Specific rotation*: [α]$_D^{24}$, +5° (in chloroform)

2.11.4   *Technical products and impurities*

Megestrol acetate is available commercially as tablets and as an oral suspension (IPPF, 2002; Editions du Vidal, 2005).

Reported impurities include: 6,17a-dimethyl-3,17-dioxo-*D*-homoandrosta-4,6-dien-17aα-yl acetate (*D-homo* megestrol acetate), 6α-methyl-3,20-dioxopregn-4-en-17-yl acetate (medroxyprogesterone acetate), 6-methyl-3,20-dioxopregna-1,4,6-trien-17-yl acetate, 6-methylene-3,20-dioxopregn-4-en-17-yl acetate (6-methylene hydroxyprogesterone acetate) and 6-methyl-17-hydroxypregna-4,6-diene-3,20-dione (megestrol) (British Pharmacopoeial Commission, 2004).

2.11.5   *Use*

Megestrol acetate has been used in a few countries as an oral contraceptive, usually in combination with ethinylestradiol, although it is believed that such usage has been discontinued. It is used for the palliative treatment of carcinoma of the breast or endometrium, in the treatment of acne, hirsutism and sexual infantilism in women and in the treatment of anorexia and cachexia in patients with acquired immunodeficiency syndrome or cancer (Reynolds, 1996; Sweetman, 2005).

Table 19 presents comparative global data on sales of megestrol acetate in 1994, 1999 and 2004 (IMS Health, 2005). The regions are broadly as those defined by WHO.

Table 19. Megestrol acetate used in combined oestrogen–progestogen contraceptives (thousands of standard units[a])

Region	1994	1999	2004
Monophasic preparations (≥ 50 µg estrogen)			
South America	185	87	0
Total	185	87	0

From IMS Health (2005)
[a] Standard units are sales in terms of standard dose units; the standard dose unit for oral products is one tablet or capsule.

2.12   Norethisterone

2.12.1   *Nomenclature*

Chem. Abstr. Serv. Reg. No.: 68-22-4
Chem. Abstr. Name: (17α)-17-Hydroxy-19-norpregn-4-en-20-yn-3-one
IUPAC Systematic Name: 17-Hydroxy-19-nor-17α-pregn-4-en-20-yn-3-one
Synonyms: Ethinylnortestosterone; 17α-ethinyl-19-nortestosterone; ethynylnortestosterone; 17-ethynyl-19-nortestosterone; 17α-ethynyl-19-nortestosterone; norethindrone; norethisteron; norethynodrone; 19-nor-17α-ethynyltestosterone; norpregneninolone

2.12.2   *Structural and molecular formulae and relative molecular mass*

$C_{20}H_{26}O_2$ Relative molecular mass: 298.4

2.12.3   *Chemical and physical properties of the pure substance*

From O'Neil (2001) and Sweetman (2005)
(*a*)   *Description*: White or yellowish white, odourless, crystalline powder
(*b*)   *Melting-point*: 203–204 °C

(c) *Solubility*: Practically insoluble in water; slightly to sparingly soluble in ethanol; slightly soluble in diethyl ether; soluble in chloroform and dioxane

(d) *Specific rotation*: $[\alpha]_D^{20}$, −31.7° (in chloroform)

2.12.4 *Technical products and impurities*

Norethisterone is available commercially as single-ingredient tablets or as a component of combination tablets with ethinylestradiol or mestranol (IPPF, 2002).

2.12.5 *Use (norethisterone and its acetate and enanthate esters)*

Norethisterone and its acetate and enanthate esters are progestogens that have weak estrogenic and androgenic properties. They are commonly used as hormonal contraceptives in monophasic, biphasic and triphasic regimens (Sweetman, 2005).

Norethisterone and norethisterone acetate are both given orally. Typical daily doses are 0.35 mg for norethisterone and 0.6 mg for norethisterone acetate when used alone, or 0.5–1 mg for norethisterone and 1–1.5 mg for norethisterone acetate when used with an estrogen. Norethisterone enanthate is given by intramuscular injection; a dose of 200 mg provides contraception for 8 weeks (Sweetman, 2005).

Norethisterone and norethisterone acetate are used as the progestogen component of hormonal menopausal therapy. Typical regimens have included either continuous daily doses of 0.7 mg norethisterone or 0.5–1 mg norethisterone acetate, or cyclical regimens of 1 mg norethisterone or norethisterone acetate daily for 10–12 days of a 28-day cycle. Norethisterone acetate is also available as transdermal patches that supply 170 or 250 µg in 24 h and are applied twice weekly for 2 weeks of a 4-week cycle; the lower dose may also be applied twice weekly on a continuous basis (Sweetman, 2005).

Table 20 presents comparative global data on sales of norethisterone in 1994, 1999 and 2004 (IMS Health, 2005). The regions are broadly as those defined by WHO.

2.13   Norethisterone acetate

2.13.1 *Nomenclature*

Chem. Abstr. Serv. Reg. No.: 51-98-9
Chem. Abstr. Name: (17α)-17-(Acetyloxy)-19-norpregn-4-en-20-yn-3-one
IUPAC Systematic Name: 17-Hydroxy-19-nor-17α-pregn-4-en-20-yn-3-one, acetate
Synonyms: 17α-Ethinyl-19-nortestosterone 17β-acetate; 17α-ethinyl-19-nortestosterone acetate; 17α-ethynyl-19-nortestosterone acetate; norethindrone acetate; norethindrone 17-acetate; norethisteron acetate; norethisterone 17-acetate; 19-norethisterone acetate; norethynyltestosterone acetate; 19-norethynyltestosterone acetate; norethysterone acetate

Table 20. Norethisterone used in combined estrogen–progestogen contraceptives and combined estrogen–progestogen menopausal therapy (thousands of standard units[a])

Region	1994	1999	2004
Combined hormonal contraceptives			
Monophasic preparations (< 50 µg estrogen)			
Africa	7	2	0
Eastern Mediterranean	52	0	0
Europe	4 462	6 107	4 654
North America	20 035	20 682	17 720 .
South America	8	85	59
South-East Asia	6 421	0	0
Western Pacific	1 094	1 819	1 698
Subtotal	32 079	28 696	24 132
Monophasic preparations (≥ 50 µg estrogen)			
Africa	94	92	42
Eastern Mediterranean	1 185	11	0
Europe	1 827	930	202
North America	3 734	1 889	1 193
South America	75	23	13
South-East Asia	1 439	892	650
Western Pacific	181	163	181
Subtotal	8 535	4 000	2 281
Biphasic preparations			
Africa	119	87	74
Europe	2 778	1 867	1 117
North America	574	250	70
South America	167	71	0
Western Pacific	0	9	0
Subtotal	3 637	2 283	1 260
Triphasic preparations			
Africa	111	63	34
Europe	6 587	4 995	3 134
North America	16 279	12 882	7 908
South America	138	135	24
Western Pacific	284	231	532
Subtotal	23 399	18 306	11 632
Total	67 650	53 285	39 305
Combined hormonal menopausal therapy			
Africa	8 687	12 325	12 960
Eastern Mediterranean	15	632	1 008
Europe	390 651	702 960	444 352
North America	409	16 506	159 294
South America	16 951	60 481	75 382
South-East Asia	4 520	8 229	22 067
Western Pacific	21 123	42 462	37 686
Total	442 356	843 594	752 747

From IMS Health (2005)

[a] Standard units are sales in terms of standard dose units; the standard dose unit for oral products is one tablet or capsule.

2.13.2   *Structural and molecular formulae and relative molecular mass*

C$_{22}$H$_{28}$O$_{3}$ Relative molecular mass: 340.5

2.13.3   *Chemical and physical properties of the pure substance*

(*a*) *Description*: White or creamy white, odourless, crystalline powder (Sweetman, 2005)

(*b*) *Melting-point*: 161–162 °C (O'Neil, 2001)

(*c*) *Solubility*: Practically insoluble in water (1 g in > 10 L); soluble in ethanol (1 part in 10), chloroform (1 part in < 1), dioxane (1 part in 2) and diethyl ether (1 part in 18) (Sweetman, 2005)

(*d*) *Specific rotation*: $[\alpha]_D^{25}$, –32° to –38° (Pharmacopeial Convention, 2004)

2.13.4   *Technical products and impurities*

Norethisterone acetate is available commercially as single-ingredient tablets or as a component of combination tablets with ethinylestradiol. For hormonal postmenopausal therapy, norethisterone acetate is used in combination with estradiol or estradiol hemi-hydrate. It is also available as a percutaneous patch with estradiol (IPPF, 2002; British Medical Association, 2004; Editions du Vidal, 2005).

Reported impurities include: 6β-acetyl-3-oxo-19-nor-17α-pregn-4-en-20-yn-17-yl acetate, 3,20-dioxo-19-nor-17α-pregn-4-en-17-yl acetate, 6β-hydroxy-3-oxo-19-nor-17α-pregn-4-en-20-yn-17-yl acetate, 3,6-dioxo-19-nor-17α-pregn-4-en-20-yn-17-yl acetate, norethisterone, 3-oxo-19-nor-17α-pregn-5(10)-en-20-yn-17-yl acetate and 3-oxo-19-nor-17α-pregn-5-en-20-yn-17-yl acetate (British Pharmacopoeial Commission, 2004).

2.13.5   *Use*

See norethisterone.

2.14 Norethisterone enanthate

2.14.1 *Nomenclature*

Chem. Abstr. Serv. Reg. No.: 3836-23-5
Chem. Abstr. Name: (17α)-17-(Heptanoyl)-19-norpregn-4-en-20-yn-3-one
IUPAC Systematic Name: 17-Hydroxy-19-nor-17α-pregn-4-en-20-yn-3-one, heptanoate
Synonyms: Norethindrone enanthate; norethindrone oenanthate; norethisterone enanthate; norethisterone heptanoate; 17β-hydroxy-19-nor-17α-pregn-4-en-20-yn-3-one heptanoate

2.14.2 *Structural and molecular formulae and relative molecular mass*

$C_{27}H_{38}O_3$ Relative molecular mass: 410.6

2.14.3 *Chemical and physical properties of the pure substance*

No information was available to the Working Group.

2.14.4 *Technical products and impurities*

Norethisterone enanthate is available commercially in an oily solution for depot injection (IPPF, 2002).

2.14.5 *Use*

See norethisterone.

2.15 Norethynodrel

2.15.1 *Nomenclature*

Chem. Abstr. Serv. Reg. No.: 68-23-5
Chem. Abstr. Name: (17α)-17-Hydroxy-19-norpregn-5(10)-en-20-yn-3-one
IUPAC Systematic Name: 17-Hydroxy-19-nor-17α-pregn-5(10)-en-20-yn-3-one
Synonyms: Enidrel; noretynodrel

2.15.2 *Structural and molecular formulae and relative molecular mass*

$C_{20}H_{26}O_2$ Relative molecular mass: 298.4

2.15.3 *Chemical and physical properties of the pure substance*

From O'Neil (2001) and Sweetman (2005)
(a) *Description*: White, odourless, crystalline powder
(b) *Melting-point*: 169–170 °C
(c) *Solubility*: Very slightly soluble in water; freely soluble in chloroform; soluble in acetone; sparingly soluble in ethanol
(d) *Optical rotation*: $[\alpha]_D^{25}$, +108° (in 1% chloroform)

2.15.4 *Technical products and impurities*

Norethynodrel was available commercially as a component of a combination tablet with mestranol. Information available in 2005 indicated that there is no usage of norethynodrel at any dose in any form of drug (Sweetman, 2005).

2.15.5 *Use*

Norethynodrel is a progestogen that is structurally related to norethisterone, which has been given orally in conjunction with an estrogen such as mestranol for the treatment of various menstrual disorders and endometriosis (Sweetman, 2005). Available information indicates that it is no longer produced or used.

Table 21 presents comparative global data on sales of norethynodrel in 1994, 1999 and 2004 (IMS Health, 2005). The regions are broadly as those defined by WHO.

Table 21. Norethynodrel used in combined estrogen–progestogen menopausal therapy (thousands of standard units[a])

Region	1994	1999	2004
Western Pacific	18	0	0
Total	18	0	0

From IMS Health (2005)
[a] Standard units are sales in terms of standard dose units; the standard dose unit for oral products is one tablet or capsule.

2.16   Norgestimate

2.16.1   *Nomenclature*

Chem. Abstr. Serv. Reg. No.: 35189-28-7
Chem. Abstr. Name: (17α)-17-(Acetyloxy)-13-ethyl-18,19-dinorpregn-4-en-20-yn-3-one, 3-oxime
IUPAC Systematic Name: 13-Ethyl-17-hydroxy-18,19-dinor-17α-pregn-4-en-20-yn-3-one oxime acetate (ester)
Synonyms: 17α-Acetoxy-13-ethyl-17-ethynylgon-4-en-3-one oxime; dexnorgestrel acetime

2.16.2   *Structural and molecular formulae and relative molecular mass*

C$_{23}$H$_{31}$NO$_3$ Relative molecular mass: 369.5

2.16.3   *Chemical and physical properties of the pure substance*

From O'Neil (2001) and Sweetman (2005), unless otherwise noted
(a) *Description*: White to pale yellow powder (a mixture of (E)- and (Z)-isomers that has a ratio of (E)- to (Z)-isomer of between 1.27 and 1.78)
(b) *Melting-point*: 214–218 °C
(c) *Solubility*: Insoluble in water; sparingly soluble in acetonitrile; freely to very soluble in dichloromethane
(d) *Specific rotation*: [α]$_D^{25}$, +110°; [α]$_D$, +40° to +46° (in chloroform) (Pharmacopeial Commission, 2004)

2.16.4   *Technical products and impurities*

Norgestimate is available commercially as a component of a combination tablet with ethinylestradiol (British Medical Association, 2004; IPPF, 2004; Editions du Vidal, 2005).

2.16.5   *Use*

Norgestimate is structurally related to levonorgestrel (to which it is partly metabolized) and is used as the progestogenic component of combined oral contraceptives and in hormonal menopausal therapy. A typical daily dose is 250 µg in monophasic contraceptive preparations and 180–250 µg in triphasic preparations. For hormonal menopausal therapy, a regimen of estradiol daily for 3 days followed by estradiol combined with 90 µg norgestimate daily for 3 days is used; this 6-day cycle is repeated continuously without interruption (Sweetman, 2005).

Table 22 presents comparative global data on sales of norgestimate in 1994, 1999 and 2004 (IMS Health, 2005). The regions are broadly as those defined by WHO.

Table 22. Norgestimate used in combined estrogen–progestogen contraceptives and combined estrogen–progestogen menopausal therapy (thousands of standard units[a])

Region	1994	1999	2004
Combined hormonal contraceptives			
Monophasic preparations (< 50 µg estrogen)			
Africa	0	0	4
Eastern Mediterranean	0	133	258
Europe	13 748	19 133	16 355
North America	2 865	6 091	5 562
South America	60	359	204
South-East Asia	0	0	172
Subtotal	16 673	25 717	22 554
Triphasic preparations			
Africa	0	12	6
Europe	907	1 421	1 732
North America	1 599	16 973	30 846
South America	56	236	171
Subtotal	2 562	18 642	32 755
Total	19 235	44 359	55 309
Combined hormonal menopausal therapy			
North America	0	0	14 095
South America	0	0	6 364
Total	0	0	20 459

From IMS Health (2005)
[a] Standard units are sales in terms of standard dose units; the standard dose unit for oral products is one tablet or capsule.

2.17   Norgestrel

2.17.1   *Nomenclature*

Chem. Abstr. Serv. Reg. No.: 6533-00-2

Chem. Abstr. Name: (17α)-dl-13-Ethyl-17-hydroxy-18,19-dinorpregn-4-en-20-yn-3-one

IUPAC Systematic Name: dl-13-Ethyl-17-hydroxy-18,19-dinor-17α-pregn-4-en-20-yn-3-one

Synonyms: (17α)-13-Ethyl-17-hydroxy-18,19-dinorpregn-4-en-20-yn-3-one; methyl-norethindrone; α-norgestrel; dl-norgestrel; DL-norgestrel

2.17.2   *Structural and molecular formulae and relative molecular mass*

$C_{21}H_{28}O_2$ Relative molecular mass: 312.5

2.17.3   *Chemical and physical properties of the pure substance*

From O'Neil (2001) and Sweetman (2005), unless otherwise noted
(*a*)   *Description*: White, practically odourless, crystalline powder
(*b*)   *Boiling-point*: 205–207 °C
(*c*)   *Solubility*: Practically insoluble in water; slightly to sparingly soluble in ethanol; sparingly soluble in dichloromethane; freely soluble in chloroform
(*d*)   *Optical rotation*: $[\alpha]_D^{25}$, –0.1° to +0.1° (in chloroform) (Pharmacopeial Convention, 2004)

2.17.4   *Technical products and impurities*

Norgestrel is available commercially as a single-ingredient tablet and as a component of combination tablets with ethinylestradiol, estradiol valerate or as combined injectable solution with ethinylestradiol (IPPF, 2002; Editions du Vidal, 2005).

2.17.5   *Use*

Uses of norgestrel in oral contraception and menopausal hormonal therapy are similar to those of levonorgestrel, with the exception of applications of the levo-enantiomer in subcutaneous implants and intrauterine devices (Sweetman, 2005).

Table 23 presents comparative global data on sales of norgestrel in 1994, 1999 and 2004 (IMS Health, 2005). The regions are broadly as those defined by WHO.

Table 23. Norgestrel used in combined estrogen–progestogen contraceptives and combined estrogen–progestogen menopausal therapy (thousands of standard units[a])

Region	1994	1999	2004
Combined hormonal contraceptives			
Monophasic preparations (< 50 μg estrogen)			
Eastern Mediterranean	0	0	3 075
Europe	227	193	361
North America	6 751	7 185	7 007
South America	8	10	52
South-East Asia	120	3 746	7 103
Western Pacific	0	0	8
Subtotal	7 105	11 134	17 605
Monophasic preparations (≥ 50 μg estrogen)			
Africa	1 912	1 539	1 359
Eastern Mediterranean	430	530	60
Europe	4 285	3 024	2 019
North America	1 814	1 165	928
South America	7 141	3 948	1 339
South-East Asia	762	1 074	1 010
Western Pacific	541	615	615
Subtotal	16 886	11 895	7 330
Total	23 991	23 029	24 935
Combined hormonal menopausal therapy			
Africa	3 308	3 213	1 797
Eastern Mediterranean	6 545	15 656	19 387
Europe	338 968	237 793	91 053
North America	14 787	13 048	12 237
South America	31 690	24 458	21 968
South East Asia	5 821	10 489	11 395
Western Pacific	53 391	49 259	29 457
Total	454 510	353 916	187 294

From IMS Health (2005)

[a] Standard units are sales in terms of standard dose units; the standard dose unit for oral products is one tablet or capsule.

2.18   Progesterone

2.18.1 *Nomenclature*

Chem. Abst. Services Reg. No.: 57-83-0
Chem. Abstr. Name: Pregn-4-ene-3,20-dione
Synonyms: Corpus luteum hormone; luteal hormone; luteine; luteohormone; Δ^4-pregnene-3,20-dione

2.18.2 *Structural and molecular formulae and relative molecular mass*

$C_{21}H_{30}O_2$ Relative molecular mass: 314.5

2.18.3 *Chemical and physical properties*

From O'Neil (2001) and Sweetman (2005), unless otherwise noted
(a)   *Description*: Exists in two readily interconvertible crystalline forms: the α form, in white orthorhombic prisms, and the β form, in white orthorhombic needles
(b)   *Melting-point*: α form, 128.5–131 °C; β form, 121–122 °C
(c)   *Solubility*: Practically insoluble in water; soluble in ethanol (1 in 8), arachis oil (1 in 60), chloroform (1 in < 1), diethyl ether (1 in 16), ethyl oleate (1 in 60) and light petroleum (1 in 100) (Wade, 1977); soluble in acetone, dioxane and concentrated sulfuric acid; sparingly soluble in vegetable oils
(d)   *Optical rotation*: α form — $[\alpha]_D^{20}$, +192°; β form — $[\alpha]_D^{20}$, +172° to +182° (in dioxane)

2.18.4 *Technical products and impurities*

Progesterone is available in an oily solution for injection, as pessaries or suppositories and as an intrauterine device (IPPF, 2002; British Medical Association, 2004; Editions du Vidal, 2005).

Reported impurities include: 21-(cyclohex-1-enyl)pregn-4-ene-3,20-dione, 21-(cyclohexylidene)pregn-4-ene-3,20-dione, (20R)-20-hydroxypregn-4-en-3-one, (20S)-20-hydroxypregn-4-en-3-one, (20R)-3-oxopregn-4-en-20-yl acetate, (20S)-3-oxopregn-4-en-20-yl acetate and pregna-4,14-diene-3,20-dione (British Pharmacopoeial Commission, 2004).

2.18.5   *Use*

Progesterone is a naturally occurring steroidal hormone found in a wide variety of tissues and biological fluids, including cow's milk. It has also been found in certain plant species (IARC, 1979).

Progesterone is used in human medicine for the treatment of secondary amenorrhoea and dysfunctional uterine bleeding, although progestational agents that are active orally are generally preferred to progesterone (Reynolds, 1996). Progesterone is usually administered as an oily intramuscular injection, a vaginal gel or pessaries or as suppositories. An oral micronized preparation of progesterone is also available. In dysfunctional uterine bleeding or amenorrhoea, 5–10 mg progesterone daily may be given by intramuscular injection for about 5–10 days until 2 days before the anticipated onset of menstruation. Alternatively, progesterone may be administered as a vaginal gel at a usual dose of 45 mg on alternate days from day 15 to 25 of the cycle or orally at a dose of 400 mg daily for 10 days (Sweetman, 2005).

Progesterone gel may be administered intravaginally at a dose of 45 mg on alternate days for 12 days of a 28-day cycle as the progestogen component of menopausal hormonal therapy. A progesterone-releasing intrauterine device has also been used as a hormonal contraceptive; the device contains 38 mg of progesterone and is effective for up to 12 months (Sweetman, 2005).

In women with a history of recurrent miscarriage and proven progesterone deficiency, twice-weekly intramuscular injections (increased to daily if necessary) of 25–100 mg progesterone, from approximately day 15 of the pregnancy until 8–16 weeks, has been used. A similar schedule has been used in in-vitro fertilization or gamete intra-fallopian transfer techniques (Sweetman, 2005).

Table 24 presents comparative global data on sales of progesterone in 1994, 1999 and 2004 (IMS Health, 2005). The regions are broadly as those defined by WHO.

Table 24. Progesterone used for combined estrogen–progestogen menopausal therapy (thousands of standard units)

Region	1994	1999	2004
Africa	837	827	1 143
Eastern Mediterranean	1 255	729	979
Europe	2 844	1 946	1 415
North America	2 824	1 438	1 005
South America	3 122	2 402	897
South-East Asia	1 231	1 764	1 806
Western Pacific	465	6 253	1 298
Total	12 578	15 358	8 543

From IMS Health (2005)
[a] Standard units are sales in terms of standard dose units; the standard dose unit for oral products is one tablet or capsule.

2.19   Regulations and guidelines

Guidelines for the use of progestogens are those found in national and international pharmacopoeias (Secretaría de Salud, 1994, 1995; Society of Japanese Pharmacopoeia, 2001; British Pharmacopoeial Commission, 2004; Pharmacopeial Convention, 2004; Swiss Pharmaceutical Society, 2004; Council of Europe, 2005; Sweetman, 2005).

3.   References

American Hospital Formulary Service (2005) *2005 AHFS Drug Information®*, Bethesda, MD, American Society of Health-System Pharmacists

APPCo (2005) *Australian Prescription Products Guide*, 34th Ed., Australian Pharmaceutical Publishing Co.

British Medical Association/Royal Pharmaceutical Society of Great Britain (2004) *British National Formulary* (No. 49), London, British Medical Association/The Pharmaceutical Press

British Pharmacopoeial Commission (2004) *British Pharmacopoeia 2004*, London, The Stationery Office

Council of Europe (2005) *European Pharmacopoeia*, 5th Ed., Strasbourg

Editions du Vidal (2005) *Vidal*, 81st Ed., Paris, OVP

Food and Drug Administration (2005) *Electronic Orange Book — Approved Drug Products with Therapeutic Equivalence Evaluations*, Rockville, MD, Center for Drug Evaluation and Research [http://www.fda.gov/]

Gennaro, A.R. (2000) *Remington: The Science and Practice of Pharmacy*, 20th Ed., Baltimore, MD, Lippincott Williams & Wilkins

IARC (1979) *IARC Monographs on the Evaluation of the Carcinogenic Risk of Chemicals to Humans*, Vol. 21, *Sex Hormones (II)*, Lyon, pp. 257–278, 365–375, 431–439, 441–460, 491–515

IMS Health (2005) *IMS Health MIDAS*, June

IPPF (2002) *Directory of Hormonal Contraceptives*, London, IPPF Medical Publications [http://contraceptive.ippf.org]

O'Neil, M.J., ed. (2001) *The Merck Index*, 13th Ed., Whitehouse Station, NJ, Merck & Co.

Pharmacopeial Convention (2004) *The 2005 US Pharmacopeia*, 28th rev./*The National Formulary*, 23rd rev., Rockville, MD

Reynolds, J.E.F., ed. (1996) *Martindale: The Extra Pharmacopoeia*, 31st Ed., London, The Pharmaceutical Press

Secretaría de Salud (1994) *Farmacopea de los Estados Unidos Mexicanos*, 6th Ed., Mexico City, Comision Permanente de la Farmacopea de los Estados Unidos Mexicanos

Secretaría de Salud (1995) *Farmacopea de los Estados Unidos Mexicanos*, 6th Ed., Suppl. 1, Mexico City, Comision Permanente de la Farmacopea de los Estados Unidos Mexicanos

Society of Japanese Pharmacopoeia (2001) *JP XIV The Japanese Pharmacopoeia*, 14th Ed., Tokyo [http://jpdb.nihs.go.jp/jp14e/]

Sweetman, S.C., ed. (2005) *Martindale: The Complete Drug Reference*, 34th Ed., London, The Pharmaceutical Press

Swiss Pharmaceutical Society, ed. (2004) *Index Nominum, International Drug Directory,* Stuttgart, Medpharm Scientific Publishers

Wade, A., ed. (1977) *Martindale, The Extra Pharmacopoeia*, 27th Ed., London, Pharmaceutical Press, pp. 1422–1424

ANNEX 2
COMPOSITION OF ORAL AND INJECTABLE
ESTROGEN–PROGESTOGEN CONTRACEPTIVES

Annex 2 lists the composition of brands of estrogen–progestogen preparations used in combined injectables (Table 1), combined oral (Table 2) and phasic oral (Table 3) contraceptives. The countries in which these formulations are used are noted. Are listed only those brands for which availability was reported. The source of these tables is the International Planned Parenthood Foundation (IPPF). Data have been taken from the IPPF 2002 website [http://contraceptive.ippf.org] at the time of the monograph meeting (June 2005). This online site is regularly updated.

Table 1. Combined injectables

Brand name	Composition	Countries of availability
Acefil	Dihydroxyprogesterone acetophenide 150 mg + estradiol enanthate 10 mg	Paraguay
Agurin	Dihydroxyprogesterone acetophenide 150 mg + estradiol enanthate 10 mg	Chile
Anafertin	Dihydroxyprogesterone acetophenide 75 mg + estradiol enanthate 5 mg	El Salvador, Mexico
Ciclofem	Medroxyprogesterone acetate 25 mg + estradiol cypionate 5 mg	Guatemala
Ciclofemina	Medroxyprogesterone acetate 25 mg + estradiol cypionate 5 mg	El Salvador
Ciclomes	Dihydroxyprogesterone acetophenide 150 mg + estradiol enanthate 10 mg	Paraguay
Ciclovular	Dihydroxyprogesterone acetophenide 150 mg + estradiol enanthate 10 mg	Brazil
Clinomin	Dihydroxyprogesterone acetophenide 150 mg + estradiol enanthate 10 mg	Paraguay
Cyclofem	Medroxyprogesterone acetate 25 mg + estradiol cypionate 5 mg	Chile, Indonesia, Malaysia, Mexico, Panama, Zimbabwe
Cyclofemina	Medroxyprogesterone acetate 25 mg + estradiol cypionate 5 mg	Brazil, Costa Rica, Mexico
Cycloven	Dihydroxyprogesterone acetophenide 150 mg + estradiol enanthate 10 mg	Paraguay

Table 1 (contd)

Brand name	Composition	Countries of availability
Deproxone	Dihydroxyprogesterone acetophenide 150 mg + estradiol enanthate 10 mg	Dominican Republic, El Salvador, Honduras, Panama
Ginestest	Dihydroxyprogesterone acetophenide 150 mg + estradiol enanthate 10 mg	Paraguay
Gynomes	Dihydroxyprogesterone acetophenide 150 mg + estradiol enanthate 10 mg	El Salvador
Listen	Dihydroxyprogesterone acetophenide 150 mg + estradiol enanthate 10 mg	Paraguay
Lunelle	Medroxyprogesterone acetate 25 mg + estradiol cypionate 5 mg	Puerto Rico, USA
Mesigyna	Norethisterone enanthate 50 mg + estradiol valerate 5 mg	Argentina, Bahamas, Barbados, Bolivia, Brazil, Chile, Colombia, Dominican Republic, Ecuador, Egypt, El Salvador, Ghana, Grenada, Guatemala, Guyana, Honduras, Jamaica, Mexico, Nicaragua, Panama, Paraguay, Peru, St. Lucia, Turkey, Uruguay, Venezuela
Neogestar	Dihydroxyprogesterone acetophenide 150 mg + estradiol enanthate 10 mg	Paraguay
Norigynon	Norethisterone enanthate 50 mg + estradiol valerate 5 mg	Ghana, Kenya, Zimbabwe
Normagest	Dihydroxyprogesterone acetophenide 150 mg + estradiol enanthate 10 mg	El Salvador, Honduras, Nicaragua, Panama
Novafem	Medroxyprogesterone acetate 25 mg + estradiol cypionate 5 mg	Chile
Novular	Dihydroxyprogesterone acetophenide 150 mg + estradiol enanthate 10 mg	El Salvador
Oterol	Dihydroxyprogesterone acetophenide 150 mg + estradiol enanthate 10 mg	Paraguay
Ovoginal	Dihydroxyprogesterone acetophenide 150 mg + estradiol enanthate 10 mg	Paraguay
Perlutal	Dihydroxyprogesterone acetophenide 150 mg + estradiol enanthate 10 mg	Argentina, Belize, Mexico, Peru
Perlutan	Dihydroxyprogesterone acetophenide 150 mg + estradiol enanthate 10 mg	Brazil
Perlutin-Unifarma	Dihydroxyprogesterone acetophenide 150 mg + estradiol enanthate 10 mg	Paraguay
Permisil	Dihydroxyprogesterone acetophenide 150 mg + estradiol enanthate 10 mg	Paraguay

Table 1 (contd)

Brand name	Composition	Countries of availability
Proter	Dihydroxyprogesterone acetophenide 150 mg + estradiol enanthate 10 mg	Costa Rica
Seguralmes	Dihydroxyprogesterone acetophenide 150 mg + estradiol enanthate 10 mg	Chile
Soluna	Dihydroxyprogesterone acetophenide 150 mg + estradiol benzoate 10 mg	Peru
Topasel	Dihydroxyprogesterone acetophenide 150 mg + estradiol enanthate 10 mg	Costa Rica, Dominican Republic, Ecuador, El Salvador, Honduras, Nicaragua, Panama, Spain
Unigalen	Dihydroxyprogesterone acetophenide 150 mg + estradiol enanthate 10 mg	Paraguay
Uno Ciclo	Dihydroxyprogesterone acetophenide 150 mg + estradiol enanthate 10 mg	Brazil
Vagital	Dihydroxyprogesterone acetophenide 150 mg + estradiol enanthate 10 mg	Paraguay
Yectames	Dihydroxyprogesterone acetophenide 75 mg + estradiol enanthate 5 mg	Costa Rica, Dominican Republic, El Salvador, Honduras, Mexico, Panama
Yectuna	Dihydroxyprogesterone acetophenide 120 mg + estradiol enanthate 10 mg	Paraguay

From IPPF (2002)

Table 2. Combined pills

Brand name	Composition	Countries of availability
Alesse	Levonorgestrel 0.1 mg + ethinylestradiol 20 µg	Canada, USA
Anfertil	Levonorgestrel 0.25 mg + ethinylestradiol 50 µg	Brazil
Anna	Levonorgestrel 0.15 mg + ethinylestradiol 30 µg	Cambodia, Laos, Myanmar, Thailand, Viet Nam
Anovlar 1mg	Norethisterone acetate 1 mg + ethinylestradiol 50 µg	Egypt, Iraq, Morocco
Anovulatorios Microdosis	Levonorgestrel 0.15 mg + ethinylestradiol 30 µg	Chile
Anuar	Cyproterone acetate 2 mg + ethinylestradiol 35 µg	Chile
Anulette 20	Levonorgestrel 0.1 mg + ethinylestradiol 20 µg	Chile

Table 2. Combined pills

Brand name	Composition	Countries of availability
Anulette C.D.	Levonorgestrel 0.15 mg + ethinylestradiol 30 µg	Chile
Anulette	Levonorgestrel 0.15 mg + ethinylestradiol 30 µg	Chile, Peru
Anulit	Levonorgestrel 0.15 mg + ethinylestradiol 30 µg	Paraguay
April	Levonorgestrel 0.1 mg + ethinylestradiol 20 µg	Uruguay
Belara	Chlormadinone acetate 2 mg + ethinylestradiol 30 µg	Ecuador, Germany
Brenda 35	Cyproterone acetate 2 mg + ethinylestradiol 35 µg	Australia
Brevicon	Norethisterone 0.5 mg + ethinylestradiol 35 µg	Puerto Rico, St. Lucia, USA
Brevicon 0.5 + 35	Norethisterone 0.5 mg + ethinylestradiol 35 µg	Canada
Brevicon 1+35	Norethisterone 1 mg + ethinylestradiol 35 µg	Canada
Brevicon 20	Norethisterone 0.5 mg + ethinylestradiol 35 µg	Mexico
Brevinor	Norethisterone 0.5 mg + ethinylestradiol 35 µg	Australia, Hong Kong, Ireland, Malaysia, Malta, Mauritius, New Zealand, South Africa, Sudan, United Kingdom
Brevinor-1	Norethisterone 1 mg + ethinylestradiol 35 µg	Australia
Ciclidon	Desogestrel 0.15 mg + ethinylestradiol 30 µg	Chile
Ciclidon 20	Desogestrel 0.15 mg + ethinylestradiol 20 µg	Chile
Ciclo 21	Levonorgestrel 0.15 mg + ethinylestradiol 30 µg	Brazil
Ciclomex	Gestodene 0.075 mg + ethinylestradiol 30 µg	Chile
Ciclomex 20	Gestodene 0.075 mg + ethinylestradiol 20 µg	Chile
Ciclon	Levonorgestrel 0.15 mg + ethinylestradiol 30 µg	Brazil

Table 2 (contd)

Brand name	Composition	Countries of availability
Cilest	Norgestimate 0.25 mg + ethinylestradiol 35 µg	Argentina, Armenia, Aruba, Austria, Barbados, Belgium, Bermuda, Bolivia, Bulgaria, Colombia, Costa Rica, Cyprus, Czech Republic, Denmark, Dominican Republic, Egypt, El Salvador, Estonia, Finland, France, Germany, Guatemala, Honduras, Hungary, Ireland, Israel, Italy, Jamaica, Kuwait, Latvia, Lithuania, Luxembourg, Macedonia, Mexico, Netherlands, Netherlands Antilles, Nicaragua, Norway, Panama, Paraguay, Poland, Qatar, Romania, Russia, Slovak Republic, Slovenia, Spain, Sudan, Sweden, Switzerland, Trinidad and Tobago, United Arab Emirates, United Kingdom, Uruguay, Yugoslavia
Conceplan M	Norethisterone 0.5 mg + ethinylestradiol 30 µg	Germany
Confiance	Levonorgestrel 0.15 mg + ethinylestradiol 30 µg	Côte D'Ivoire
Conova	Ethynodiol diacetate 2 mg + ethinylestradiol 30 µg	Bermuda
Conova 30	Ethynodiol diacetate 2 mg + ethinylestradiol 30 µg	Belgium, Luxembourg, Malawi, St. Vincent and the Grenadines, Tanzania, Trinidad and Tobago
Cycleane 30	Desogestrel 0.15 mg + ethinylestradiol 30 µg	Djibouti, France
Cycleane-20	Desogestrel 0.15 mg + ethinylestradiol 20 µg	France
Demulen	Ethynodiol diacetate 1 mg + ethinylestradiol 50 µg	Russia, Trinidad and Tobago
Demulen 1/35	Ethynodiol diacetate 1 mg + ethinylestradiol 35 µg	Jamaica, Netherlands Antilles, Puerto Rico, USA
Demulen 1/50	Ethynodiol diacetate 1 mg + ethinylestradiol 50 µg	Russia, USA
Demulen 30	Ethynodiol diacetate 2 mg + ethinylestradiol 30 µg	Canada, Puerto Rico
Denoval	Levonorgestrel 0.25 mg + ethinylestradiol 50 µg	Belize, Dominican Republic, El Salvador, Guatemala, Honduras, Nicaragua
Denoval-Wyeth	Levonorgestrel 0.25 mg + ethinylestradiol 50 µg	Costa Rica
Desmin 20	Desogestrel 0.15 mg + ethinylestradiol 20 µg	Germany

Table 2 (contd)

Brand name	Composition	Countries of availability
Desmin 30	Desogestrel 0.15 mg + ethinylestradiol 30 µg	Germany
Desogen	Desogestrel 0.15 mg + ethinylestradiol 30 µg	USA
Desolett	Desogestrel 0.15 mg + ethinylestradiol 30 µg	Sweden, Turkey
Desoran	Desogestrel 0.15 mg + ethinylestradiol 30 µg	Chile
Desorelle	Desogestrel 0.15 mg + ethinylestradiol 30 µg	Denmark, Romania
Desoren 20	Desogestrel 0.15 mg + ethinylestradiol 20 µg	Chile
Diane	Cyproterone acetate 2 mg + ethinylestradiol 35 µg	Albania, Armenia, Australia, Azerbaijan, Bahrain, Barbados, Belarus, Belgium, Bermuda, Brazil, Bulgaria, Canada, Colombia, Croatia, Cyprus, Czech Republic, Egypt, France, Georgia, Germany, Hungary, Ireland, Israel, Italy, Jordan, Kazakhstan, Kenya, Kuwait, Kyrgyzstan, Lebanon, Luxembourg, Macedonia, Malawi, Malaysia, Malta, Mauritius, Mexico, Moldova, Morocco, Netherlands, New Zealand, Nigeria, Norway, Oman, Pakistan, Peru, Philippines, Poland, Portugal, Qatar, Romania, Russia, Saudi Arabia, Singapore, Slovak Republic, Slovenia, South Africa, Spain, Sri Lanka, St. Lucia, Sweden, Switzerland, Taiwan (China), Tajikistan, Thailand, Trinidad and Tobago, Tunisia, Turkey, Turkmenistan, Ukraine, United Arab Emirates, Uruguay, Uzbekistan, Venezuela, Viet Nam, Yemen, Yugoslavia, Zimbabwe
Diane 35 DIARIO	Cyproterone acetate 2 mg + ethinylestradiol 35 µg	Spain
Diane Mite	Cyproterone acetate 2 mg + ethinylestradiol 35 µg	Austria, Denmark, Iceland
Diane Nova	Cyproterone acetate 2 mg + ethinylestradiol 35 µg	Finland

Table 2 (contd)

Brand name	Composition	Countries of availability
Diane-35	Cyproterone acetate 2 mg + ethinylestradiol 35 µg	Albania, Algeria, Argentina, Australia, Bahrain, Belgium, Bermuda, Bolivia, Brazil, Chile, Colombia, Croatia, Czech Republic, Côte D'Ivoire, Dominican Republic, Ecuador, El Salvador, Estonia, France, Germany, Guatemala, Guyana, Hong Kong, Indonesia, Jamaica, Kenya, Kuwait, Latvia, Lebanon, Lithuania, Madagascar, Mauritius, Morocco, Netherlands Antilles, New Zealand, Nicaragua, Pakistan, Paraguay, Peru, Philippines, Portugal, Qatar, Romania, Russia, Saudi Arabia, Serbia, Slovak Republic, Slovenia, South Africa, Spain, Sri Lanka, St. Lucia, Switzerland, Taiwan (China), Thailand, Togo, Trinidad and Tobago, Tunisia, Turkey, Uganda, Ukraine, United Arab Emirates, Uruguay, Venezuela, Zimbabwe
Dianette	Cyproterone acetate 2 mg + ethinylestradiol 35 µg	Ireland
Dianette Generic	Cyproterone acetate 2 mg + ethinylestradiol 35 µg	Ireland
Diminut	Gestodene 0.075 mg + ethinylestradiol 20 µg	Brazil
Dixi 35	Cyproterone acetate 2 mg + ethinylestradiol 35 µg	Chile
Duofem	Levonorgestrel 0.15 mg + ethinylestradiol 30 µg	Bolivia, Cameroon, Democratic Republic of Congo, Dominican Republic, Ecuador, Zimbabwe
Duoluton	Levonorgestrel 0.25 mg + ethinylestradiol 50 µg	Argentina, Hong Kong, Japan, Luxembourg, Taiwan (China)
Duoluton L	Levonorgestrel 0.25 mg + ethinylestradiol 50 µg	India, Nepal
Dystrol	Levonorgestrel 0.25 mg + ethinylestradiol 50 µg	Denmark
EVE 20	Norethisterone 0.5 mg + ethinylestradiol 20 µg	Germany
Econ	Norethisterone acetate 2 mg + ethinylestradiol 50 µg	Denmark
Econ Mite	Norethisterone acetate 1 mg + ethinylestradiol 30 µg	Denmark

Table 2 (contd)

Brand name	Composition	Countries of availability
Effiprev	Norgestimate 0.25 mg + ethinylestradiol 35 µg	France
Effiprev 35	Norgestimate 0.25 mg + ethinylestradiol 35 µg	France
Egestrenol	Acetomepreginol 0.5 mg + ethinylestradiol 40 µg	Russia
Eugynon	Levonorgestrel 0.25 mg + ethinylestradiol 50 µg	Algeria, Angola, Argentina, Brunei, Burkina Faso, Bénin, Cameroon, Central African Republic, Congo, Cook Islands, Cuba, Dominican Republic, El Salvador, Equatorial Guinea, Ethiopia, Fiji, Greece, Guinea-Bissau, Guinea-Conakry, Haiti, Hong Kong, Iraq, Italy, Kenya, Kuwait, Lesotho, Libya, Malawi, Malaysia, Maldives, Mali, Malta, Mauritania, Mauritius, Mexico, Mozambique, Nicaragua, Niger, Norway, Qatar, Saudi Arabia, Sierra Leone, Solomon Islands, Sri Lanka, St. Lucia, St. Vincent and the Grenadines, Swaziland, Syria, Sénégal, Tanzania, Trinidad and Tobago, Turkey, Vanuatu, Zambia
Eugynon 30	Levonorgestrel 0.25 mg + ethinylestradiol 30 µg	Fiji, United Kingdom
Eugynon CD	Levonorgestrel 0.25 mg + ethinylestradiol 50 µg	Mexico
Evacin	Gestodene 0.075 mg + ethinylestradiol 30 µg	Uruguay
Evanor	Levonorgestrel 0.25 mg + ethinylestradiol 50 µg	Brazil, Italy
Evanor-d	Levonorgestrel 0.25 mg + ethinylestradiol 50 µg	Italy
Evilin	Cyproterone acetate 2 mg + ethinylestradiol 35 µg	Chile
FMP	Levonorgestrel 0.25 mg + ethinylestradiol 50 µg	Cambodia, Laos, Myanmar, Thailand, Viet Nam
Fedra	Gestodene 0.075 mg + ethinylestradiol 20 µg	Italy
Femiane	Gestodene 0.075 mg + ethinylestradiol 20 µg	Argentina, Bolivia, Brazil, Colombia, Dominican Republic, Ecuador, El Salvador, Guatemala, Guyana, Honduras, Panama, Paraguay, Peru, Trinidad and Tobago, Uruguay, Venezuela

Table 2 (contd)

Brand name	Composition	Countries of availability
Femigoa	Levonorgestrel 0.15 mg + ethinylestradiol 30 µg	Germany
Femilon	Desogestrel 0.15 mg + ethinylestradiol 20 µg	India, Nepal
Femina	Desogestrel 0.15 mg + ethinylestradiol 20 µg	Brazil
Feminol	Gestodene 0.075 mg + ethinylestradiol 30 µg	Chile
Feminol-20	Gestodene 0.075 mg + ethinylestradiol 20 µg	Chile
Femodeen	Gestodene 0.075 mg + ethinylestradiol 30 µg	Netherlands
Femoden	Gestodene 0.075 mg + ethinylestradiol 30 µg	Albania, Armenia, Australia, Azerbaijan, Belarus, Bulgaria, Croatia, Czech Republic, Estonia, Finland, Georgia, Hungary, Kazakhstan, Kyrgyzstan, Latvia, Lithuania, Poland, Romania, Russia, Serbia, Slovak Republic, Slovenia, Tajikistan, Turkmenistan, Ukraine, United Kingdom, Uzbekistan
Femodene	Gestodene 0.075 mg + ethinylestradiol 30 µg	Belgium, Democratic Republic of Congo, Ireland, Luxembourg, New Zealand, South Africa, United Kingdom
Femodene ED	Gestodene 0.075 mg + ethinylcstradiol 30 µg	United Kingdom
Femodette	Gestodene 0.075 mg + ethinylestradiol 20 µg	United Kingdom
Femovan	Gestodene 0.075 mg + ethinylestradiol 30 µg	Germany, Lebanon
Femranette mikro	Levonorgestrel 0.15 mg + ethinylestradiol 30 µg	Germany
Follimin	Levonorgestrel 0.15 mg + ethinylestradiol 30 µg	Norway, Sweden
Follinette	Levonorgestrel 0.25 mg + ethinylestradiol 50 µg	Sweden
Frilavon	Desogestrel 0.15 mg + ethinylestradiol 30 µg	Serbia, Slovenia
Genora 1/35	Norethisterone 1 mg + ethinylestradiol 35 µg	USA
Genora 1/50	Norethisterone 1 mg + mestranol 50 µg	USA

Table 2 (contd)

Brand name	Composition	Countries of availability
Gestamestrol N	Chlormadinone acetate 2 mg + mestranol 50 µg	Germany
Gestodeno	Gestodene 0.075 mg + ethinylestradiol 30 µg	Chile
Gestrelan	Levonorgestrel 0.15 mg + ethinylestradiol 30 µg	Brazil
Ginera	Gestodene 0.075 mg + ethinylestradiol 30 µg	Turkey
Ginoden	Gestodene 0.075 mg + ethinylestradiol 30 µg	Italy
Gravistat	Levonorgestrel 0.25 mg + ethinylestradiol 50 µg	Bulgaria, Poland
Gravistat 125	Levonorgestrel 0.125 mg + ethinylestradiol 50 µg	Bulgaria, Germany, Slovak Republic
Gynatrol	Levonorgestrel 0.15 mg + ethinylestradiol 30 µg	Denmark, Iceland
Gynera	Gestodene 0.075 mg + ethinylestradiol 30 µg	Bahrain, Barbados, Belize, Bermuda, Brazil, Brunei, Cape Verde, Chile, Cyprus, Denmark, Ecuador, Egypt, Greece, Guyana, Haiti, Hong Kong, Iceland, Indonesia, Israel, Jamaica, Jordan, Kuwait, Malaysia, Malta, Netherlands Antilles, Oman, Palestine, Peru, Philippines, Portugal, Qatar, Saudi Arabia, Singapore, St. Lucia, St. Vincent and the Grenadines, Switzerland, Taiwan (China), Thailand, Trinidad and Tobago, United Arab Emirates, Uruguay, Venezuela, Western Sahara, Yemen
Gynera 75/20	Gestodene 0.075 mg + ethinylestradiol 20 µg	Chile
Gynofen 35	Cyproterone acetate 2 mg + ethinylestradiol 35 µg	Greece
Gynostat	Desogestrel 0.15 mg + ethinylestradiol 30 µg	Chile
Gynostat-20	Desogestrel 0.15 mg + ethinylestradiol 20 µg	Chile
Gynovin	Gestodene 0.075 mg + ethinylestradiol 30 µg	Argentina, Austria, Bolivia, Colombia, Dominican Republic, El Salvador, Guatemala, Honduras, Mexico, Nicaragua, Panama, Paraguay, Spain
Gynovin 20	Gestodene 0.075 mg + ethinylestradiol 20 µg	Mexico

Table 2 (contd)

Brand name	Composition	Countries of availability
Gynovin CD	Gestodene 0.075 mg + ethinylestradiol 30 µg	Mexico
Gynovlane	Norethisterone acetate 2 mg + ethinylestradiol 50 µg	Côte D'Ivoire, Djibouti, France, Togo
Gynovlar	Norethisterone acetate 3 mg + ethinylestradiol 50 µg	Argentina, Brunei, Lesotho, Libya, Malawi, Morocco, Saudi Arabia, St. Lucia, Tanzania
Harmonet	Gestodene 0.075 mg + ethinylestradiol 20 µg	Argentina, Aruba, Austria, Bahamas, Barbados, Belgium, Bolivia, Brazil, Bulgaria, Chile, Colombia, Costa Rica, Czech Republic, Democratic Republic of Congo, Denmark, Djibouti, Ecuador, El Salvador, Estonia, Finland, France, Greece, Guatemala, Honduras, Hong Kong, Hungary, Iceland, Ireland, Israel, Italy, Jamaica, Latvia, Lithuania, Luxembourg, Mexico, Netherlands, Netherlands Antilles, Nicaragua, Panama, Paraguay, Poland, Portugal, Singapore, Slovak Republic, Spain, Sweden, Switzerland, Trinidad and Tobago, Uruguay, Venezuela
Innova CD	Levonorgestrel 0.15 mg + ethinylestradiol 30 µg	Chile
Jeanine	Dienogest 2 mg + ethinylestradiol 30 µg	Czech Republic, Slovak Republic
Juliet-35 ED	Cyproterone acetate 2 mg + ethinylestradiol 35 µg	Australia
Lady-Ten 35	Cyproterone acetate 2 mg + ethinylestradiol 35 µg	Chile
Leios	Levonorgestrel 0.1 mg + ethinylestradiol 20 µg	Germany
Lerogin	Gestodene 0.075 mg + ethinylestradiol 30 µg	Paraguay
Lerogin 20	Gestodene 0.075 mg + ethinylestradiol 20 µg	Paraguay
Levlen	Levonorgestrel 0.15 mg + ethinylestradiol 30 µg	Australia, New Zealand, USA
Levlite	Levonorgestrel 0.1 mg + ethinylestradiol 20 µg	USA
Levora	Levonorgestrel 0.15 mg + ethinylestradiol 30 µg	USA

Table 2 (contd)

Brand name	Composition	Countries of availability
Lo-Femenal	Levonorgestrel 0.15 mg + ethinylestradiol 30 µg	Antigua, Bahamas, Belize, Burkina Faso, Burundi, Bénin, Cameroon, Cape Verde, Central African Republic, Chad, Chile, Congo, Côte D'Ivoire, Democratic Republic of Congo, Dominica, Dominican Republic, Ecuador, El Salvador, Eritrea, Ethiopia, Ghana, Grenada, Guatemala, Guinea-Conakry, Guyana, Haiti, Jamaica, Jordan, Lebanon, Lesotho, Liberia, Madagascar, Mali, Mauritius, Nepal, Netherlands Antilles, Nicaragua, Niger, Nigeria, Oman, Pakistan, Peru, Rwanda, Sierra Leone, St. Lucia, St. Vincent and the Grenadines, Swaziland, Sénégal, Thailand, The Gambia, Togo, Tonga, Turkey, Uganda, Uruguay, Vanuatu, Zambia, Zimbabwe
Lo-Gentrol	Levonorgestrel 0.15 mg + ethinylestradiol 30 µg	Philippines
Lo-Ovral	Levonorgestrel 0.15 mg + ethinylestradiol 30 µg	Puerto Rico, Turkey, USA
Lo-Rondal	Levonorgestrel 0.15 mg + ethinylestradiol 30 µg	Costa Rica, Kenya
Loestrin	Norethisterone acetate 1 mg + ethinylestradiol 20 µg	Bermuda
Loestrin 1.5/30	Norethisterone acetate 1.5 mg + ethinylestradiol 30 µg	Canada
Loestrin 1/20	Norethisterone acetate 1 mg + ethinylestradiol 20 µg	El Salvador
Loestrin 20	Norethisterone acetate 1 mg + ethinylestradiol 20 µg	Bahrain, Kuwait, Saudi Arabia, United Arab Emirates, United Kingdom
Loestrin 21 1.5/30	Norethisterone acetate 1.5 mg + ethinylestradiol 30 µg	USA
Loestrin 21 1/20	Norethisterone acetate 1 mg + ethinylestradiol 20 µg	USA
Loestrin 30	Norethisterone acetate 1 mg + ethinylestradiol 30 µg	Bahrain, Saudi Arabia, United Arab Emirates, United Kingdom
Loestrin Fe 1.5/30+	Norethisterone acetate 1.5 mg + ethinylestradiol 30 µg	USA
Loestrin Fe 1/20+	Norethisterone acetate 1 mg + ethinylestradiol 20 µg	USA

Table 2 (contd)

Brand name	Composition	Countries of availability
Loette	Levonorgestrel 0.1 mg + ethinylestradiol 20 µg	Australia, Canada, Chile, Germany, India, Italy, Malaysia, Netherlands, New Zealand, Puerto Rico, Singapore
Loette 21	Levonorgestrel 0.1 mg + ethinylestradiol 20 µg	Bulgaria
Logest	Gestodene 0.075 mg + ethinylestradiol 20 µg	Bulgaria, Czech Republic, Estonia, Georgia, Kazakhstan, Latvia, Lithuania
Lorsax	Levonorgestrel 0.15 mg + ethinylestradiol 30 µg	Mexico
Lovelle	Desogestrel 0.15 mg + ethinylestradiol 20 µg	Germany
Lovette	Levonorgestrel 0.1 mg + ethinylestradiol 20 µg	Netherlands
Lovina 20	Desogestrel 0.15 mg + ethinylestradiol 20 µg	Germany
Lovina 30	Desogestrel 0.15 mg + ethinylestradiol 30 µg	Germany
Lyn-ratiopharm	Lynestrenol 2.5 mg + ethinylestradiol 50 µg	Germany
Mactex	Norgestimate 0.25 mg + ethinylestradiol 35 µg	Chile
Marvelon	Desogestrel 0.15 mg + ethinylestradiol 30 µg	Albania, Algeria, Angola, Anguilla, Antigua, Argentina, Australia, Austria, Bahrain, Bangladesh, Barbados, Belgium, Bermuda, Botswana, Brazil, Bulgaria, Burkina Faso, Bénin, Canada, Central African Republic, Chile, China, Colombia, Cook Islands, Cuba, Cyprus, Czech Republic, Côte D'Ivoire, Democratic People's Republic of Korea, Democratic Republic of Congo, Denmark, Dominica, Ecuador, Egypt, Estonia, Ethiopia, Finland, France, Georgia, Germany, Ghana, Greece, Guatemala, Guyana, Hong Kong, Hungary, Iceland, Indonesia, Iraq, Jordan, Kenya, Kuwait, Latvia, Lebanon, Lesotho, Libya, Lithuania, Luxembourg, Malaysia, Malta, Mexico, Myanmar, Netherlands, Netherlands Antilles, New Zealand, Nicaragua, Norway, Oman, Palestine, Paraguay, Peru, Philippines, Poland, Portugal, Qatar, Romania, Russia, Saudi Arabia, Seychelles, Singapore, Slovak Republic, South Africa, St. Lucia, St. Vincent and

Table 2 (contd)

Brand name	Composition	Countries of availability
Marvelon (contd)		the Grenadines, Sudan, Sweden, Switzerland, Syria, Taiwan (China), Tanzania, Thailand, Tonga, Tunisia, Ukraine, United Arab Emirates, United Kingdom, Uruguay, Venezuela, Viet Nam, Yemen, Zambia, Zimbabwe
Marvelon 20	Desogestrel 0.15 mg + ethinylestradiol 20 µg	Chile
Marvelon 28	Levonorgestrel 0.15 mg + ethinylestradiol 30 µg	Myanmar
Marviol	Desogestrel 0.15 mg + ethinylestradiol 30 µg	Ireland
Meliane	Gestodene 0.075 mg + ethinylestradiol 20 µg	Austria, Belgium, Côte D'Ivoire, Finland, France, Greece, Hong Kong, Hungary, Israel, Luxembourg, Madagascar, Malta, Netherlands, Philippines, Singapore, Spain, Thailand
Meliane Light	Gestodene 0.06 mg + ethinylestradiol 15 µg	Colombia
Meloden	Gestodene 0.075 mg + ethinylestradiol 20 µg	Denmark, Switzerland
Melodene	Gestodene 0.075 mg + ethinylestradiol 20 µg	New Zealand, South Africa
Melodene 15	Gestodene 0.06 mg + ethinylestradiol 15 µg	Spain
Melodia	Gestodene 0.06 mg + ethinylestradiol 15 µg	France
Mercilon	Desogestrel 0.15 mg + ethinylestradiol 20 µg	Argentina, Austria, Belgium, Bermuda, Brazil, Canada, Colombia, Czech Republic, Côte D'Ivoire, Democratic Republic of Congo, Denmark, Djibouti, Ecuador, Estonia, Finland, France, Georgia, Greece, Hong Kong, Hungary, Iceland, Indonesia, Ireland, Israel, Italy, Kenya, Latvia, Lithuania, Luxembourg, Malaysia, Mexico, Morocco, Netherlands, Netherlands Antilles, New Zealand, Peru, Philippines, Poland, Portugal, Republic of Korea, Romania, Russia, Singapore, Slovak Republic, South Africa, St. Lucia, Sweden, Switzerland, Taiwan (China), Thailand, Ukraine, United Kingdom, Uruguay
Microdiol	Desogestrel 0.15 mg + ethinylestradiol 30 µg	Algeria, Brazil, Denmark, Israel, Morocco, Palestine, Spain, Western Sahara

Table 2 (contd)

Brand name	Composition	Countries of availability
Microfemin	Levonorgestrel 0.15 mg + ethinylestradiol 30 μg	Chile, Colombia
Microfemin Cd	Levonorgestrel 0.15 mg + ethinylestradiol 30 μg	Colombia
Microgen	Gestodene 0.075 mg + ethinylestradiol 20 μg	Chile
Microgest	Levonorgestrel 0.15 mg + ethinylestradiol 30 μg	Cuba, Portugal, Sri Lanka, Thailand
Microgyn	Levonorgestrel 0.15 mg + ethinylestradiol 30 μg	Denmark
Microgynon	Levonorgestrel 0.15 mg + ethinylestradiol 30 μg	Albania, Argentina, Armenia, Azerbaijan, Bangladesh, Belarus, Bolivia, Brunei, Bulgaria, Chile, Colombia, Cook Islands, Croatia, Cyprus, Czech Republic, Democratic Republic of Congo, Djibouti, Dominican Republic, Ecuador, El Salvador, Eritrea, Estonia, Finland, Gabon, Georgia, Germany, Guatemala, Guyana, Hong Kong, Iceland, Iraq, Italy, Kazakhstan, Kenya, Kyrgyzstan, Latvia, Lithuania, Madagascar, Malaysia, Mauritius, Moldova, Mongolia, Morocco, Nicaragua, Nigeria, Norway, Panama, Paraguay, Peru, Poland, Romania, Russia, Singapore, Slovak Republic, Slovenia, Solomon Islands, Spain, Sri Lanka, Syria, Tajikistan, The Gambia, Turkey, Turkmenistan, Ukraine, Uruguay, Uzbekistan, Yugoslavia
Microgynon 20	Levonorgestrel 0.1 mg + ethinylestradiol 20 μg	Australia, New Zealand
Microgynon 21	Levonorgestrel 0.15 mg + ethinylestradiol 30 μg	Germany, Turkey
Microgynon 30 ED	Levonorgestrel 0.15 mg + ethinylestradiol 30 μg	Antigua, Cape Verde, Jamaica, New Zealand, United Kingdom
Microgynon 50 ED	Levonorgestrel 0.125 mg + ethinylestradiol 50 μg	New Zealand
Microgynon CD	Levonorgestrel 0.15 mg + ethinylestradiol 30 μg	Chile, Mexico
Microgynon ED	Levonorgestrel 0.15 mg + ethinylestradiol 30 μg	Cambodia, Comoros
Microgynon ED 28	Levonorgestrel 0.15 mg + ethinylestradiol 30 μg	Papua New Guinea

Table 2 (contd)

Brand name	Composition	Countries of availability
Microgynon Suave	Levonorgestrel 0.1 mg + ethinylestradiol 20 µg	Colombia
Microgynon-28	Levonorgestrel 0.15 mg + ethinylestradiol 30 µg	Colombia
Microgynon-30	Levonorgestrel 0.15 mg + ethinylestradiol 30 µg	Albania, Algeria, Angola, Anguilla, Australia, Austria, Bahamas, Bahrain, Barbados, Belgium, Belize, Bermuda, Bolivia, Bulgaria, Burkina Faso, Burundi, Bénin, Cameroon, Central African Republic, Chad, Congo, Cook Islands, Costa Rica, Cyprus, Côte D'Ivoire, Democratic People's Republic of Korea, Democratic Republic of Congo, Dominica, Equatorial Guinea, Ethiopia, Fiji, Ghana, Greece, Grenada, Guinea-Bissau, Guinea-Conakry, Honduras, Hong Kong, Indonesia, Ireland, Israel, Jamaica, Jordan, Kenya, Kuwait, Lebanon, Lesotho, Liberia, Luxembourg, Malawi, Maldives, Mali, Malta, Mauritania, Mauritius, Mexico, Montserrat, Morocco, Mozambique, Netherlands, Netherlands Antilles, Nevis and St. Kitts, New Zealand, Oman, Pakistan, Palestine, Philippines, Portugal, Qatar, Rwanda, Samoa, Saudi Arabia, Serbia, Seychelles, Sierra Leone, Singapore, Slovak Republic, Solomon Islands, Somalia, St. Lucia, Sudan, Suriname, Switzerland, Sénégal, Tanzania, Thailand, Togo, Tonga, Trinidad and Tobago, Tunisia, Uganda, Ukraine, United Arab Emirates, United Kingdom, Vanuatu, Venezuela, Viet Nam, Yemen, Zambia
Microgynon-50	Levonorgestrel 0.125 mg + ethinylestradiol 50 µg	Albania, Australia, Austria, Belgium, Luxembourg, Malaysia, Netherlands, New Zealand, St. Lucia, Switzerland
Microlite	Levonorgestrel 0.1 mg + ethinylestradiol 20 µg	Ireland
Microvlar	Levonorgestrel 0.15 mg + ethinylestradiol 30 µg	Argentina, Brazil, Egypt
Milli-Anovlar	Norethisterone acetate 1 mg + ethinylestradiol 50 µg	Cameroon, Chad, Côte D'Ivoire, France, Madagascar, Togo
Min-Ovral	Levonorgestrel 0.15 mg + ethinylestradiol 30 µg	Canada, Puerto Rico, Turkey, United Kingdom
Minerva	Cyproterone acetate 2 mg + ethinylestradiol 35 µg	South Africa

Table 2 (contd)

Brand name	Composition	Countries of availability
Minesse	Gestodene 0.06 mg + ethinylestradiol 15 µg	Argentina, Austria, Belgium, Chile, Colombia, Czech Republic, France, Ireland, South Africa, Spain, Switzerland
Minestril-20	Norethisterone acetate 1 mg + ethinylestradiol 20 µg	Belgium, Democratic Republic of Congo, Luxembourg
Minestril-30	Norethisterone acetate 1.5 mg + ethinylestradiol 30 µg	Belgium, Democratic. Republic of Congo, Luxembourg
Minestrin 1/20	Norethisterone acetate 1 mg + ethinylestradiol 20 µg	Canada
Mini Pregnon	Lynestrenol 0.75 mg + ethinylestradiol 37.5 µg	Netherlands
Minidril	Levonorgestrel 0.15 mg + ethinylestradiol 30 µg	Algeria, Bénin, Cameroon, Côte D'Ivoire, Djibouti, France, Gabon, Guinea-Conakry, Madagascar, Morocco, Niger, Romania, St. Lucia, Togo
Minifem	Gestodene 0.075 mg + ethinylestradiol 20 µg	Uruguay
Minigeste	Gestodene 0.075 mg + ethinylestradiol 20 µg	Portugal
Minigynon	Levonorgestrel 0.15 mg + ethinylestradiol 30 µg	Bolivia, Peru, Venezuela
Minigynon 30	Levonorgestrel 0.15 mg + ethinylestradiol 30 µg	Haiti, Jamaica, St. Vincent and the Grenadines, Taiwan (China), Trinidad and Tobago
Minisiston	Levonorgestrel 0.125 mg + ethinylestradiol 30 µg	Bulgaria, Czech Republic, Estonia, Germany, Kazakhstan, Latvia, Lithuania, Poland, Russia, Slovak Republic, Ukraine
Minivlar	Levonorgestrel 0.15 mg + ethinylestradiol 30 µg	Republic of Korea
Minovlar	Norethisterone acetate 1 mg + ethinylestradiol 50 µg	Guinea-Bissau, Swaziland

Table 2 (contd)

Brand name	Composition	Countries of availability
Minulet	Gestodene 0.075 mg + ethinylestradiol 30 µg	Argentina, Aruba, Australia, Austria, Bahamas, Bahrain, Bangladesh, Barbados, Belgium, Belize, Bermuda, Bolivia, Brazil, Bulgaria, Chile, China, Colombia, Congo, Dem. Republic, Costa Rica, Cyprus, Czech Republic, Côte D'Ivoire, Denmark, Djibouti, Dominican Republic, Ecuador, Egypt, El Salvador, Estonia, Finland, France, Gabon, Germany, Greece, Guatemala, Haiti, Honduras, Hong Kong, Hungary, Ireland, Israel, Italy, Jamaica, Jordan, Korea, Republic of, Kuwait, Latvia, Lithuania, Luxembourg, Macedonia, Malaysia, Malta, Mauritius, Mexico, Moldova, Morocco, Netherlands, Netherlands Antilles, New Zealand, Nicaragua, Oman, Palestine, Panama, Philippines, Poland, Portugal, Qatar, Romania, Samoa, Saudi Arabia, Singapore, Slovak Republic, Slovenia, South Africa, Spain, Sri Lanka, St. Lucia, Switzerland, Taiwan (China), Thailand, Trinidad and Tobago, Turkey, United Arab Emirates, United Kingdom, Uruguay, Venezuela, Zimbabwe
Minulette	Gestodene 0.075 mg + ethinylestradiol 30 µg	South Africa
Miranova	Levonorgestrel 0.1 mg + ethinylestradiol 20 µg	Argentina, Germany, Ireland, Italy, New Zealand, Turkey, Uruguay
Mirelle	Gestodene 0.06 mg + ethinylestradiol 15 µg	Argentina, Austria, Belgium, Chile, Czech Republic, Denmark, Finland, Luxembourg, Slovak Republic, South Africa, Switzerland, Uruguay
Modicon	Norethisterone 0.5 mg + ethinylestradiol 35 µg	Luxembourg, Netherlands, USA
Moneva	Gestodene 0.075 mg + ethinylestradiol 30 µg	Côte D'Ivoire, Djibouti, France, Gabon, Madagascar, Morocco
Mono Step	Levonorgestrel 0.125 mg + ethinylestradiol 30 µg	Germany
Monofeme	Levonorgestrel 0.15 mg + ethinylestradiol 30 µg	New Zealand
Myralon	Desogestrel 0.15 mg + ethinylestradiol 20 µg	Turkey

Table 2 (contd)

Brand name	Composition	Countries of availability
Myvlar	Gestodene 0.075 mg + ethinylestradiol 30 µg	Republic of Korea
Neo-Ovulen	Ethynodiol diacetate 1 mg + mestranol 50 µg	Iceland
Neo-Stediril	Levonorgestrel 0.125 mg + ethinylestradiol 50 µg	Albania, Australia, Austria, Belgium, Germany, Luxembourg, Netherlands, Switzerland
Neocon	Norethisterone 1 mg + ethinylestradiol 35 µg	Australia, Ireland, Luxembourg, Netherlands, United Kingdom
Neocon 1/35	Norethisterone 1 mg + ethinylestradiol 35 µg	Bermuda, Jamaica
Neofam	Norgestimate 0.25 mg + ethinylestradiol 35 µg	Chile
Neogentrol	Levonorgestrel 0.25 mg + ethinylestradiol 50 µg	Denmark
Neogynon	Levonorgestrel 0.25 mg + ethinylestradiol 50 µg	Albania, Algeria, Angola, Antigua, Argentina, Austria, Bahrain, Barbados, Belgium, Belize, Bénin, Cameroon, Colombia, Congo, Cook Islands, Costa Rica, Croatia, Côte D'Ivoire, Democratic People's Republic of Korea, Democratic Republic of Congo, Denmark, Djibouti, Dominica, Dominican Republic, Ecuador, El Salvador, Ethiopia, Gabon, Germany, Greece, Grenada, Guatemala, Guinea-Bissau, Guinea-Conakry, Haiti, Honduras, Hong Kong, Iceland, Iraq, Israel, Italy, Jordan, Kenya, Kuwait, Lebanon, Libya, Luxembourg, Malawi, Malaysia, Malta, Mauritania, Mauritius, Mexico, Morocco, Netherlands, Netherlands Antilles, Nicaragua, Nigeria, Palestine, Papua New Guinea, Paraguay, Qatar, Rwanda, Samoa, Saudi Arabia, Serbia, Seychelles, Sierra Leone, Slovenia, Solomon Islands, Somalia, St. Lucia, St. Vincent and the Grenadines, Sudan, Suriname, Switzerland, Syria, Sénégal, The Gambia, Togo, Trinidad and Tobago, Tunisia, Uganda, United Arab Emirates, Uruguay, Vanuatu, Venezuela, Yemen, Zambia
Neogynon 21	Levonorgestrel 0.25 mg + ethinylestradiol 50 µg	Germany
Neogynon 30	Levonorgestrel 0.25 mg + ethinylestradiol 30 µg	Central African Republic, United Kingdom

Table 2 (contd)

Brand name	Composition	Countries of availability
Neogynon CD	Levonorgestrel 0.25 mg + ethinylestradiol 50 µg	Mexico
Neogynon ED	Levonorgestrel 0.15 mg + Ethinylestradiol 50 µg	Comoros
Neogynona	Levonorgestrel 0.25 mg + ethinylestradiol 50 µg	Spain
Neomonovar	Levonorgestrel 0.15 mg + ethinylestradiol 30 µg	Portugal
Neorlest 21	Norethisterone acetate 0.6 mg + ethinylestradiol 30 µg	Germany
Neovlar	Levonorgestrel 0.25 mg + ethinylestradiol 50 µg	Brazil, Taiwan (China)
Neovletta	Levonorgestrel 0.15 mg + ethinylestradiol 30 µg	Sweden
Nociclin	Levonorgestrel 0.15 mg + ethinylestradiol 30 µg	Brazil
Non-Ovlon	Norethisterone 1 mg + ethinylestradiol 50 µg	Estonia, Germany, Iraq, Libya, Russia
Nonovlon	Norethisterone acetate 1 mg + ethinylestradiol 50 µg	Bulgaria, Czech Republic, Latvia
Nora-ratiopharm	Norethisterone 0.5 mg + ethinylestradiol 30 µg	Germany
Noral	Levonorgestrel 0.25 mg + ethinylestradiol 50 µg	Colombia
Nordet	Levonorgestrel 0.15 mg + ethinylestradiol 30 µg	Mexico
Nordette	Levonorgestrel 0.15 mg + ethinylestradiol 30 µg	Angola, Argentina, Aruba, Australia, Austria, Bahamas, Bahrain, Bangladesh, Barbados, Belgium, Belize, Bermuda, Bolivia, Botswana, Brazil, Bulgaria, Bénin, Canada, Cayman Islands, Chile, Colombia, Cook Islands, Costa Rica, Croatia, Cyprus, Denmark, Dominica, Dominican Republic, Ecuador, Egypt, El Salvador, Eritrea, Estonia, Ethiopia, Fiji, Finland, France, Germany, Gibraltar, Greece, Grenada, Guatemala, Guinea-Bissau, Guyana, Haiti, Honduras, Hong Kong, Iceland, India, Indonesia, Iraq, Israel, Italy, Jamaica, Jordan, Kenya, Kuwait, Lebanon, Lesotho, Liberia, Libya, Macedonia, Malaysia, Malta, Mauritius, Mexico, Namibia, Nepal, Netherlands, Netherlands Antilles,

Table 2 (contd)

Brand name	Composition	Countries of availability
Nordette (contd)		Nevis and St. Kitts, New Zealand, Nicaragua, Norway, Oman, Pakistan, Palestine, Panama, Peru, Philippines, Poland, Portugal, Puerto Rico, Qatar, Samoa, Saudi Arabia, Sierra Leone, Singapore, Slovak Republic, Slovenia, Solomon Islands, South Africa, Spain, Sri Lanka, St. Lucia, St. Vincent and the Grenadines, Sudan, Suriname, Sweden, Switzerland, Syria, Taiwan (China), Tanzania, Thailand, Trinidad and Tobago, United Arab Emirates, United Kingdom, USA, Uruguay, Vanuatu, Venezuela, Viet Nam, Zambia, Zimbabwe
Nordette 150/30	Levonorgestrel 0.15 mg + ethinylestradiol 30 µg	Uruguay
Nordette 28	Levonorgestrel 0.15 mg + ethinylestradiol 30 µg	Bangladesh, Papua New Guinea
Nordette 50	Levonorgestrel 0.125 mg + ethinylestradiol 50 µg	Australia, St. Lucia
Nordiol	Levonorgestrel 0.25 mg + ethinylestradiol 50 µg	Argentina, Aruba, Australia, Austria, Bahamas, Bahrain, Barbados, Belgium, Belize, Bermuda, Brazil, Brunei, Chile, Colombia, Cook Islands, Costa Rica, Croatia, Cyprus, Denmark, Dominican Republic, El Salvador, Fiji, Germany, Greece, Guatemala, Guyana, Haiti, Honduras, Hong Kong, Italy, Jordan, Kuwait, Lebanon, Lesotho, Macedonia, Malawi, Malaysia, Malta, Mauritius, Mexico, Netherlands, Netherlands Antilles, New Zealand, Nicaragua, Nigeria, Palestine, Panama, Philippines, Poland, Qatar, Samoa, Saudi Arabia, Slovenia, South Africa, Spain, St. Lucia, St. Vincent and the Grenadines, Sweden, Switzerland, Syria, Taiwan (China), Tanzania, Thailand, Trinidad and Tobago, United Kingdom, Uruguay, Vanuatu, Venezuela
Nordiol 21	Levonorgestrel 0.25 mg + ethinylestradiol 50 µg	Chile, Cyprus, Papua New Guinea
Norgylen	Levonorgestrel 0.15 mg + ethinylestradiol 50 µg	Dominican Republic
Norimin	Norethisterone 1 mg + ethinylestradiol 35 µg	Australia, Bermuda, Hong Kong, Mauritius, New Zealand, Thailand, United Kingdom

Table 2 (contd)

Brand name	Composition	Countries of availability
Norinyl	Norethisterone 1 mg + mestranol 50 μg	Bolivia, Botswana, Costa Rica, Mauritius, St. Lucia
Norinyl 1+35	Norethisterone 1 mg + ethinylestradiol 35 μg	USA
Norinyl 1+50	Norethisterone 1 mg + mestranol 50 μg	Canada, Costa Rica, USA
Norinyl 1/35	Norethisterone 1 mg + ethinylestradiol 35 μg	Puerto Rico
Norinyl 1/50	Norethisterone 1 mg + mestranol 50 μg	Dominican Republic, El Salvador, Nicaragua, Puerto Rico
Norinyl 28	Norethisterone 1 mg + ethinylestradiol 50 μg	Mexico
Norinyl-1	Norethisterone 1 mg + mestranol 50 μg	Australia, Bermuda, Brunei, Hong Kong, Lesotho, Malta, Mexico, Saudi Arabia, South Africa, Sudan, United Kingdom
Norlestrin	Norethisterone acetate 2.5 mg + ethinylestradiol 50 μg	Argentina, Jordan, St. Vincent and the Grenadines
Normamor	Levonorgestrel 0.25 mg + ethinylestradiol 50 μg	Brazil
Norminest	Norethisterone 0.5 mg + ethinylestradiol 35 μg	Dominican Republic, Egypt, Honduras, Malaysia
Norquest	Norethisterone 1 mg + ethinylestradiol 35 μg	Bangladesh, Uganda, Zimbabwe
Norvetal	Levonorgestrel 0.15 mg + ethinylestradiol 30 μg	Bolivia, Chile
Nouvelle Duo	Levonorgestrel 0.15 mg + ethinylestradiol 30 μg	Cameroon
Novelon	Desogestrel 0.15 mg + ethinylestradiol 30 μg	India, Nepal
Novogyn 21	Levonorgestrel 0.25 mg + ethinylestradiol 50 μg	Italy
Novynette	Desogestrel 0.15 mg + ethinylestradiol 20 μg	Armenia, Azerbaijan, Belarus, Bulgaria, Czech Republic, Denmark, Estonia, Georgia, Hungary, Jamaica, Kazakhstan, Kyrgyzstan, Latvia, Lithuania, Malaysia, Moldova, Poland, Romania, Russia, Slovak Republic, Turkmenistan, Ukraine, Uzbekistan
Ologyn	Levonorgestrel 0.25 mg + ethinylestradiol 50 μg	Jordan, Switzerland, Yemen
Ologyn-micro	Levonorgestrel 0.15 mg + ethinylestradiol 30 μg	Switzerland, Yemen

Table 2 (contd)

Brand name	Composition	Countries of availability
Ortho 0.5 + 35	Norethisterone 0.5 mg + ethinylestradiol 35 μg	Canada
Ortho 1/35	Norethisterone 1 mg + ethinylestradiol 35 μg	Canada
Ortho Novin 1/50	Norethisterone 1 mg + mestranol 50 μg	Bahrain, Iceland, Ireland, Jamaica, Malawi, Malta, Palestine, Portugal, Qatar, United Kingdom, Western Sahara
Ortho Novum 1/35	Norethisterone 1 mg + ethinylestradiol 35 μg	Armenia, Aruba, Central African Republic, Dominican Republic, Finland, France, Haiti, Jamaica, Mexico, USA
Ortho Novum 1/50	Norethisterone 1 mg + mestranol 50 μg	Aruba, Bahrain, Belgium, Canada, Cyprus, Dominican Republic, El Salvador, Germany, Greece, Haiti, Jordan, Korea, Dem. People's Rep of, Kuwait, Luxembourg, Netherlands, Netherlands Antilles, Puerto Rico, St. Lucia, St. Vincent and the Grenadines, Switzerland, Taiwan (China), Tanzania, Trinidad and Tobago, United Arab Emirates, USA
Ortho-Cept	Desogestrel 0.15 mg + ethinylestradiol 30 μg	Canada, Puerto Rico, USA
Ortho-Cyclen	Norgestimate 0.25 mg + ethinylestradiol 35 μg	Canada, Puerto Rico, Slovenia, USA
Orthonett Novum	Norethisterone 0.5 mg + ethinylestradiol 35 μg	Sweden
Orthonovum	Norethisterone 1 mg + ethinylestradiol 35 μg	France, Mexico
Ovcon 35	Norethisterone 0.4 mg + ethinylestradiol 35 μg	Puerto Rico, USA
Ovcon 50	Norethisterone 1 mg + ethinylestradiol 50 μg	Puerto Rico, USA
Ovidon	Levonorgestrel 0.25 mg + ethinylestradiol 50 μg	Algeria, Angola, Armenia, Azerbaijan, Belarus, Bulgaria, Ethiopia, Hungary, Jamaica, Kazakhstan, Kyrgyzstan, Latvia, Maldives, Moldova, Mongolia, Russia, Syria, Thailand, Turkmenistan, Ukraine, Uzbekistan, Zimbabwe
Oviprem	Norethisterone 0.4 mg + ethinylestradiol 35 μg	Mexico
Ovoplex	Levonorgestrel 0.25 mg + ethinylestradiol 50 μg	Spain
Ovoplex 3	Levonorgestrel 0.15 mg + ethinylestradiol 30 μg	Spain

Table 2 (contd)

Brand name	Composition	Countries of availability
Ovoplex 30/50	Levonorgestrel 0.15 mg + ethinylestradiol 30 µg	Spain
Ovral	Levonorgestrel 0.25 mg + ethinylestradiol 50 µg	Argentina, Aruba, Bahamas, Bahrain, Bangladesh, Barbados, Belgium, Belize, Bermuda, Brazil, Brunei, Burkina Faso, Bénin, Canada, Cayman Islands, Chad, Cook Islands, Costa Rica, Croatia, Cyprus, Czech Republic, Democratic Republic of Congo, Dominica, Dominican Republic, Ecuador, El Salvador, France, Georgia, Germany, Greece, Guatemala, Guyana, Haiti, Honduras, Hong Kong, India, Iraq, Jamaica, Japan, Jordan, Kuwait, Latvia, Lebanon, Lesotho, Liberia, Libya, Macedonia, Maldives, Mali, Malta, Mauritius, Mexico, Namibia, Nepal, Netherlands Antilles, New Zealand, Nicaragua, Oman, Pakistan, Panama, Peru, Philippines, Puerto Rico, Qatar, Réunion, Saudi Arabia, Sierra Leone, Slovak Republic, Slovenia, South Africa, Sri Lanka, St. Lucia, St. Vincent and the Grenadines, Swaziland, Syria, Sénégal, Tanzania, Thailand, The Gambia, Trinidad and Tobago, Turkey, United Kingdom, USA, Uruguay, Venezuela, Zambia, Zimbabwe
Ovran	Levonorgestrel 0.25 mg + ethinylestradiol 50 µg	Ireland, United Kingdom
Ovran 30	Levonorgestrel 0.25 mg + ethinylestradiol 30 µg	India, Ireland, Nepal, Poland, United Kingdom
Ovranet	Levonorgestrel 0.15 mg + ethinylestradiol 30 µg	Italy
Ovranette	Levonorgestrel 0.15 mg + ethinylestradiol 30 µg	Austria, Ireland, United Kingdom
Ovranette 30	Levonorgestrel 0.15 mg + ethinylestradiol 30 µg	Austria, Ireland, United Kingdom
Ovulen	Ethynodiol diacetate 1 mg + ethinylestradiol 50 µg	El Salvador, Pakistan, Puerto Rico, Sierra Leone, St. Lucia, Thailand
Ovulen 1/50	Ethynodiol diacetate 1 mg + mestranol 50 µg	Singapore
Ovulen 50	Ethynodiol diacetate 1 mg + mestranol 50 µg	Angola, Argentina, Bahrain, Belize, Iraq, Libya, Malawi, Malaysia, Malta, Mauritius, Netherlands, Qatar, Saudi Arabia, St. Vincent and the Grenadines, Tanzania, Thailand, Turkey, United Arab Emirates

Table 2 (contd)

Brand name	Composition	Countries of availability
Ovysmen	Norethisterone 0.5 mg + ethinylestradiol 35 µg	Belgium, Bermuda, Dominican Republic, Egypt, Ethiopia, Ghana, Iceland, Ireland, Israel, Jordan, Kuwait, Lebanon, Malta, Sierra Leone, United Arab Emirates, United Kingdom, Zimbabwe
Ovysmen 0.5/35	Norethisterone 0.5 mg + ethinylestradiol 35 µg	Austria, Bahrain, Germany, Iceland, Ireland, Kenya, Mauritius, Palestine, Qatar, Sierra Leone, Switzerland, United Kingdom
Ovysmen 1/35	Norethisterone 1 mg + ethinylestradiol 35 µg	Austria, Belgium, France, Germany, Kuwait, Luxembourg, Puerto Rico
Perle Ld	Levonorgestrel 0.15 mg + ethinylestradiol 30 µg	Jamaica
Petibelle	Drospirenone 3 mg + ethinylestradiol 30 µg	Germany
Planor	Norgestrienone 2 mg + ethinylestradiol 50 µg	France
Practil 21	Desogestrel 0.15 mg + ethinylestradiol 30 µg	Italy
Preme	Cyproterone acetate 2 mg + ethinylestradiol 35 µg	Cambodia, Laos, Myanmar, Thailand, Viet Nam
Prevenon	Desogestrel 0.15 mg + ethinylestradiol 30 µg	Thailand
Primera	Desogestrel 0.15 mg + ethinylestradiol 20 µg	Brazil
Primovlar	Levonorgestrel 0.25 mg + ethinylestradiol 50 µg	Brazil, Costa Rica, Ecuador, Egypt, Taiwan (China)
R-den	Levonorgestrel 0.15 mg + ethinylestradiol 30 µg	Thailand
Regulon	Desogestrel 0.15 mg + ethinylestradiol 30 µg	Armenia, Azerbaijan, Belarus, Bulgaria, Czech Republic, Estonia, Georgia, Hungary, Kazakhstan, Kyrgyzstan, Latvia, Lithuania, Moldova, Poland, Russia, Slovak Republic, Turkmenistan, Ukraine, Uzbekistan
Regunon	Levonorgestrel 0.125 mg + ethinylestradiol 50 µg	Sweden
Riget	Levonorgestrel 0.15 mg + ethinylestradiol 30 µg	Malaysia, Thailand

Table 2 (contd)

Brand name	Composition	Countries of availability
Rigevidon	Levonorgestrel 0.15 mg + ethinylestradiol 30 μg	Albania, Algeria, Angola, Armenia, Azerbaijan, Belarus, Bulgaria, Chile, Dominican Republic, Georgia, Hong Kong, Hungary, Jordan, Kazakhstan, Kyrgyzstan, Latvia, Lithuania, Malaysia, Maldives, Mexico, Moldova, Mongolia, Papua New Guinea, Poland, Romania, Russia, Sudan, Syria, Thailand, Turkmenistan, Ukraine, Uzbekistan, Viet Nam, Yemen, Zimbabwe
Secure	Norethisterone 1 mg + ethinylestradiol 35 μg	Ghana
Securgin	Desogestrel 0.15 mg + ethinylestradiol 20 μg	Italy
Selene	Cyproterone acetate 2 mg + ethinylestradiol 35 μg	Brazil
Sinovula mikro	Norethisterone 0.5 mg + ethinylestradiol 30 μg	Germany
Stediril	Levonorgestrel 0.25 mg + ethinylestradiol 50 μg	Algeria, Bénin, Cameroon, Chad, Congo, Croatia, Côte D'Ivoire, Djibouti, France, Gabon, Germany, Luxembourg, Madagascar, Morocco, Niger, Serbia, Slovenia, Togo
Stediril 30	Levonorgestrel 0.15 mg + ethinylestradiol 30 μg	Belgium, Bulgaria, Czech Republic, Germany, Latvia, Luxembourg, Netherlands, Poland, Slovak Republic, Slovenia, Switzerland
Stediril-d	Levonorgestrel 0.25 mg + ethinylestradiol 50 μg	Afghanistan, Austria, Belgium, Croatia, Germany, Luxembourg, Netherlands, Serbia, Slovenia, Switzerland
Suavuret	Desogestrel 0.15 mg + ethinylestradiol 20 μg	Spain
Tina	Cyproterone acetate 2 mg + ethinylestradiol 35 μg	Thailand
Trentovlane	Norethisterone acetate 1 mg + ethinylestradiol 30 μg	France
Trust Pill	Levonorgestrel 0.125 mg + ethinylestradiol 30 μg	Philippines
Valette	Dienogest 2 mg + ethinylestradiol 30 μg	Germany, Mexico
Varnoline	Desogestrel 0.15 mg + ethinylestradiol 30 μg	Cameroon, Côte D'Ivoire, Djibouti, France, Gabon, Mauritius, Togo

Table 2 (contd)

Brand name	Composition	Countries of availability
Yasmin	Drospirenone 3 mg + ethinylestradiol 30 µg	Austria, Belgium, Denmark, France, Germany, Iceland, Ireland, Luxembourg, Netherlands, Norway, Sweden, Switzerland, United Kingdom
Yermonil	Lynestrenol 2 mg + ethinylestradiol 40 µg	Austria, Costa Rica, Czech Republic, Germany

From IPPF (2002)

Table 3. Phasic pills

Brand name	Composition	Countries of availability
Adépal	Levonorgestrel 0.15/0.2 mg + ethinylestradiol 30/40 µg	Algeria, Bénin, Cameroon, Chad, Congo, Côte D'Ivoire, Democratic Republic of Congo, Djibouti, France, Gabon, Guinea- Conakry, Madagascar, Togo
Anteovin	Levonorgestrel 0.05/0.125 mg + ethinylestradiol 50 µg	Algeria, Armenia, Azerbaijan, Belarus, Bulgaria, Czech Republic, Hungary, Jamaica, Kazakhstan, Kyrgyzstan, Latvia, Lithuania, Moldova, Mongolia, Poland, Romania, Russia, Slovak Republic, Thailand, Turkmenistan, Ukraine, Uzbekistan, Zimbabwe
Binordiol	Levonorgestrel 0.05/0.125 mg + ethinylestradiol 50 µg	Belgium, Italy, Luxembourg, Switzerland
Binovum	Norethisterone 0.5/1 mg + ethinylestradiol 35 µg	Colombia, Ireland, Peru, Puerto Rico, United Kingdom
Biphasil	Levonorgestrel 0.05/0.125 mg + ethinylestradiol 50 µg	Australia, Austria, Belgium, Germany, Lesotho, Netherlands, New Zealand, South Africa, Switzerland
Biviol	Desogestrel 0.025/0.125 mg + ethinylestradiol 40/30 µg	Germany
Bivlar	Levonorgestrel 0.05/0.125 mg + ethinylestradiol 50 µg	Italy
Cyclosa	Desogestrel 0/0.125 mg + ethinylestradiol 50 µg	Germany
Dueva	Desogestrel 0.025/0.125 mg + ethinylestradiol 40/30 µg	Italy
Estrostep 21	Norethisterone 1/0.03/0.035 mg + ethinylestradiol 20 µg	USA

Table 3 (contd)

Brand name	Composition	Countries of availability
Estrostep Fe+	Norethisterone 1/0.03/0.035 mg + ethinylestradiol 20 µg	USA
Femilar	Cyproterone acetate 1/2 mg + estradiol valerate 1/2 mg	Finland
Fironetta	Levonorgestrel 0.05/0.075/0.125 mg + ethinylestradiol 30/40/30 µg	Denmark
Gracial	Desogestrel 0.025/0.125 mg + ethinylestradiol 40/30 µg	Austria, Bahrain, Belgium, Brazil, Chile, Cyprus, Denmark, Estonia, Finland, Hong Kong, Indonesia, Italy, Kuwait, Lithuania, Luxembourg, Netherlands, Peru, Portugal, Spain, Switzerland, Syria
Gynophase	Norethisterone acetate 1/2 mg + ethinylestradiol 50 µg	Bénin, France, St. Lucia
Improvil	Norethisterone 0.5/1.0/0.5 mg + ethinylestradiol 35 µg	Australia
Jenest-28	Norethisterone 0.5/1 mg + ethinylestradiol 35 µg	USA
Laurina	Desogestrel 0.05/0.1/0.15 mg + ethinylestradiol 35/30 µg	Sweden
Levordiol	Levonorgestrel 0.05/0.075/0.125 mg + ethinylestradiol 30/40/30 µg	Brazil
Libian	Levonorgestrel 0.05/0.05/0.125 mg + ethinylestradiol 30/50/40 µg	Japan
Logynon	Levonorgestrel 0.05/0.075/0.125 mg + ethinylestradiol 30/40/30 µg	Australia, Bahrain, Barbados, Belize, Bermuda, Cyprus, Guyana, Haiti, Ireland, Israel, Jamaica, Jordan, Kenya, Kuwait, Lesotho, Malawi, Malta, Mauritius, Netherlands Antilles, Nigeria, Oman, Palestine, Philippines, Qatar, Saudi Arabia, South Africa, St. Lucia, St. Vincent and the Grenadines, Syria, Taiwan (China), Tanzania, Thailand, Trinidad and Tobago, Uganda, United Arab Emirates, United Kingdom, Western Sahara, Zambia, Zimbabwe
Logynon 21	Levonorgestrel 0.05/0.075/0.125 mg + ethinylestradiol 30/40/30 µg	Papua New Guinea, Philippines
Logynon ED	Levonorgestrel 0.05/0.075/0.125 mg + ethinylestradiol 30/40/30 µg	United Kingdom
Lyn-ratiopharm Sequenz	Lynestrenol 0/2.5 mg + ethinylestradiol 50 µg	Germany

Table 3 (contd)

Brand name	Composition	Countries of availability
Milvane	Gestodene 0.05/0.07/0.1 mg + ethinylestradiol 30/40/30 µg	Denmark, Italy, Poland, Russia, Slovak Republic, Switzerland
Miniphase	Norethisterone acetate 1/2 mg + ethinylestradiol 30/40 µg	Bénin, Cameroon, Chad, Côte D'Ivoire, Djibouti, France, Gabon, Madagascar, Togo
Mircette	Desogestrel 0.15/0.01 mg + ethinylestradiol 20 µg	USA
Neo-Eunomin	Chlormadinone acetate 1/2 mg + ethinylestradiol 50 µg	Germany, Switzerland
Normovlar	Levonorgestrel 0.05/0.125 mg + ethinylestradiol 50 µg	Lesotho, South Africa
NovaStep	Levonorgestrel 0.05/0.075/0.125 mg + ethinylestradiol 30/40/30 µg	Germany
Nuriphasic	Lynestrenol 0/2.5 mg + ethinylestradiol 50 µg	Germany
Ortho 10/11	Norethisterone 0.5/1 mg + ethinylestradiol 35 µg	Canada, Jamaica, Trinidad and Tobago
Ortho 7/7/7	Norethisterone 0.5/0.75/1.0 mg + ethinylestradiol 35 µg	Canada, Dominican Republic, India, Jamaica, Trinidad and Tobago
Ortho 777-28	Norethisterone 0.5/0.75/1.0 mg + ethinylestradiol 35 µg	Japan
Ortho Novum 10/11	Norethisterone 0.5/1 mg + ethinylestradiol 35 µg	USA
Ortho Novum 7/7/7	Norethisterone 0.5/0.75/1.0 mg + ethinylestradiol 35 µg	Dominican Republic, Jamaica, Nepal, USA
Ortho Tri-Cyclen	Norgestimate 0.18/0.215/0.25 mg + ethinylestradiol 35 µg	Canada, Puerto Rico, USA
Ovidol	Desogestrel 0/0.125 mg + ethinylestradiol 50 µg	Belgium, Netherlands, Switzerland
Oviol 22	Desogestrel 0/0.125 mg + ethinylestradiol 50 µg	Germany
Oviol 28	Desogestrel 0/0.125 mg + ethinylestradiol 50 µg	Germany
Perikursal	Levonorgestrel 0.05/0.125 mg + ethinylestradiol 50 µg	Austria
Perikursal 21	Levonorgestrel 0.05/0.125 mg + ethinylestradiol 50 µg	Austria, Germany
Phaeva	Gestodene 0.05/0.07/0.1 mg + ethinylestradiol 30/40/30 µg	Côte D'Ivoire, Djibouti, France, Gabon, Madagascar, Morocco
Pramino	Norgestimate 0.18/0.215/0.25 mg + ethinylestradiol 35 µg	Czech Republic, Germany

Table 3 (contd)

Brand name	Composition	Countries of availability
Sequilar	Levonorgestrel 0.05/0.125 mg + ethinylestradiol 50 μg	Australia, Austria, Germany
Sequostat	Norethisterone acetate 0/5 mg + ethinylestradiol 50 μg	Germany
Synfase	Norethisterone 0.5/1.0/0.5 mg + ethinylestradiol 35 μg	Norway, Sweden
Synphase	Norethisterone 0.5/1.0/0.5 mg + ethinylestradiol 35 μg	Hong Kong, Malta, Mauritius, Qatar, United Kingdom
Synphasec	Norethisterone 0.5/1.0/0.5 mg + ethinylestradiol 35 μg	Germany
Synphasic	Norethisterone 0.5/1.0/0.5 mg + ethinylestradiol 35 μg	Australia, Canada, New Zealand
Tri Femoden	Gestodene 0.05/0.07/0.1 mg + ethinylestradiol 30/40/30 μg	Finland
Tri-Cilest	Norgestimate 0.18/0.215/0.25 mg + ethinylestradiol 35 μg	Bolivia, Slovak Republic
Tri-Gynera	Gestodene 0.05/0.07/0.1 mg + ethinylestradiol 30/40/30 μg	Cape Verde, Portugal
Tri-Levlen	Levonorgestrel 0.05/0.075/0.125 mg + ethinylestradiol 30/40/30 μg	Puerto Rico, USA
Tri-Mactex	Norgestimate 0.18/0.215/0.25 mg + ethinylestradiol 35 μg	Chile
Tri-Minulet	Gestodene 0.05/0.07/0.1 mg + ethinylestradiol 30/40/30 μg	Australia, Austria, Belgium, Czech Republic, Denmark, Djibouti, Estonia, Finland, France, Gabon, Germany, Greece, Hungary, Ireland, Italy, Latvia, Lithuania, Luxembourg, Morocco, Netherlands, Poland, Portugal, Romania, Slovak Republic, South Africa, Spain, Switzerland, United Kingdom
Tri-Norinyl	Norethisterone 0.5/1.0/0.5 mg + ethinylestradiol 35 μg	Puerto Rico, USA
Tri-Regol	Levonorgestrel 0.05/0.075/0.125 mg + ethinylestradiol 30/40/30 μg	Albania, Algeria, Armenia, Azerbaijan, Belarus, Bulgaria, Czech Republic, Estonia, Hong Kong, Hungary, Jamaica, Kazakhstan, Kyrgyzstan, Latvia, Lithuania, Malaysia, Moldova, Philippines, Poland, Romania, Russia, Slovak Republic, Syria, Trinidad and Tobago, Turkmenistan, Ukraine, Uzbekistan, Viet Nam, Yemen

Table 3 (contd)

Brand name	Composition	Countries of availability
Tri-Stediril	Levonorgestrel 0.05/0.075/0.125 mg + ethinylestradiol 30/40/30 µg	Slovenia
TriStep	Levonorgestrel 0.05/0.05/0.125 mg + ethinylestradiol 30/50/40 µg	Bulgaria, Germany
Triadene	Gestodene 0.05/0.07/0.1 mg + ethinylestradiol 30/40/30 µg	United Kingdom
Triagynon	Levonorgestrel 0.05/0.075/0.125 mg + ethinylestradiol 30/40/30 µg	Spain
Triciclomex	Gestodene 0.05/0.07/0.1 mg + ethinylestradiol 30/40/30 µg	Chile, Paraguay
Triciclor	Levonorgestrel 0.05/0.075/0.125 mg + ethinylestradiol 30/40/30 µg	Spain
Tricilest	Norgestimate 0.18/0.215/0.25 mg + ethinylestradiol 35 µg	Austria, Belgium, Finland, Hungary, Italy, Mexico, South Africa, Spain
Tridestan	Levonorgestrel 0.05/0.075/0.125 mg + mestranol 30/40/30 µg	Argentina
Tridette	Norgestimate 0.18/0.215/0.25 mg + ethinylestradiol 35 µg	Bolivia, Paraguay, Uruguay
Triella	Norethisterone 0.5/0.75/1.0 mg + ethinylestradiol 35 µg	Côte D'Ivoire, Djibouti, France, Guinea-Conakry, Morocco
Triette 21	Levonorgestrel 0.05/0.075/0.125 mg + ethinylestradiol 30/40/30 µg	Germany
Trievacin	Gestodene 0.05/0.07/0.1 mg + ethinylestradiol 30/40/30 µg	Uruguay
Trifas	Levonorgestrel 0.05/0.075/0.125 mg + ethinylestradiol 30/40/30 µg	Chile, Paraguay
Trifeme	Levonorgestrel 0.05/0.075/0.125 mg + ethinylestradiol 30/40/30 µg	Australia, New Zealand
Trifeminal	Levonorgestrel 0.05/0.075/0.125 mg + ethinylestradiol 30/40/30 µg	Colombia
Trigoa 21	Levonorgestrel 0.05/0.075/0.125 mg + ethinylestradiol 30/40/30 µg	Bulgaria, Germany
Trigynera	Gestodene 0.05/0.07/0.1 mg + ethinylestradiol 30/40/30 µg	Greece
Trigynon	Levonorgestrel 0.05/0.075/0.125 mg + ethinylestradiol 30/40/30 µg	Albania, Austria, Belgium, Democratic Republic of Congo, Italy, Luxembourg, Morocco, Netherlands
Trigynovin	Gestodene 0.05/0.07/0.1 mg + ethinylestradiol 30/40/30 µg	Spain
Trikvilar	Levonorgestrel 0.05/0.075/0.125 mg + ethinylestradiol 30/40/30 µg	Finland

Table 3 (contd)

Brand name	Composition	Countries of availability
Trimiron	Desogestrel 0.05/0.1/0.15 mg + ethinylestradiol 35/30 µg	Sweden
Trinordiol	Levonorgestrel 0.05/0.075/0.125 mg + ethinylestradiol 30/40/30 µg	Argentina, Australia, Austria, Bahamas, Bahrain, Barbados, Belgium, Belize, Bermuda, Bolivia, Brazil, Brunei, Bulgaria, Canada, Chile, Congo, Costa Rica, Cuba, Cyprus, Czech Republic, Côte D'Ivoire, Democratic Republic of Congo, Denmark, Djibouti, Dominica, Dominican Republic, Ecuador, Egypt, El Salvador, Estonia, Finland, France, Gabon, Georgia, Germany, Gibraltar, Grenada, Guadeloupe, Guatemala, Guinea-Conakry, Haiti, Honduras, Hong Kong, Hungary, Iceland, Indonesia, Israel, Italy, Jamaica, Japan, Jordan, Kenya, Kuwait, Lebanon, Luxembourg, Madagascar, Malaysia, Malta, Mauritius, Mexico, Moldova, Mongolia, Morocco, Netherlands, Netherlands Antilles, New Zealand, Nicaragua, Norway, Oman, Palestine, Panama, Peru, Philippines, Poland, Portugal, Puerto Rico, Qatar, Romania, Sierra Leone, Singapore, Slovak Republic, Slovenia, South Africa, Spain, Sri Lanka, St. Lucia, St. Vincent and the Grenadines, Sweden, Switzerland, Taiwan (China), Thailand, Togo, Trinidad and Tobago, Turkey, United Arab Emirates, United Kingdom, USA, Uruguay, Venezuela, Western Sahara, Zimbabwe
Trinordiol 21	Levonorgestrel 0.05/0.075/0.125 mg + mestranol 30/40/30 µg	Austria, Bahrain, Belgium, Bulgaria, Cyprus, Czech Republic, Denmark, Egypt, Finland, France, Germany, Greece, Hungary, Iceland, Ireland, Israel, Italy, Jordan, Kuwait, Lebanon, Luxembourg, Malta, Netherlands, Norway, Oman, Peru, Poland, Portugal, Qatar, Slovak Republic, Sweden, Switzerland, Turkey, United Arab Emirates, United Kingdom
Trinordiol 28	Levonorgestrel 0.05/0.075/0.125 mg + mestranol 30/40/30 µg	Germany, Norway, Sweden

Table 3 (contd)

Brand name	Composition	Countries of availability
Trinovum	Norethisterone 0.5/0.75/1.0 mg + ethinylestradiol 35 µg	Armenia, Austria, Barbados, Belgium, Bermuda, Brazil, Bulgaria, Croatia, Czech Republic, Denmark, Dominican Republic, France, Germany, Hong Kong, Iran, Ireland, Israel, Italy, Jamaica, Jordan, Kazakhstan, Kenya, Lesotho, Libya, Lithuania, Luxembourg, Mexico, Netherlands, Netherlands Antilles, Palestine, Peru, Poland, Puerto Rico, Qatar, Romania, Serbia, Singapore, Slovak Republic, Slovenia, South Africa, Sweden, Switzerland, Taiwan (China), Tanzania, Trinidad and Tobago, United Arab Emirates, United Kingdom, Western Sahara, Yemen, Yugoslavia, Zimbabwe
Triodeen	Gestodene 0.05/0.07/0.1 mg + ethinylestradiol 30/40/30 µg	Netherlands
Trioden	Gestodene 0.05/0.07/0.1 mg + ethinylestradiol 30/40/30 µg	Australia
Triodena	Gestodene 0.05/0.07/0.1 mg + ethinylestradiol 30/40/30 µg	Austria, Hungary
Triodene	Gestodene 0.05/0.07/0.1 mg + ethinylestradiol 30/40/30 µg	Belgium, Ireland, Luxembourg, South Africa
Trionetta	Levonorgestrel 0.05/0.075/0.125 mg + ethinylestradiol 30/40/30 µg	Norway, Sweden
Triovalet	Levonorgestrel 0.05/0.075/0.125 mg + ethinylestradiol 30/40/30 µg	Belgium
Triovlar	Levonorgestrel 0.05/0.075/0.125 mg + ethinylestradiol 30/40/30 µg	Egypt
Triphasil	Levonorgestrel 0.05/0.075/0.125 mg + ethinylestradiol 30/40/30 µg	Australia, Canada, Lesotho, New Zealand, Papua New Guinea, Puerto Rico, South Africa, United Kingdom, USA
Triquilar	Levonorgestrel 0.05/0.075/0.125 mg + ethinylestradiol 30/40/30 µg	Albania, Argentina, Armenia, Australia, Azerbaijan, Belarus, Bolivia, Brazil, Bulgaria, Canada, Chile, Cook Islands, Costa Rica, Croatia, Cuba, Czech Republic, Denmark, Dominican Republic, Ecuador, El Salvador, Estonia, Georgia, Germany, Greece, Guatemala, Honduras, Hong Kong, Hungary, Iceland, India, Indonesia, Japan, Kazakhstan, Kyrgyzstan, Latvia, Lithuania, Malaysia, Mexico, Moldova, Morocco, Mozambique, Nepal, New Zealand, Nicaragua, Panama, Paraguay, Peru, Philippines, Poland,

Table 3 (contd)

Brand name	Composition	Countries of availability
Triquilar (contd)		Portugal, Republic of Korea, Romania, Russia, Samoa, Seychelles, Singapore, Slovak Republic, Suriname, Switzerland, Syria, Tajikistan, Thailand, Tonga, Turkey, Turkmenistan, Ukraine, Uruguay, Uzbekistan, Venezuela
Trisiston	Levonorgestrel 0.05/0.075/0.125 mg + ethinylestradiol 30/40/30 µg	Bulgaria, Czech Republic, Estonia, Germany, Kazakhstan, Latvia, Lithuania, Poland, Russia, Slovak Republic, Syria, Ukraine
Trolit	Levonorgestrel 0.05/0.075/0.125 mg + ethinylestradiol 30/40/30 µg	Chile, Peru

From IPPF (2002)

ANNEX 3
BRANDS OF ESTROGEN–PROGESTOGEN CONTRACEPTIVES

Annex 3 lists the brands of hormonal contraceptives that contain the estrogens and progestogens that are listed and described in Annex 1. The type of contraceptives in which it is used is also noted (Table 1). The source of this listing is the Directory of Hormonal Contraceptives of the International Parenthood Foundation (IPPF, 2002). Data have been taken from the IPPF 2002 website [http://contraceptive.ippf.org] at the time of the monograph meeting (June 2005). This online site is regularly updated.

Table 1. Brands of estrogen–progestogen contraceptives

Common name of ingredient	Brand name	Type of contraceptive
Chlormadinone acetate	Belara	Combined pills
	Gestamestrol N	Combined pills
	Neo-Eunomin	Phasic pills
Cyproterone acetate	Anuar	Combined pills
	Brenda 35	Combined pills
	Diane	Combined pills
	Diane 35 DIARIO	Combined pills
	Diane Mite	Combined pills
	Diane Nova	Combined pills
	Diane-35	Combined pills
	Dianette	Combined pills
	Dianette Generic	Combined pills
	Dixi 35	Combined pills
	Evilin	Combined pills
	Femilar	Phasic pills
	Gynofen 35	Combined pills
	Juliet-35 ED	Combined pills
	Lady-Ten 35	Combined pills
	Minerva	Combined pills
	Preme	Combined pills
	Selene	Combined pills
	Tina	Combined pills

Table 1 (contd)

Common name of ingredient	Brand name	Type of contraceptive
Desogestrel	Biviol	Phasic pills
	Ciclidon	Combined pills
	Ciclidon 20	Combined pills
	Cycleane 30	Combined pills
	Cycleane-20	Combined pills
	Cyclosa	Phasic pills
	Desmin 20	Combined pills
	Desmin 30	Combined pills
	Desogen	Combined pills
	Desolett	Combined pills
	Desoran	Combined pills
	Desorelle	Combined pills
	Desoren 20	Combined pills
	Dueva	Phasic pills
	Femilon	Combined pills
	Femina	Combined pills
	Frilavon	Combined pills
	Gracial	Phasic pills
	Gynostat	Combined pills
	Gynostat-20	Combined pills
	Laurina	Phasic pills
	Lovelle	Combined pills
	Lovina 20	Combined pills
	Lovina 30	Combined pills
	Marvelon	Combined pills
	Marvelon 20	Combined pills
	Marviol	Combined pills
	Mercilon	Combined pills
	Microdiol	Combined pills
	Mircette	Phasic pills
	Myralon	Combined pills
	Novelon	Combined pills
	Novynette	Combined pills
	Ortho-Cept	Combined pills
	Ovidol	Phasic pills
	Oviol 22	Phasic pills
	Oviol 28	Phasic pills
	Practil 21	Combined pills
	Prevenon	Combined pills
	Primera	Combined pills
	Regulon	Combined pills
	Securgin	Combined pills
	Suavuret	Combined pills
	Trimiron	Phasic pills
	Varnoline	Combined pills

Table 1 (contd)

Common name of ingredient	Brand name	Type of contraceptive
Dienogest	Jeanine	Combined pills
	Valette	Combined pills
Drospirenone	Petibelle	Combined pills
	Yasmin	Combined pills
Estradiol	No. 2 injectable	Combined injectables
Estradiol benzoate	Protegin	Combined injectables
	Soluna	Combined injectables
	Unijab	Combined injectables
	Vermagest	Emergency contraception
Estradiol cypionate	Ciclofem	Combined injectables
	Ciclofemina	Combined injectables
	Cyclofem	Combined injectables
	Cyclofemina	Combined injectables
	Cycloprovera	Combined injectables
	Lunelle	Combined injectables
	Novafem	Combined injectables
Estradiol valerate	Femilar	Phasic pills
	No. 1 injectable	Combined injectables
Ethinylestradiol	Adépal	Phasic pills
	Alesse	Combined pills
	Anfertil	Combined pills
	Anna	Combined pills
	Anovlar 1mg	Combined pills
	Anovulatorios Microdosis	Combined pills
	Anteovin	Phasic pills
	Anuar	Combined pills
	Anulette 20	Combined pills
	Anulette C.D.	Combined pills
	Anulette	Combined pills
	Anulit	Combined pills
	April	Combined pills
	Belara	Combined pills
	Binordiol	Phasic pills
	Binovum	Phasic pills
	Biphasil	Phasic pills
	Biviol	Phasic pills
	Bivlar	Phasic pills
	Brenda 35	Combined pills
	Brevicon	Combined pills
	Brevicon 0.5 + 35	Combined pills
	Brevicon 1+35	Combined pills
	Brevicon 20	Combined pills
	Brevinor	Combined pills
	Brevinor-1	Combined pills
	Ciclidon	Combined pills

Table 1 (contd)

Common name of ingredient	Brand name	Type of contraceptive
Ethinylestradiol (contd)	Ciclidon 20	Combined pills
	Ciclo 21	Combined pills
	Ciclomex	Combined pills
	Ciclomex 20	Combined pills
	Ciclon	Combined pills
	Cilest	Combined pills
	Combination 3	Combined pills
	Conceplan M	Combined pills
	Confiance	Combined pills
	Conova	Combined pills
	Conova 30	Combined pills
	Contraceptive H.D.	Combined pills
	Contraceptive L.D.	Combined pills
	Cycleane 30	Combined pills
	Cycleane-20	Combined pills
	Cyclen	Combined pills
	Cyclosa	Phasic pills
	D-Norginor	Combined pills
	Demulen	Combined pills
	Demulen 1/35	Combined pills
	Demulen 1/50	Combined pills
	Demulen 30	Combined pills
	Denoval	Combined pills
	Denoval-Wyeth	Combined pills
	Desmin 20	Combined pills
	Desmin 30	Combined pills
	Desogen	Combined pills
	Desolett	Combined pills
	Desoran	Combined pills
	Desorelle	Combined pills
	Desoren 20	Combined pills
	Diane	Combined pills
	Diane 35 DIARIO	Combined pills
	Diane Mite	Combined pills
	Diane Nova	Combined pills
	Diane-35	Combined pills
	Dianette	Combined pills
	Dianette Generic	Combined pills
	Diminut	Combined pills
	Dixi 35	Combined pills
	Dueva	Phasic pills
	Duofem	Combined pills
	Duoluton	Combined pills
	Duoluton L	Combined pills
	Dystrol	Combined pills
	E Gen C	Emergency contraception
	EVE 20	Combined pills

Table 1 (contd)

Common name of ingredient	Brand name	Type of contraceptive
Ethinylestradiol (contd)	Econ	Combined pills
	Econ Mite	Combined pills
	Effiprev	Combined pills
	Effiprev 35	Combined pills
	Egestrenol	Combined pills
	Estrostep 21	Phasic pills
	Estrostep Fe+	Phasic pills
	Eugynon	Combined pills
	Eugynon 30	Combined pills
	Eugynon CD	Combined pills
	Evacin	Combined pills
	Evanor	Combined pills
	Evanor-d	Combined pills
	Evilin	Combined pills
	FMP	Combined pills
	Fedra	Combined pills
	Femenal	Combined pills
	Femiane	Combined pills
	Femigoa	Combined pills
	Femilon	Combined pills
	Femina	Combined pills
	Feminol	Combined pills
	Feminol-20	Combined pills
	Femodeen	Combined pills
	Femoden	Combined pills
	Femodene	Combined pills
	Femodene ED	Combined pills
	Femodette	Combined pills
	Femovan	Combined pills
	Femranette mikro	Combined pills
	Fertilan	Emergency contraception
	Fironetta	Combined pills
	Follimin	Combined pills
	Follinette	Combined pills
	Frilavon	Combined pills
	Genora 1/35	Combined pills
	Gestodeno	Combined pills
	Gestrelan	Combined pills
	Ginera	Combined pills
	Ginoden	Combined pills
	Gracial	Phasic pills
	Gravistat	Combined pills
	Gravistat 125	Combined pills
	Gynatrol	Combined pills
	Gynera	Combined pills
	Gynera 75/20	Combined pills

Table 1 (contd)

Common name of ingredient	Brand name	Type of contraceptive
Ethinylestradiol (contd)	Gynofen 35	Combined pills
	Gynophase	Phasic pills
	Gynostat	Combined pills
	Gynostat-20	Combined pills
	Gynovin	Combined pills
	Gynovin 20	Combined pills
	Gynovin CD	Combined pills
	Gynovlane	Combined pills
	Gynovlar	Combined pills
	Harmonet	Combined pills
	Improvil	Phasic pills
	Innova CD	Combined pills
	Jeanine	Combined pills
	Jenest-28	Phasic pills
	Juliet-35 ED	Combined pills
	Kanchan	Combined pills
	Lady-Ten 35	Combined pills
	Laurina	Phasic pills
	Leios	Combined pills
	Lerogin	Combined pills
	Lerogin 20	Combined pills
	Levlen	Combined pills
	Levlite	Combined pills
	Levonorgestrel Pill	Combined pills
	Levora	Combined pills
	Levordiol	Phasic pills
	Libian	Phasic pills
	Lo-Femenal	Combined pills
	Lo-Gentrol	Combined pills
	Lo-Ovral	Combined pills
	Lo-Rondal	Combined pills
	Loestrin	Combined pills
	Loestrin 1.5/30	Combined pills
	Loestrin 1/20	Combined pills
	Loestrin 20	Combined pills
	Loestrin 21 1.5/30	Combined pills
	Loestrin 21 1/20	Combined pills
	Loestrin 30	Combined pills
	Loestrin Fe 1.5/30+	Combined pills
	Loestrin Fe 1/20+	Combined pills
	Loette	Combined pills
	Loette 21	Combined pills
	Logest	Combined pills
	Logynon	Phasic pills
	Logynon 21	Phasic pills
	Logynon ED	Phasic pills

Table 1 (contd)

Common name of ingredient	Brand name	Type of contraceptive
Ethinylestradiol (contd)	Lorsax	Combined pills
	Lovelle	Combined pills
	Loveston	Combined pills
	Lovette	Combined pills
	Lovina 20	Combined pills
	Lovina 30	Combined pills
	Lyn-ratiopharm	Combined pills
	Lyn-ratiopharm Sequenz	Phasic pills
	Mactex	Combined pills
	Mala D	Combined pills
	Mala N	Combined pills
	Marvelon	Combined pills
	Marvelon 20	Combined pills
	Marvelon 28	Combined pills
	Marviol	Combined pills
	Meliane	Combined pills
	Meliane Light	Combined pills
	Meloden	Combined pills
	Melodene	Combined pills
	Melodene 15	Combined pills
	Melodia	Combined pills
	Mercilon	Combined pills
	Mesigyna	Combined injectables
	Microdiol	Combined pills
	Microfemin	Combined pills
	Microfemin Cd	Combined pills
	Microgen	Combined pills
	Microgest	Combined pills
	Microgyn	Combined pills
	Microgynon	Combined pills
	Microgynon 20	Combined pills
	Microgynon 21	Combined pills
	Microgynon 30 ED	Combined pills
	Microgynon 50 ED	Combined pills
	Microgynon CD	Combined pills
	Microgynon ED	Combined pills
	Microgynon ED 28	Combined pills
	Microgynon Suave	Combined pills
	Microgynon-28	Combined pills
	Microgynon-30	Combined pills
	Microgynon-50	Combined pills
	Microlite	Combined pills
	Micropil	Combined pills
	Microvlar	Combined pills
	Milli-Anovlar	Combined pills
	Milvane	Phasic pills

Table 1 (contd)

Common name of ingredient	Brand name	Type of contraceptive
Ethinylestradiol (contd)	Min-Ovral	Combined pills
	Minerva	Combined pills
	Minesse	Combined pills
	Minestril-20	Combined pills
	Minestril-30	Combined pills
	Minestrin 1/20	Combined pills
	Mini Pregnon	Combined pills
	Minidril	Combined pills
	Minifem	Combined pills
	Minigeste	Combined pills
	Minigynon	Combined pills
	Minigynon 30	Combined pills
	Miniphase	Phasic pills
	Minisiston	Combined pills
	Minivlar	Combined pills
	Minovlar	Combined pills
	Minulet	Combined pills
	Minulette	Combined pills
	Miranova	Combined pills
	Mircette	Phasic pills
	Mirelle	Combined pills
	Mithuri	Combined pills
	Modicon	Combined pills
	Modutrol	Phasic pills
	Moneva	Combined pills
	Mono Step	Combined pills
	Monofeme	Combined pills
	Myralon	Combined pills
	Myvlar	Combined pills
	Nelova 0.5/35 E	Combined pills
	Nelova 1+35 E	Combined pills
	Nelova 1/35	Combined pills
	Nelova 10/11	Phasic pills
	Neo-Eunomin	Phasic pills
	Neo-Stediril	Combined pills
	Neocon	Combined pills
	Neocon 1/35	Combined pills
	Neofam	Combined pills
	Neogentrol	Combined pills
	Neogynon	Combined pills
	Neogynon 21	Combined pills
	Neogynon 30	Combined pills
	Neogynon CD	Combined pills
	Neogynon ED	Combined pills
	Neogynona	Combined pills

Table 1 (contd)

Common name of ingredient	Brand name	Type of contraceptive
Ethinylestradiol (contd)	Neomonovar	Combined pills
	Neorlest 21	Combined pills
	Neovlar	Combined pills
	Neovletta	Combined pills
	Nilocan	Combined pills
	No. 0 oral Pill	Combined pills
	No. 1 oral Pill	Combined pills
	No. 2 oral Pill	Combined pills
	No. 3 injectable	Combined injectables
	Nociclin	Combined pills
	Non-Ovlon	Combined pills
	Nonovlon	Combined pills
	Nora-ratiopharm	Combined pills
	Noral	Combined pills
	Nordet	Combined pills
	Nordette	Combined pills
	Nordette 150/30	Combined pills
	Nordette 28	Combined pills
	Nordette 50	Combined pills
	Nordiol	Combined pills
	Nordiol 21	Combined pills
	Norethin 1/50M	Combined pills
	Norgylen	Combined pills
	Norgylene	Combined pills
	Norigynon	Combined injectables
	Norimin	Combined pills
	Norinyl 1+35	Combined pills
	Norinyl 1/35	Combined pills
	Norinyl 28	Combined pills
	Norlestrin	Combined pills
	Normanor	Combined pills
	Norminest	Combined pills
	Normovlar	Phasic pills
	Norquest	Combined pills
	Norvetal	Combined pills
	Nouvelle Duo	Combined pills
	NovaStep	Phasic pills
	Novelon	Combined pills
	Novogyn 21	Combined pills
	Novynette	Combined pills
	Nuriphasic	Phasic pills
	Ologyn	Combined pills
	Ologyn-micro	Combined pills
	Orgalutin	Combined pills
	Ortho 0.5 + 35	Combined pills
	Ortho 1/35	Combined pills

Table 1 (contd)

Common name of ingredient	Brand name	Type of contraceptive
Ethinylestradiol (contd)	Ortho 10/11	Phasic pills
	Ortho 7/7/7	Phasic pills
	Ortho 777-28	Phasic pills
	Ortho Novum 1/35	Combined pills
	Ortho Novum 10/11	Phasic pills
	Ortho Novum 7/7/7	Phasic pills
	Ortho Tri-Cyclen	Phasic pills
	Ortho-Cept	Combined pills
	Ortho-Cyclen	Combined pills
	Orthonett Novum	Combined pills
	Orthonovum	Combined pills
	Ovacon	Combined pills
	Ovcon 35	Combined pills
	Ovcon 50	Combined pills
	Ovidol	Phasic pills
	Ovidon	Combined pills
	Oviol 22	Phasic pills
	Oviol 28	Phasic pills
	Oviprem	Combined pills
	Ovoplex	Combined pills
	Ovoplex 3	Combined pills
	Ovoplex 30/50	Combined pills
	Ovral	Combined pills
	Ovran	Combined pills
	Ovran 30	Combined pills
	Ovranet	Combined pills
	Ovranette	Combined pills
	Ovranette 30	Combined pills
	Ovulen	Combined pills
	Ovysmen	Combined pills
	Ovysmen 0.5/35	Combined pills
	Ovysmen 1/35	Combined pills
	Perikursal	Phasic pills
	Perikursal 21	Phasic pills
	Perle LD	Combined pills
	Perle Ld	Combined pills
	Petibelle	Combined pills
	Phaeva	Phasic pills
	Planor	Combined pills
	Practil 21	Combined pills
	Pramino	Phasic pills
	Preme	Combined pills
	Preven	Emergency contraception
	Prevenon	Combined pills
	Primera	Combined pills
	Primovlar	Combined pills
	R-den	Combined pills

Table 1 (contd)

Common name of ingredient	Brand name	Type of contraceptive
Ethinylestradiol (contd)	Regulon	Combined pills
	Regunon	Combined pills
	Riget	Combined pills
	Rigevidon	Combined pills
	Secure	Combined pills
	Securgin	Combined pills
	Selene	Combined pills
	Sequilar	Phasic pills
	Sequostat	Phasic pills
	Sexcon	Combined pills
	Sinovula mikro	Combined pills
	Stediril	Combined pills
	Stediril 30	Combined pills
	Stediril-d	Combined pills
	Suavuret	Combined pills
	Suginor	Combined pills
	Sukhi	Combined pills
	Synfase	Phasic pills
	Synphase	Phasic pills
	Synphasec	Phasic pills
	Synphasic	Phasic pills
	Tetragynon	Emergency contraception
	Tina	Combined pills
	Trentovlane	Combined pills
	Tri Femoden	Phasic pills
	Tri-Cilest	Phasic pills
	Tri-Gynera	Phasic pills
	Tri-Levlen	Phasic pills
	Tri-Mactex	Phasic pills
	Tri-Minulet	Phasic pills
	Tri-Norinyl	Phasic pills
	Tri-Regol	Phasic pills
	Tri-Stediril	Phasic pills
	TriStep	Phasic pills
	Triadene	Phasic pills
	Triagynon	Phasic pills
	Triciclomex	Phasic pills
	Triciclor	Phasic pills
	Tricilest	Phasic pills
	Tridette	Phasic pills
	Triella	Phasic pills
	Triette 21	Phasic pills
	Trievacin	Phasic pills
	Trifas	Phasic pills
	Trifeme	Phasic pills
	Trifeminal	Phasic pills

Table 1 (contd)

Common name of ingredient	Brand name	Type of contraceptive
Ethinylestradiol (contd)	Trigoa 21	Phasic pills
	Trigynera	Phasic pills
	Trigynon	Phasic pills
	Trigynovin	Phasic pills
	Trikvilar	Phasic pills
	Trimiron	Phasic pills
	Trinordiol	Phasic pills
	Trinovum	Phasic pills
	Triodeen	Phasic pills
	Triodcn	Phasic pills
	Triodena	Phasic pills
	Triodene	Phasic pills
	Trionetta	Phasic pills
	Triovalet	Phasic pills
	Triovlar	Phasic pills
	Triphasil	Phasic pills
	Triquilar	Phasic pills
	Trisiston	Phasic pills
	Trolit	Phasic pills
	Trust Pill	Combined pills
	Valette	Combincd pills
	Varnoline	Combined pills
	Yasmin	Combined pills
	Yermonil	Combined pills
Ethynodiol diacetate	Conova	Combined pills
	Conova 30	Combined pills
	Continuin	Progestagen-only Pills
	Demulen	Combined pills
	Demulen 1/35	Combined pills
	Demulen 1/50	Combined pills
	Demulen 30	Combined pills
	Femulen	Progestagen-only Pills
	Neo-Ovulen	Combined pills
	Ovulen	Combined pills
	Ovulen 1/50	Combined pills
	Ovulen 50	Combined pills
Etonogestrel	Implanon	Implants
Gestodene	Ciclomex	Combined pills
	Ciclomex 20	Combined pills
	Diminut	Combined pills
	Evacin	Combined pills
	Fedra	Combined pills
	Femiane	Combined pills
	Feminol	Combined pills
	Feminol-20	Combined pills

Table 1 (contd)

Common name of ingredient	Brand name	Type of contraceptive
Gestodene	Femodeen	Combined pills
	Femoden	Combined pills
	Femodene	Combined pills
	Femodene ED	Combined pills
	Femodette	Combined pills
	Femovan	Combined pills
	Gestodeno	Combined pills
	Ginera	Combined pills
	Ginoden	Combined pills
	Gynera	Combined pills
	Gynera 75/20	Combined pills
	Gynovin	Combined pills
	Gynovin 20	Combined pills
	Gynovin CD	Combined pills
	Harmonet	Combined pills
	Lerogin	Combined pills
	Lerogin 20	Combined pills
	Logest	Combined pills
	Meliane	Combined pills
	Meliane Light	Combined pills
	Meloden	Combined pills
	Melodene	Combined pills
	Melodene 15	Combined pills
	Melodia	Combined pills
	Microgen	Combined pills
	Milvane	Phasic pills
	Minesse	Combined pills
	Minifem	Combined pills
	Minigeste	Combined pills
	Minulet	Combined pills
	Minulette	Combined pills
	Mirelle	Combined pills
	Moneva	Combined pills
	Myvlar	Combined pills
	Phaeva	Phasic pills
	Tri Femoden	Phasic pills
	Tri-Gynera	Phasic pills
	Tri-Minulet	Phasic pills
	Triadene	Phasic pills
	Triciclomex	Phasic pills
	Trievacin	Phasic pills
	Trigynera	Phasic pills
	Trigynovin	Phasic pills
	Triodeen	Phasic pills
	Trioden	Phasic pills
	Triodena	Phasic pills
	Triodene	Phasic pills

Table 1 (contd)

Common name of ingredient	Brand name	Type of contraceptive
Levonorgestrel	Adépal	Phasic pills
	Alesse	Combined pills
	Anfertil	Combined pills
	Anna	Combined pills
	Anovulatorios Microdosis	Combined pills
	Anteovin	Phasic pills
	Anulette 20	Combined pills
	Anulette C.D.	Combined pills
	Anulette	Combined pills
	Anulit	Combined pills
	April	Combined pills
	Binordiol	Phasic pills
	Biphasil	Phasic pills
	Bivlar	Phasic pills
	Ciclo 21	Combined pills
	Ciclon	Combined pills
	Combination 3	Combined pills
	Confiance	Combined pills
	Contraceptive H.D.	Combined pills
	Contraceptive L.D.	Combined pills
	D-Norginor	Combined pills
	Denoval	Combined pills
	Denoval-Wyeth	Combined pills
	Duofem (ECP)	Emergency contraception
	Duofem	Combined pills
	Duoluton	Combined pills
	Duoluton L	Combined pills
	Dystrol	Combined pills
	E Gen C	Emergency contraception
	Estinor	Emergency contraception
	Eugynon	Combined pills
	Eugynon 30	Combined pills
	Eugynon CD	Combined pills
	Evanor	Combined pills
	Evanor-d	Combined pills
	FMP	Combined pills
	Femenal	Combined pills
	Femigoa	Combined pills
	Femranette mikro	Combined pills
	Fertilan	Emergency contraception
	Fironetta	Phasic pills
	Follimin	Combined pills
	Follinette	Combined pills
	Gestrelan	Combined pills
	Gravistat	Combined pills

Table 1 (contd)

Common name of ingredient	Brand name	Type of contraceptive
Levonorgestrel (contd)	Gravistat 125	Combined pills
	Gynatrol	Combined pills
	Innova CD	Combined pills
	Jadelle	Implants
	Leios	Combined pills
	Levlen	Combined pills
	Levlite	Combined pills
	Levonelle	Emergency contraception
	Levonorgestrel Pill	Combined pills
	Levora	Combined pills
	Levordiol	Phasic pills
	Libian	Phasic pills
	Lo-Femenal	Combined pills
	Lo-Gentrol	Combined pills
	Lo-Ovral	Combined pills
	Lo-Rondal	Combined pills
	Loette	Combined pills
	Loette 21	Combined pills
	Logynon	Phasic pills
	Logynon 21	Phasic pills
	Logynon ED	Phasic pills
	Lorsax	Combined pills
	Lovette	Combined pills
	Madonna	Emergency contraception
	Mala D	Combined pills
	Microfemin	Combined pills
	Microfemin Cd	Combined pills
	Microgest	Combined pills
	Microgyn	Combined pills
	Microgynon	Combined pills
	Microgynon 20	Combined pills
	Microgynon 21	Combined pills
	Microgynon 30 ED	Combined pills
	Microgynon 50 ED	Combined pills
	Microgynon CD	Combined pills
	Microgynon ED	Combined pills
	Microgynon ED 28	Combined pills
	Microgynon Suave	Combined pills
	Microgynon-28	Combined pills
	Microgynon-30	Combined pills
	Microgynon-50	Combined pills
	Microlite	Combined pills
	Microvlar	Combined pills
	Min-Ovral	Combined pills
	Minidril	Combined pills
	Minigynon	Combined pills

Table 1 (contd)

Common name of ingredient	Brand name	Type of contraceptive
Levonorgestrel (contd)	Minigynon 30	Combined pills
	Minisiston	Combined pills
	Minivlar	Combined pills
	Miranova	Combined pills
	Mithuri	Combined pills
	Modutrol	Phasic pills
	Mono Step	Combined pills
	Monofeme	Combined pills
	Neo-Stediril	Combined pills
	Neogentrol	Combined pills
	Neogynon	Combined pills
	Neogynon 21	Combined pills
	Neogynon 30	Combined pills
	Neogynon CD	Combined pills
	Neogynon ED	Combined pills
	Neogynona	Combined pills
	Neomonovar	Combined pills
	Neovlar	Combined pills
	Neovletta	Combined pills
	Nociclin	Combined pills
	Noral	Combined pills
	Nordet	Combined pills
	Nordette	Combined pills
	Nordette 150/30	Combined pills
	Nordette 28	Combined pills
	Nordette 50	Combined pills
	Nordiol	Combined pills
	Nordiol 21	Combined pills
	Norgylen	Combined pills
	Norgylene	Combined pills
	Norlevo	Emergency contraception
	Normanor	Combined pills
	Normovlar	Phasic pills
	Norplant	Implants
	Norvetal	Combined pills
	Nouvelle Duo	Combined pills
	NovaStep	Phasic pills
	Novogyn 21	Combined pills
	Ologyn	Combined pills
	Ologyn-micro	Combined pills
	Ovidon	Combined pills
	Ovoplex	Combined pills
	Ovoplex 3	Combined pills
	Ovoplex 30/50	Combined pills
	Ovral	Combined pills
	Ovran	Combined pills

Table 1 (contd)

Common name of ingredient	Brand name	Type of contraceptive
Levonorgestrel (contd)	Ovran 30	Combined pills
	Ovranet	Combined pills
	Ovranette	Combined pills
	Ovranette 30	Combined pills
	Perikursal	Phasic pills
	Perikursal 21	Phasic pills
	Perle Ld	Combined pills
	Plan B	Emergency contraception
	Postinor	Emergency contraception
	Postinor-2	Emergency contraception
	Preven	Emergency contraception
	Primovlar	Combined pills
	R-den	Combined pills
	Regunon	Combined pills
	Rigesoft	Emergency contraception
	Riget	Combined pills
	Rigevidon	Combined pills
	Sequilar	Phasic pills
	Sexcon	Combined pills
	Sino implant (2 rods)	Implants
	Stediril	Combined pills
	Stediril 30	Combined pills
	Stediril-d	Combined pills
	Subdermal implant (6 rods)	Implants
	Suginor	Combined pills
	Tetragynon	Emergency contraception
	Tri-Levlen	Phasic pills
	Tri-Regol	Phasic pills
	Tri-Stediril	Phasic pills
	TriStep	Phasic pills
	Triagynon	Phasic pills
	Triciclor	Phasic pills
	Tridestan	Phasic pills
	Triette 21	Phasic pills
	Trifas	Phasic pills
	Trifeme	Phasic pills
	Trifeminal	Phasic pills
	Trigoa 21	Phasic pills
	Trigynon	Phasic pills
	Trikvilar	Phasic pills
	Trinordiol	Phasic pills
	Trinordiol 21	Phasic pills
	Trinordiol 28	Phasic pills
	Trionetta	Phasic pills
	Triovalet	Phasic pills
	Triovlar	Phasic pills

Table 1 (contd)

Common name of ingredient	Brand name	Type of contraceptive
Levonorgestrel (contd)	Triphasil	Phasic pills
	Triquilar	Phasic pills
	Trisiston	Phasic pills
	Trolit	Phasic pills
	Trust Pill	Combined pills
	Vikela	Emergency contraception
Lynestrenol	Lyn-ratiopharm	Combined pills
	Lyn-ratiopharm Sequenz	Phasic pills
	Minette	Progestagen-only Pills
	Mini Pregnon	Combined pills
	Nuriphasic	Phasic pills
	Orgalutin	Combined pills
	Sukhi	Combined pills
	Yermonil	Combined pills
Medroxyprogesterone acetate	Ciclofem	Combined injectables
	Ciclofemina	Combined injectables
	Cyclofem	Combined injectables
	Cyclofemina	Combined injectables
	Cycloprovera	Combined injectables
	Lunelle	Combined injectables
	Novafem	Combined injectables
Megestrol acetate	No. 2 injectable	Combined injectables
	No. 2 oral pill	Combined pills
Mestranol	Combiginor	Combined pills
	Genora 1/50	Combined pills
	Gestamestrol N	Combined pills
	Gulaf	Combined pills
	Nelova 1/50 M	Combined pills
	Neo-Ovulen	Combined pills
	Norace	Phasic pills
	Norinyl	Combined pills
	Norinyl 1+50	Combined pills
	Norinyl 1/50	Combined pills
	Norinyl-1	Combined pills
	Ortho Novin 1/50	Combined pills
	Ortho Novum 1/50	Combined pills
	Ovulen 1/50	Combined pills
	Ovulen 50	Combined pills
	Perle	Combined pills
	Regovar	Combined pills
	Tridestan	Phasic pills
	Trinordiol 21	Phasic pills
	Trinordiol 28	Phasic pills

Table 1 (contd)

Common name of ingredient	Brand name	Type of contraceptive
Norethisterone	Binovum	Phasic pills
	Brevicon	Combined pills
	Brevicon 0.5 + 35	Combined pills
	Brevicon 1+35	Combined pills
	Brevicon 20	Combined pills
	Brevinor	Combined pills
	Brevinor-1	Combined pills
	Combiginor	Combined pills
	Conceplan M	Combined pills
	EVE 20	Combined pills
	Estrostep 21	Phasic pills
	Estrostep Fe+	Phasic pills
	Genora 1/35	Combined pills
	Genora 1/50	Combined pills
	Gulaf	Combined pills
	Improvil	Phasic pills
	Jenest-28	Phasic pills
	Kanchan	Combined pills
	Micropil	Combined pills
	Modicon	Combined pills
	Nelova 0.5/35 E	Combined pills
	Nelova 1+35 E	Combined pills
	Nelova 1/35	Combined pills
	Nelova 1/50 M	Combined pills
	Nelova 10/11	Phasic pills
	Neocon	Combined pills
	Neocon 1/35	Combined pills
	Nilocan	Combined pills
	No. 0 oral Pill	Combined pills
	No. 1 oral Pill	Combined pills
	Non-Ovlon	Combined pills
	Nora-ratiopharm	Combined pills
	Norace	Phasic pills
	Norethin 1/50M	Combined pills
	Norimin	Combined pills
	Norinyl	Combined pills
	Norinyl 1+35	Combined pills
	Norinyl 1+50	Combined pills
	Norinyl 1/35	Combined pills
	Norinyl 1/50	Combined pills
	Norinyl 28	Combined pills
	Norinyl-1	Combined pills
	Norminest	Combined pills
	Norquest	Combined pills
	Ortho 0.5 + 35	Combined pills
	Ortho 1/35	Combined pills

Table 1 (contd)

Common name of ingredient	Brand name	Type of contraceptive
Norethisterone (contd)	Ortho 10/11	Phasic pills
	Ortho 7/7/7	Phasic pills
	Ortho 777-28	Phasic pills
	Ortho Novin 1/50	Combined pills
	Ortho Novum 1/35	Combined pills
	Ortho Novum 1/50	Combined pills
	Ortho Novum 10/11	Phasic pills
	Ortho Novum 7/7/7	Phasic pills
	Orthonett Novum	Combined pills
	Orthonovum	Combined pills
	Ovacon	Combined pills
	Ovcon 35	Combined pills
	Ovcon 50	Combined pills
	Oviprem	Combined pills
	Ovysmen	Combined pills
	Ovysmen 0.5/35	Combined pills
	Ovysmen 1/35	Combined pills
	Perle	Combined pills
	Perle LD	Combined pills
	Regovar	Combined pills
	Secure	Combined pills
	Sequostat	Phasic pills
	Sinovula mikro	Combined pills
	Synfase	Phasic pills
	Synphase	Phasic pills
	Synphasec	Phasic pills
	Synphasic	Phasic pills
	Tri-Norinyl	Phasic pills
	Triella	Phasic pills
	Trinovum	Phasic pills
Norethisterone acetate	Anovlar 1mg	Combined pills
	Econ	Combined pills
	Econ Mite	Combined pills
	Gynophase	Phasic pills
	Gynovlane	Combined pills
	Gynovlar	Combined pills
	Loestrin	Combined pills
	Loestrin 1.5/30	Combined pills
	Loestrin 1/20	Combined pills
	Loestrin 20	Combined pills
	Loestrin 21 1.5/30	Combined pills
	Loestrin 21 1/20	Combined pills
	Loestrin 30	Combined pills
	Loestrin Fe 1.5/30+	Combined pills
	Loestrin Fe 1/20+	Combined pills
	Loveston	Combined pills

Table 1 (contd)

Common name of ingredient	Brand name	Type of contraceptive
Norethisterone acetate (contd)	Mala N	Combined pills
	Milli-Anovlar	Combined pills
	Minestril-20	Combined pills
	Minestril-30	Combined pills
	Minestrin 1/20	Combined pills
	Miniphase	Phasic pills
	Minovlar	Combined pills
	Neorlest 21	Combined pills
	Nonovlon	Combined pills
	Norlestrin	Combined pills
	Trentovlane	Combined pills
Norethisterone enanthate	Mesigyna	Combined injectables
	No 3 injectable	Combined injectables
	Norigynon	Combined injectables
Norgestimate	Cilest	Combined pills
	Cyclen	Combined pills
	Effiprev	Combined pills
	Effiprev 35	Combined pills
	Mactex	Combined pills
	Neofam	Combined pills
	Ortho Tri-Cyclen	Phasic pills
	Ortho-Cyclen	Combined pills
	Pramino	Phasic pills
	Tri-Cilest	Phasic pills
	Tri-Mactex	Phasic pills
	Tricilest	Phasic pills
	Tridette	Phasic pills
Progesterone	Vermagest	Emergency contraception

From IPPF (2002)

ANNEX 4
COMPOSITION OF COMBINED ESTROGEN–PROGESTOGEN MENOPAUSAL THERAPY

Annex 4 lists the composition of brands of combined hormonal menopausal therapy preparations that are used continuously (Table 1) or sequentially (Table 2).

Table 1. Combined continuous preparations

Trade name	Preparation	Active ingredient/dose
Activella, Kliovance	Tablet	Estradiol, 1 mg + norethisterone acetate, 500 µg
Climesse	Tablet	Estradiol valerate, 2 mg + norethisterone, 700 µg
CombiPatch	Patch	Estradiol, 50 µg/24 h + norethisterone acetate, 0.14 mg/24 h
Elleste-Duet Conti, Kliofem, Nuvelle Continuous	Tablet	Estradiol, 2 mg + norethisterone acetate, 1 mg
Evorel Conti	Patch	Estradiol, 50 µg/24 h + norethisterone acetate, 170 µg/24 h
Femhrt	Tablet	Ethinylestradiol, 5 µg + norethisterone acetate, 1 mg
Femoston Conti	Tablet	Estradiol, 1 mg + dydrogesterone, 5 mg
FemSeven Conti	Patch	Ethinylestradiol, 50 µg/24 h + levonorgestrel, 25 µg/24 h
Indivina	Tablet	Estradiol valerate, 1 mg + medroxyprogesterone acetate, 2.5 mg (also 1 mg/5 mg and 2 mg/5 mg)
Premique, Prempro	Tablet	Conjugated equine estrogen, 625 µg + medroxyprogesterone acetate, 5 mg
Premfest	Tablet	Estradiol, 1 mg + norgestimate, 90 µg

From Sturdee (2004)

Table 2. Combined sequential preparations

Trade name	Preparation	Active ingredient/dose
Adgyn Combi	Tablet	White tablet: estradiol, 2 mg; pink tablet: estradiol, 2 mg + norethisterone, 1 mg
Climagest	Tablet	Grey-blue tablet: estradiol valerate, 1 mg (also 2 mg strength); white tablet: estradiol valerate, 1 mg + norethisterone, 1 mg
Cyclo-Progynova	Tablet	Beige tablet: estradiol valerate, 1 mg; brown tablet: estradiol valerate, 1 mg + levonorgestrel, 250 µg (also 2 mg strength with estradiol valerate, 2 mg + norgestrel, 500 µg)
Elleste-Duet	Tablet	White tablet: estradiol, 1 mg (also 2 mg strength); green tablet: estradiol, 1 mg + norethisterone acetate, 1 mg
Estracombi	Patch	Estraderm TTS 50: estradiol, 50 µg/24 h; Estragest TTS: estradiol, 50 µg/24 h + norethisterone acetate, 250 µg/24 h
Estrapak 50	Patch and tablet	Patch: estradiol, 50 µg/24 h; tablet: norethisterone acetate, 1 mg
Evorel Pak	Patch and tablet	Patch: estradiol, 50 µg/24 h; tablet: norethisterone, 1 mg
Evorel Sequi	Patch	Evorel 50: estradiol, 50 µg/24 h; Evorel Conti: estradiol, 50 µg/24 h + norethisterone, 0.17 mg/24 h
Femapak	Patch and tablet	Patch: estradiol, 40 µg/24 h (also 80 µg strength); tablet: dydrogesterone, 10 mg
Femoston	Tablet	White tablet: estradiol, 1 mg (also 2 mg strength); grey tablet: estradiol, 1 mg + dydrogesterone, 10 mg
FemSeven Sequi	Patch	Phase I patch: estradiol, 50 µg/24 h; phase II patch: estradiol, 50 µg/24 h + levonorgestrel, 25 µg/24 h
NovoFem	Tablet	Red tablet: estradiol, 1 mg; white tablet: estradiol, 1 mg + norethisterone acetate, 1 mg
Nuvelle	Tablet	White tablet: estradiol valerate, 2 mg; pink tablet: estradiol valerate, 2 mg + levonorgestrel 75 µg
Nuvelle TS	Patch	Phase I patch: estradiol, 80 µg/24 h; phase II patch: estradiol, 50 µg/24 h + levonorgestrel, 20 µg/24 h
Premique Cycle	Tablet	White tablet: conjugated equine estrogen, 625 µg; green tablet: conjugated equine estrogen, 625 µg + medroxy-progesterone acetate, 10 mg
Prempak-C	Tablet	Maroon tablet: conjugated equine estrogen, 625 µg; brown tablet: norgestrel, 150 µg (also 1.25 mg tablet)
Premphase	Tablet	Maroon tablet: conjugated equine estrogen, 625 µg; blue tablet: conjugated equine estrogen, 625 µg + medroxyprogesterone acetate, 5 mg

Table 2 (contd)

Trade names	Preparation	Active ingredient/dose
Tridestra	Tablet	White tablet: estradiol valerate, 2 mg; blue tablet: estradiol valerate, 2 mg + medroxyprogesterone acetate, 20 mg; yellow tablet: inactive
Trisequens	Tablet	Blue tablet: estradiol, 2 mg; white tablet: estradiol, 2 mg + norethisterone acetate, 1 mg; red tablet: estradiol, 1 mg

From Sturdee (2004)

Reference

Sturdee, D.W. (2004) *The Facts of Hormone Therapy for Menopausal Women*, London, The Parthenon Publishing Group, pp. 37–51, 174–180

LIST OF ABBREVIATIONS

AhR	Aryl hydrocarbon receptor
AP-1	Activator protein 1
AR	Androgen receptor
AUC	Area under the curve
BCDDP	Breast Cancer Detection Demonstration Project
BRCA	Breast cancer gene
CARE	Contraceptive and Reproductive Experiences
CASH	Cancer and Steroid Hormone
CAT	Chloramphenicol acetyl transferase
CBG	Corticoid-binding globulin
CEE	Conjugated equine estrogen
CI	Confidence interval
CIN	Cervical intraepithelial neoplasia
CMM	Cutaneous malignant melanoma
CoA	Coenzyme A
COMT	Catechol-*O*-methyltransferase
CYP	Cytochrome P450
DMBA	7,12-Dimethylbenz[*a*]anthracene
DOM	Diagnostisch Onderzoek Mammacarcinoom
E_2	Estradiol
EE	Ethinylestradiol
ENNG	*N*-Ethyl-*N′*-nitro-*N*-nitrosoguanidine
ENU	*N*-Ethyl-*N*-nitrosourea
EPIC	European Prospective Investigation into Cancer and Nutrition
ER	Estrogen receptor
GC	Gas chromatography
GR	Glucocorticoid receptor
GSH	Glutathione
GST	Glutathione *S*-transferase
GT	Glucuronyltransferase
GTD	Gestational trophoblastic disease
HBsAg	Hepatitis B virus surface antigen
HBV	Hepatitis B virus
HDL	High-density lipoprotein

HERS	Heart and Estrogen/Progestin Replacement Study
HPLC	High-performance liquid chromatography
HPV	Human papillomavirus
HSD	Hydroxysteroid dehydrogenase
HSIL	High-grade squamous intraepithelial lesions
K14	Keratin 14
K_m	Michaelis-Menten constant
KPMCP	Kaiser Permanente Medical Care Program
LDL	Low-density lipoprotein
LSIL	Low-grade squamous intraepithelial lesions
LTED	Long-term estrogen-deprived
$MeOE_2$	Methoxyestradiol
MILTS	Multicentre International Liver Tumour Study
MONICA	WHO Monitoring Trends and Determinants in Cardiovascular Disease
MP	Micronized progesterone
MPA	Medroxyprogesterone acetate
MR	Mineralocorticoid receptor
MS	Mass spectrometry
MXC	Methoxychlor
NA	Not available
NOWAC	Norwegian Women and Cancer
NR	Not reported
NS	Not significant
OFPA	Oxford Family Planning Association
OH	Hydroxy
8-OH-dG	8-Hydroxy-2'-deoxyguanosine
OHE_2	Hydroxyestradiol
Pap	Papanicolaou
PCR	Polymerase chain reaction
PEPI	Postmenopausal Estrogen/Progestin Interventions
PR	Progesterone receptor
Q	Quinine
RCGP	Royal College of General Practitioners
RCGPOCS	Royal College of General Practitioners' Oral Contraceptive Study
SD	Standard deviation
SEER	Surveillance, Epidemiology and End Results
SG	S-Glutathione
SHBG	Sex hormone-binding globulin
SIR	Standardized incidence ratio
SMM	Superficial malignant melanoma

SQ	Semiquinone
SULT	Sulfotransferase
TGF	Transforming growth factor
UDP	Uridine-5′-diphosphate
UGT	Uridine-5′-diphosphate glucuronyltransferase
V_{max}	Maximum velocity of an enzymatic reaction
WHI	Women's Health Initiative

CUMULATIVE CROSS INDEX TO *IARC MONOGRAPHS ON THE EVALUATION OF CARCINOGENIC RISKS TO HUMANS*

The volume, page and year of publication are given. References to corrigenda are given in parentheses.

A

A-α-C	*40*, 245 (1986); *Suppl. 7*, 56 (1987)
Acetaldehyde	*36*, 101 (1985) (*corr. 42*, 263);
	Suppl. 7, 77 (1987); *71*, 319 (1999)
Acetaldehyde formylmethylhydrazone (*see* Gyromitrin)	
Acetamide	*7*, 197 (1974); *Suppl. 7*, 56, 389
	(1987); *71*, 1211 (1999)
Acetaminophen (*see* Paracetamol)	
Aciclovir	*76*, 47 (2000)
Acid mists (*see* Sulfuric acid and other strong inorganic acids, occupational exposures to mists and vapours from)	
Acridine orange	*16*, 145 (1978); *Suppl. 7*, 56 (1987)
Acriflavinium chloride	*13*, 31 (1977); *Suppl. 7*, 56 (1987)
Acrolein	*19*, 479 (1979); *36*, 133 (1985);
	Suppl. 7, 78 (1987); *63*, 337 (1995)
	(*corr. 65*, 549)
Acrylamide	*39*, 41 (1986); *Suppl. 7*, 56 (1987);
	60, 389 (1994)
Acrylic acid	*19*, 47 (1979); *Suppl. 7*, 56 (1987);
	71, 1223 (1999)
Acrylic fibres	*19*, 86 (1979); *Suppl. 7*, 56 (1987)
Acrylonitrile	*19*, 73 (1979); *Suppl. 7*, 79 (1987);
	71, 43 (1999)
Acrylonitrile-butadiene-styrene copolymers	*19*, 91 (1979); *Suppl. 7*, 56 (1987)
Actinolite (*see* Asbestos)	
Actinomycin D (*see also* Actinomycins)	*Suppl. 7*, 80 (1987)
Actinomycins	*10*, 29 (1976) (*corr. 42*, 255)
Adriamycin	*10*, 43 (1976); *Suppl. 7*, 82 (1987)
AF-2	*31*, 47 (1983); *Suppl. 7*, 56 (1987)
Aflatoxins	*1*, 145 (1972) (*corr. 42*, 251);
	10, 51 (1976); *Suppl. 7*, 83 (1987);
	56, 245 (1993); *82*, 171 (2002)
Aflatoxin B₁ (*see* Aflatoxins)	
Aflatoxin B₂ (*see* Aflatoxins)	
Aflatoxin G₁ (*see* Aflatoxins)	
Aflatoxin G₂ (*see* Aflatoxins)	
Aflatoxin M₁ (*see* Aflatoxins)	
Agaritine	*31*, 63 (1983); *Suppl. 7*, 56 (1987)
Alcohol drinking	*44* (1988)
Aldicarb	*53*, 93 (1991)

Aldrin	*5*, 25 (1974); *Suppl. 7*, 88 (1987)
Allyl chloride	*36*, 39 (1985); *Suppl. 7*, 56 (1987); *71*, 1231 (1999)
Allyl isothiocyanate	*36*, 55 (1985); *Suppl. 7*, 56 (1987); *73*, 37 (1999)
Allyl isovalerate	*36*, 69 (1985); *Suppl. 7*, 56 (1987); *71*, 1241 (1999)
Aluminium production	*34*, 37 (1984); *Suppl. 7*, 89 (1987)
Amaranth	*8*, 41 (1975); *Suppl. 7*, 56 (1987)
5-Aminoacenaphthene	*16*, 243 (1978); *Suppl. 7*, 56 (1987)
2-Aminoanthraquinone	*27*, 191 (1982); *Suppl. 7*, 56 (1987)
para-Aminoazobenzene	*8*, 53 (1975); *Suppl. 7*, 56, 390 (1987)
ortho-Aminoazotoluene	*8*, 61 (1975) (*corr. 42*, 254); *Suppl. 7*, 56 (1987)
para-Aminobenzoic acid	*16*, 249 (1978); *Suppl. 7*, 56 (1987)
4-Aminobiphenyl	*1*, 74 (1972) (*corr. 42*, 251); *Suppl. 7*, 91 (1987)
2-Amino-3,4-dimethylimidazo[4,5-*f*]quinoline (*see* MeIQ)	
2-Amino-3,8-dimethylimidazo[4,5-*f*]quinoxaline (*see* MeIQx)	
3-Amino-1,4-dimethyl-5*H*-pyrido[4,3-*b*]indole (*see* Trp-P-1)	
2-Aminodipyrido[1,2-*a*:3′,2′-*d*]imidazole (*see* Glu-P-2)	
1-Amino-2-methylanthraquinone	*27*, 199 (1982); *Suppl. 7*, 57 (1987)
2-Amino-3-methylimidazo[4,5-*f*]quinoline (*see* IQ)	
2-Amino-6-methyldipyrido[1,2-*a*:3′,2′-*d*]imidazole (*see* Glu-P-1)	
2-Amino-1-methyl-6-phenylimidazo[4,5-*b*]pyridine (*see* PhIP)	
2-Amino-3-methyl-9*H*-pyrido[2,3-*b*]indole (*see* MeA-α-C)	
3-Amino-1-methyl-5*H*-pyrido[4,3-*b*]indole (*see* Trp-P-2)	
2-Amino-5-(5-nitro-2-furyl)-1,3,4-thiadiazole	*7*, 143 (1974); *Suppl. 7*, 57 (1987)
2-Amino-4-nitrophenol	*57*, 167 (1993)
2-Amino-5-nitrophenol	*57*, 177 (1993)
4-Amino-2-nitrophenol	*16*, 43 (1978); *Suppl. 7*, 57 (1987)
2-Amino-5-nitrothiazole	*31*, 71 (1983); *Suppl. 7*, 57 (1987)
2-Amino-9*H*-pyrido[2,3-*b*]indole (*see* A-α-C)	
11-Aminoundecanoic acid	*39*, 239 (1986); *Suppl. 7*, 57 (1987)
Amitrole	*7*, 31 (1974); *41*, 293 (1986) (*corr. 52*, 513; *Suppl. 7*, 92 (1987); *79*, 381 (2001)
Ammonium potassium selenide (*see* Selenium and selenium compounds)	
Amorphous silica (*see also* Silica)	*42*, 39 (1987); *Suppl. 7*, 341 (1987); *68*, 41 (1997) (*corr. 81*, 383)
Amosite (*see* Asbestos)	
Ampicillin	*50*, 153 (1990)
Amsacrine	*76*, 317 (2000)
Anabolic steroids (*see* Androgenic (anabolic) steroids)	
Anaesthetics, volatile	*11*, 285 (1976); *Suppl. 7*, 93 (1987)
Analgesic mixtures containing phenacetin (*see also* Phenacetin)	*Suppl. 7*, 310 (1987)
Androgenic (anabolic) steroids	*Suppl. 7*, 96 (1987)
Angelicin and some synthetic derivatives (*see also* Angelicins)	*40*, 291 (1986)
Angelicin plus ultraviolet radiation (*see also* Angelicin and some synthetic derivatives)	*Suppl. 7*, 57 (1987)
Angelicins	*Suppl. 7*, 57 (1987)
Aniline	*4*, 27 (1974) (*corr. 42*, 252); *27*, 39 (1982); *Suppl. 7*, 99 (1987)

Benz[c]acridine	3, 241 (1973); 32, 129 (1983); Suppl. 7, 58 (1987)
Benzal chloride (see also α-Chlorinated toluenes and benzoyl chloride)	29, 65 (1982); Suppl. 7, 148 (1987); 71, 453 (1999)
Benz[a]anthracene	3, 45 (1973); 32, 135 (1983); Suppl. 7, 58 (1987)
Benzene	7, 203 (1974) (corr. 42, 254); 29, 93, 391 (1982); Suppl. 7, 120 (1987)
Benzidine	1, 80 (1972); 29, 149, 391 (1982); Suppl. 7, 123 (1987)
Benzidine-based dyes	Suppl. 7, 125 (1987)
Benzo[b]fluoranthene	3, 69 (1973); 32, 147 (1983); Suppl. 7, 58 (1987)
Benzo[j]fluoranthene	3, 82 (1973); 32, 155 (1983); Suppl. 7, 58 (1987)
Benzo[k]fluoranthene	32, 163 (1983); Suppl. 7, 58 (1987)
Benzo[ghi]fluoranthene	32, 171 (1983); Suppl. 7, 58 (1987)
Benzo[a]fluorene	32, 177 (1983); Suppl. 7, 58 (1987)
Benzo[b]fluorene	32, 183 (1983); Suppl. 7, 58 (1987)
Benzo[c]fluorene	32, 189 (1983); Suppl. 7, 58 (1987)
Benzofuran	63, 431 (1995)
Benzo[ghi]perylene	32, 195 (1983); Suppl. 7, 58 (1987)
Benzo[c]phenanthrene	32, 205 (1983); Suppl. 7, 58 (1987)
Benzo[a]pyrene	3, 91 (1973); 32, 211 (1983) (corr. 68, 477); Suppl. 7, 58 (1987)
Benzo[e]pyrene	3, 137 (1973); 32, 225 (1983); Suppl. 7, 58 (1987)
1,4-Benzoquinone (see para-Quinone)	
1,4-Benzoquinone dioxime	29, 185 (1982); Suppl. 7, 58 (1987); 71, 1251 (1999)
Benzotrichloride (see also α-Chlorinated toluenes and benzoyl chloride)	29, 73 (1982); Suppl. 7, 148 (1987); 71, 453 (1999)
Benzoyl chloride (see also α-Chlorinated toluenes and benzoyl chloride)	29, 83 (1982) (corr. 42, 261); Suppl. 7, 126 (1987); 71, 453 (1999)
Benzoyl peroxide	36, 267 (1985); Suppl. 7, 58 (1987); 71, 345 (1999)
Benzyl acetate	40, 109 (1986); Suppl. 7, 58 (1987); 71, 1255 (1999)
Benzyl chloride (see also α-Chlorinated toluenes and benzoyl chloride)	11, 217 (1976) (corr. 42, 256); 29, 49 (1982); Suppl. 7, 148 (1987); 71, 453 (1999)
Benzyl violet 4B	16, 153 (1978); Suppl. 7, 58 (1987)
Bertrandite (see Beryllium and beryllium compounds)	
Beryllium and beryllium compounds	1, 17 (1972); 23, 143 (1980) (corr. 42, 260); Suppl. 7, 127 (1987); 58, 41 (1993)
Beryllium acetate (see Beryllium and beryllium compounds)	
Beryllium acetate, basic (see Beryllium and beryllium compounds)	
Beryllium-aluminium alloy (see Beryllium and beryllium compounds)	
Beryllium carbonate (see Beryllium and beryllium compounds)	
Beryllium chloride (see Beryllium and beryllium compounds)	
Beryllium-copper alloy (see Beryllium and beryllium compounds)	
Beryllium-copper-cobalt alloy (see Beryllium and beryllium compounds)	

Butylated hydroxytoluene	*40*, 161 (1986); *Suppl. 7*, 59 (1987)
Butyl benzyl phthalate	*29*, 193 (1982) (*corr. 42*, 261);
	Suppl. 7, 59 (1987); *73*, 115 (1999)
β-Butyrolactone	*11*, 225 (1976); *Suppl. 7*, 59
	(1987); *71*, 1317 (1999)
γ-Butyrolactone	*11*, 231 (1976); *Suppl. 7*, 59
	(1987); *71*, 367 (1999)

C

Cabinet-making (*see* Furniture and cabinet-making)	
Cadmium acetate (*see* Cadmium and cadmium compounds)	
Cadmium and cadmium compounds	*2*, 74 (1973); *11*, 39 (1976)
	(*corr. 42*, 255); *Suppl. 7*, 139
	(1987); *58*, 119 (1993)
Cadmium chloride (*see* Cadmium and cadmium compounds)	
Cadmium oxide (*see* Cadmium and cadmium compounds)	
Cadmium sulfate (*see* Cadmium and cadmium compounds)	
Cadmium sulfide (*see* Cadmium and cadmium compounds)	
Caffeic acid	*56*, 115 (1993)
Caffeine	*51*, 291 (1991)
Calcium arsenate (*see* Arsenic in drinking-water)	
Calcium chromate (*see* Chromium and chromium compounds)	
Calcium cyclamate (*see* Cyclamates)	
Calcium saccharin (*see* Saccharin)	
Cantharidin	*10*, 79 (1976); *Suppl. 7*, 59 (1987)
Caprolactam	*19*, 115 (1979) (*corr. 42*, 258);
	39, 247 (1986) (*corr. 42*, 264);
	Suppl. 7, 59, 390 (1987); *71*, 383
	(1999)
Captafol	*53*, 353 (1991)
Captan	*30*, 295 (1983); *Suppl. 7*, 59 (1987)
Carbaryl	*12*, 37 (1976); *Suppl. 7*, 59 (1987)
Carbazole	*32*, 239 (1983); *Suppl. 7*, 59
	(1987); *71*, 1319 (1999)
3-Carbethoxypsoralen	*40*, 317 (1986); *Suppl. 7*, 59 (1987)
Carbon black	*3*, 22 (1973); *33*, 35 (1984);
	Suppl. 7, 142 (1987); *65*, 149
	(1996)
Carbon tetrachloride	*1*, 53 (1972); *20*, 371 (1979);
	Suppl. 7, 143 (1987); *71*, 401
	(1999)
Carmoisine	*8*, 83 (1975); *Suppl. 7*, 59 (1987)
Carpentry and joinery	*25*, 139 (1981); *Suppl. 7*, 378
	(1987)
Carrageenan	*10*, 181 (1976) (*corr. 42*, 255); *31*,
	79 (1983); *Suppl. 7*, 59 (1987)
Cassia occidentalis (*see* Traditional herbal medicines)	
Catechol	*15*, 155 (1977); *Suppl. 7*, 59
	(1987); *71*, 433 (1999)
CCNU (*see* 1-(2-Chloroethyl)-3-cyclohexyl-1-nitrosourea)	
Ceramic fibres (*see* Man-made vitreous fibres)	

Cyclamates   *22*, 55 (1980); *Suppl. 7*, 178 (1987);
                                                    73, 195 (1999)

Cyclamic acid (*see* Cyclamates)
Cyclochlorotine   *10*, 139 (1976); *Suppl. 7*, 61 (1987)
Cyclohexanone   *47*, 157 (1989); *71*, 1359 (1999)
Cyclohexylamine (*see* Cyclamates)
Cyclopenta[*cd*]pyrene   *32*, 269 (1983); *Suppl. 7*, 61 (1987)
Cyclopropane (*see* Anaesthetics, volatile)
Cyclophosphamide   *9*, 135 (1975); *26*, 165 (1981);
                                                    Suppl. 7, 182 (1987)
Cyproterone acetate   *72*, 49 (1999)

D

2,4-D (*see also* Chlorophenoxy herbicides; Chlorophenoxy   *15*, 111 (1977)
    herbicides, occupational exposures to)
Dacarbazine   *26*, 203 (1981); *Suppl. 7*, 184
                                                    (1987)
Dantron   *50*, 265 (1990) (*corr. 59*, 257)
D&C Red No. 9   *8*, 107 (1975); *Suppl. 7*, 61 (1987);
                                                    57, 203 (1993)
Dapsone   *24*, 59 (1980); *Suppl. 7*, 185 (1987)
Daunomycin   *10*, 145 (1976); *Suppl. 7*, 61 (1987)
DDD (*see* DDT)
DDE (*see* DDT)
DDT   *5*, 83 (1974) (*corr. 42*, 253);
                                                    Suppl. 7, 186 (1987); *53*, 179
                                                    (1991)
Decabromodiphenyl oxide   *48*, 73 (1990); *71*, 1365 (1999)
Deltamethrin   *53*, 251 (1991)
Deoxynivalenol (*see* Toxins derived from *Fusarium graminearum,*
    F. culmorum and *F. crookwellense*)
Diacetylaminoazotoluene   *8*, 113 (1975); *Suppl. 7*, 61 (1987)
N,N-Diacetylbenzidine   *16*, 293 (1978); *Suppl. 7*, 61 (1987)
Diallate   *12*, 69 (1976); *30*, 235 (1983);
                                                    Suppl. 7, 61 (1987)
2,4-Diaminoanisole and its salts   *16*, 51 (1978); *27*, 103 (1982);
                                                    Suppl. 7, 61 (1987); *79*, 619 (2001)
4,4'-Diaminodiphenyl ether   *16*, 301 (1978); *29*, 203 (1982);
                                                    Suppl. 7, 61 (1987)
1,2-Diamino-4-nitrobenzene   *16*, 63 (1978); *Suppl. 7*, 61 (1987)
1,4-Diamino-2-nitrobenzene   *16*, 73 (1978); *Suppl. 7*, 61 (1987);
                                                    57, 185 (1993)
2,6-Diamino-3-(phenylazo)pyridine (*see* Phenazopyridine hydrochloride)
2,4-Diaminotoluene (*see also* Toluene diisocyanates)   *16*, 83 (1978); *Suppl. 7*, 61 (1987)
2,5-Diaminotoluene (*see also* Toluene diisocyanates)   *16*, 97 (1978); *Suppl. 7*, 61 (1987)
ortho-Dianisidine (*see* 3,3'-Dimethoxybenzidine)
Diatomaceous earth, uncalcined (*see* Amorphous silica)
Diazepam   *13*, 57 (1977*); Suppl. 7*, 189
                                                    (1987); *66*, 37 (1996)
Diazomethane   *7*, 223 (1974); *Suppl. 7*, 61 (1987)
Dibenz[*a,h*]acridine   *3*, 247 (1973); *32*, 277 (1983);
                                                    Suppl. 7, 61 (1987)

1,3-Dichloropropene (technical-grade)	*41*, 113 (1986); *Suppl. 7*, 195 (1987); *71*, 933 (1999)
Dichlorvos	*20*, 97 (1979); *Suppl. 7*, 62 (1987); *53*, 267 (1991)
Dicofol	*30*, 87 (1983); *Suppl. 7*, 62 (1987)
Dicyclohexylamine (*see* Cyclamates)	
Didanosine	*76*, 153 (2000)
Dieldrin	*5*, 125 (1974); *Suppl. 7*, 196 (1987)
Dienoestrol (*see also* Nonsteroidal oestrogens)	*21*, 161 (1979); *Suppl. 7*, 278 (1987)
Diepoxybutane (*see also* 1,3-Butadiene)	*11*, 115 (1976) (*corr. 42*, 255); *Suppl. 7*, 62 (1987); *71*, 109 (1999)
Diesel and gasoline engine exhausts	*46*, 41 (1989)
Diesel fuels	*45*, 219 (1989) (*corr. 47*, 505)
Diethanolamine	*77*, 349 (2000)
Diethyl ether (*see* Anaesthetics, volatile)	
Di(2-ethylhexyl) adipate	*29*, 257 (1982); *Suppl. 7*, 62 (1987); *77*, 149 (2000)
Di(2-ethylhexyl) phthalate	*29*, 269 (1982) (*corr. 42*, 261); *Suppl. 7*, 62 (1987); *77*, 41 (2000)
1,2-Diethylhydrazine	*4*, 153 (1974); *Suppl. 7*, 62 (1987); *71*, 1401 (1999)
Diethylstilboestrol	*6*, 55 (1974); *21*, 173 (1979) (*corr. 42*, 259); *Suppl. 7*, 273 (1987)
Diethylstilboestrol dipropionate (*see* Diethylstilboestrol)	
Diethyl sulfate	*4*, 277 (1974); *Suppl. 7*, 198 (1987); *54*, 213 (1992); *71*, 1405 (1999)
N,N'-Diethylthiourea	*79*, 649 (2001)
Diglycidyl resorcinol ether	*11*, 125 (1976); *36*, 181 (1985); *Suppl. 7*, 62 (1987); *71*, 1417 (1999)
Dihydrosafrole	*1*, 170 (1972); *10*, 233 (1976) *Suppl. 7*, 62 (1987)
1,8-Dihydroxyanthraquinone (*see* Dantron)	
Dihydroxybenzenes (*see* Catechol; Hydroquinone; Resorcinol)	
1,3-Dihydroxy-2-hydroxymethylanthraquinone	*82*, 129 (2002)
Dihydroxymethylfuratrizine	*24*, 77 (1980); *Suppl. 7*, 62 (1987)
Diisopropyl sulfate	*54*, 229 (1992); *71*, 1421 (1999)
Dimethisterone (*see also* Progestins; Sequential oral contraceptives)	*6*, 167 (1974); *21*, 377 (1979))
Dimethoxane	*15*, 177 (1977); *Suppl. 7*, 62 (1987)
3,3'-Dimethoxybenzidine	*4*, 41 (1974); *Suppl. 7*, 198 (1987)
3,3'-Dimethoxybenzidine-4,4'-diisocyanate	*39*, 279 (1986); *Suppl. 7*, 62 (1987)
para-Dimethylaminoazobenzene	*8*, 125 (1975); *Suppl. 7*, 62 (1987)
para-Dimethylaminoazobenzenediazo sodium sulfonate	*8*, 147 (1975); *Suppl. 7*, 62 (1987)
trans-2-[(Dimethylamino)methylimino]-5-[2-(5-nitro-2-furyl)-vinyl]-1,3,4-oxadiazole	*7*, 147 (1974) (*corr. 42*, 253); *Suppl. 7*, 62 (1987)
4,4'-Dimethylangelicin plus ultraviolet radiation (*see also* Angelicin and some synthetic derivatives)	*Suppl. 7*, 57 (1987)
4,5'-Dimethylangelicin plus ultraviolet radiation (*see also* Angelicin and some synthetic derivatives)	*Suppl. 7*, 57 (1987)
2,6-Dimethylaniline	*57*, 323 (1993)
N,N-Dimethylaniline	*57*, 337 (1993)

cis-9,10-Epoxystearic acid	*11*, 153 (1976); *Suppl. 7*, 63 (1987); *71*, 1443 (1999)
Epstein-Barr virus	*70*, 47 (1997)
d-Equilenin	*72*, 399 (1999)
Equilin	*72*, 399 (1999)
Erionite	*42*, 225 (1987); *Suppl. 7*, 203 (1987)
Estazolam	*66*, 105 (1996)
Ethinyloestradiol	*6*, 77 (1974); *21*, 233 (1979); *Suppl. 7*, 286 (1987); *72*, 49 (1999)
Ethionamide	*13*, 83 (1977); *Suppl. 7*, 63 (1987)
Ethyl acrylate	*19*, 57 (1979); *39*, 81 (1986); *Suppl. 7*, 63 (1987); *71*, 1447 (1999)
Ethylbenzene	*77*, 227 (2000)
Ethylene	*19*, 157 (1979); *Suppl. 7*, 63 (1987); *60*, 45 (1994); *71*, 1447 (1999)
Ethylene dibromide	*15*, 195 (1977); *Suppl. 7*, 204 (1987); *71*, 641 (1999)
Ethylene oxide	*11*, 157 (1976); *36*, 189 (1985) (*corr. 42*, 263); *Suppl. 7*, 205 (1987); *60*, 73 (1994)
Ethylene sulfide	*11*, 257 (1976); *Suppl. 7*, 63 (1987)
Ethylenethiourea	*7*, 45 (1974); *Suppl. 7*, 207 (1987); *79*, 659 (2001)
2-Ethylhexyl acrylate	*60*, 475 (1994)
Ethyl methanesulfonate	*7*, 245 (1974); *Suppl. 7*, 63 (1987)
N-Ethyl-*N*-nitrosourea	*1*, 135 (1972); *17*, 191 (1978); *Suppl. 7*, 63 (1987)
Ethyl selenac (*see also* Selenium and selenium compounds)	*12*, 107 (1976); *Suppl. 7*, 63 (1987)
Ethyl tellurac	*12*, 115 (1976); *Suppl. 7*, 63 (1987)
Ethynodiol diacetate	*6*, 173 (1974); *21*, 387 (1979); *Suppl. 7*, 292 (1987); *72*, 49 (1999)
Etoposide	*76*, 177 (2000)
Eugenol	*36*, 75 (1985); *Suppl. 7*, 63 (1987)
Evans blue	*8*, 151 (1975); *Suppl. 7*, 63 (1987)
Extremely low-frequency electric fields	*80* (2002)
Extremely low-frequency magnetic fields	*80* (2002)

F

Fast Green FCF	*16*, 187 (1978); *Suppl. 7*, 63 (1987)
Fenvalerate	*53*, 309 (1991)
Ferbam	*12*, 121 (1976) (*corr. 42*, 256); *Suppl. 7*, 63 (1987)
Ferric oxide	*1*, 29 (1972); *Suppl. 7*, 216 (1987)
Ferrochromium (*see* Chromium and chromium compounds)	
Fluometuron	*30*, 245 (1983); *Suppl. 7*, 63 (1987)
Fluoranthene	*32*, 355 (1983); *Suppl. 7*, 63 (1987)
Fluorene	*32*, 365 (1983); *Suppl. 7*, 63 (1987)
Fluorescent lighting (exposure to) (*see* Ultraviolet radiation)	

Guinea Green B	*16*, 199 (1978); *Suppl. 7*, 64 (1987)
Gyromitrin	*31*, 163 (1983); *Suppl. 7*, 64, 391 (1987)

H

Haematite	*1*, 29 (1972); *Suppl. 7*, 216 (1987)
Haematite and ferric oxide	*Suppl. 7*, 216 (1987)
Haematite mining, underground, with exposure to radon	*1*, 29 (1972); *Suppl. 7*, 216 (1987)
Hairdressers and barbers (occupational exposure as)	*57*, 43 (1993)
Hair dyes, epidemiology of	*16*, 29 (1978); *27*, 307 (1982)
Halogenated acetonitriles	*52*, 269 (1991); *71*, 1325, 1369, 1375, 1533 (1999)
Halothane (*see* Anaesthetics, volatile)	
HC Blue No. 1	*57*, 129 (1993)
HC Blue No. 2	*57*, 143 (1993)
α-HCH (*see* Hexachlorocyclohexanes)	
β-HCH (*see* Hexachlorocyclohexanes)	
γ-HCH (*see* Hexachlorocyclohexanes)	
HC Red No. 3	*57*, 153 (1993)
HC Yellow No. 4	*57*, 159 (1993)
Heating oils (*see* Fuel oils)	
Helicobacter pylori (infection with)	*61*, 177 (1994)
Hepatitis B virus	*59*, 45 (1994)
Hepatitis C virus	*59*, 165 (1994)
Hepatitis D virus	*59*, 223 (1994)
Heptachlor (*see also* Chlordane/Heptachlor)	*5*, 173 (1974); *20*, 129 (1979)
Hexachlorobenzene	*20*, 155 (1979); *Suppl. 7*, 219 (1987); *79*, 493 (2001)
Hexachlorobutadiene	*20*, 179 (1979); *Suppl. 7*, 64 (1987); *73*, 277 (1999)
Hexachlorocyclohexanes	*5*, 47 (1974); *20*, 195 (1979) (*corr. 42*, 258); *Suppl. 7*, 220 (1987)
Hexachlorocyclohexane, technical-grade (*see* Hexachlorocyclohexanes)	
Hexachloroethane	*20*, 467 (1979); *Suppl. 7*, 64 (1987); *73*, 295 (1999)
Hexachlorophene	*20*, 241 (1979); *Suppl. 7*, 64 (1987)
Hexamethylphosphoramide	*15*, 211 (1977); *Suppl. 7*, 64 (1987); *71*, 1465 (1999)
Hexoestrol (*see also* Nonsteroidal oestrogens)	*Suppl. 7*, 279 (1987)
Hormonal contraceptives, progestogens only	*72*, 339 (1999)
Human herpesvirus 8	*70*, 375 (1997)
Human immunodeficiency viruses	*67*, 31 (1996)
Human papillomaviruses	*64* (1995) (*corr. 66*, 485); *90* (2007)
Human T-cell lymphotropic viruses	*67*, 261 (1996)
Hycanthone mesylate	*13*, 91 (1977); *Suppl. 7*, 64 (1987)
Hydralazine	*24*, 85 (1980); *Suppl. 7*, 222 (1987)
Hydrazine	*4*, 127 (1974); *Suppl. 7*, 223 (1987); *71*, 991 (1999)
Hydrochloric acid	*54*, 189 (1992)
Hydrochlorothiazide	*50*, 293 (1990)

J

Jacobine	*10*, 275 (1976); *Suppl. 7*, 65 (1987)
Jet fuel	*45*, 203 (1989)
Joinery (*see* Carpentry and joinery)	

K

Kaempferol	*31*, 171 (1983); *Suppl. 7*, 65 (1987)
Kaposi's sarcoma herpesvirus	*70*, 375 (1997)
Kepone (*see* Chlordecone)	
Kojic acid	*79*, 605 (2001)

L

Lasiocarpine	*10*, 281 (1976); *Suppl. 7*, 65 (1987)
Lauroyl peroxide	*36*, 315 (1985); *Suppl. 7*, 65 (1987); *71*, 1485 (1999)
Lead acetate (*see* Lead and lead compounds)	
Lead and lead compounds (*see also* Foreign bodies)	*1*, 40 (1972) (*corr. 42*, 251); *2*, 52, 150 (1973); *12*, 131 (1976); *23*, 40, 208, 209, 325 (1980); *Suppl. 7*, 230 (1987); *87* (2006)
Lead arsenate (*see* Arsenic and arsenic compounds)	
Lead carbonate (*see* Lead and lead compounds)	
Lead chloride (*see* Lead and lead compounds)	
Lead chromate (*see* Chromium and chromium compounds)	
Lead chromate oxide (*see* Chromium and chromium compounds)	
Lead compounds, inorganic and organic	*Suppl. 7*, 230 (1987); *87* (2006)
Lead naphthenate (*see* Lead and lead compounds)	
Lead nitrate (*see* Lead and lead compounds)	
Lead oxide (*see* Lead and lead compounds)	
Lead phosphate (*see* Lead and lead compounds)	
Lead subacetate (*see* Lead and lead compounds)	
Lead tetroxide (*see* Lead and lead compounds)	
Leather goods manufacture	*25*, 279 (1981); *Suppl. 7*, 235 (1987)
Leather industries	*25*, 199 (1981); *Suppl. 7*, 232 (1987)
Leather tanning and processing	*25*, 201 (1981); *Suppl. 7*, 236 (1987)
Ledate (*see also* Lead and lead compounds)	*12*, 131 (1976)
Levonorgestrel	*72*, 49 (1999)
Light Green SF	*16*, 209 (1978); *Suppl. 7*, 65 (1987)
d-Limonene	*56*, 135 (1993); *73*, 307 (1999)
Lindane (*see* Hexachlorocyclohexanes)	
Liver flukes (*see Clonorchis sinensis, Opisthorchis felineus* and *Opisthorchis viverrini*)	
Lucidin (*see* 1,3-Dihydro-2-hydroxymethylanthraquinone)	
Lumber and sawmill industries (including logging)	*25*, 49 (1981); *Suppl. 7*, 383 (1987)
Luteoskyrin	*10*, 163 (1976); *Suppl. 7*, 65 (1987)

Methoxychlor	*5*, 193 (1974); *20*, 259 (1979); *Suppl. 7*, 66 (1987)
Methoxyflurane (*see* Anaesthetics, volatile)	
5-Methoxypsoralen	*40*, 327 (1986); *Suppl. 7*, 242 (1987)
8-Methoxypsoralen (*see also* 8-Methoxypsoralen plus ultraviolet radiation)	*24*, 101 (1980)
8-Methoxypsoralen plus ultraviolet radiation	*Suppl. 7*, 243 (1987)
Methyl acrylate	*19*, 52 (1979); *39*, 99 (1986); *Suppl. 7*, 66 (1987); *71*, 1489 (1999)
5-Methylangelicin plus ultraviolet radiation (*see also* Angelicin and some synthetic derivatives)	*Suppl. 7*, 57 (1987)
2-Methylaziridine	*9*, 61 (1975); *Suppl. 7*, 66 (1987); *71*, 1497 (1999)
Methylazoxymethanol acetate (*see also* Cycasin)	*1*, 164 (1972); *10*, 131 (1976); *Suppl. 7*, 66 (1987)
Methyl bromide	*41*, 187 (1986) (*corr. 45*, 283); *Suppl. 7*, 245 (1987); *71*, 721 (1999)
Methyl *tert*-butyl ether	*73*, 339 (1999)
Methyl carbamate	*12*, 151 (1976); *Suppl. 7*, 66 (1987)
Methyl-CCNU (*see* 1-(2-Chloroethyl)-3-(4-methylcyclohexyl)-1-nitrosourea)	
Methyl chloride	*41*, 161 (1986); *Suppl. 7*, 246 (1987); *71*, 737 (1999)
1-, 2-, 3-, 4-, 5- and 6-Methylchrysenes	*32*, 379 (1983); *Suppl. 7*, 66 (1987)
N-Methyl-*N*,4-dinitrosoaniline	*1*, 141 (1972); *Suppl. 7*, 66 (1987)
4,4′-Methylene bis(2-chloroaniline)	*4*, 65 (1974) (*corr. 42*, 252); *Suppl. 7*, 246 (1987); *57*, 271 (1993)
4,4′-Methylene bis(*N*,*N*-dimethyl)benzenamine	*27*, 119 (1982); *Suppl. 7*, 66 (1987)
4,4′-Methylene bis(2-methylaniline)	*4*, 73 (1974); *Suppl. 7*, 248 (1987)
4,4′-Methylenedianiline	*4*, 79 (1974) (*corr. 42*, 252); *39*, 347 (1986); *Suppl. 7*, 66 (1987)
4,4′-Methylenediphenyl diisocyanate	*19*, 314 (1979); *Suppl. 7*, 66 (1987); *71*, 1049 (1999)
2-Methylfluoranthene	*32*, 399 (1983); *Suppl. 7*, 66 (1987)
3-Methylfluoranthene	*32*, 399 (1983); *Suppl. 7*, 66 (1987)
Methylglyoxal	*51*, 443 (1991)
Methyl iodide	*15*, 245 (1977); *41*, 213 (1986); *Suppl. 7*, 66 (1987); *71*, 1503 (1999)
Methylmercury chloride (*see* Mercury and mercury compounds)	
Methylmercury compounds (*see* Mercury and mercury compounds)	
Methyl methacrylate	*19*, 187 (1979); *Suppl. 7*, 66 (1987); *60*, 445 (1994)
Methyl methanesulfonate	*7*, 253 (1974); *Suppl. 7*, 66 (1987); *71*, 1059 (1999)
2-Methyl-1-nitroanthraquinone	*27*, 205 (1982); *Suppl. 7*, 66 (1987)
N-Methyl-*N*′-nitro-*N*-nitrosoguanidine	*4*, 183 (1974); *Suppl. 7*, 248 (1987)
3-Methylnitrosaminopropionaldehyde [*see* 3-(*N*-Nitrosomethylamino)-propionaldehyde]	

N

Nafenopin	*24*, 125 (1980); *Suppl. 7*, 67 (1987)
Naphthalene	*82*, 367 (2002)
1,5-Naphthalenediamine	*27*, 127 (1982); *Suppl. 7*, 67 (1987)
1,5-Naphthalene diisocyanate	*19*, 311 (1979); *Suppl. 7*, 67 (1987); *71*, 1515 (1999)
1-Naphthylamine	*4*, 87 (1974) (*corr. 42*, 253); *Suppl. 7*, 260 (1987)
2-Naphthylamine	*4*, 97 (1974); *Suppl. 7*, 261 (1987)
1-Naphthylthiourea	*30*, 347 (1983); *Suppl. 7*, 263 (1987)
Neutrons	*75*, 361 (2000)
Nickel acetate (*see* Nickel and nickel compounds)	
Nickel ammonium sulfate (*see* Nickel and nickel compounds)	
Nickel and nickel compounds (*see also* Implants, surgical)	*2*, 126 (1973) (*corr. 42*, 252); *11*, 75 (1976); *Suppl. 7*, 264 (1987) (*corr. 45*, 283); *49*, 257 (1990) (*corr. 67*, 395)
Nickel carbonate (*see* Nickel and nickel compounds)	
Nickel carbonyl (*see* Nickel and nickel compounds)	
Nickel chloride (*see* Nickel and nickel compounds)	
Nickel-gallium alloy (*see* Nickel and nickel compounds)	
Nickel hydroxide (*see* Nickel and nickel compounds)	
Nickelocene (*see* Nickel and nickel compounds)	
Nickel oxide (*see* Nickel and nickel compounds)	
Nickel subsulfide (*see* Nickel and nickel compounds)	
Nickel sulfate (*see* Nickel and nickel compounds)	
Niridazole	*13*, 123 (1977); *Suppl. 7*, 67 (1987)
Nithiazide	*31*, 179 (1983); *Suppl. 7*, 67 (1987)
Nitrilotriacetic acid and its salts	*48*, 181 (1990); *73*, 385 (1999)
5-Nitroacenaphthene	*16*, 319 (1978); *Suppl. 7*, 67 (1987)
5-Nitro-*ortho*-anisidine	*27*, 133 (1982); *Suppl. 7*, 67 (1987)
2-Nitroanisole	*65*, 369 (1996)
9-Nitroanthracene	*33*, 179 (1984); *Suppl. 7*, 67 (1987)
7-Nitrobenz[*a*]anthracene	*46*, 247 (1989)
Nitrobenzene	*65*, 381 (1996)
6-Nitrobenzo[*a*]pyrene	*33*, 187 (1984); *Suppl. 7*, 67 (1987); *46*, 255 (1989)
4-Nitrobiphenyl	*4*, 113 (1974); *Suppl. 7*, 67 (1987)
6-Nitrochrysene	*33*, 195 (1984); *Suppl. 7*, 67 (1987); *46*, 267 (1989)
Nitrofen (technical-grade)	*30*, 271 (1983); *Suppl. 7*, 67 (1987)
3-Nitrofluoranthene	*33*, 201 (1984); *Suppl. 7*, 67 (1987)
2-Nitrofluorene	*46*, 277 (1989)
Nitrofural	*7*, 171 (1974); *Suppl. 7*, 67 (1987); *50*, 195 (1990)
5-Nitro-2-furaldehyde semicarbazone (*see* Nitrofural)	
Nitrofurantoin	*50*, 211 (1990)
Nitrofurazone (*see* Nitrofural)	
1-[(5-Nitrofurfurylidene)amino]-2-imidazolidinone	*7*, 181 (1974); *Suppl. 7*, 67 (1987)
N-[4-(5-Nitro-2-furyl)-2-thiazolyl]acetamide	*1*, 181 (1972); *7*, 185 (1974); *Suppl. 7*, 67 (1987)
Nitrogen mustard	*9*, 193 (1975); *Suppl. 7*, 269 (1987)

N-Nitrosopyrrolidine   *17*, 313 (1978); *Suppl. 7*, 68 (1987)
N-Nitrososarcosine   *17*, 327 (1978); *Suppl. 7*, 68 (1987)
Nitrosoureas, chloroethyl (*see* Chloroethyl nitrosoureas)
5-Nitro-*ortho*-toluidine   *48*, 169 (1990)
2-Nitrotoluene   *65*, 409 (1996)
3-Nitrotoluene   *65*, 409 (1996)
4-Nitrotoluene   *65*, 409 (1996)
Nitrous oxide (*see* Anaesthetics, volatile)
Nitrovin   *31*, 185 (1983); *Suppl. 7*, 68 (1987)
Nivalenol (*see* Toxins derived from *Fusarium graminearum*,
    F. culmorum and *F. crookwellense*)
NNK (*see* 4-(*N*-Nitrosomethylamino)-1-(3-pyridyl)-1-butanone)
NNN (*see N*-Nitrosonornicotine)
Nonsteroidal oestrogens   *Suppl. 7*, 273 (1987)
Norethisterone   *6*, 179 (1974); *21*, 461 (1979);
                                                        Suppl. 7, 294 (1987); *72*, 49
                                                        (1999)
Norethisterone acetate   *72*, 49 (1999)
Norethynodrel   *6*, 191 (1974); *21*, 461 (1979)
                                                        (*corr. 42*, 259); *Suppl. 7*, 295
                                                        (1987); *72*, 49 (1999)
Norgestrel   *6*, 201 (1974); *21*, 479 (1979);
                                                        Suppl. 7, 295 (1987); *72*, 49 (1999)
Nylon 6   *19*, 120 (1979); *Suppl. 7*, 68 (1987)

O

Ochratoxin A   *10*, 191 (1976); *31*, 191 (1983)
                                                        (*corr. 42*, 262); *Suppl. 7*, 271
                                                        (1987); *56*, 489 (1993)
Oestradiol   *6*, 99 (1974); *21*, 279 (1979);
                                                        Suppl. 7, 284 (1987); *72*, 399
                                                        (1999)
Oestradiol-17β (*see* Oestradiol)
Oestradiol 3-benzoate (*see* Oestradiol)
Oestradiol dipropionate (*see* Oestradiol)
Oestradiol mustard   *9*, 217 (1975); *Suppl. 7*, 68 (1987)
Oestradiol valerate (*see* Oestradiol)
Oestriol   *6*, 117 (1974); *21*, 327 (1979);
                                                        Suppl. 7, 285 (1987); *72*, 399
                                                        (1999)
Oestrogen replacement therapy (*see* Post-menopausal oestrogen
    therapy)
Oestrogens (*see* Oestrogens, progestins and combinations)
Oestrogens, conjugated (*see* Conjugated oestrogens)
Oestrogens, nonsteroidal (*see* Nonsteroidal oestrogens)
Oestrogens, progestins (progestogens) and combinations *6* (1974); *21* (1979); *Suppl. 7*, 272
                                                        (1987); *72*, 49, 339, 399, 531
                                                        (1999)
Oestrogens, steroidal (*see* Steroidal oestrogens)
Oestrone   *6*, 123 (1974); *21*, 343 (1979)
                                                        (*corr. 42*, 259); *Suppl. 7*, 286
                                                        (1987); *72*, 399 (1999)

Phenoxyacetic acid herbicides (*see* Chlorophenoxy herbicides)

Phenoxybenzamine hydrochloride	*9*, 223 (1975); *24*, 185 (1980); *Suppl. 7*, 70 (1987)
Phenylbutazone	*13*, 183 (1977); *Suppl. 7*, 316 (1987)
meta-Phenylenediamine	*16*, 111 (1978); *Suppl. 7*, 70 (1987)
para-Phenylenediamine	*16*, 125 (1978); *Suppl. 7*, 70 (1987)
Phenyl glycidyl ether (*see also* Glycidyl ethers)	*71*, 1525 (1999)
N-Phenyl-2-naphthylamine	*16*, 325 (1978) (*corr. 42*, 257); *Suppl. 7*, 318 (1987)
ortho-Phenylphenol	*30*, 329 (1983); *Suppl. 7*, 70 (1987); *73*, 451 (1999)
Phenytoin	*13*, 201 (1977); *Suppl. 7*, 319 (1987); *66*, 175 (1996)
Phillipsite (*see* Zeolites)	
PhIP	*56*, 229 (1993)
Pickled vegetables	*56*, 83 (1993)
Picloram	*53*, 481 (1991)
Piperazine oestrone sulfate (*see* Conjugated oestrogens)	
Piperonyl butoxide	*30*, 183 (1983); *Suppl. 7*, 70 (1987)
Pitches, coal-tar (*see* Coal-tar pitches)	
Polyacrylic acid	*19*, 62 (1979); *Suppl. 7*, 70 (1987)
Polybrominated biphenyls	*18*, 107 (1978); *41*, 261 (1986); *Suppl. 7*, 321 (1987)
Polychlorinated biphenyls	*7*, 261 (1974); *18*, 43 (1978) (*corr. 42*, 258); *Suppl. 7*, 322 (1987)
Polychlorinated camphenes (*see* Toxaphene)	
Polychlorinated dibenzo-*para*-dioxins (other than 2,3,7,8-tetrachlorodibenzodioxin)	*69*, 33 (1997)
Polychlorinated dibenzofurans	*69*, 345 (1997)
Polychlorophenols and their sodium salts	*71*, 769 (1999)
Polychloroprene	*19*, 141 (1979); *Suppl. 7*, 70 (1987)
Polyethylene (*see also* Implants, surgical)	*19*, 164 (1979); *Suppl. 7*, 70 (1987)
Poly(glycolic acid) (*see* Implants, surgical)	
Polymethylene polyphenyl isocyanate (*see also* 4,4′-Methylenediphenyl diisocyanate)	*19*, 314 (1979); *Suppl. 7*, 70 (1987)
Polymethyl methacrylate (*see also* Implants, surgical)	*19*, 195 (1979); *Suppl. 7*, 70 (1987)
Polyoestradiol phosphate (*see* Oestradiol-17β)	
Polypropylene (*see also* Implants, surgical)	*19*, 218 (1979); *Suppl. 7*, 70 (1987)
Polystyrene (*see also* Implants, surgical)	*19*, 245 (1979); *Suppl. 7*, 70 (1987)
Polytetrafluoroethylene (*see also* Implants, surgical)	*19*, 288 (1979); *Suppl. 7*, 70 (1987)
Polyurethane foams (*see also* Implants, surgical)	*19*, 320 (1979); *Suppl. 7*, 70 (1987)
Polyvinyl acetate (*see also* Implants, surgical)	*19*, 346 (1979); *Suppl. 7*, 70 (1987)
Polyvinyl alcohol (*see also* Implants, surgical)	*19*, 351 (1979); *Suppl. 7*, 70 (1987)
Polyvinyl chloride (*see also* Implants, surgical)	*7*, 306 (1974); *19*, 402 (1979); *Suppl. 7*, 70 (1987)
Polyvinyl pyrrolidone	*19*, 463 (1979); *Suppl. 7*, 70 (1987); *71*, 1181 (1999)
Ponceau MX	*8*, 189 (1975); *Suppl. 7*, 70 (1987)
Ponceau 3R	*8*, 199 (1975); *Suppl. 7*, 70 (1987)
Ponceau SX	*8*, 207 (1975); *Suppl. 7*, 70 (1987)
Post-menopausal oestrogen therapy	*Suppl. 7*, 280 (1987); *72*, 399 (1999)

Q

Quercetin (*see also* Bracken fern)   *31*, 213 (1983); *Suppl. 7*, 71
                                                       (1987); *73*, 497 (1999)

para-Quinone   *15*, 255 (1977); *Suppl. 7*, 71
                                                       (1987); *71*, 1245 (1999)

Quintozene   *5*, 211 (1974); *Suppl. 7*, 71 (1987)

R

Radiation (*see* gamma-radiation, neutrons, ultraviolet radiation,
    X-radiation)
Radionuclides, internally deposited   *78* (2001)
Radon   *43*, 173 (1988) (*corr. 45*, 283)
Refractory ceramic fibres (*see* Man-made vitreous fibres)
Reserpine   *10*, 217 (1976); *24*, 211 (1980)
                                                       (*corr. 42*, 260); *Suppl. 7*, 330
                                                       (1987)
Resorcinol   *15*, 155 (1977); *Suppl. 7*, 71
                                                       (1987); *71*, 1119 (1990)
Retrorsine   *10*, 303 (1976); *Suppl. 7*, 71 (1987)
Rhodamine B   *16*, 221 (1978); *Suppl. 7*, 71 (1987)
Rhodamine 6G   *16*, 233 (1978); *Suppl. 7*, 71 (1987)
Riddelliine   *10*, 313 (1976); *Suppl. 7*, 71
                                                       (1987); *82*, 153 (2002)
Rifampicin   *24*, 243 (1980); *Suppl. 7*, 71 (1987)
Ripazepam   *66*, 157 (1996)
Rock (stone) wool (*see* Man-made vitreous fibres)
Rubber industry   *28* (1982) (*corr. 42*, 261); *Suppl. 7*,
                                                       332 (1987)
Rubia tinctorum (*see also* Madder root, Traditional herbal medicines)   *82*, 129 (2002)
Rugulosin   *40*, 99 (1986); *Suppl. 7*, 71 (1987)

S

Saccharated iron oxide   *2*, 161 (1973); *Suppl. 7*, 71 (1987)
Saccharin and its salts   *22*, 111 (1980) (*corr. 42*, 259);
                                                       Suppl. 7, 334 (1987); *73*, 517 (1999)
Safrole   *1*, 169 (1972); *10*, 231 (1976);
                                                       Suppl. 7, 71 (1987)
Salted fish   *56*, 41 (1993)
Sawmill industry (including logging) (*see* Lumber and
    sawmill industry (including logging))
Scarlet Red   *8*, 217 (1975); *Suppl. 7*, 71 (1987)
Schistosoma haematobium (infection with)   *61*, 45 (1994)
Schistosoma japonicum (infection with)   *61*, 45 (1994)
Schistosoma mansoni (infection with)   *61*, 45 (1994)
Selenium and selenium compounds   *9*, 245 (1975) (*corr. 42*, 255);
                                                       Suppl. 7, 71 (1987)
Selenium dioxide (*see* Selenium and selenium compounds)
Selenium oxide (*see* Selenium and selenium compounds)
Semicarbazide hydrochloride   *12*, 209 (1976) (*corr. 42*, 256);
                                                       Suppl. 7, 71 (1987)
Senecio jacobaea L. (*see also* Pyrrolizidine alkaloids)   *10*, 333 (1976)

Streptozotocin   *4*, 221 (1974); *17*, 337 (1978);
                                                                Suppl. 7, 72 (1987)

Strobane® (*see* Terpene polychlorinates)
Strong-inorganic-acid mists containing sulfuric acid (*see* Mists and
    vapours from sulfuric acid and other strong inorganic acids)
Strontium chromate (*see* Chromium and chromium compounds)
Styrene   *19*, 231 (1979) (*corr. 42*, 258);
                                                                Suppl. 7, 345 (1987); *60*, 233
                                                                (1994) (*corr. 65*, 549); *82*, 437
                                                                (2002)

Styrene–acrylonitrile copolymers   *19*, 97 (1979); *Suppl. 7*, 72 (1987)
Styrene–butadiene copolymers   *19*, 252 (1979); *Suppl. 7*, 72 (1987)
Styrene-7,8-oxide   *11*, 201 (1976); *19*, 275 (1979);
                                                                36, 245 (1985); *Suppl. 7*, 72
                                                                (1987); *60*, 321 (1994)

Succinic anhydride   *15*, 265 (1977); *Suppl. 7*, 72 (1987)
Sudan I   *8*, 225 (1975); *Suppl. 7*, 72 (1987)
Sudan II   *8*, 233 (1975); *Suppl. 7*, 72 (1987)
Sudan III   *8*, 241 (1975); *Suppl. 7*, 72 (1987)
Sudan Brown RR   *8*, 249 (1975); *Suppl. 7*, 72 (1987)
Sudan Red 7B   *8*, 253 (1975); *Suppl. 7*, 72 (1987)
Sulfadimidine (*see* Sulfamethazine)
Sulfafurazole   *24*, 275 (1980); *Suppl. 7*, 347
                                                                (1987)
Sulfallate   *30*, 283 (1983); *Suppl. 7*, 72 (1987)
Sulfamethazine and its sodium salt   *79*, 341 (2001)
Sulfamethoxazole   *24*, 285 (1980); *Suppl. 7*, 348
                                                                (1987); *79*, 361 (2001)

Sulfites (*see* Sulfur dioxide and some sulfites, bisulfites and metabisulfites)
Sulfur dioxide and some sulfites, bisulfites and metabisulfites *54*, 131 (1992)
Sulfur mustard (*see* Mustard gas)
Sulfuric acid and other strong inorganic acids, occupational exposures   *54*, 41 (1992)
    to mists and vapours from
Sulfur trioxide   *54*, 121 (1992)
Sulphisoxazole (*see* Sulfafurazole)
Sunset Yellow FCF   *8*, 257 (1975); *Suppl. 7*, 72 (1987)
Symphytine   *31*, 239 (1983); *Suppl. 7*, 72 (1987)

T

2,4,5-T (*see also* Chlorophenoxy herbicides; Chlorophenoxy   *15*, 273 (1977)
    herbicides, occupational exposures to)
Talc   *42*, 185 (1987); *Suppl. 7*, 349
                                                                (1987)
Tamoxifen   *66*, 253 (1996)
Tannic acid   *10*, 253 (1976) (*corr. 42*, 255);
                                                                Suppl. 7, 72 (1987)
Tannins (*see also* Tannic acid)   *10*, 254 (1976); *Suppl. 7*, 72 (1987)
TCDD (*see* 2,3,7,8-Tetrachlorodibenzo-*para*-dioxin)
TDE (*see* DDT)
Tea   *51*, 207 (1991)
Temazepam   *66*, 161 (1996)
Teniposide   *76*, 259 (2000)

ortho-Toluidine	*16*, 349 (1978); *27*, 155 (1982) (*corr. 68*, 477); *Suppl. 7*, 362 (1987); *77*, 267 (2000)
Toremifene	*66*, 367 (1996)
Toxaphene	*20*, 327 (1979); *Suppl. 7*, 72 (1987); *79*, 569 (2001)
T-2 Toxin (*see* Toxins derived from *Fusarium sporotrichioides*)	
Toxins derived from *Fusarium graminearum, F. culmorum* and *F. crookwellense*	*11*, 169 (1976); *31*, 153, 279 (1983); *Suppl. 7*, 64, 74 (1987); *56*, 397 (1993)
Toxins derived from *Fusarium moniliforme*	*56*, 445 (1993)
Toxins derived from *Fusarium sporotrichioides*	*31*, 265 (1983); *Suppl. 7*, 73 (1987); *56*, 467 (1993)
Traditional herbal medicines	*82*, 41 (2002)
Tremolite (*see* Asbestos)	
Treosulfan	*26*, 341 (1981); *Suppl. 7*, 363 (1987)
Triaziquone (*see* Tris(aziridinyl)-*para*-benzoquinone)	
Trichlorfon	*30*, 207 (1983); *Suppl. 7*, 73 (1987)
Trichlormethine	*9*, 229 (1975); *Suppl. 7*, 73 (1987); *50*, 143 (1990)
Trichloroacetic acid	*63*, 291 (1995) (*corr. 65*, 549); *84* (2004)
Trichloroacetonitrile (*see also* Halogenated acetonitriles)	*71*, 1533 (1999)
1,1,1-Trichloroethane	*20*, 515 (1979); *Suppl. 7*, 73 (1987); *71*, 881 (1999)
1,1,2-Trichloroethane	*20*, 533 (1979); *Suppl. 7*, 73 (1987); *52*, 337 (1991); *71*, 1153 (1999)
Trichloroethylene	*11*, 263 (1976); *20*, 545 (1979); *Suppl. 7*, 364 (1987); *63*, 75 (1995) (*corr. 65*, 549)
2,4,5-Trichlorophenol (*see also* Chlorophenols; Chlorophenols, occupational exposures to; Polychlorophenols and their sodium salts)	*20*, 349 (1979)
2,4,6-Trichlorophenol (*see also* Chlorophenols; Chlorophenols, occupational exposures to; Polychlorophenols and their sodium salts)	*20*, 349 (1979)
(2,4,5-Trichlorophenoxy)acetic acid (*see* 2,4,5-T)	
1,2,3-Trichloropropane	*63*, 223 (1995)
Trichlorotriethylamine-hydrochloride (*see* Trichlormethine)	
T₂-Trichothecene (*see* Toxins derived from *Fusarium sporotrichioides*)	
Tridymite (*see* Crystalline silica)	
Triethanolamine	*77*, 381 (2000)
Triethylene glycol diglycidyl ether	*11*, 209 (1976); *Suppl. 7*, 73 (1987); *71*, 1539 (1999)
Trifluralin	*53*, 515 (1991)
4,4′,6-Trimethylangelicin plus ultraviolet radiation (*see also* Angelicin and some synthetic derivatives)	*Suppl. 7*, 57 (1987)
2,4,5-Trimethylaniline	*27*, 177 (1982); *Suppl. 7*, 73 (1987)
2,4,6-Trimethylaniline	*27*, 178 (1982); *Suppl. 7*, 73 (1987)
4,5′,8-Trimethylpsoralen	*40*, 357 (1986); *Suppl. 7*, 366 (1987)
Trimustine hydrochloride (*see* Trichlormethine)	
2,4,6-Trinitrotoluene	*65*, 449 (1996)
Triphenylene	*32*, 447 (1983); *Suppl. 7*, 73 (1987)

Tris(aziridinyl)-*para*-benzoquinone	9, 67 (1975); *Suppl. 7*, 367 (1987)
Tris(1-aziridinyl)phosphine-oxide	9, 75 (1975); *Suppl. 7*, 73 (1987)
Tris(1-aziridinyl)phosphine-sulphide (*see* Thiotepa)	
2,4,6-Tris(1-aziridinyl)-*s*-triazine	9, 95 (1975); *Suppl. 7*, 73 (1987)
Tris(2-chloroethyl) phosphate	48, 109 (1990); 71, 1543 (1999)
1,2,3-Tris(chloromethoxy)propane	15, 301 (1977); *Suppl. 7*, 73 (1987); 71, 1549 (1999)
Tris(2,3-dibromopropyl) phosphate	20, 575 (1979); *Suppl. 7*, 369 (1987); 71, 905 (1999)
Tris(2-methyl-1-aziridinyl)phosphine-oxide	9, 107 (1975); *Suppl. 7*, 73 (1987)
Trp-P-1	31, 247 (1983); *Suppl. 7*, 73 (1987)
Trp-P-2	31, 255 (1983); *Suppl. 7*, 73 (1987)
Trypan blue	8, 267 (1975); *Suppl. 7*, 73 (1987)
Tussilago farfara L. (*see also* Pyrrolizidine alkaloids)	10, 334 (1976)

U

Ultraviolet radiation	40, 379 (1986); 55 (1992)
Underground haematite mining with exposure to radon	1, 29 (1972); *Suppl. 7*, 216 (1987)
Uracil mustard	9, 235 (1975); *Suppl. 7*, 370 (1987)
Uranium, depleted (*see* Implants, surgical)	
Urethane	7, 111 (1974); *Suppl. 7*, 73 (1987)

V

Vanadium pentoxide	86, 227 (2006)
Vat Yellow 4	48, 161 (1990)
Vinblastine sulfate	26, 349 (1981) (*corr. 42*, 261); *Suppl. 7*, 371 (1987)
Vincristine sulfate	26, 365 (1981); *Suppl. 7*, 372 (1987)
Vinyl acetate	19, 341 (1979); 39, 113 (1986); *Suppl. 7*, 73 (1987); 63, 443 (1995)
Vinyl bromide	19, 367 (1979); 39, 133 (1986); *Suppl. 7*, 73 (1987); 71, 923 (1999)
Vinyl chloride	7, 291 (1974); 19, 377 (1979) (*corr. 42*, 258); *Suppl. 7*, 373 (1987)
Vinyl chloride-vinyl acetate copolymers	7, 311 (1976); 19, 412 (1979) (*corr. 42*, 258); *Suppl. 7*, 73 (1987)
4-Vinylcyclohexene	11, 277 (1976); 39, 181 (1986) *Suppl. 7*, 73 (1987); 60, 347 (1994)
4-Vinylcyclohexene diepoxide	11, 141 (1976); *Suppl. 7*, 63 (1987); 60, 361 (1994)
Vinyl fluoride	39, 147 (1986); *Suppl. 7*, 73 (1987); 63, 467 (1995)
Vinylidene chloride	19, 439 (1979); 39, 195 (1986); *Suppl. 7*, 376 (1987); 71, 1163 (1999)
Vinylidene chloride-vinyl chloride copolymers	19, 448 (1979) (*corr. 42*, 258); *Suppl. 7*, 73 (1987)

Vinylidene fluoride   *39*, 227 (1986); *Suppl. 7*, 73
                                             (1987); *71*, 1551 (1999)
N-Vinyl-2-pyrrolidone   *19*, 461 (1979); *Suppl. 7*, 73
                                             (1987); *71*, 1181 (1999)
Vinyl toluene   *60*, 373 (1994)
Vitamin K substances   *76*, 417 (2000)

W

Welding   *49*, 447 (1990) (*corr. 52*, 513)
Wollastonite   *42*, 145 (1987); *Suppl. 7*, 377
                                             (1987); *68*, 283 (1997)
Wood dust   *62*, 35 (1995)
Wood industries   *25* (1981); *Suppl. 7*, 378 (1987)

X

X-radiation   *75*, 121 (2000)
Xylenes   *47*, 125 (1989); *71*, 1189 (1999)
2,4-Xylidine   *16*, 367 (1978); *Suppl. 7*, 74 (1987)
2,5-Xylidine   *16*, 377 (1978); *Suppl. 7*, 74 (1987)
2,6-Xylidine (*see* 2,6-Dimethylaniline)

Y

Yellow AB   *8*, 279 (1975); *Suppl. 7*, 74 (1987)
Yellow OB   *8*, 287 (1975); *Suppl. 7*, 74 (1987)

Z

Zalcitabine   *76*, 129 (2000)
Zearalenone (*see* Toxins derived from *Fusarium graminearum*,
    F. culmorum and *F. crookwellense*)
Zectran   *12*, 237 (1976); *Suppl. 7*, 74 (1987)
Zeolites other than erionite   *68*, 307 (1997)
Zidovudine   *76*, 73 (2000)
Zinc beryllium silicate (*see* Beryllium and beryllium compounds)
Zinc chromate (*see* Chromium and chromium compounds)
Zinc chromate hydroxide (*see* Chromium and chromium compounds)
Zinc potassium chromate (*see* Chromium and chromium compounds)
Zinc yellow (*see* Chromium and chromium compounds)
Zineb   *12*, 245 (1976); *Suppl. 7*, 74 (1987)
Ziram   *12*, 259 (1976); *Suppl. 7*, 74
                                             (1987); *53, 423* (1991)

List of IARC Monographs on the Evaluation of Carcinogenic Risks to Humans*

Volume 1
Some Inorganic Substances, Chlorinated Hydrocarbons, Aromatic Amines, N-Nitroso Compounds, and Natural Products
1972; 184 pages (out-of-print)

Volume 2
Some Inorganic and Organo-metallic Compounds
1973; 181 pages (out-of-print)

Volume 3
Certain Polycyclic Aromatic Hydrocarbons and Heterocyclic Compounds
1973; 271 pages (out-of-print)

Volume 4
Some Aromatic Amines, Hydra-zine and Related Substances, N-Nitroso Compounds and Miscellaneous Alkylating Agents
1974; 286 pages (out-of-print)

Volume 5
Some Organochlorine Pesticides
1974; 241 pages (out-of-print)

Volume 6
Sex Hormones
1974; 243 pages (out-of-print)

Volume 7
Some Anti-Thyroid and Related Substances, Nitrofurans and Industrial Chemicals
1974; 326 pages (out-of-print)

Volume 8
Some Aromatic Azo Compounds
1975; 357 pages (out-of-print)

Volume 9
Some Aziridines, N-, S- and O-Mustards and Selenium
1975; 268 pages (out-of-print)

Volume 10
Some Naturally Occurring Substances
1976; 353 pages (out-of-print)

Volume 11
Cadmium, Nickel, Some Epoxides, Miscellaneous Industrial Chemicals and General Considerations on Volatile Anaesthetics
1976; 306 pages (out-of-print)

Volume 12
Some Carbamates, Thio-carbamates and Carbazides
1976; 282 pages (out-of-print)

Volume 13
Some Miscellaneous Pharmaceutical Substances
1977; 255 pages

Volume 14
Asbestos
1977; 106 pages (out-of-print)

Volume 15
Some Fumigants, the Herbicides 2,4-D and 2,4,5-T, Chlorinated Dibenzodioxins and Miscella-neous Industrial Chemicals
1977; 354 pages (out-of-print)

Volume 16
Some Aromatic Amines and Related Nitro Compounds—Hair Dyes, Colouring Agents and Miscellaneous Industrial Chemicals
1978; 400 pages

Volume 17
Some N-Nitroso Compounds
1978; 365 pages

Volume 18
Polychlorinated Biphenyls and Polybrominated Biphenyls
1978; 140 pages (out-of-print)

Volume 19
Some Monomers, Plastics and Synthetic Elastomers, and Acrolein
1979; 513 pages (out-of-print)

Volume 20
Some Halogenated Hydrocarbons
1979; 609 pages (out-of-print)

Volume 21
Sex Hormones (II)
1979; 583 pages

Volume 22
Some Non-Nutritive Sweetening Agents
1980; 208 pages

Volume 23
Some Metals and Metallic Compounds
1980; 438 pages (out-of-print)

Volume 24
Some Pharmaceutical Drugs
1980; 337 pages

Volume 25
Wood, Leather and Some Associated Industries
1981; 412 pages

Volume 26
Some Antineoplastic and Immunosuppressive Agents
1981; 411 pages (out-of-print)

Volume 27
Some Aromatic Amines, Anthraquinones and Nitroso Compounds, and Inorganic Fluorides Used in Drinking-water and Dental Preparations
1982; 341 pages (out-of-print)

Volume 28
The Rubber Industry
1982; 486 pages (out-of-print)

Volume 29
Some Industrial Chemicals and Dyestuffs
1982; 416 pages (out-of-print)

Volume 30
Miscellaneous Pesticides
1983; 424 pages (out-of-print)

---

*High-quality photocopies of all out-of-print volumes may be purchased from University Microfilms International, 300 North Zeeb Road, Ann Arbor, MI 48106-1346, USA (Tel.: +1 313-761-4700, +1 800-521-0600).

Supplement No. 2
Long-term and Short-term Screening Assays for Carcinogens: A Critical Appraisal
1980; 426 pages (out-of-print)
(updated as IARC Scientific
Publications No. 83, 1986)

Supplement No. 3
Cross Index of Synonyms and Trade Names in Volumes 1 to 26 of the *IARC Monographs*
1982; 199 pages (out-of-print)

Supplement No. 4
Chemicals, Industrial Processes and Industries Associated with Cancer in Humans (*IARC Monographs*, Volumes 1 to 29)
1982; 292 pages (out-of-print)

Supplement No. 5
Cross Index of Synonyms and Trade Names in Volumes 1 to 36 of the *IARC Monographs*
1985; 259 pages (out-of-print)

Supplement No. 6
Genetic and Related Effects: An Updating of Selected *IARC Monographs* from Volumes 1 to 42
1987; 729 pages (out-of-print)

Supplement No. 7
Overall Evaluations of Carcinogenicity: An Updating of *IARC Monographs* Volumes 1–42
1987; 440 pages (out-of-print)

Supplement No. 8
Cross Index of Synonyms and Trade Names in Volumes 1 to 46 of the *IARC Monographs*
1990; 346 pages (out-of-print)

Achevé d'imprimer sur rotative par l'imprimerie Darantiere
à Dijon-Quetigny en avril 2007

Dépôt légal : avril 2007 - N° d'impression : 27-1474

Imprimé en France

4. Most people use the terms *Web* and *Internet* interchangeably, but techni-cally the Internet and the Web are two different beasts. The Internet is a global network of millions of computers that began in the late 1960s as a tool for university research and national defense. Information that travels over the Internet does so in a variety of languages (known as *protocols*). Think of the many languages that are spoken over the telephone wires. In order to have true communication with the person on the other end, you both need to speak the same language. Technically, the Web (and its HTTP protocol) is just one of the languages spoken on the Internet. Others include e-mail, FTP (file transfer protocol), and Usenet news groups. So the Web is just a portion (albeit[1] a large one) of the Internet. It consists of multimedia (pictures, sounds, movies, and words) viewed through a browser such as Netscape Navigator or Internet Explorer.*

The author's primary purpose is to

a. entertain.
b. inform.
c. persuade.

5. No doubt you've heard something recently about carbohydrates and their role in diet and weight loss. With a long history of providing science-based weight-loss programs that are safe, healthy, and focused on the long term, you can count on Weight Watchers to give you sound information. No- and low-carb diets may be the latest "craze" in weight loss, but they've taken the sound idea of cutting back on empty calories and hijacked it into extreme, flawed thinking. If you need to cut calories to lose weight, should you cut out all carbs? No! Many carbs—including fruits, vegetables, whole grains, and nonfat dairy—provide essential nutrients and are vital to your health and well-being. On the other hand, excess consumption of saturated fat and trans fat has been repeatedly shown to hurt your long-term health. So, although weight loss is an important health goal, finding a smart, healthy way to lose the weight and keep it off is what counts.†

The author's primary purpose is to

a. entertain.
b. inform.
c. persuade.

1. **albeit:** although

* Adapted from Barbara J. Feldman, "What's the Difference Between the Web and the Internet?" iVillage.com.

† Adapted from Weight Watchers, "The Truth About Carbs," WeightWatchers.com, October 21, 2003.

Question #2: Does the Author Reveal Bias or a Certain Tone?

One of the main reasons to determine an author's purpose is so that you can detect any bias the author might have about his or her subject. **Bias** is an in-clination toward a particular opinion or viewpoint. The term describes our tendency to feel strongly that something is right or wrong, positive or nega-tive. Even authors who try to present information neutrally, without reveal-ing any of their own feelings about the topic, will often allow their own prej-udices to creep into their writing. Conversely, authors can also make their bias perfectly clear. They often do so in hopes that they will influence the reader to agree with them.

Authors communicate their bias by using words that urge the reader to feel a certain way about a topic. Many of these words are emotional, and they provoke strong reactions in readers, encouraging them to feel either positive or negative. For example, the word *psychiatrist* is a respectful term, but the word *shrink* is negative and disrespectful. In the following pairs of sentences, the first sentence includes words that are relatively neutral. Notice how the substitution of a few more emotional words injects bias into the statement.

Neutral:	Our desire to own private property is the motivation that drives humans to want to achieve.
Emotional:	Our materialistic natures are the only thing preventing us all from becoming fat and lazy couch potatoes.
Neutral:	The recording industry should not sell records that con-tain objectionable lyrics to children.
Emotional:	The money-hungry recording industry is guilty of destroy-ing children's morals with lewd and violent song lyrics.
Neutral:	The Egyptian pyramids are interesting for many reasons.
Emotional:	The awe-inspiring Egyptian pyramids will no doubt fasc? nate and astonish modern visitors.

In the second sentence of each pair, you can see that the choice of w makes the author's opinion more emotionally forceful.

Exercise 9.6

In each of the following statements, underline the words or p' veal the author's bias. Then, on the blank provided, write ?

words encourage you to feel positive about the subject or *NEGATIVE* if they urge you to feel negative.

1. Like a <u>fox</u> in a hen house, <u>ruthless</u> collectors are <u>plundering</u>[1] Africa's cultural heritage by encouraging <u>poor</u> Africans to sell stolen treasures. __NEGATIVE__

2. Ken Burns's <u>spectacular</u> outline of jazz history will surprise no one; in *Jazz*, his <u>beautiful</u> miniseries on the subject, Burns <u>delights</u> in the details. __POSITIVE__

3. Tyler Chicken turns your dinners into something to talk about—where ordinary meals become <u>masterpieces</u>. __POSITIVE__

4. Critics say that the McMahon family—the founders and gatekeepers of the World Wrestling Federation—are a <u>menace to society</u>. __NEGATIVE__

5. The artificial heart may just be the most <u>momentous</u>[2] invention of the late twentieth century because of its ability to prolong the lives of those who suffer from heart ailments. __POSITIVE__

6. Many people who engage in skydiving describe the event as <u>exhilarating, heart pounding, and just plain fun</u>. __POSITIVE__

7. A <u>ferocious and vicious</u> pit bull was responsible for the <u>damage</u> to my front tire. __NEGATIVE__

8. <u>Lovely bright</u> purple and white flowers <u>blanketed</u> the <u>peaceful</u> landscape. __POSITIVE__

9. There's no <u>better</u> place to watch TV sports than leaning back in a <u>nice, comfy</u> recliner. __POSITIVE__

10. Many recliners are <u>ugly—bulky and overstuffed</u>—sort of like football linemen. __NEGATIVE__

1. **plundering:** robbing   2. **momentous:** important

---

rocks, they need to send my wife and have her take a whiff of the Martian atmosphere. If there's a single one-celled organism anywhere on the planet, she'll smell it. And if the other astronauts don't stop her, she'll kill it with Lysol. This is why her approach to leftovers baffles me. I am opposed to leftovers. I believe the only food that should be kept around is takeout Chinese, which contains a powerful preservative chemical called "kung pao" that enables it to remain edible for several football seasons. All other leftover foods should be thrown away immediately.*

The author's primary purpose is to

  (a.) entertain.
  b. inform.
  c. persuade.

3. President George Bush seems to want to minimize the suffering of our military family to help his election chances in the fall. And his Democratic opponents seem eager to exploit every dead and wounded soldier to defeat him. Neither side seems genuinely interested in the human cost and sacrifice. Maybe this is because some of the people who run for national office these days, or who manage their campaigns, do not have a child deployed[1] in harm's way. I find that the whole debate about how to treat the subject of our war dead is mostly being carried on by people with no skin in the game. This is hypocritical.[2] Each side wants to use the war on terrorism and the fighting in Iraq and Afghanistan for political ends. They should earn the right in lost sleep over a child sent to war before they speak to the issue. And they should stop trying to find military parents or personnel to quote to support their political agendas.†

The author's primary purpose is to

  a. entertain.
  b. inform.
  (c.) persuade.

1. **deployed:** sent into combat or action   2. **hypocritical:** professing to have feelings or virtues that one does not actually possess

* Adapted from Dave Barry, "Forget Mars, Just Open the Refrigerator," *Miami Herald*, March 14, 2004.

† Adapted from Frank Schaeffer, "For War Families, It's Not Political," *USA Today*, May 6, 2004, 13A.

9

Exercise 9.7

Read each of the following passages and then decide whether the author is neutral or communicates positive or negative bias. Then, circle the letter of the correct answer to the question that follows.

1. It has become clear that despite mounting evidence of a massive terrorist attack against the United States, President Bush and his team failed to grasp the significance of intelligence signaling imminent[1] danger. Bush, the National Security Council, the Justice Department, and the Pentagon could have taken steps to tighten leaky airport security, track known al Qaeda[2] operatives[3] in this country, alert local law enforcement, and ready our military defense systems. For heaven's sake, the CIA knew of possible plans to hijack airliners, and the FBI knew of Mideastern nationals taking flying lessons! I am a high school teacher. If I had assembled my brightest students prior to 9-11,[4] given them all the information we now know existed within our government, and asked them to imagine possible scenarios, I guarantee that one or more could have formulated an airborne suicide attack against prominent targets. This says something about the colossal[5] lack of imagination infecting every level of our national security apparatus under Bush.*

The author of this passage communicates

a. no bias (neutral).
b. positive bias.
c. negative bias.

2. Hired by the U.S. Bureau of Fisheries to write radio scripts during the Depression, Rachel Carson became worried about the widespread use of synthetic[6] chemical pesticides. She wanted to warn the public. After a New England birdwatcher noticed that sprays used to kill mosquitoes and gypsy moths were also killing birds, Carson started writing *Silent Spring,* which came out in 1962. The chemical industry and some in government attacked it. However, President John Kennedy demanded that all of the

1. **imminent:** about to happen
2. **al Qaeda:** a terrorist group
3. **operatives:** secret agents; spies
4. **9-11:** September 11, 2001, the day terrorists attacked the U.S.

5. **colossal:** huge
6. **synthetic:** prepared or made artificially, not naturally

9

* Excerpted from Michael S. Weiss (Matthews, NC), "The Observer Forum," *The Charlotte Observer,* April 18, 2004, 2E.

chemicals mentioned in the book be tested and studied. His Science Advisory Committee later backed up Carson's claims, causing a major shift in public consciousness about the environment. By the end of the year, more than 40 bills regulating pesticides came up for vote, eventually leading to a ban of DDT.[1] The creation of the Environmental Protection Agency followed.*

The author of this passage communicates

(a.) no bias (neutral).
b. positive bias.
c. negative bias.

3. If Betsy Ross stitching together the first American flag is one of the few images that comes to mind when conjuring[2] Revolution-era women, a new book by Cokie Roberts adds a few more to the mix. An impressively researched work of women's lives and activities during the fourteen-year period of the American Revolution, *Founding Mothers: The Women Who Raised Our Nation* offers a lesson in a history that few of us would recognize. Exploring a wide range of historical evidence from military records to recipes, private correspondence, pamphlets, and songs, Roberts succeeds in presenting something entirely new on a topic seemingly otherwise exhausted.[3] *Founding Mothers* is a welcome addition to American Revolution biography, which is saturated[4] by the lives of the Founding Fathers.[5] It fills in blanks and adds substance, detail, and dimension to what until now has seemed a strangely distant and totally masculine mythology.†

The author of this passage communicates

a. no bias (neutral).
(b.) positive bias.
c. negative bias.

1. **DDT:** an insecticide banned in 1972
2. **conjuring:** bringing forth
3. **exhausted:** thoroughly explored
4. **saturated:** full of

5. **Founding Fathers:** the men who formed the new American republic in the late 18th century

* Excerpted from Ida Tarbell, "Stories That Directly Changed How We Live (and Die)," http://www.ksg.harvard.edu/ksgpress/bulletin/autumn2002/features/journal_side.html.

† Adapted from Maria Fish, "'Founding Mothers' Get Their Place in the Birth of American History," *USA Today*, May 6, 2004, 4D.

9

4. Florida's governor and legislature have no right to intervene in a family tragedy nor to trample over the judicial process. That was the case when Governor Jeb Bush ordered Terri Schiavo's feeding tube reinserted last year in contravention[1] of a court order, and it remains so today. Ms. Schiavo has been in a coma since suffering a heart attack fourteen years ago at age twenty-six. Her husband, Michael Schiavo, legally speaks for her. He has said that she didn't want to be kept alive by artificial means and would have wanted to be removed from life support. Her parents, who hope for a recovery, want her to be kept alive. The courts have agreed with Mr. Schiavo in years of litigation.[2] Governor Bush encroached on judicial power by ignoring years of court proceedings to order Ms. Schiavo's feeding tube reinserted. The job of the governor and legislature is to make policy and pass laws that apply fairly to Floridians, not to tailor one law for one case in which they don't agree with the legal outcome. A ruling last week by Pinellas County Circuit Judge W. Douglas Baird affirms just how inappropriate the action was. He declared it unconstitutional.*

The author of this passage communicates

a. no bias (neutral).

b. positive bias.

c. negative bias.

5. This Memorial Day weekend, we will join in celebrating the opening of the National World War II Memorial honoring the great generation of Americans who saved the world from fascist[3] aggression and secured the blessings of liberty for hundreds of millions of people around the world. Today, their descendants are fighting the global war against terrorism, serving and sacrificing in Afghanistan and Iraq and at other outposts on the front lines of freedom. The life of each and every one of them is precious to their loved ones and to our nation. And each life given in the name of liberty is a life that has not been lost in vain. Do not hasten through Memorial Day. Take the time to remember the good souls whose memories are a blessing to you and your family. Take your children to our memorial parks and monuments. Above all, take the time to honor our

1. **in contravention:** in violation
2. **litigation:** legal proceedings

3. **fascist:** related to a government run by a dictator (an absolute ruler)

9

* Adapted from "Respect Separation of Powers, Privacy Rights," *Miami Herald,* May 9, 2004.

fellow Americans who have given their last full measure of devotion to our country and for the freedoms we cherish.*

The author of this passage communicates

a. no bias (neutral).
b. positive bias.
c. negative bias.

In addition to communicating either an overall positive or an overall negative view about a subject, an author can also reveal a more specific attitude, or **tone**. For example, the author may be angry, critical, or sarcastic about his subject. These attitudes express more particular types of negative bias. Or an author might be excited, sympathetic, amused, or awed. These are some examples of positive bias. Of course, authors can present their ideas and information with a neutral, objective tone, too. The following series of passages illustrates how changing a few words here and there results in a very different tone.

This passage illustrates a **neutral tone:**

> The Immigration and Naturalization Service ranks among the worst managed federal agencies rated by *Government Executive* magazine. It charges immigrants for doing basic paperwork and even for some informational phone calls. Additionally, its facilities aren't equipped to handle the volume of people it serves.†

This passage illustrates a **critical tone:**

> The *bureaucratic[1] nightmare* we call the Immigration and Naturalization Service ranks among the worst managed federal agencies rated by *Government Executive* magazine. It *robs poor immigrants of their hard-earned money* by charging them for basic paperwork, and it *even has the nerve* to require these people to pay for informational phone calls. Additionally, its *embarrassingly substandard[2]* facilities aren't equipped to handle the volumes of people it serves.

1. **bureaucratic:** related to a government with many different departments

2. **substandard:** below standard; inadequate

---

* Adapted from Colin Powell, "Of Memory and Our Democracy," *USA Weekend,* April 30–May 2, 2004, 9.

† Adapted from "Amnesty Debate Only Skirts U.S. Immigration Troubles," *USA Today,* August 6, 2001, 12A.

This passage illustrates a **sympathetic tone:**

> The *overworked and struggling* Immigration and Naturalization Service ranks among the *worst* managed federal agencies rated by *Government Executive* magazine. Its *meager[1] resources force it* to charge immigrants for doing basic paperwork, and its *pitiful lack of funding leaves it no choice* but to charge people for informational phone calls. *The agency has been ignored for so long that its cramped and outdated* facilities just aren't equipped to handle the volumes of people it serves.

The first paragraph is relatively neutral. It includes one opinion and two facts, all of which are free of emotional words. Therefore, the reader is not encouraged toward any particular feeling or attitude. The second version, however, is clearly critical and angry. Words and phrases like *nightmare, robs,* and *embarrassingly substandard* leave no doubt in the reader's mind about the author's attitude, and they encourage the reader to blame the agency for its problems. Notice, though, how the tone changes to one of sympathy in the third version. In that paragraph, the boldfaced, italicized words and phrases suggest that we should feel sorry for the "ignored" agency, which is not to blame for its troubles.

The following is a list of some words that can be used to describe tone.

admiring	praising, favoring, or supportive
amused	humorous of playful
angry	feeling displeased or hostile
arrogant	boastful; feeling of being superior to others
bitter	very angry
concerned	troubled and anxious
critical	expressing disapproval or strong disagreement
disgusted	feeling sickened or irritated
enthusiastic	excited and supportive
frightened	apprehensive, fearful
insulted	offended and angry
insulting	being rude or offensive
ironic	saying the opposite of what you really mean
irreverent	disrespectful
joyful	cheerful, glad, pleased
lighthearted	not serious; carefree

Continued

9

1. **meager:** deficient; scanty

outraged	extremely angry
passionate	expressing very strong feelings
sad	feeling down, depressed, or hurt
sarcastic	mean and hurtful
scolding	openly criticizing or reprimanding
sentimental	very emotional
serious	with deep concern about important matters
sympathetic	understanding the feelings of others
worried	concerned or frightened about what will happen

Exercise 9.8

Read each of the following paragraphs and then use the boldfaced, italicized words to help you circle the letter of the word that best describes its tone.

1. John Buell, a former high school history teacher who coauthored the book *The End of Homework: How Homework Disrupts Families, Overburdens Children and Limits Learning,* has finally proven once and for all that the benefits of homework assignments are ***terribly overrated.*** For one thing, homework is ***useless*** for the many students who don't go home to a quiet house with the required reference materials or support. For these kids, who are just like the fairy tale princess asked to spin straw into gold, homework is just another ***misery.*** It's ***ridiculous,*** too, to believe that homework teaches kids responsibility and discipline. Schools and teachers have no business taking over those lessons from parents, who can achieve the same results by assigning chores. Homework's ***worst fault,*** though, is its ***shameful takeover*** of limited family time. Families certainly have better things to do than supervise some teacher's agenda.*

   (a.) critical   c. neutral
   b. amused

2. Your body has a way of telling you to chill out. When you're ***overworked*** and ***overtired,*** you can feel ***tension*** in ***vulnerable areas*** such as the neck, back, and shoulders. If you don't relax, your ***stress zones*** can become ***chronically¹ tight,*** which can lead to strength imbalances and even more

1. **chronically:** continually or
   frequently

---

* Adapted from Greg Toppo, "How Much Is Too Much?" *News Herald* (Morganton, NC), August 2, 2001, 5A.

tension as other muscles work to compensate, says Greg Roskopf, a Denver-based exercise physiologist who works with the Utah Jazz and Denver Broncos. For fast relief in your most *stress-prone spots,* do some stretching activities.*

(a.) neutral   c. sarcastic
b. amused

3. In the beginning, there was Lucy. Long before Marlo, Mary, Rhoda, Roseanne, Ellen, and other one-name TV women, Lucille Ball, the *queen of funny women, blazed a trail.* Whether packing chocolates or stomping grapes, she traveled a *wacky path* that has never been surpassed. Lucy, born ninety years ago this month in Jamestown, NY, died in 1989 after heart surgery. Her *escapades¹* on *I Love Lucy,* which debuted on CBS fifty years ago this fall, and later series still *delight* viewers. What do you know about this *zany redhead?*†

(a.) admiring   c. neutral
b. outraged

4. Ireland has no shortage of *charming villages* and *spectacular scenery.* Go almost anywhere, and you're bound to come upon *wonderful vacation spots.* My first stop is always Kenmare, a town of about 1,200 that sits at the head of the bay separating the thirty-mile-long Beara from a peninsula to the north, more commonly known as the Ring of Kerry. If it seems to have been designed by a tourism board—*immaculate, colorful, timeless,* situated on the sea and ringed by mountains—there's a reason for it: Kenmare is one of only two planned towns in Ireland. Last year it won the country's annual Tidy Town competition, and it really is hard to understand why it does not *win by default* every year.‡

a. insulting   (c.) admiring
b. neutral

5. Thank God the Democrats are no longer in the White House. We had eight years of *scandal, impropriety,² shady dealings,* and general *amorality.³* I used to be a Democrat, but now I am a Republican. You just can't trust

1. **escapades:** adventures
2. **impropriety:** improper behavior
3. **amorality:** lack of concern about right and wrong

9

* Adapted from Martica K. Heaner, "Delete Stress in 4 Minutes," *Glamour,* September 2001, 140.
† Adapted from Kenneth C. Davis, "Don't Know Much About Lucille Ball," *USA Weekend,* August 26, 2001, 22.
‡ Adapted from Thomas Kelly, "Island in the Stream," *Daily News/Travel,* August 26, 2001, 4.

Democrats. Remember the old joke, "A Republican is a Democrat who has been mugged"? Well, I think it should be "A Republican is a Democrat who has seen the light." ***Thank goodness I've come to my senses.***

a. neutral   c. admiring

b. critical

Exercise 9.9

Read each of the following passages and then circle the letter of the word that best describes its tone.

1. Sport-utility vehicles (SUVs) are big and wasteful, the very emblem[1] of contemporary selfishness. They emit far more smog-forming pollutants and greenhouse gases than regular cars. And SUVs are more dangerous than regular cars: it is a common myth that the occupants inside SUVs are safer than they would be in ordinary cars, and these Godzillas[2] are instruments of death for non-SUV-driving motorists. Advertising has created the illusion that owning an SUV has something to do with being outdoorsy and adventurous, yet hardly any of these vehicles are used off-road, and they are nearly worthless in normal driving conditions, even in snow. They have blackout windows, mammoth[3] grill guards, dazzling headlights, and other features designed to make the vehicles as aggressive and hostile as possible.*

a. ironic   c. disgusted

b. joyful   d. worried

2. As a research instrument, the Hubble telescope has been a staggering success. Launched in 1991, it has helped astronomers confirm black holes, document the life cycle of stars, and age-date the universe. As a call to space, Hubble has been even more triumphant. The spectacular images it sent back of galaxies and our neighboring planets pique[4] the human imagination. Hubble's accomplishments convey the awesomeness of space and render space exploration immediate, meaningful, and

---

1. **emblem:** symbol   3. **mammoth:** huge
2. **Godzilla:** monster in Japanese films   4. **pique:** stimulate, arouse

*Adapted from Gregg Easterbrook, "Axle of Evil," *New Republic*, January 20, 2003.

9

captivating.[1] The telescope may be getting old and creaky, but it still serves admirably as the public's collective presence in space.*

a. enthusiastic c. frightened
b. outraged d. sad

3. One in three Americans is either overweight or at risk of becoming obese. Incredibly, the government has done nothing to address this growing crisis. Fortunately, though, successful anti-smoking campaigns offer a model for how an anti-sweets campaign ought to proceed. To reduce the risk of second-hand calories in the workplace, snackers should be forced to stand outside while they satisfy their filthy habit. No more munching at the desk or in the lunchroom. Desserts must be banned from restaurants and vending machines cast out of our public places. A surgeon general's warning must be placed on all snack products. For cakes, pies, cookies, candy, and sweet bread, those selling the items—waiters, waitresses, checkout counter attendants—must issue the warning verbally before making the sale. Customers must sign a form attesting[2] that they've received the warning. One can't be too careful where calories are concerned. And as every public health campaign needs a slogan, we must perpetually[3] remind all Americans: "Friends don't let friends eat junk food."†

a. serious c. bitter
b. lighthearted d. arrogant

4. We call it heartless and inhumane when in some faraway country children are beaten, raped, and kept virtually homeless and often hungry. Yet here in the United States 896,000 children faced the same fate in 2002, and as many or more face it today. Where is the outrage for the abused and neglected children among us? If we really are the responsible adults we so often profess ourselves to be, that is the question each of us should be asking ourselves. And we should follow that question with an answer to this one: What are we going to do about it? Children nationwide are living through daily horrors because we have failed to do all we can to ensure their safety and well-being. Worse, some are no longer living at all. An estimated 1,400 were killed in 2002, the latest statistics available.

1. **captivating:** interesting or charming   3. **perpetually:** without stopping
2. **attesting:** affirming or certifying

* Excerpted from "NASA's Lost Vision," *USA Today,* January 19, 2004, 14A.
† Adapted from James R. Edwards Jr., "Thank You For Not Eating," *American Outlook,* May 30, 2002.

9

These statistics should be enough to bring tears to your eyes. They also should be enough to spur[1] you to act.*

a. joyful   (c.) scolding
b. amused   d. worried

5. Buying a TV today is complicated. It's not like in the 1950s, when I was a boy, and the glaciers were receding, and electricity had just been invented. Back then there was only one kind of TV, which was a refrigerator-sized mass of walnut with two knobs and a tiny screen. In fact, some of the early TVs had no screen at all: People would just sit and stare at the walnut. That's how starved we were for entertainment. I remember when we got our first TV. Dad set it up, then climbed up onto our roof to try to aim the antenna at New York City. Then he yelled down to us, and we turned the "ON" knob, and the tiny screen started to glow, and then we saw it, right in our living room, an incredible miracle: static. Oh, sure, we'd HEARD static before, but this was the first time we'd ever actually SEEN it. And this static was coming *all the way from New York.* Back then we watched a lot of static, although sometimes, if Dad was having an unusually good aiming day up on the roof, we saw some actual programming, which mainly consisted of silent black-and-white cartoons of mice running around. That was the entire plot. There were these mice, and they ran around. I'm not saying it was as stupid as *Fear Factor,* but it was pretty stupid. Sometimes we'd yell up to Dad to turn the antenna back to the static. Today, of course, TV technology is extremely sophisticated, to the point where most of your higher-end TV sets can be operated only by children.†

a. insulting   c. concerned
b. serious   (d.) amused

Question #3: What Is the Main Point, and What Evidence Is Offered to Support It?

A second essential question for critical readers concerns the author's main point or position and the evidence that supports it. A critical reader carefully scrutinizes both to make a determination about the text's validity.

9

1. **spur:** urge

* Excerpt from "Prevent Child Abuse" from *The Charlotte Observer,* April 18, 2004, p. 2E. Reprinted with permission of The Charlotte Observer. Copyright owned by The Charlotte Observer.
† "So Many Screens, So Little Time" by Dave Barry. Reprinted by permission of TMS Reprints.

In Chapters 2 and 3, you learned to recognize stated and unstated main ideas. A critical reader not only identifies this point but also examines it further to decide whether it is valid or not. In particular, you should evaluate these characteristics of a main idea:

- **Is it significant?** Does the main idea seem important? Does it impact a lot of people? Not every point has to have huge or far-reaching implications, of course, but some ideas are obviously more worthy of attention than others.

- **Is it reasonable?** Does the idea seem logical, or does it seem weird or far-fetched? Even if an idea seems outlandish, you should not necessarily reject it. Some innovative thoughts probably seemed ridiculous at first, so you should reserve judgment until you've given the author an opportunity to explain. However, an idea that seems particularly dubious should put you on the alert, causing you to pay even more careful attention to the evidence offered as proof.

- **Is it appropriately qualified, or limited?** Beware of ideas that are expressed in absolute terms, as though they apply to everyone in every situation, with no exceptions. Authors are free to make generalizations, of course, but if they insist that the idea is universal, it may not be as valid as when they limit it with words like *most, many, several, a lot, quite a few,* and so forth.

- **Does it allow for other possibilities?** There are many different interpretations of the world around us, so reasonable authors often admit to that by using words such as *possibly, may be, could be, seems, appears, apparently,* and *seemingly* that suggest that their idea offers *one* viewpoint, not the *only* viewpoint.

After you evaluate the main point of a reading selection, you're ready to examine the evidence offered in support of that idea. Evidence comes in many forms, including facts, statistics, examples, expert testimony, observation, experience, and opinions. A critical reader weighs all of the evidence presented to decide whether it provides a firm basis of support for accepting an idea. Weighing the evidence involves looking at two qualities.

First of all, consider this question: ***Is the evidence adequate?*** Does the author provide enough support, or is he or she trying to convince you on the basis of insufficient evidence or simply more opinions instead of offering solid proof? Some opinions or ideas are **informed**; that is, they are supported by a sound body of factual information. The following passage, for example, offers an idea that is supported with sound evidence.

> The more television infants and toddlers watch, the more likely they are to have trouble paying attention and concentrating during their early school years. Pediatrician Dimitri Christakis used a government

9

database to see how much TV one- to three-year-old children watched, as reported by their mothers, and then related that to their scores on a behavior checklist showing attention problems at age seven. His report on about 1,300 kids is in *Pediatrics*. Frequent TV viewers in early childhood were most likely to score in the highest 10 percent for concentration problems, impulsiveness, and restlessness. Scoring within that 10 percent doesn't mean a child has attention deficit hyperactivity disorder (ADHD), but many would have it, and the others could face major learning problems, Christakis says. Every added hour of watching TV increased a child's odds of having attention problems by about 10 percent. Kids watching three hours a day were 30 percent more likely to have attention trouble than those viewing no TV. The researchers accounted for many factors beside television that might predict problems concentrating, but the TV-attention link remained.*

The first sentence of this paragraph offers the opinion that watching television causes shorter attention spans in kids. Then, it explains the results of a pediatrician's study, which were published in the *Pediatrics* journal. To support the opinion, the author provides data from the study. Would you agree, then, that it gives adequate and accurate evidence to prove the main idea? Does it convince you to agree? Each reader must decide for himself or herself, but most people would probably agree that the evidence presented here seems convincing. The study was conducted by an expert on kids, its findings were published in a reputable medical journal, and the author provides factual information that does indeed seem to support the link between TV-viewing and shorter attention spans.

Other opinions, however, are **uninformed**, meaning they lack enough support. Earlier in this chapter, you learned to distinguish between facts and opinions. Some uninformed paragraphs contain too many opinions and not enough facts. Others contain generalizations that are not supported with any factual evidence. The following paragraph, for example, offers little convincing support for the main idea.

American university education is still the best in the world. Many talented foreign students come to this country to earn their college degrees. Why would they do that if they didn't think they'd learn more here than they would in their homelands? Also, most American students choose to attend college in their own country rather than

* "Short Attention Span Linked to TV," by Marilyn Elias, from *USA Today*, April 5, 2004. Copyright © 2004 *USA Today*. Reprinted with permission.

studying abroad. If institutions outside the United States were as good, more students would choose to go to them.

This passage begins with an opinion that American universities are superior to those in the rest of the world. However, it offers very little evidence in support of that opinion. The two reasons given are not nearly enough to prove that American education is the "best." To do that, you'd have to add more evidence about the United States' educational resources and its "products," such as its graduates' and faculties' contributions to society. Also, you'd want to add the specific data—the numbers and other statistics—that would back up those points. As it stands now, though, the evidence in this paragraph is inadequate, so the reader has no reason to accept the author's opinion as true.

Other uninformed opinions may be supported with only the author's personal experiences or observations, or they may not offer any real evidence at all because they merely repeat the main point or offer irrelevant information that doesn't even support the point. For example, consider the following paragraph.

Many mothers banded together to urge Congress to renew the federal ban on assault weapons. They said that if this ban was allowed to expire, terrorists and mentally unbalanced people would be able to stockpile these weapons and wipe out a whole playground full of children in seconds. In reality, though, criminals mostly use guns against other criminals. Very few domestic violence cases involve assault weapons. As a matter of fact, only 4 percent of rapes and sexual assaults involve guns of any kind. Abusers are much more likely to strangle, stab, or beat their victims to death.

An alert reader will note that although the main point of this paragraph seems to be supported with factual evidence, the evidence and the point don't exactly match. The author provides information about guns' role in domestic violence, but she is supposed to be responding to the criticism that assault weapons can be used for more general acts of violence such as gunning down kids in a schoolyard.

The second question you should ask when weighing the evidence is ***Does the evidence seem accurate?*** Where did the author get the information? Are the sources well known? Are they generally considered to be reputable? If you are provided with any details about the sources of the evidence, you should examine those details to decide how trustworthy the information is. Even facts can be misrepresented or misinterpreted, so it's important to know who collected them and what methods they used.

9

Exercise 9.10

Read each of the following passages and then decide whether the author's opinion is informed or uninformed. Then, circle the letter of each correct answer.

1. Scientists employed by the Exxon oil company claim that Alaska's Prince William Sound has recovered from the 11 million gallons of oil that were spilled in 1989 when the tanker *Exxon Valdez* hit a reef there. However, this is far from true. To the naked eye, Prince William Sound may appear "normal," but a decade later, the ecosystem still suffers. Several bird and animal populations, including sea otters, killer whales, and seabirds, have not recovered. From the 1989 to 1997, for example, the population of harbor seals declined 35 percent and continues to decrease. According to the Exxon Valdez Oil Spill Trustee Council, only two out of twenty-six species studied are back to normal. The spill has resulted in profound physiological[1] effects to fish and wildlife, including reproductive failure, lowered growth and body weights, liver damage, and eye tumors.*

   a. informed
   b. uninformed

2. The videos of rap music superstars like Nelly are degrading to women. I am appalled at videos that show bikini-clad women behaving in disgusting ways. Rap videos are now so explicit that they are almost X-rated, and this is demeaning to women. It's true that the women in the videos let the rappers portray them in vulgar ways. But they should realize that they are helping to perpetuate[2] offensive stereotypes. Also, the rappers who make these videos should realize that they are being terribly insensitive. Their mothers and sisters should try to talk some sense into them. The rest of us should get angry and demand that rappers clean up their act.

   a. informed
   b. uninformed

3. Most Americans greet April 15 with the same enthusiasm that a fourth grader reserves for two hours' worth of homework. Filing an income-tax

---

1. **physiological:** related to the body   2. **perpetuate:** cause to continue

---

* Adapted from Pamela A. Miller, "Exxon Valdez Oil Spill: Ten Years Later," March 1999. Reprinted by permission of the author.

return is considered a grim duty rather than support for our democratic government. But every tax dollar we pay gives our government the ability to perform vital functions for us. You may not always like the things the government spends your money on, but it also pays for a lot of things that you're glad to have when you really need them. Thus, it's unpatriotic to gripe when it's time to help support these services. We should cheerfully mail in our returns and be proud and thankful that we have the best government in the world, one that has to pay its bills just like the rest of us do.

a. informed
b. uninformed

4. You should think twice before deciding to go under the knife to become more beautiful because plastic surgery, just like any surgery, is inherently[1] risky. According to Harvard Medical School psychologist Nancy Etcoff, "It isn't someone waving a magic wand and you look better. You're subjecting yourself to potential dangers." Rod Rohrich, president of the American Society of Plastic Surgeons, says, "It is real surgery to be done by real surgeons in a real operating room. With that is the potential for inherent real risks." Looking youthful is important in our society; consequently, about 6.6 million Americans underwent plastic surgery in 2002.*

a. informed
b. uninformed

5. It simply isn't safe for infants to sleep in a bed with adults. According to a new study conducted by the Consumer Product Safety Commission (CPSC), along with Loyola College and the St. Louis University School of Medicine, infants are twenty times more at risk of suffocation while sleeping with their parents than they are in a crib. As more parents have begun sleeping with their infant children, the number of babies who have died after getting trapped or suffocated has increased dramatically in the past ten years. Over the past three years, at least 180 babies died while sleeping in the same beds as their parents. The CPSC has documented cases of children getting trapped between the bed and the wall or the bed and another object, being suffocated by a pillow or pile of clothing, and being

1. inherently: naturally or essentially

9

* Adapted from Janet Kornblum, "There's a Risk to the Beauty of Surgery," *USA Today*, January 22, 2004, 10D.

suffocated when a child or adult accidentally lies on top of them. Consequently, the CPSC strongly recommends that babies under twenty-four months of age sleep in cribs.*

a. informed
b. uninformed

Exercise 9.11

Read each of the following passages and then respond to the questions that follow by circling the letter of each correct answer.

A. The bull shark usually grows no longer than ten feet and weighs up to 500 pounds, but what it lacks in size it makes up for in aggressiveness. Experts regard it as the most pugnacious[1] of sharks. It has, according to Robert Heuter, director of the Center of Shark Research at the Mote Marine Laboratory in Sarasota, Florida, the highest level of testosterone[2] in any animal, including lions and elephants. Its jaws are a steel trap: lower spiked teeth are designed to hold prey while the upper triangular serrated[3] teeth gouge out flesh. "The bull is an ambush type of predator. It makes this big mortal wound," says Heuter. It is fearless, taking on prey as large as it is.†

1. The main point of this passage can be paraphrased:
    a. The bull shark has spiked teeth.
    b. The bull shark shares some similarities with elephants and lions.
    c. The bull shark is the most aggressive shark.

2. What is the purpose of this passage?
    a. to entertain
    b. to inform
    c. to persuade

3. Is the evidence mostly facts or mostly opinions?
    a. mostly facts
    b. mostly opinions

1. **pugnacious:** ready to fight   3. **serrated:** saw-toothed
2. **testosterone:** a male hormone

---

* Adapted from "The Family Bed," no author credited, ABCNews.com, May 14, 2002; Michele Hatty, "15 New Findings on Caring For Your Baby," *USA Weekend,* January 9–11, 2004, 6.
† Adapted from Terry McCarthy, "Why Can't We Be Friends?" *Time,* July 30, 2001, 39.

9

4. Would you say that this opinion is informed or uninformed?

  (a.) informed
  b. uninformed

B. I hope we've finally stopped glorifying the supposedly godlike Middle Eastern soldier. During the Gulf War, everyone was worried about Saddam Hussein's[1] "elite" Republican Guard in Iraq. These soldiers were supposed to be fierce fighters who would ruthlessly snuff out large numbers of American lives. But they were really just cowards who threw up their hands in surrender as soon as they saw us coming. It is time to recognize that the American soldier is the best-trained, best-equipped, and best-motivated warrior this world has to offer. The American military is by far more powerful than any other country's military, and we don't need to romanticize the power of the enemy.

5. The main point of this passage can be paraphrased:

  (a.) American soldiers are better than Middle Eastern soldiers.
  b. Middle Eastern soldiers are fierce fighters.
  c. The Gulf War was a severe test of American bravery.
  d. The military is no place for cowards.

6. What is the purpose of this passage?

  a. to entertain
  b. to inform
  (c.) to persuade

7. Is the evidence mostly facts or mostly opinions?

  a. mostly facts
  (b.) mostly opinions

8. Would you say that this opinion is informed or uninformed?

  a. informed
  (b.) uninformed

C. American Indians on and off reservations in the 1960s called for changes in federal and state policies. Increasingly militant[2] Indian leaders demanded the protection and restoration of their ancient burial grounds, along with fishing and timber rights. They asked museums to return the remains of dead Indians on display. The National Indian Youth Council called for Indians to resist further loss of Indian lands. Vine DeLoria's[3] popular *Custer Died for Your*

1. **Saddam Hussein:** former dictator of Iraq
2. **militant:** fighting; aggressive
3. **Vine DeLoria:** a Lakota Sioux Indian and a well-known spokesperson on Native American rights

9

Sins (1969) informed readers that Indians asked "only to be freed of cultural oppression."[1] "The white does not understand the Indian," he wrote, "and the Indian does not wish to understand the white." The central issue was not equality and assimilation,[2] DeLoria explained, but Indian self-determination. Indians wanted economic prosperity and opportunity, but on terms that would ensure their continued tribal existence.*

9. The main point of this passage can be paraphrased:
   a. Vine DeLoria was the voice of the American Indian in the 1960s.
   b. "Indian self-determination" was a catch phrase in the 1960s.
   c. The government resisted change when it came to the American Indians in the 1960s.
   d. In the 1960s, American Indians fought for changes in government policy with the hope of keeping their tribal existence intact.

10. What is the purpose of this passage?
   a. to entertain
   b. to inform
   c. to persuade

11. Is the evidence mostly facts or mostly opinions?
   a. mostly facts
   b. mostly opinions

12. Would you say that this opinion is informed or uninformed?
   a. informed
   b. uninformed

D. Where I live, although the speed limit is 55 miles per hour, people who drive large cars, vans, and SUVs go in excess of 75 miles an hour. I am always very careful not to exceed the speed limit, and it really burns me up that so many people are careless with their lives and the lives of fellow drivers. Speeding is one thing, but the same crazy drivers also tailgate, pulling right up to and sometimes bumping my bumper as I drive in the left lane. They flash their lights and zoom up next to me to show their displeasure with the fact that I am driving in the "fast" lane and not going fast enough for their liking. What is the point of posting speed limits if nobody is going to drive the limit posted?

1. **oppression:** kept down by unfair use of power

2. **assimilation:** absorption of a minority group into the majority

---

* From Carol Berkin et al., *Making America,* 2nd ed. (Boston: Houghton Mifflin Co., 2001), 674–675.

9

13. The main point of this passage can be paraphrased:
    a. People do not pay attention to speed limits.
    (b.) Many drivers have bad manners.
    c. Tailgating should be illegal.
    d. There are many cars on the road today.

14. What is the purpose of this passage?
    a. to entertain
    b. to inform
    (c.) to persuade

15. Is the evidence mostly facts or mostly opinions?
    a. mostly facts
    (b.) mostly opinions

16. Would you say that this opinion is informed or uninformed?
    a. informed
    (b.) uninformed

Deciding for Yourself

Once you are able to separate fact from opinion, detect bias and different types of tone, and evaluate the main point and the evidence, you should be better able to evaluate whether a text is valid or worthy. Then, you can determine what you should do about the new ideas or information. Should you accept them as true? Should you change your own opinions in response? Should you reject the text outright? Or should you resolve to gather more information before you make up your mind? Critical readers know how to scrutinize a text so they can decide for themselves.

CHAPTER 9 REVIEW

Write the correct answers in the blanks provided in the following statements.

1. ___Critical___ reading means noticing certain techniques that the writer is using to convince you of the validity and worth of his or her ideas or information.

2. ___Facts___ are information that is verifiably true.

9

3. __Opinions__ are statements that express beliefs, feelings, judgments, attitudes, and preferences.

4. Certain __clue__ words—such as relative terms, qualifying terms, absolute terms, or terms that admit other possibilities—often appear in statements of opinion.

5. You can use three critical reading __questions__ to guide your interpretation and evaluation of a text. These questions focus on the author's __purpose__, the presence of bias or a certain __tone__, and the main point and __evidence__ offered to support it.

6. The three purposes for writing are to __entertain__, to __inform__, and to __persuade__.

7. __Bias__ is an inclination toward a particular opinion or viewpoint.

8. __Tone__ is the author's specific attitude about his or her subject.

9. A sound main point is usually __significant__, reasonable, __limited__, and mindful of other __possibilities__.

10. __Evidence__ includes facts, statistics, examples, expert testimony, observations, experiences, and opinions.

11. Sound evidence is both __adequate__ and __accurate__.

12. Some opinions or ideas are __informed__; that is, they are supported by a sound body of factual information.

13. Some opinions or ideas are __uninformed__; that is, they lack adequate support.

Reading Selection

Practicing the Active Reading Strategy:
Before and As You Read

You can use active reading strategies before, as, and after you read a selection. The following are some suggestions for active reading strategies that you can employ before you read and as you are reading.

1. Skim the selection for any unfamiliar words. Circle or highlight any words you do not know.

2. As you read, underline, highlight, or circle important words or phrases.

3. Write down any questions about the selection if you are confused by the information presented.

4. Jot notes in the margin to help you understand the material.

If ER Nurses Crash, Will Patients Follow?
by Paul Duke

1 I was sprinting down the hall when a patient waiting to be seen by a doctor asked me for a blanket. She was in her mid-seventies, cold, scared, and without any family or friends nearby. Did I have time to get her that blanket, or even stop to say a few words to let her know she wasn't alone? No, I didn't.

2 As an emergency-room nurse, I'm constantly forced to shuffle the needs of the sick and injured. At that particular moment, half of my twelve patients were screaming for pain medication, most of the others needed to be rushed off to tests, and one was desperately trying not to die on me.

3 Was that blanket important in the grand scheme of things? Not really. She wasn't going to die without it. So it got tossed on the back burner, along with my compassion.

4 I often find myself hopping from task to task just to keep everyone alive. By the end of the shift I often wonder, did I kill anyone today? I go home tired and beaten down, praying like mad that I didn't make any mistakes that hurt anyone.

5 For five years I have worked in one of the busiest emergency rooms in southeastern Michigan. For the last two I have picked up overtime by working in four other hospitals, including the busiest emergency room in inner-city Detroit. No matter where I am, I experience the same problem—too many patients, not enough staff.

6 When I started emergency-room nursing five years ago, I would typically have four or five patients. I could spend a few minutes chatting with them and answering their questions. Let's face it, when you are in a drafty[1] emergency room in just a flimsy paper gown and your underwear, it is nice to have someone actually talk to you. It's a scary experience to get poked and prodded in various parts of your anatomy.

7 But now on an average day I have ten to twelve patients. Once I even had twenty-two. On that night I was feeling swamped, so I went to the charge nurse for help. She was as busy as I was, so she told me to take the five sickest patients and keep them alive, and get to the rest when I could. Now, here's a question: do you want to be one of the five sickest who get attention right away, or one of the others who have to wait maybe seven, eight or even ten hours before someone gets to you?

8 That night I staggered home grateful that nobody had died. But I wondered, do I really want to do this job? I love the emergency room, but I was so damn frustrated. Was it just me?

9 I did an informal survey of the emergency rooms where I work. Every nurse I spoke to said the patient load had at least doubled in the last three years. None of them expected the situation to get better soon.

1. **drafty:** exposed to drafts (currents) of air

10   Troubling, but hardly scientific, so I did a little digging for some real statistics. According to the Centers for Disease Control and Prevention, from 1997 through 2000, the annual number of emergency-room visits went from 95 million to 108 million while the number of ERs decreased. So who picked up the slack? The staff at emergency rooms, like mine, that are still standing.

11   The journal *Nursing 2003* reports that approximately three out of ten RNs believe their hospital has enough nurses to provide excellent care. Not exactly what you want to hear from the people responsible for your loved ones' health.

12   The future doesn't look any brighter. Studies show that by 2010, 40 percent of all registered nurses will be over fifty. That's when most of us are getting ready to cut back our hours or switch from direct patient care to chart review. By 2020, there will be an estimated shortfall of 808,400 nurses, partly because many will have retired or become so dissatisfied that they've quit, but also because fewer people are entering the profession. Yet the number of Americans older than sixty-five is expected to double from 35 million to 70 million over the next two decades. As someone who knows just how often the elderly visit ERs due to heart attacks, strokes, and falls, I see trouble ahead.

13   Don't get me wrong—my colleagues are some of the hardest-working and most professional nurses you will find. But when you're given twenty patients when you should have six, well, you're only so good.

14   After all this you must wonder why I don't quit. The truth is [that] I love nursing. It's what I am good at. I love the challenge of not knowing what will come crashing through the doors. Emergency-room nurses rise to the occasion. But we are being steamrolled, stretched thin, and beaten down, and the best of us are frustrated.

15   At the end of my eighteen-hour shift I got that little old lady her blanket and spent a few minutes talking to her. She took my hand, smiled, and said thank you.

16   I'm frustrated, but I'll be back.*

VOCABULARY

Read the following questions about some of the vocabulary words that appear in the previous selection. Then circle the letter of each correct answer.

1. "Let's face it, when you are in a drafty emergency room in just a *flimsy* paper gown and your underwear, it is nice to have someone actually talk to you" (paragraph 6). What does *flimsy* mean?
   a. thin; insubstantial
   b. bulky
   c. colorful
   d. dark

* "If ER Nurses Crash, Will Patients Follow?" by Paul S. Duke from *Newsweek*, February 2, 2004. Copyright © 2004 Newsweek. All rights reserved. Reprinted by permission.

9

2. "By 2020, there will be an *estimated* shortfall of 808,400 nurses, partly because many will have retired . . . " (paragraph 12) What does *estimated* mean?

    a. excused
    b. projected
    c. deliberate
    d. related to money

3. "Don't get me wrong—my *colleagues* are some of the hardest-working and most professional nurses you will find." (paragraph 13) What are *colleagues?*

    a. friends
    b. patients
    c. coworkers
    d. relatives

CRITICAL READING

A. Are the following sentences (1–6) from the reading selection facts (*F*) or opinions (*O*)? Write your answer on the blank next to each sentence.

1. "For five years I have worked in one of the busiest emergency rooms in southeastern Michigan." ___F___

2. "The future doesn't look any brighter." ___O___

3. "Don't get me wrong—my colleagues are some of the hardest-working and most professional nurses you will find." ___O___

4. "It's what I'm good at." ___O___

5. "At the end of my eighteen-hour shift I got that little old lady her blanket and spent a few minutes talking to her." ___F___

6. "She took my hand, smiled, and said thank you." ___F___

B. Circle the letter of each correct answer.

7. What is Paul Duke's tone in this essay?

    a. amused
    b. delighted
    c. lighthearted
    d. serious

9

8. The main point of this selection can be paraphrased:
   a. Nurses work hard.
   b. The nursing shortage is causing the quality of care in hospitals to suffer.
   c. Paul Duke is going to remain a nurse.
   d. Paul Duke is a great nurse.

9. The purpose of this selection is
   a. to entertain.
   b. to inform.
   c. to persuade.

10. Is the evidence mostly facts, opinions, or a combination of both?
   a. facts
   b. opinions
   c. a combination of both

11. Would you say this evidence is adequate and accurate? Why?
   Answers will vary.

12. The tone of this selection could be described as
   a. amused.
   b. outraged.
   c. sarcastic.
   d. concerned.

Practicing the Active Reading Strategy:
After You Read

Now that you have read the selection, answer the following questions, using the active reading strategies that you learned in Chapter 1.

1. Identify and write down the point and purpose of this reading selection.
2. Besides the vocabulary words included in the exercise on pages 450–451, are there any other vocabulary words that are unfamiliar to you? If so, write a list of them. When you have finished writing your list, look up each word in a dictionary and write the definition that best describes the word as it is used in the selection.
3. Predict any possible test questions that may be used on a test about the content of this selection.

9

4. How could you use the information contained in this selection? Does the information contained in the selection reinforce or contradict your ideas and experiences? Explain.

QUESTIONS FOR DISCUSSION AND WRITING

Answer the following questions based on your reading of the selection. Write your answers on the blanks provided.

1. Why do you think fewer people are choosing to become nurses?

   Answers will vary.

   _____

2. What do you think of the frustrations and stresses that Paul Duke has to deal with on a daily basis as an emergency room nurse? In your own words, discuss why you think his job is particularly stressful.

   Answers will vary.

   _____

3. Nursing is a fairly well-paying job with many rewards. Would you consider nursing as a career? Why or why not? Answers will vary.

   _____

▶ Vocabulary: Figures of Speech

Figures of speech are creative comparisons between things that have something in common. An author uses figures of speech because they are clever, interesting, vivid, and imagistic. In other words, they tend to create pictures, or images, in the reader's mind. An author also includes figures of speech because they help readers understand something new and unfamiliar by comparing it to something already known or understood. Four types of figures of speech are analogies, metaphors, similes, and personification.

An **analogy** is an extended comparison between two things or ideas. Analogies can aid readers in grasping new concepts. For example, look at the following analogy:

There are much better ways to get the acceptance we crave from other people. One of the easiest is what I call "tossing fish." If you've ever

9

been to Sea World, you've probably seen trainers reward the dolphins and seals by feeding them fish. Sea mammals will do anything for anyone who's carrying a bucket of what they love most. They're a lot like people that way—and you just happen to have a bottomless bucket of what humans love most: approval.*

In this passage, humans who seek approval are compared to dolphins and seals who perform for fish. This analogy helps the reader better understand the author's point about the nature of seeking approval from others.

A **simile** is much like an analogy, but briefer. Rather than being developed over several sentences, a simile is usually just a phrase inserted into a sentence. It compares one thing or idea to another by using the word *like* or *as*. For example, look at this example from this chapter:

> *Like a fox in a hen house,* ruthless collectors are plundering Africa's cultural heritage by encouraging poor Africans to sell stolen treasures.

This simile compares collectors to a fox to express the idea that they are stealing and causing havoc just like a hungry predator does.

A **metaphor** makes a more direct comparison by stating that something actually *is* something else rather than just *like* it. For example, read this next sentence:

> Its jaws *are a steel trap:* lower spiked teeth are designed to hold prey while the upper triangular serrated teeth gouge out flesh.

A shark's jaws are not actually a steel trap, but this metaphor says they are to create an interesting and informative comparison.

One last type of figure of speech is **personification**, which compares nonhuman objects or animals to humans by giving them human abilities or characteristics. When we say the wind is *whistling* through the trees or the fire engine's siren *screams* in the night, we are giving the wind and the siren human abilities. Here's another example, which comes from Chapter 8:

> It was an unusual ceremony because all the graduates were convicted felons, and it took place in a gym *embraced* by locked metal gates and razor wire at the Bedford Hills Correctional Facility, a maximum security prison.

In this sentence, the gates and razor wire are given the human ability to embrace.

9

---

* Adapted from Martha Beck, "Equal Encounters of the Human Kind," *O* Magazine, September 2001, 118.

Vocabulary Exercise

The following sentences all come from this chapter and previous chapters. In each one, underline the figure of speech. Then, on the blank provided, write the two things or ideas that are being compared.

1. For these kids, who are just like the fairy tale princess asked to spin straw into gold, homework is just another misery. _Kids doing homework are compared to the fairy tale princess asked to spin straw into gold._

2. On the bank of the Ottawa River, at 6 AM, Colorado Avalanche hockey coach Bob Hartley removed the championship Stanley Cup trophy from its case like a father cradling a baby out of a crib, joking that he thought it was still sleeping. _Trophy is compared to a baby in a crib._

3. About sixty showed up at the docks starting at 5:30 AM to fish with Hartley and the Cup, or at least to help launch his official day with what is arguably professional sports' most storied trophy and the Holy Grail of hockey. _Stanley Cup is compared to the Holy Grail._

4. I love feeling empty, like a hollow gourd. _A person is compared to a gourd._

5. Mother England made the mistake of withholding liberty too long from her "children" in the American colonies. They grew to be rebellious "teenagers" who demanded their freedom. In response, their "mother" refused to release them. As a result, a war had to be fought. _England and America are compared to a mother with children who grow to be rebellious teenagers._

6. When attention dropped, Escalante would begin the "wave," a cheer in which row after row of students, in succession, stood, raising their hands, then sat quickly, creating a ripple across the room like a pennant billowing in victory. _People doing the wave are compared to a pennant billowing in victory._

9

7. <u>The University of Life also requires you to take general education courses.</u>
   Its courses are a little different, however. <u>These courses are offered by
   the Department of Adversities and include subjects like Problems 101,
   Obstacles 203, Mistakes 305, Failures 410, and, for some, a graduate
   course called Catastrophes 599.</u> Life and its hardships are compared to taking
   college courses.

8. You can fake a smile, not admitting to yourself or the group that you have
   any concerns about speaking—ever though <u>your legs have turned to rubber bands</u> and <u>your mind is jelly.</u> The nervous feeling in your legs and your
   state of mind are compared to rubber bands and jelly.

READING STRATEGY: Skimming

When you look at an Internet website for the first time, do you read
every word on your computer screen? Of course not. Instead, your eyes
probably flick around over the pictures and text, reading individual
words or phrases as you try to form a general impression of the site and
its content. You do the same thing when you're standing in a store, deciding whether to buy a magazine. You flip through the pages, glancing
at the titles of the articles and at the pictures as you try to determine if
the magazine is worth your money. This is called *skimming*, and it's also
a useful strategy for reading printed materials.

When you skim a text or a passage, you're not looking for specific
details or information (that's called *scanning*, which is discussed in another chapter). Instead, you're trying to get some sense of the content
and organization. In particular, you skim a reading selection to get an
idea of the author's subject, main point, overall focus, or purpose.

Skimming should never be a substitute for reading. It will not give
you a full understanding of a text or a passage. However, skimming is
useful for three particular purposes: previewing, evaluating a source's
worth or relevancy, and reviewing.

Previewing. Skimming a reading selection—for instance, a chapter in
a textbook or a journal article—will provide you with a "big picture" of
what you're about to read. As a result, when you do finally read the
text, you'll have a framework for understanding the specific details.

Evaluating. Skimming is also useful for research. You don't have time to read every single article you find when you're looking for information about a research topic. Skimming gives you a way to determine if a particular book or article relates to your project and is worth reading in detail later.

Reviewing. Finally, you can skim a text after reading it as a way of reviewing the information. Therefore, skimming can be a valuable technique for studying and remembering information.

To skim a text or a passage, follow these steps:

1. Glance over the title and all of the headings.

2. Quickly read the first sentence of each paragraph. Authors often state their main ideas at the beginnings of paragraphs, so reading these first sentences can help you get a sense of the major points.

3. Quickly move your eyes in a zigzag pattern over the words in the text. At the same time, ask yourself, *What's this about?* and *What's the point?* Try to answer those questions by noticing words or phrases that are highlighted with bold print, italics, or some other kind of distinctive typeface. As you practice skimming, you'll become better at noticing key words or concepts even when they're not highlighted. You'll find that after a while, these words will begin to jump out at you as you run your eyes over the passage.

Follow the three steps described above to skim the following passage from a textbook. Then, answer the questions that follow the passage. Write your answers on the blanks provided.

Understanding Emotional Intelligence

For most of us, life presents bumpy roads now and then. We fail a college course. The job we want goes to someone else. The person we love doesn't return our affections. Our health gives way to sickness. How we handle the resulting emotional distress is critical to the outcomes of our lives.

Success depends on much more than high IQs and academic success. Karen Arnold and Terry Denny at the University of Illinois studied eighty-one valedictorians and salutatorians[1] from the 1981 graduating classes

Continued

9

1. **valedictorians and salutatorians:**
   students with the first and second
   highest academic rank in their class

from Illinois high schools. They found that ten years after graduation, only 25 percent were at the highest level of those of similar age and chosen professions. Actually, many were doing significantly less well. What seems to be missing for these academic stars is **emotional intelligence.**

An experiment during the 1960s shows just how important emotional control is to success. Four-year-old children at a preschool were told that they could have one marshmallow immediately, or if they could wait for about twenty minutes, they could have two. More than a dozen years later, experimenters examined the differences in the lives of the one-marshmallow (emotionally impulsive) children and the two-marshmallow (emotionally intelligent) children. The adolescents who as children were able to delay gratification[1] were found to be superior to their counterparts[2] as high school students and to score an average of 210 points higher on SAT tests. Additionally, the two-marshmallow teenagers had borne fewer children out of wedlock and had experienced fewer problems with the law. Clearly, the ability to endure some emotional discomfort in the present in exchange for greater rewards in the future is a key to success.

Components of Emotional Intelligence

In his book *Emotional Intelligence,* psychologist Daniel Goleman suggests that mastery of our emotions requires the ability to do the following:

1. **Recognize our emotions as they occur.** This ability might seem easy; surprisingly, for many, it is difficult. As children, many of us learned to minimize, maximize, or substitute our emotions. These three emotional patterns will be explained below.

2. **Manage our distressing emotions in a positive way.** This ability allows us to shake off or soothe our emotional upsets so that we can bring reason and purpose to our decisions.

3. **Control impulses and motivate ourselves.** This ability gives us the self-control and willpower necessary to delay gratification, as the two-marshmallow kids did. We learn to sacrifice immediate pleasure for future achievement.

4. **Recognize others' emotions (empathy).** Empathy is demonstrated by such responses as listening actively, respecting differences, and having compassion for others.

1. **gratification:** satisfaction of desires
2. **counterparts:** people in similar situations

5. **Handle feelings that come up in a relationship.** This ability (along with empathy) allows us to develop the relationships that are essential to achieving our greatest success. We demonstrate this ability by positively resolving disagreements, avoiding defensiveness, negotiating compromises, cooperating with others, and avoiding self-righteous judgments.

Knowing Your Own Emotions

The foundation of emotional intelligence is a keen awareness of our emotions as they rise and fall. None of the other abilities can exist without this one. However, three self-defeating patterns learned in childhood too often thwart this ability. *Minimizing* emotions causes people to become numb to their current emotions; minimizers typically say they aren't feeling anything, or they state what they are thinking and, inappropriately, label it a feeling. *Maximizing* emotions causes people to exaggerate their feelings; maximizers become overwhelmed by the flood of their strong emotions. *Substituting* emotions causes people to replace an "unacceptable" emotion with an "acceptable" emotion; substitutors, for example, may express inappropriate anger instead of sadness upon the loss of someone or something important to them.

Here are some steps toward becoming more attuned to your emotions:

- **Build a vocabulary of feelings.** Learn the names of emotions you might experience. There are dozens. How many can you name beyond anger, fear, sadness, and happiness?

- **Be mindful of emotions as they are happening.** Learn to identify and express emotions in the moment. Be aware of the subtleties[1] of emotion, learning to make fine distinctions between similar feelings such as sadness and depression.

- **Understand what is causing your emotion.** Look behind the emotion. See when anger is caused by hurt feelings. Notice when anxiety is caused by irrational thoughts. Realize when sadness is caused by disappointments.

- **Recognize the difference between a feeling and resulting actions.** Feeling an emotion is one thing; acting on the emotion is quite

Continued

9

1. **subtleties:** fine distinctions or characteristics

another. Emotions and behaviors are separate experiences, one internal, one external. Note when you tend to confuse the two, as a student did who said, "My teacher made me so upset [that] I had to drop the class." One can be upset with a teacher and remain enrolled in the class.

You will never reach your full potential without emotional intelligence. No matter how academically bright you may be, emotional illiteracy will limit how much you achieve. Emotions that run wild can destroy you; emotions that fuel motivation and guide your wise choices can propel you successfully to your goals and dreams.*

1. What is the topic of this entire passage? <u>Emotional intelligence</u>

2. According to the headings, what two aspects of the topic are discussed in this passage? <u>Components of emotional intelligence and knowing your own emotions</u>

3. How many components of emotional intelligence are covered in this passage? <u>5</u>

4. Skim the first paragraph of the section labeled "Knowing Your Own Emotions" by reading the topic sentence and then running your eyes in a zigzag pattern over the rest of the paragraph. Then answer this question: What are the self-defeating patterns that interfere with emotional intelligence? <u>Minimizing, maximizing, and substituting</u>

5. How many steps should you complete in order to become more attuned to your own emotions? <u>4</u>

9

* From *On Course,* 4th ed., by Skip Downing, 195–197. Copyright © 2005. Reprinted by permission of Houghton Mifflin Company.

Name _____ Date _____

TEST 1

A. Read the following questions carefully and then respond to them by circling the letter of each correct answer.

1. Which of the following is a fact?

   a. Most computers use Microsoft Windows.
   b. Microsoft has too much power over computers.
   c. Microsoft is the computer user's best friend.
   d. Everybody uses Microsoft Windows.

2. Which of the following is an opinion?

   a. Tiger Woods is one of today's best golfers.
   b. Tiger Woods worked hard to develop his championship skills.
   c. Tiger Woods is the best golfer who ever lived.
   d. Tiger Woods has a lot of commercial endorsements.

3. Which of the following is a fact?

   a. Ashley's abnormal liking for seafood is disgusting.
   b. Nobody eats seafood more often than Ashley.
   c. Ashley must get her seafood for free.
   d. Ashley usually eats seafood twice a week.

4. Which of the following is an opinion?

   a. Cell phones are dangerous.
   b. One study has shown that the normal radiation emitted by cell phones has been harmful to rats.
   c. Other studies in humans have shown no difference in cancer rates between those who use cell phones and those who don't.
   d. Many people regularly use cell phones these days.

5. Which of the following is a fact?

   a. I just hate it when it's really hot outside.
   b. It was 95 degrees in the shade yesterday.

For additional tests, see the Test Bank.

9

   c. I prefer to stay inside when it's super-hot outside.
   d. Air conditioning was mankind's greatest invention.

B. Read the following passages and then respond to the questions that follow by circling the letter of each correct answer.

I. Sunlight may be a key prescription for easing surgical pain and saving millions of dollars in hospital pharmacy costs, according to a new study. Surgery patients in rooms with lots of natural light took less pain medication, and their drug costs ran 21 percent less than those for equally ill patients assigned to darker rooms. Those in the brighter rooms also had lower stress levels and said they felt less pain the day after surgery and at discharge, says Bruce Rabin, a physician and immunologist[1] at the University of Pittsburgh. It's thought to be the first evidence that sunlight can affect the perception of pain. Bright light has been shown to improve mood, says Russell Portenoy, chairman of the department of pain medicine at Beth Israel Medical Center in New York, "so mood may be what's leading them to use less pain medication." Bright light triggers the release of "feel good" brain chemicals such as serotonin, some research has found.*

6. The purpose of this passage is

   (a.) to inform.
    b. to persuade.

7. The author's idea or opinion is

    a. informed.
   (b.) uninformed.

   II. (1) The role of deer predator is an apt[2] one for humans. (2) We are biologically specialized for hunting game and can do it accurately and well. (3) When it comes to the predation[3] of small animals, we are not so well equipped. (4) Our ears aren't attuned to grubs chewing on a root. (5) Our noses are too dull to sniff mice hiding in a hole. (6) I really hate those bug zappers that buzz and blink near swimming pools and patios, creating unnecessary holes in the nocturnal[4] community of insects. (7) They kill insects that navigate by

---

9

1. **immunologist:** one who studies the immune system
2. **apt:** suitable; appropriate
3. **predation:** killing and eating
4. **nocturnal:** active at night

---

* Adapted from Marilyn Elias, "Sunlight Reduces Need for Pain Medication," *USA Today,* March 3, 2004, 7D.

celestial[1] light or orient toward brightness, such as moths that guide their course by moonlight or search for pale blossoms blooming in the night. (8) Mosquitoes out for blood are guided by the exhalations[2] of their victims. (9) They don't fly to light, so they aren't electrocuted by zappers.*

8. The purpose of this passage is

    a. to inform.
    (b.) to persuade.

9. The author's idea or opinion is

    a. informed.
    (b.) uninformed.

III. (1) Our city block has become a much more pleasant place in the last few years. (2) I think it's because some of us in the block association made a big push to plant trees on the block. (3) I'm also pleased that the trees we planted are steadily growing and seem to be very healthy. (4) We deliberately selected the types of trees that have proven to withstand and even flourish[3] in an urban environment. (5) In fact, now that we know this has been a success, I think we should plant even more trees on the block to fill in the gaps.

10. The purpose of this passage is

    a. to inform.
    (b.) to persuade.

11. The author's idea or opinion is

    a. informed.
    (b.) uninformed.

IV. All cultures in this country need to realize that Native Americans should not be forgotten. They are a proud people whose heritage means a lot to them. Most Americans forget that it was the Native Americans who were here first. As our immigrant ancestors dealt with them, there was a lot of fighting and bloodshed. Still, though, Native Americans contributed much to our history and our country. Who has taken the time to visit an Indian reservation today? If people did, they would see Native Americans living in poverty and unhealthy conditions. Native Americans deserve so much better, and we should not stand by and do nothing.

1. **celestial:** related to the sky or heavens   3. **flourish:** thrive
2. **exhalations:** acts of breathing out
   and expelling air

9

* From Sara Stein, *Noah's Garden* (Boston: Houghton Mifflin Co., 1993), 83.

12. The purpose of this passage is

   a. to inform.
   b. to persuade.

13. The author's idea or opinion is

   a. informed.
   b. uninformed.

TEST 2

A. Read each of the following statements and then respond to the questions that follow by circling the letter of each correct answer.

Many schools in our district are unruly and even dangerous.

1. Which of the following words indicates the author's bias?

   a. schools   c. dangerous
   b. district   d. even

2. Does the author's choice of words make you feel positive or negative about the subject?

   a. positive   b. negative

The dancers in our local ballet company are highly trained and beautiful to watch when they perform.

3. Which of the following words indicates the author's bias?

   a. dancer   c. beautiful
   b. local   d. perform

4. Does the author's choice of words make you feel positive or negative about the subject?

   a. positive   b. negative

Rebuilding a 100-story building on the World Trade Center[1] site would lead to economic destruction to the downtown New York City area

1. **World Trade Center:** buildings that were destroyed when terrorists attacked the United States on September 11, 2001

9

because nobody will want to rent out the higher, and more vulnerable, floors of the building.

5. Which of the following word or words indicate(s) the author's bias?

a. destruction   c. rebuilding
b. downtown   d. would lead to

6. Does the author's choice of words make you feel positive or negative about the subject?

a. positive   b. negative

B. Select the statement that reveals the author's bias by circling the letter of the correct answer.

7. a. Our country is dependent on fossil fuels for energy.
b. Our country relies much too heavily on fossil fuels for energy.
c. Our country must import a substantial portion of the oil it uses.
d. Our country used to produce all the fossil fuels it needed.

8. a. The property taxes in our town primarily go toward paying for our local schools' expenses and educators' salaries.
b. The property taxes in our town have gone up every year for the past eight years.
c. The property taxes in our town are determined by our town council.
d. The property taxes in our town are ridiculously high and keep going up with no end in sight.

9. a. Many people do not like to receive telemarketing calls.
b. Donna is normally very polite and friendly to telemarketers when they call.
c. Joan gets justifiably angry when a rude telemarketer calls during dinner.
d. People have different ways of saying "no" to a telemarketer.

C. Read the following passages and then respond to the questions that follow by circling the letter of each correct answer.

10. The great Hollywood film mogul[1] Samuel Goldwyn was the owner of the Goldwyn Picture Company. But the company was not in fact named for Goldwyn, but rather he for it. His real name was Schmuel Gelbfisz, though for his first thirty years in America he had called himself—perhaps a little unwisely—Samuel Goldfish. "Goldwyn" was a combination

9

1. **mogul:** rich or powerful person

of the names of the studio's two founders: Samuel Goldfish and Edgar Selwyn. It wasn't until 1918, tired of being the butt of endless fishbowl jokes, that he named himself after his corporation.*

What is the tone of the passage?

a. critical
b. sarcastic

c. insulting
d. neutral (circled)

11. Boot camp was actually one of the most enjoyable experiences of my life. I think I liked it so much because it was so well organized. The first week we were there, we ran everywhere, even to and from the bathroom and the shower. At the cafeteria, we'd wait in the chow line for several minutes until we finally were able to get some food on our plates; then one minute after we sat down to eat, our company commander would say we had to get started running to our next class. Even sleeping was highly organized. Our beds were closely inspected every day for wrinkles and improper folds. The problem was that we didn't have time to fold everything properly, and who knew how to fold it anyway? So we all got to experience the pleasure of sleeping on the floor under our beds.

What is the tone of the passage?

a. critical
b. sarcastic (circled)

c. insulting
d. neutral

12. You men know you need a bigger TV. And you know who is standing in your way: your wife. The instant you tell her you need a new TV, she's going to start coming up with nit-picky legalistic arguments like "But our current TV works fine!" Or "But we bought a new TV yesterday!" Or "But we're broke and we live in a homeless shelter!"

Women! Always ruled by their emotions. But you CAN overcome your wife's resistance, men, if you (a) take the time to listen—really listen—to her objections; then (b) respond patiently and sincerely, without resorting to browbeating; then (c) when she falls asleep, smash your current TV screen with a brick.†

What is the tone of the passage?

a. angry
b. worried

c. amused (circled)
d. frightened

9

* Adapted from Bill Bryson, *Made in America* (New York: Avon Books, 1994), 255.
† "How to Negotiate Way to a Bigger TV" by Dave Barry. Reprinted by permission of TMS Reprints.

CHAPTER 10
Reading Longer Selections

GOALS FOR CHAPTER 10

▶ Define the term *thesis statement*.

▶ Recognize the topic and thesis statement of longer reading selections.

▶ Define the term *headings* and explain the purpose of headings.

▶ Identify major and minor supporting details in longer reading selections.

▶ Determine implied main ideas in longer reading selections.

▶ Recognize patterns of organization in longer reading selections.

▶ Identify transitions in longer reading selections.

▶ Explain the difference between skimming and scanning, and scan a text for information.

Now that you've practiced improving your comprehension of paragraphs, you are ready to move on to reading longer passages. To see how well you already comprehend longer selections, complete the following test.

TEST YOURSELF

As you continue in your academic career, you will be asked to read longer and more challenging selections, most of which will come from textbooks. Take some time to do this test and warm up for the longer, more challenging readings you will encounter in the rest of this chapter. Read the passage that follows and then respond to the questions by circling the letter of each correct answer. If you come across any difficult or unfamiliar words, consult your dictionary.

10

ELIMINATE SEXUAL HARASSMENT

1 One of the most sensitive problems between men and women in organizations is **sexual harassment**, or unwelcome verbal or physical behavior that affects a person's job performance or work environment. Most people believe sexual harassment is a problem for women only, but each year a large number of sexual harassment cases are filed by men. Research indicates that 90 percent of Fortune 500 companies have dealt with sexual harassment complaints from their workers. It is estimated that the problem costs the average large corporation $6.7 million a year in increased absenteeism, staff turnover, low morale, and low productivity.

2 Under the law, sexual harassment may take one of two forms. The first is *quid pro quo* (something for something), which occurs when a person in a powerful position threatens the job security or a potential promotion of a worker who refuses to submit to sexual advances. These kinds of threats are absolutely prohibited, and employers are liable for damages under the Fair Employment Practices section of the Civil Rights Act. These behaviors can take the form of comments of a personal or sexual nature, unwanted touching and feeling, or demands for sexual favors.

3 The second form of sexual harassment involves the existence of a **hostile work environment**. Supreme Court decisions have held that sexual harassment exists if a "reasonable person" believes that the behavior is sufficiently severe or pervasive to create an abusive working environment, even if the victim does not get fired or held back from a promotion. A hostile work environment exists when supervisors or coworkers use sexual innuendo,[1] tell sexually oriented jokes, display sexually explicit photos in the work area, discuss sexual exploits,[2] and so on. Unlike *quid pro quo* harassment, hostile work environment claims tend to fall in a gray area: What is offensive to one person may not be offensive to another. The bottom line is that most kinds of sexually explicit language, conduct, and behavior are inappropriate in the workplace, regardless of whether such conduct constitutes sexual harassment within the legal meaning of the term.*

1. What is the topic of this selection?

   a. *quid pro quo*   c. hostile work environments
   b. sexual harassment   d. the workplace

1. **innuendo:** suggestion or hint   2. **exploits:** experiences or adventures

---

* Excerpted from Barry L. Reece and Rhonda Brandt, *Effective Human Relations in Organizations*, 7th ed. (Boston: Houghton Mifflin Co., 1999), 437.

10

2. Which of the following is a *major* supporting detail from the selection?

 a. "Under the law, sexual harassment may take one of two forms." (paragraph 2)
 b. "The first is *quid pro quo* (something for something), which occurs when a person in a powerful position threatens the job security or a potential promotion of a worker who refuses to submit to sexual advances." (paragraph 2)
 c. "These behaviors can take the form of comments of a personal or sexual nature, unwanted touching and feeling, or demands for sexual favors." (paragraph 2)
 d. "A hostile work environment exists when supervisors or coworkers use sexual innuendo, tell sexually oriented jokes, display sexually explicit photos in the work area, discuss sexual exploits, and so on." (paragraph 3)

3. Which of the following is a *minor* supporting detail from the selection?

 a. "Under the law, sexual harassment may take one of two forms." (paragraph 2)
 b. "The first is *quid pro quo* (something for something), which occurs when a person in a powerful position threatens the job security or a potential promotion of a worker who refuses to submit to sexual advances." (paragraph 2)
 c. "These kinds of threats are absolutely prohibited, and employers are liable for damages under the Fair Employment Practices section of the Civil Rights Act." (paragraph 2)
 d. "The second form of sexual harassment involves the existence of a hostile work environment." (paragraph 3)

4. What pattern organizes the *major* supporting details in this selection?

 a. cause/effect   c. time order
 b. comparison/contrast   d. series

5. What is the tone of this selection?

 a. annoyed   c. amused
 b. neutral   d. sarcastic

So far, this book has focused mainly on helping you improve your reading comprehension by awareness and understanding of important features in *paragraphs*. But what about longer selections, those that are composed of multiple paragraphs? You may be wondering if you'll have to learn a whole new set of concepts in order to understand long selections such as chapters or articles. Fortunately, the answer is no. Many of the same principles apply to

10

reading longer passages. This chapter, therefore, will focus on applying the information you've already learned in previous chapters to help you get more out of a reading composed of more than one paragraph.

Topic, Main Idea, and Thesis

In Chapter 2 of this book, you learned about topics, main ideas, and topic sentences. Like paragraphs, longer reading selections contain all three of these elements. A longer selection such as an essay or an article will be about a topic, and it will make a point about that topic just as a paragraph's topic sentence states the main idea.

However, in a longer reading selection, the main point is usually referred to as a thesis. The **thesis** is the one idea or opinion the author wants readers to know or to believe after they have read the piece. Just like the paragraph's topic sentence, the thesis includes the subject plus what is being said about that subject. You'll notice when you read the following thesis statements that they sound a lot like topic sentences.

> Although memory lapses[1] are normal, following certain strategies will help improve your ability to recall information.

> Modern archeologists[2] are making discoveries that affirm the historical truth of biblical stories in both the Old and New Testaments.

> People in drug or alcohol detoxification[3] programs, chemotherapy patients, and patients suffering from chronic pain can all benefit from acupuncture.[4]

Rather than being developed in one paragraph, however, a thesis statement generally presents an idea that needs several paragraphs of explanation. It is often a point that is broader than one you would see in a topic sentence. That is why it takes longer to explain.

The thesis statement almost always appears near the beginning of the selection, most often in the opening paragraph. It is the main idea that will be developed throughout the rest of the piece. It may be useful here to recall what you learned about the terms *general* and *specific*. These concepts apply to longer readings, too. Just as paragraphs include a general topic and a specific point about that topic, longer selections also focus on one particular idea about a broader subject.

1. **lapses:** failures
2. **archaeologists:** people who study the remains of past human life and culture
3. **detoxification:** process of removing the poisons from something or someone
4. **acupuncture:** inserting needles into the body at certain points to relieve pain

10

To find the thesis statement, determine first what the subject is. What does the opening paragraph seem to be about? Then look for a sentence that includes both this topic and a particular point about that topic.

A longer selection will still include topic sentences, too. Each paragraph will present a particular idea, just like those you studied in Chapter 2, and many of these paragraphs will state the point in a topic sentence that appears at the beginning, in the middle, or at the end of the paragraph. The major difference, however, is that these paragraphs do not stand alone; instead, they are smaller units within a larger whole.

For an illustration of how a longer selection includes a topic, a thesis statement, and topic sentences, read the following passage.

Will Your Hotel Be Super-safe?

If your summer vacation plans include a hotel stay, you have a lot of company. Americans spent over $300 billion on hotels last year. And, of course, you want to stay in (the safest hotel.) Well, you can make sure you do by asking some simple questions when you call for reservations. The safest hotels (those where crime rarely happens) have five features.   **TOPIC / THESIS**

Magnetic cards or cards with punch holes are much safer than room keys, say experts. Management changes these cards every time someone checks out, and with them, the hotel can track who goes in and out. Plus, they don't show your room number like most keys do, so potential thieves won't see where you're staying.   **TOPIC SENTENCE**

The second floor is definitely the safest, so try to get a room on that level. The first floor makes your room accessible from the windows while higher floors can present problems if there's a fire. And avoid rooms around corners and at the end of dead-end hallways. You want a room with lots of traffic, lots of light, and more than one direction to go in case you need to get out fast.   **TOPIC SENTENCE**

Safe hotels include some type of deadbolt lock on the inside of room doors. Just like in your home, they add extra protection at night while you're asleep.   **TOPIC SENTENCE**

The safest hotels staff their premises with more than just one employee during the night shift. You want a security guard working there at all times, not just a manager doubling as security.   **TOPIC SENTENCE**

In a safe hotel, you can get to your room only through the lobby. Staying in a hotel with only one entrance cuts your risk of robbery by half because intruders can't slip in unnoticed.*   **TOPIC SENTENCE**

In longer selections, sections of the text will often be labeled with headings. **Headings** are like mini-titles that identify the topic of one part of a

* Adapted from Rosemarie Lenner, "Will Your Hotel Room Be Super-safe?" *Woman's Day,* June 19, 2001, 17. Reprinted by permission of *Woman's Day.*

10

longer work like a chapter or an article. They help the reader understand the focus of a particular section of text, and they also reveal how various sections are related to each other. For example, look at the following passage.

Help Children Succeed at School

Parenting children through their school years requires a balancing act between what's best for family dynamics and for a child's academic success.

Dr. Andrea Pastorok, an educational psychologist with Kumon Math and Reading Centers, offers these tips to help parents avoid five common mistakes when dealing with a child's scholastic achievement:

1. **Expecting perfection instead of progress.** If you only praise your child when he completes a task or reaches a goal, he may give up long before he ever gets there. Demonstrate to your child that you believe in him by giving genuine and frequent praise for progress and effort.

2. **Allowing your child to quit whenever the work gets hard.** Encourage your child to persevere when schoolwork becomes challenging by becoming her coach to get her through the tough spots. Help her to take a one-step-at-a-time approach. Work with her to identify the information needed to solve problems and pinpoint places where she gets "stuck."

3. **Underestimating your child's ability.** Don't assume your child will be weak in a subject because you were, and don't underestimate his abilities. Expect your child to reach his potential in all subjects, not just the ones that are easiest. If your child is struggling in math but loves reading, help your child discover new ways to enjoy math. However, keep your expectations realistic.

4. **Allowing your child to be disorganized.** To ensure that children will become successful students, parents must help them acquire good study habits and strong organizational skills. Start by creating a special learning area at home; set aside time for homework and reading. For older children, teach them to organize their time by using a calendar or planner.

5. **Refusing to admit that your child is capable of wrongdoing.** Children are individuals, and no matter how hard we try to raise smart, honest, and caring children, they will make mistakes or poor decisions. If a teacher, friend, or parent brings to your attention your child's behavior, don't deny it. Listen. Depending on the

10

situation, speak to your child about the incident in the privacy of your home and decide the best way to handle it.*

The previous passage describes five common mistakes parents make. Each mistake is numbered and discussed in a separate paragraph. Each of these paragraphs has a mini-title, in bold print, that reveals its topic.

Exercise 10.1

Read the selection below and then respond to the questions that follow by circling the letter of each correct answer.

Ford's Road Map for a Healthier Environment

1　Henry Ford knew that environmental protection is a journey, not a destination. A nature lover as well as an industrialist, the founder of Ford Motor Company was a firm believer in conserving the planet's resources. As early as the 1920s, he was showing concern for the environment by recycling wood scraps and sawdust for fuel and selectively harvesting trees to prevent deforestation.[1] Today's environmental challenges are even more complex, yet all over the world Ford is finding ways to control pollution and recycle materials.

2　One challenge is to meet government mandates[2] for reducing harmful fuel emissions[3] by developing alternative-fuel vehicles and electric vehicles. In response, Ford has created the Flexible Fuel Taurus car, the Ecostar electric van, the Ranger EV electric vehicle, and other experimental vehicles. Long-term tests are underway to determine whether these fuel-efficient vehicles can live up to real-world driving conditions.

3　A second challenge is to put recycling to work throughout the entire life cycle of a vehicle. In the manufacturing phase, Ford is incorporating more and more parts made from recycled materials. The company has also established a recycling research center in Cologne, Germany, where experts study ways of building cars that can be easily dismantled[4] for recycling. Because each model line must meet increasingly stricter internal standards for recoverability of parts, recycling has become an integral[5] part of the design and manufacturing process of every Ford vehicle.

1. **deforestation:** cutting down of trees
2. **mandates:** requirements
3. **emissions:** substances released into the air
4. **dismantled:** taken apart
5. **integral:** essential or necessary

* Adapted from "Help Children Succeed at School," as viewed in *The Charlotte Observer,* February 11, 2004, 2A.

10

4   In Europe, recycling is a major cornerstone of Ford's corporate citizenship program. The company's "Clean and Safe" campaign was the first to offer German customers cash in exchange for older cars without catalysts;[1] the vehicles go to a network of dismantlers who have been trained to remove fluids and recyclable parts without damaging the environment. A similar program in Belgium offers financial incentives[2] to customers who turn in old cars and buy new Ford cars.

5   A third challenge is to reduce or recycle wastes in factories around the world. Ford plants in North America have found innovative[3] ways of recycling wastes. For example, plants in Cleveland, Ohio, and Windsor, Ontario, use sand for casting molds to make engine blocks and other car components.[4] In the past, the factories sent the sand to landfills once the casting process was complete; these days, the factories recycle the sand for use in paving and building materials.

6   Given Ford's long and active role in safeguarding the environment, the company is not about to put on the brakes. Indeed, its socially responsible environmental programs are only going to pick up speed as Ford drives into the new millennium.[5]*

1. What is the topic of this selection?
   a. Henry Ford
   b. environmental challenges
   (c.) environmental programs at Ford Motor Company
   d. electric cars

2. Which of the following sentences states the thesis of this selection?
   a. "Henry Ford knew that environmental protection is a journey, not a destination." (paragraph 1)
   (b.) "Today's environmental challenges are even more complex, yet all over the world Ford is finding ways to control pollution and recycle materials." (paragraph 1)
   c. "A second challenge is to put recycling to work throughout the entire life cycle of a vehicle." (paragraph 3)
   d. "Given Ford's long and active role in safeguarding the environment, the company is not about to put on the brakes." (paragraph 6)

1. **catalysts:** devices that convert the pollution in automotive exhaust to carbon dioxide and water
2. **incentives:** rewards

3. **innovative:** new
4. **components:** parts
5. **millennium:** period spanning 1,000 years

---

* Adapted from William Pride, Robert Hughes, Jack Kapoor, *Business*, 6th ed. (Boston: Houghton Mifflin Co., 1999), 30.

10

3. Which of the following functions as a topic sentence in this selection?

   a. "Henry Ford knew that environmental protection is a journey, not a destination." (paragraph 1)

   b. "Long-term tests are underway to determine whether these fuel-efficient vehicles can live up to real-world driving conditions." (paragraph 2)

   c. "Today's environmental challenges are even more complex, yet all over the world Ford is finding ways to control pollution and recycle materials." (paragraph 1)

   (d.) "A third challenge is to reduce or recycle wastes in factories around the world." (paragraph 5)

Supporting Details

Longer reading selections also contain both major and minor supporting details, just as paragraphs do. The following diagram summarizes how the parts of a paragraph correspond to those of many longer selections. Each box represents a different paragraph.

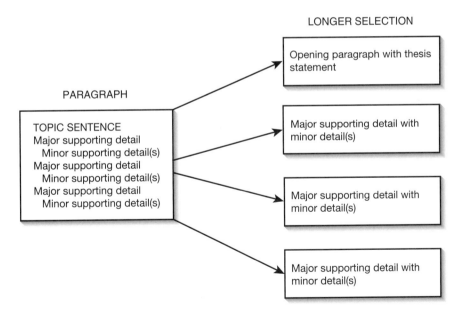

In other words, a longer selection spreads the major supporting details over several paragraphs. Each of these major details is the topic of a separate paragraph, and each is developed with the examples, anecdotes, explanations, or other information that functions as minor details. Here is an example of a longer selection that labels the major and minor details.

10

Add Ten Years to Your Life Just by Loving a Pet

Almost 60 percent of us house, feed, and care for a furry, finned, or feathered friend—and in return they give us unconditional love. But pet ownership brings more than just warm fuzzies: studies have documented that caring for a pet relieves stress, depression, and even pain.

THESIS

"Now the latest research suggests that the health benefits go even deeper than that," says animal ecologist Alan Beck, ScD, at Purdue University. In fact, experts now say just having a pet in the house can improve your health in several more significant ways.

MAJOR DETAIL

First of all, pet ownership can lower your blood pressure and cholesterol. In one National Institutes of Health (NIH) study, just interacting with animals caused an eight-point drop in blood pressure—enough to reduce the risk of stroke 15 percent. And another NIH study showed that animal owners have 13 percent lower cholesterol than those without pets! "We believe these benefits are due to the fact that pets help lower our production of damaging stress hormones," says Beck, author of *Between Pets and People.*

Minor Details

The health payoff can be dramatic: in one study, pet owners were four times less likely to have a heart attack—and 78 percent less likely to have a second one if they'd already had one.

MAJOR DETAIL

Owning a pet can also get you in better shape—effortlessly. Only one in four Americans gets enough exercise, but research shows pet owners—especially dog owners—are twice as likely to exercise regularly. "Walking a dog on a leash actually burns 75 more calories per hour than walking alone because dogs keep people moving at a more energetic pace," says Beck.

Minor Details

MAJOR DETAIL

Finally, pets can strengthen your immune system—and lengthen your life. Studies show that 74 percent of people feel healthier if they have a pet, and need to see their doctor 21 percent less often. Doctors believe that's because by reducing depression and anxiety and lowering stress hormones like cortisol, pets help strengthen our immune defenses against colds, flu, infections—even major diseases.

Minor Details

Research suggests even gazing at goldfish helps reduce stress-related headaches, cold sores, and other chronic[1] infections. Toss in the benefits of pet-lowered blood pressure and cholesterol, and doctors say that could add up to ten years to your life!*

Minor Details

1. **chronic:** continuing or occurring frequently

* Adapted from Caitlin Castro, "Add 10 Years to Your Life by Loving a Pet!" *Woman's Day*, June 26, 2001, 16. Reprinted by permission of *Woman's Day*.

10

In this selection, three of the topic sentences announce major supporting details, the three health benefits mentioned in the thesis statement. Then, each major detail is developed with one or two paragraphs of minor details.

Exercise 10.2

Read the selection below and then respond to the questions that follow by circling the letter of each correct answer.

McGregor's Theory X and Theory Y

1   In most organizations, day-to-day operations are significantly influenced by the relationship between workers and managers. One management consultant, Douglas McGregor, believes that many managers do not understand or accept the idea that workers are motivated by different kinds of needs. McGregor's influential book *The Human Side of Enterprise* outlines a set of assumptions that he says influence the thinking of most managers. He divides these assumptions into two categories: Theory X and Theory Y.

2   Theory X represents a pessimistic[1] view of human nature. According to this theory, people do not really want to work. They have to be pushed, closely supervised, and prodded into doing things, either with incentives[2] such as pay or with punishments for not working. Because they have little or no ambition, workers prefer to avoid responsibility and do only as much work as they have to. The general belief of management under this theory is that workers are paid to do a good job and that management's function is to supervise the work and correct employees if they go off course.

3   Theory Y reflects an optimistic[3] view of human behavior. According to this theory, work is as natural to people as play or rest. People are capable of self-direction and can learn both to accept and seek responsibility if they are committed to the objectives[4] of the organization. Another Theory Y assumption is that people will become committed to organizational objectives if they are rewarded for doing so.

4   A healthy, mutually supportive relationship based on trust, openness, and respect can create a work climate in which employees want to give more of themselves. Goethe, the German poet and philosopher, may have said it best: "Trust people as if they were what they ought to be and you help them become what they are capable of being."*

1. **pessimistic:** tending to stress the negative or take a gloomy view
2. **incentives:** motivators
3. **optimistic:** tending to expect the best possible outcome
4. **objectives:** goals

* Adapted from Barry L. Reece and Rhonda Brandt, *Effective Human Relations in Organizations,* 7th ed. (Boston: Houghton Mifflin Co., 1999), 183.

10

1. What is the topic of this selection?

    a. Douglas McGregor
    b. Theory X and Theory Y
    c. management
    d. optimism and pessimism

2. Which of the following sentences states the thesis of this selection?

    a. "He divides these assumptions into two categories: Theory X and Theory Y." (paragraph 1)
    b. "Theory X represents a pessimistic view of human nature." (paragraph 2)
    c. "Goethe, the German poet and philosopher, may have said it best: 'Trust people as if they were what they ought to be and you help them become what they are capable of being.'" (paragraph 4)
    d. "Because they have little or no ambition, workers prefer to avoid responsibility and do only as much work as they have to." (paragraph 2)

3. Which of the following sentences offers a *major* supporting detail?

    a. "He divides these assumptions into two categories: Theory X and Theory Y." (paragraph 1)
    b. "Theory Y reflects an optimistic view of human behavior." (paragraph 3)
    c. "Another Theory Y assumption is that people will become committed to organizational objectives if they are rewarded for doing so." (paragraph 3)
    d. "People are capable of self-direction and can learn both to accept and seek responsibility if they are committed to the objectives of the organization." (paragraph 3)

4. Which of the following is a *minor* supporting detail?

    a. "He divides these assumptions into two categories: Theory X and Theory Y." (paragraph 1)
    b. "Theory X represents a pessimistic view of human nature." (paragraph 2)
    c. "The general belief of management under this theory is that workers are paid to do a good job and that management's function is to supervise the work and correct employees if they go off course." (paragraph 2)
    d. "Theory Y reflects an optimistic view of human behavior." (paragraph 3)

Implied Main Ideas

In Chapter 4 of this book, you learned to determine the main idea of a paragraph when it is not actually stated. Longer selections, too, will occasionally ask you to infer the author's overall point. You do this using the same procedure you used for paragraphs; however, you make adjustments for the multiple

10

paragraphs. Instead of examining the topic of each sentence, for instance, you study the topic and point of each *topic sentence* and then add up those details to draw your conclusion. For example, read the following passage.

The Awesome Power of Volcanoes

A volcanic explosion can spew[1] rocks into the air up to 800 mph, and toss large boulders like pebbles—for miles. When Indonesia's Tambora volcano exploded in 1815, for example, it killed over 10,000 people. Then the ash falling from the sky piled so thick that it ruined crops, and more than 80,000 people perished[2] from famine and disease. The gases and dust emitted into the atmosphere brought the "year without a summer" in New England and may have inspired the red skies painted by J. M. W. Turner.[3]

Seven decades later, Krakatau, another Indonesian volcano, erupted and much of the island collapsed. The explosion produced a 100-foot-high tsunami[4] that wiped out some 36,000 people on nearby shores. As recently as 1985, the relatively small eruption of Nevado del Ruiz in Colombia dropped some 20 million cubic meters of hot ash and rocks on its ice cap. This melting ice created massive mudflows that buried the nearby town of Armero, killing more than 23,000 people.

It can take 10,000 years for molten[5] rock to inch its way to the earth's surface, but once it does, volcano building can be surprisingly rapid. One day in 1943, volcanic steam began rising from a cornfield in Mexico. Within 24 hours, a 150-foot volcano punctuated the field. A year later it had grown to more than 1,000 feet. Closer to home, the blast of Mount St. Helens, Washington, in 1980 killed 57 people—a comparatively low number of deaths—but it made up in property damage what it spared in lives. The eruption cost nearby residents, businesses, and industries an estimated $1 billion.*

This selection never actually states a thesis, but you can infer that it means to suggest that volcanic eruptions can cause devastating losses in property and human lives. You arrive at that conclusion by looking first at the topic of each

---

1. **spew:** force out; eject forcefully
2. **perished:** died
3. **J.M.W. Turner:** 19th century British painter
4. **tsunami:** very large ocean wave caused by an earthquake or volcanic eruption
5. **molten:** melted

---

* Excerpted from "The Awesome Power of Volcanoes" by William Garvey. Reprinted with permission from *Reader's Digest*, May 2001. Copyright © 2001 by The Reader's Digest Assn., Inc.

10

paragraph. Each topic is a different volcano. Next, what is being said about each one? The details presented all relate to the specific kinds of damage these volcanoes caused when they erupted. Therefore, you can conclude that the whole passage says that volcanic eruptions can be very destructive.

Exercise 10.3

Read the passage below and then respond to the questions that follow by circling the letter of each correct answer.

A Very Lucky Daughter

1   I should have been just another face in the hotel lobby in Zhangjiajie, a city in central China. But my words singled me out.

2   "*Yun dou*," I repeated to the clerk. Maybe he understood English: "Do you have a gym here?"

3   The clerk blinked, and then reached behind the counter and pulled out an iron.

4   I smiled blankly. My brain rooted through my limited Chinese vocabulary. Just then my dad strolled up, his eyebrows arched in amused triangles.

5   "She wants to know where the gym is," he supplied in rapid Mandarin Chinese, his native language. He turned to me and explained gently, "*Yun dong* is exercise, Sharon. *Yun dou* means iron."

6   I mumbled a sheepish[1] apology to the laughing clerk and glanced at my dad. A look of recognition flashed through his eyes. We'd gone through this before. Only this time, the tables were turned.

7   When I was younger, I would try to imagine my parents growing up in China and Taiwan. But I could only envision them in the grainy black-and-white of their faded childhood pictures. Their childhood stories didn't match the people I knew. I couldn't picture my domestic mom, unsure of her halting English, studying international economics at a Taiwanese university. I laughed at the image of my stern father, an electrical engineer, chasing after chickens in his Chinese village.

8   I related to my parents' pre-American lives as only a series of events, like facts for some history exam. My dad fled to Taiwan in 1949 as a 14-year-old, after the Communists[2] won the civil war. His father fought for the losing side, the Nationalists.[3] My mom's father, a Nationalist navy captain, also retreated

---

1. **sheepish:** embarrassed
2. **Communists:** people who support government control of the economy
3. **Nationalists:** people who want their country to remain independent from foreign influence

10

to Taiwan. My mom, who was born in Taiwan, grew up thinking that her family would eventually return to China, after the Nationalists reclaimed their homeland.

9   But that didn't happen. As young adults, my parents moved to the United States to lead better lives. They did not step onto Chinese soil for more than 50 years. Then their friends arranged a trip to China. And they asked me to join them on the six-city tour.

10   My list of why-nots was jam-packed. And yet something inside—I could not explain what—urged me to go.

11   When the plane jerked to a stop in Shanghai, our first destination, all of those reasons I decided to go materialized in the expression on my parents' faces. My mom folded and unfolded her hands impatiently in her lap. I was surprised and slightly scared to see my stoic[1] dad's eyes glimmering with emotion. He slipped his hand, soft and spotted with age, in mine.

12   "Last time I was here," he said, "my parents going from north to south, away from the Communists. So much bombing. A lot of people starving." He leaned close. "You very lucky, Sharon."

13   That was my dad's line. When I would whine as a child, my dad's response was inevitable: "Some people not as lucky as you."

14   But I never cared about being lucky. I just wanted to be like the other American kids.

15   My parents, however, intended me to become a model Chinese American. Starting when I was six, they would drag me away from Saturday cartoons to a Chinese church. I would squirm like a worm in my seat while a teacher recited Chinese vocabulary. I dutifully recited my *bo po mo fos*—the ABCs of speaking Mandarin. But in my head, I rearranged the chalk marks that made up the characters into pictures of houses and trees.

16   When I turned nine, I declared I wasn't going to Chinese school anymore. "This stinks," I yelled. "None of my friends have to go to extra school. Why do I have to go?"

17   "Because you Chinese," my mom replied coolly.

18   "Then I don't want to be Chinese," I shouted back. "It's not fair. I just want to be normal. Why can't you and Dad be like everybody else's parents? I wish I were somebody else's kid."

19   I waited for my mom to shout, but she just stared at me with tired eyes. "If you don't want to go, don't have to," she said.

20   Though my parents had lived in the United States for decades, they still led a Chinese life at home. They spoke to each other in Chinese and read a Taiwanese paper. Chinese food covered our dinner table. Breakfast consisted

---

1. **stoic:** unemotional

10

of watery rice with pickled vegetables and meat, or fried eggs with soy sauce. At dinner I would douse my rice with ketchup and remind my parents that Sara's family ate hamburgers.

21   I envied my friends' relationships with their parents. My friends didn't have to worry that their parents would embarrass them with questions like "Is this good price?" and "What's this meaning?"

22   My friends' parents chatted easily with each other and our teachers. Their parents understood dating, and what it was like to grow up with the pressures of drinking, drugs, and sex. My parents discussed only my grades, career, and prospective salary.

23   My mom speaks English like I speak Chinese: slowly and punctuated by ums and ahs. When someone speaks English too rapidly, my mom's eyes cloud with confusion. I instantly recognize her I-don't-get-it look, and I know it's time to explain something.

24   About a month before we left for China, I helped my mom return a purchase to Wal-Mart.

25   The clerk rudely ignored my mom's slow English, speaking to me instead.

26   Later my mom thanked me for my help. "*Xie xie,* Sharon," she said, patting my shoulder. "I have good American daughter."

27   "It's nothing, Mom," I said.

28   In the airport before we departed for China, my parents' friends herded around me. "Your parents so proud of you," said one man. "Always talking about you."

29   His words surprised me. I felt like I barely spoke with my parents. Did they really know who I was? Then another question, the one I always managed to skirt, surfaced in my conscience: did I even come close to understanding *them?*

30   The tour was a 17-day whirlwind. We visited lakes laden with lotus flowers, snapped pictures of jagged mountains rising out of the Yellow River, and hiked up stone stairs to intricately painted temples.

31   I saw rice paddies[1] cut like square emeralds into the mountainside. I toured a factory where the employees spun silk into sheets of gloss.

32   But the best part of the trip was watching my parents. They carried themselves with an ease unfamiliar to me. They blended into the throngs of Chinese people instead of sticking out in the crowd. Their voices swelled with authority. My mom translated the tour guide's Chinese in her unwavering voice, whispering historical anecdotes[2] she'd learned in school.

33   Often during the tour, my own face resembled my mom's I-don't-get-it look. At meals, my parents answered my constant questions about each colorful bowl that would rotate by on the Lazy Susan.[3]

---

1. **paddies:** fields where rice is grown   3. **Lazy Susan:** a revolving tray for food
2. **anecdotes:** stories

10

34   My parents chuckled at my response when a waiter put a bowl of soup on our table. While the other diners shouted with excitement, I was horrified to see the remnants[1] of a turtle floating in the clear yellow broth.

35   My table cried in dismay when I let the soup circle past me. "Strange," said one man, shaking his head. "Such good soup."

36   A few days after "the iron incident," as my run-in with the hotel clerk became known in our tour group, my parents and I sat on a bench overlooking stone monoliths.[2] "Too bad I don't speak fluent Chinese," I said. "I should have listened when you tried to teach me."

37   My dad looked at me with understanding. "It's okay," he said. "You learning it now."

38   My mom smiled supportively. "Never too late," she said.*

1. What is the implied main idea of this entire longer selection?

   (a.) A trip to China helped the author understand her parents and her heritage.
   b. The author wanted to be American, not Chinese.
   c. The author's parents never liked America because they were treated badly there.
   d. Everyone should visit China as soon as he or she gets a chance.

2. Which of the following supporting details helps the reader figure out the implied main idea?

   a. "Breakfast consisted of watery rice with pickled vegetables and meat, or fried eggs with soy sauce." (paragraph 20)
   b. "The tour was a 17-day whirlwind." (paragraph 30)
   c. "My dad fled to Taiwan in 1949 as a 14-year-old, after the Communists won the civil war." (paragraph 8)
   (d.) "Often during the tour, my own face resembled my mom's I-don't-get-it look." (paragraph 33)

3. Many of the supporting details are in the form of

   a. steps and reasons.
   (b.) events and points of comparison and contrast.
   c. causes and effects.
   d. reasons and examples.

___

1. **remnants:** pieces   2. **monoliths:** huge rocks or stones

___

* From Sharon Liao, "A Very Lucky Daughter," *Reader's Digest,* June 2001, 81–87, originally appeared as "A Daughter's Journey" in *Washingtonian,* January 2001. Reprinted with permission from the June 2001 *Reader's Digest* and the January 2001 *Washingtonian.*

10

Patterns of Organization

Chapter 6 of this book explained five common patterns of organization (series, time order, cause/effect, comparison/contrast, and definition) used to arrange supporting details within paragraphs. Conveniently, longer selections are organized according to the very same patterns. Here is an example of a passage that's organized with a series of types:

THESIS

The fossil record is vital to the understanding of geologic[1] time. A **fossil** is any remnant[2] or indication of prehistoric life preserved in rock. The study of fossils is called **paleontology**, an area of interest to both biologists and geologists. Evidence of ancient plants and animals can be preserved in several ways.

Type #1

Some fossils are in the form of original remains. Ancient insects have been preserved by the sticky tree resin, in which they were trapped. The hardened resin, called *amber* and often used for jewelry, is found in Eastern Europe and the Dominican Republic. The entire bodies of woolly mammoths[3] have been found frozen in the permafrost[4] of Alaska and Siberia. More often, only the hardest parts of organisms are preserved, such as bones. Shark teeth and the shells of shallow-water marine organisms endure well, are easily buried in sediment,[5] and are thus common types of fossils.

Type #2

Other fossils are in the form of replaced remains. The hard parts (bone, shell, etc.) of a buried organism can be slowly replaced by minerals such as silica (SiO_2), calcite ($CaCO_3$), and pyrite (FeS_2) in circulating groundwater. A copy of the original plant or animal material results. Petrified wood, such as the beautiful samples from Arizona's Petrified National Forest, is a common type of replacement fossil. *Carbonization* occurs when plant remains are decomposed by bacteria under anaerobic (airless) conditions. The hydrogen, nitrogen, and oxygen are driven off, leaving a carbon residue that may retain many of the features of the original plant. In this way, coal was formed.

Type #3

Still other fossils are molds and casts of remains. When an embedded shell or bone is dissolved completely out of a rock, it leaves a hollow depression called a *mold*. If new mineral material fills the mold, it forms a *cast* of the original shell or bone. Molds and casts can only show the original shape of the remains.

1. **geologic:** related to the earth
2. **remnant:** leftover piece or reminder
3. **mammoths:** large, hairy extinct elephants
4. **permafrost:** permanently frozen ground
5. **sediment:** material that settles to the bottom of a liquid

10

One final type of fossil is the trace fossil, a fossil imprint made by the movement of an animal. Examples are tracks, borings, and burrows.* Type #4

The preceding selection offers a series of four types of fossils in support of the thesis. Each type of fossil is stated and explained in a separate paragraph.

The major supporting details of this next passage are organized with the time order pattern.

The first wiring of the world began in 1850, only six years after Samuel Morse demonstrated the reality of telegraphy. British engineers made a copper-wire cable, insulated it with gutta-percha (a rubberlike Malayan tree sap), and laid it across the English Channel.

Soon came a cable across the Atlantic. On August 16, 1858, Queen Victoria sent a hundred-word message to President James Buchanan. Some of the royal words reached Washington that day; the rest came through on the 17th. Agonizingly slow and chronically[1] unreliable, the cable went dead after three weeks.

The problem was the behavior of electricity in cables. Convinced that they had found the solution, engineers tried again, this time with the world's largest ship, the *Great Eastern.* In July 1865, she set out from England with a crew of 500, a dozen oxen for hauling, a cow for fresh milk, a herd of pigs for bacon—and a thickly insulated 2,800-mile cable that weighed 5,000 tons. They had almost finished laying it when the cable snapped. The next year they succeeded.

Cable laying continued through the nineteenth century and into the twentieth. Words were humming along at more than 200 a minute, compared with twelve a minute in 1866. But cable met competition when wireless telegraphs, in 1901, and commercial telephone calls, in 1927, began crackling across the Atlantic on radio waves. Not until 1956 did a telephone cable span the Atlantic. Then in 1965, the first Early Bird Satellite went into orbit, and again cable became a has-been.[2]

But by the mid-1990s, thank to fiber optics, cable was making a comeback, carrying most telephone calls between the United States and Europe, Japan, and Australia. Pulsing with Internet data packets, cables connect more than 80 nations, carrying far more telephone

1. **chronically:** happening again and again

2. **has-been:** something that is no longer popular or useful

* Adapted from James T. Shipman et al., *An Introduction to Physical Science,* 9th ed. (Boston: Houghton Mifflin Co., 2000), 634.

10

calls than satellites or mobile phones. But those mobile phones and satellites are bridging the digital divide, using wireless networks as a way to connect the unconnected.*

Longer passages are more likely to use a combination of patterns to organize details. This next selection from a textbook, for example, combines time order and cause/effect to explain the events and results of the California Gold Rush.

The market economy[1] provided a great impetus[2] for expansion. Early on, the fur trapper system brought the Far West—way beyond settlement—into a market system that extended through St. Louis, Montreal, and New York to the hat merchants of Europe. Then, in the late 1840s, settlement jumped over the trapping areas to the West Coast of the American continent, when the promise of instant wealth in the form of gold sparked a gold rush.

Gold stimulated a mass migration to the West Coast. The United States had acquired Alta California in the Treaty of Guadalupe Hidalgo from Mexico, and the province was inhabited mostly by native peoples, some Mexicans living on large estates, and a chain of small settlements around military forts (presidios) and missions. That changed almost overnight after James Marshall, a carpenter, spotted gold particles in the millrace[3] at Sutter's Mill (now Coloma, California, northwest of Sacramento) in January. Word of the discovery spread, and other Californians rushed in like ants to a picnic to scrabble for instant fortunes. When John C. Fremont reached San Francisco five months later, he found that "all or nearly all its male inhabitants had gone to the mines." The town, "which a few months before was so busy and thriving, was then almost deserted."

By 1849, the news had spread around the world, and hundreds of thousands of fortune seekers, mostly young men, streamed in from Mexico, England, Germany, France, Ireland, and all over the United States. The newcomers came for one reason: instant wealth. In search of gold and silver, they mined the lodes[4] and washed away the surface soil with hydraulic[5] mining, leaving the land unsuitable for anything after they abandoned it.

1. **market economy:** buying and selling of goods and services
2. **impetus:** stimulus; cause
3. **millrace:** fast-moving stream of water
4. **lodes:** sources of mineral ore
5. **hydraulic:** related to fluids, especially water

* Excerpt from "The Future Is Calling" by Thomas B. Allen from *National Geographic*, December 2001, 82–83. Reprinted by permission of the National Geographic Society.

10

Success in the market economy required capital, hard labor, and time; by contrast, gold mining seemed to promise instant riches. Most "forty-niners,"[1] however, never found enough gold to pay their expenses. "The stories you hear frequently in the States," one gold seeker wrote home, "are the most extravagant lies imaginable—the mines are a humbug[2]. . . . The almost universal feeling is to get home." But many stayed, either unable to afford the passage home or tempted by the growing labor shortage in California's cities and agricultural districts.

San Francisco, the former presidio and mission of Yerba Buena, the gateway from the West Coast to the interior, became an instant city, ballooning to 35,000 people in 1850. In 1848, it had been a small settlement of about a thousand Mexicans, Anglos, soldiers, friars,[3] and Indians. Ships bringing people and supplies continuously jammed the harbor, a scene that artist Frank Marryat captured in an 1849 painting. A French visitor in that year wrote, "At San Francisco, where fifteen months ago one found only a half dozen large cabins, one finds today a stock exchange, a theater, churches of all Christian cults, and a large number of quite beautiful homes."*

This passage covers the events of 1848 to 1850 related to the Gold Rush, and it presents some of the results of those events, too.

Exercise 10.4

Read the passage below and then respond to the questions that follow by circling the letter of each correct answer.

The Moral Lessons of Harry Potter

1   For adults who haven't read them, the frenzy over the Harry Potter books— and now the movie version of *Harry Potter and the Sorcerer's Stone*—can seem perplexing.[4] What, after all, could be so special about a boy wizard and his friends? Some parents have expressed concern about author J. K. Rowling's use of magic and what they believe to be elements of witchcraft in the books. But a variety of academic experts believe that Harry's life and adventures offer valuable lessons to his young fans.

1. **forty-niners:** people who took part in the 1849 California Gold Rush
2. **humbug:** fraud; nonsense
3. **friars:** members of a religious order
4. **perplexing:** confusing

---

* Adapted from Peggy Norton et al., *A People and a Nation*, Vol. 1, 5th ed. (Boston: Houghton Mifflin Co., 1998), 279–280.

10

2   **Adversity[1] can be overcome through perseverance[2] and hard work.** Despite the circumstances surrounding his early life, Harry is hopeful and able to thrive. "He isn't bitter," says Leah J. Dickstein, MD, professor of psychiatry at the University of Louisville in Kentucky and a former sixth-grade teacher. "He gets the opportunity to go to the Hogwarts School, and while it's risky to try something new, he does it." Life improves at Hogwarts, but he still faces plenty of frightening obstacles, such as battling the evil and powerful Professor Quirrell and Voldemort, the terrible wizard who killed his parents. But even though he and his friends are only first-year students of magic, they never consider giving up.

3   "Harry is always having to confront his fears," says Kylene Beers, assistant professor of reading at the University of Houston and author of Scholastic's online Harry Potter discussion guide. It is his wise teacher, the wizard Dumbledore, who advises Harry to name those fears. "Fear of the name increases fear of the thing itself," Dumbledore tells him. Part of the genius of Rowling's story is that it allows children to confront their own fears in a manageable way.

4   **It's important to be accepting of differences in others and to treat everyone equally.** Having been rejected by his own relatives, Harry is particularly sensitive to others' suffering, whether it's Ron's embarrassment that his family doesn't have much money or Hagrid's large size, which makes him something of an outcast. "J. K. Rowling appears to be creating a caste system so readers can explore the notion of what it means to be different and how much surface differences matter in our lives," says Beers. A good example is Harry's nemesis,[3] Draco Malfoy, who hails from a family with elite bloodlines. Rather than befriending Malfoy, which could have assured Harry's popularity, he distances himself from the mean snob. From then on, Malfoy taunts[4] Harry about being an orphan and makes cracks about Ron's financial hardships. Racism, classism,[5] and other biases also emerge, such as a prejudice against Muggles (non-wizards), something Harry won't stand for since his friend Hermione is Muggle-born.

5   **You don't have to be perfect.** Harry's not your standard hero. In fact, he's rather gawky,[6] and his hair won't even stay in place. "He has a scar on his forehead. He's not perfect," says Dr. Dickstein. Nonetheless, he prevails, using logic, kindness, patience, and bravery when strength or special powers fail him. "There are so many negative messages out in society—that you're too fat or you're not smart enough—and children are very aware of that," Dr. Dickstein says. "These characters gain self-acceptance, which is something parents can discuss with their children."

1. **adversity:** hardship; misfortune
2. **perseverance:** not giving up
3. **nemesis:** source of harm or ruin; enemy based
4. **taunts:** insults or mocks
5. **classism:** bias (preference) based on social or economic class
6. **gawky:** awkward

10

6   **Education and knowledge are essential.** School plays a prominent role in all the Harry Potter books. "There is nothing wrong with being smart in the book," says Dr. Elizabeth Schafer, a specialist in children's literature and author of *Exploring Harry Potter*. Harry admires his friend Hermione for her intelligence and hard work. Often, it is her knowledge that helps them get out of a predicament,[1] whether it's using logic to determine which liquid is poisonous or casting a spell on an evil wizard who has put a curse on Harry. The friends spend a great deal of time in the immense Hogwarts library researching questions such as the contents of a mysterious package hidden in the school. Dr. Dickstein also points to the fabulous use of language throughout the story. Rowling employs rich vocabulary words, such as *flouted, prudent*, and *abashed*, and also incorporates other languages. For example, the murderous Voldemort's name borrows from the French word for *death*, and the name of Harry's nemesis, Draco, means "serpent" or "dragon" in Latin. So consider the story something of an early SAT prep class!

7   **Loyalty to friends is important.** From the moment Harry and Ron meet on the train to Hogwarts, they're inseparable. And after a few rocky encounters, they forge a strong friendship with Hermione as well. "Even though the characters are strong as individuals, it's as a team that they solve all their problems," such as when they band together to support their awkward friend Neville, says Dr. Schafer. She suggests using the characters' friendship as a starting point to talk with kids about whom they want to emulate[2] in life and why. "It might also help children identify negative behaviors [like Draco's] that they don't want to continue," she adds.

8   Though parents may be concerned that parts of the story are too scary, the key—after gauging your child's maturity—is to share the books and movie as a family. "The lessons offered by the Harry Potter books are ones that readers can use throughout their lives and build upon as they gain life experiences and acquire new insights about familial, social, cultural, intellectual, and professional situations," Dr. Schafer says.*

1. Which of the following sentences states the thesis of this selection?

   a. "Some parents have expressed concern about author J. K. Rowling's use of magic and what they believe to be elements of witchcraft in the books." (paragraph 1)

   b. "But a variety of academic experts believe that Harry's life and adventures offer valuable lessons to his young fans." (paragraph 1)

---

1. predicament: unpleasant situation; problem   **2. emulate:** copy, imitate

---

* Adapted from Michelle Holcenberg, *Child*, November 2001. Copyright © 2002. Originally published by Gruner + Jahr USA Publishing in the Dec./Jan. 2002 issue of *Child* Magazine. Used with permission. For subscription information, please call 1-800-777-0222.

10

(c.) "Adversity can be overcome through perseverance and hard work." (paragraph 2)

d. "Despite the circumstances surrounding his early life, Harry is hopeful and able to thrive." (paragraph 2)

2. What pattern of organization organizes the *major* supporting details?

   a. time order
   b. definition
   c. cause/effect
   (d.) series

3. How many supporting points develop the thesis statement?

   a. two
   b. three
   c. four
   (d.) five

Transitions

As you learned in Chapter 5 of this book, paragraphs include transitions, words that signal relationships between sentences. Longer reading selections employ transitions for the very same purpose, but they also show how whole *paragraphs* are related to one another. As you read the following example of a time order (process) paragraph, notice how the boldfaced, italicized transition words help you understand the relationships among major details.

Time Out the Right Way

Time Out is probably the most widely researched technique for dealing with unwanted behavior in young children. Unfortunately, it is often used incorrectly. It is therefore worth knowing that Time Out means removing the child from all rewarding activities for a short period. The common practice of sending a child to his room, where he can play computer games, watch TV, or talk with friends on the telephone, is not Time Out behavior. Time Out means exposing the child to a very boring, unrewarding environment. For the sake of illustration, let's assume that your child has bitten someone. THESIS STATEMENT Here is a simple, highly effective way of discouraging this behavior.

First, say to her: "We do not bite." Say nothing more than this—give no further description of the behavior, no explanation of what you are doing. Say nothing except, "We do not bite."

Second, take her by the hand and seat her in a small chair facing a blank wall. Stand close enough so that if she attempts to leave the chair you can immediately return her to it.

10

Next, keep her in the chair for three minutes. (Do not tell her how long she will be in the chair. Say nothing.) If she screams, kicks the wall, asks questions, or says she has to go to the bathroom, ignore her. It is absolutely essential that you say nothing.

Then, at the end of three minutes, keep her in the chair until she has been quiet and well behaved for five more seconds. When she does so, tell her she has been good and may now leave the chair. Never let her leave until she has been well behaved for at least a few seconds.

Finally, following Time Out, say nothing about it. Do not discuss the punished behavior or the fairness of the punishment. Say nothing except, "We do not bite."

Once the child realizes that you mean business, that she cannot manipulate you into providing attention for bad behavior, Time Out will proceed more smoothly and quickly, and there will be far fewer times when you need to use it.*

Exercise 10.5

Read the passage below and then respond to the questions that follow by circling the letter of each correct answer.

Technostress

1   The computer revolution has created a form of stress that is causing mental and physical health problems among many workers. Craig Brod, a consultant specializing in stress reduction, was one of the first people to use the term *technostress* to describe this source of stress. Technostress is the inability to cope with computer and related technologies in a healthy manner. It may take several forms.

2   One type of technostress is known as "upgrade anxiety." As the processing speed of new computers increases, it is often necessary to acquire new equipment every one or two years in order to keep up with the demands of customers, suppliers, and communications in general. With each upgrade, workers are forced to adapt to new technology just as they were adjusting to the previous system.

* "Why Our Kids Are Out of Control" by Jacob Azerrad. Reprinted with permission from *Psychology Today* Magazine, September/October 2001. Copyright © 2001 Sussex Publishers, Inc.

10

3   Another kind of technostress takes the form of addiction to computers. Many computer users develop deep feelings of dependency on their machines and thereby lose the capacity to feel or relate to other people. Some workers have adopted a machinelike mind-set that reflects the characteristics of the computer itself. Signs of the techno-centered state include a high degree of factual thinking, poor access to feelings, and low tolerance for the ambiguities[1] of human behavior and communication.

4   Information overload, too, is a kind of technostress. It is easy to experience sensory overload as you sort through the hundreds of messages that come to you daily by means of the Internet, e-mail, pagers, commercial advertising, and many other sources. With the aid of pagers and cellular phones, messages can reach you at the beach or during the backyard barbecue. *Data smog,* the term that David Shenk uses to describe the information-dense society we live in, is a problem because it crowds out quiet moments, obstructs[2] much-needed contemplation,[3] and often leaves us feeling confused.

5   Finally, the computer workstation can cause technostress. Many employees spend their entire workday confined to a computer terminal. Carpal tunnel syndrome, a repetitive-stress wrist injury, is often caused by constant computer keyboarding and is one of the fastest-growing occupational hazards. Computer-related vision problems are also very common.*

1. What pattern of organization is used to arrange the major supporting details?

   a. cause/effect
   b. time order
   c. series
   d. definition

2. Which of the following sentences begins with a series transition?

   a. "One type of technostress is known as 'upgrade anxiety.'" (paragraph 2)
   b. "Signs of the techno-centered state include a high degree of factual thinking, poor access to feelings, and low tolerance for the ambiguities of human behavior and communication." (paragraph 3)
   c. "Information overload, too, is a kind of technostress." (paragraph 4)
   d. "Computer-related vision problems are also very common." (paragraph 5)

1. **ambiguities:** uncertainties   3. **contemplation:** thinking
2. **obstructs:** blocks

---

* Adapted from Barry L. Reece and Rhonda Brandt, *Effective Human Relations in Organizations,* 7th ed. (Boston: Houghton Mifflin Co., 1999), 365–366.

10

3. Which of the following transitions from the selection is NOT a series transition?

   a. another (paragraph 3)
   b. too (paragraph 4)
   c. because (paragraph 4)
   d. finally (paragraph 5)

CHAPTER 10 REVIEW

Write the correct answers in the blanks in the following statements.

1. Like paragraphs, longer reading selections include a ____topic____ and a ____main idea____.

2. The main idea of a longer passage is usually called a ____thesis____.

3. ____Headings____ are mini-titles that identify the topic of one section of a longer work like a chapter or an article.

4. Though not as common, a longer reading selection can offer an ____implied____ main idea.

5. Longer reading selections, like paragraphs, organize supporting details according to common ____patterns____, and they include ____transitions____ to show how paragraphs are related to one another.

▶ Vocabulary: Review

You've covered many important vocabulary concepts in Chapters 1 through 9 of this book. The following exercise, which draws sentences from examples in Chapter 10, will give you practice reviewing several of these concepts.

Vocabulary Exercise

A. On the blanks following each paragraph, write in the synonym(s) that the sentence or passage includes for the boldfaced, italicized word or phrase.

1. A volcanic explosion can spew *rocks* into the air up to 800 mph, and toss large boulders like pebbles—for miles.

   Two synonyms for italicized word: _Boulders, pebbles_

2. My dad *fled* to Taiwan in 1949 as a 14-year-old, after the Communists won the civil war. His father fought for the losing side, the Nationalists.

10

My mom's father, a Nationalist navy captain, also retreated to Taiwan.

One synonym for italicized word: <u>Retreated</u>

B. In the sentences that follow, look up the boldfaced, italicized words in a dictionary and determine which definition best describes how each word is being used. Write that definition on the blank provided.

3. I couldn't picture my ***domestic*** mom, unsure of her halting English, studying international economics at a Taiwanese university.

<u>Of or relating to the family household</u>

4. Success in the market economy required ***capital,*** hard labor, and time; by contrast, gold mining seemed to promise instant riches.

<u>Money or investment</u>

C. In each of the following sentences, underline the context clue that helps you understand the meaning of the boldfaced, italicized word, and then write what kind of context clue (definition/restatement, example, explanation, or contrast) it is on the blank provided.

5. Racism, classism, and other ***biases*** also emerge, <u>such as a prejudice against Muggles (non-wizards)</u>, something Harry won't stand for since his friend Hermione is Muggle-born. <u>Example</u>

6. She suggests using the characters' friendship as a starting point to talk with kids about whom they want to ***emulate*** in life and why. "It might also help children identify <u>negative behaviors [like Draco's] that they don't want to continue</u>," she adds. <u>Contrast</u>

7. The explosion produced a <u>100-foot-high</u> ***tsunami*** that <u>wiped out</u> some 36,000 people on nearby <u>shores</u>. <u>Explanation</u>

D. In each of the following sentences, underline the figure of speech (analogy, metaphor, simile, or personification).

8. I saw rice paddies cut <u>like square emeralds</u> into the mountainside.

9. Word of the discovery spread, and other Californians rushed in <u>like ants to a picnic</u> to scrabble for instant fortunes.

10. Given Ford's long and active role in safeguarding the environment, the company is not about <u>to put on the brakes.</u>

10

READING STRATEGY: Scanning

The last time you went to a restaurant hungry for a particular dish, like fried chicken, did you read every word of the menu before placing your order? You probably didn't. Instead, you glanced over the lists and descriptions of the items available until you found the ones that included fried chicken, and you probably ignored most of the other sections of the menu. This is called **scanning**, and it is a useful strategy to use when you are searching for a particular piece of information. You also scan when you look for a certain topic in a book's table of contents or index or when you read a visual aid like a table. You are scanning when you look at classified ads, telephone books, dictionaries, or a list of websites generated by an Internet search engine.

When you scan a text, you don't read the whole thing; rather, you run your eyes over the page, reading words or phrases here and there until you discover what you are looking for. Though this seems like skimming, the strategy explained in Chapter 9, it is different because when you scan, you know what you are looking for. When you skim, you don't; you are just trying to gain a general understanding of a text and/or its main features.

When might scanning be appropriate for longer texts such as chapters or articles? If you are looking for an answer to a particular question, or if you are searching for a specific fact, name, or other type of detail, scan the text to find what you need. Scanning is often useful, then, for completing assignments or for refreshing your memory about some piece of information you remember reading about. If you need to form a complete understanding of the ideas in a text, however, you'll have to read it more thoroughly.

On page 496 is a page from a textbook's index. Scan it to answer the questions that follow.

1. On what page can you find information about the organization of interest groups? ____71____
2. On how many different pages is Jesse Jackson mentioned? __6__
3. If you want to find information about ideology, to what topic in the index must you turn? ____Political ideology____
4. How many figures in the text relate to immigration? ____2____
5. If you want to learn about the assassination attempt on Andrew Jackson, to which page should you turn? ____362____

10

Source: From James Q. Wilson and John J. Dilulio, Jr., *American Government,* 9th ed. (Boston: Houghton Mifflin Co., 2004), I12. Copyright © 2004 by Houghton Mifflin Company. Reprinted with permission.

10

Name _____ Date _____

COMBINED SKILLS TEST 1

Read the essay below and then respond to the questions that follow by circling the letter of each correct answer.

The Ones Who Turn Up Along the Way

1 Not long ago my building super,[1] Walter, stopped by my apartment. He rang the bell saying, "Super," in a way to which I had grown accustomed, dragging out the "u" and adding a slight roll to the "r." I imagined that he was coming to fix something or maybe to bring me a package. But when I opened the door, he was holding the spare set of keys that he kept to my place.

2   Walter told me he had come to return the keys because he would no longer be working in my building. His family had gotten too big for the basement apartment that came with the job, he explained. Walter had been there for 11 years, ever since coming to the United States from Colombia. He had been available at all hours for the occasional maintenance crisis, but, more important, he always gave me the sense that he looked out for me—which is a great comfort when you're living alone in Manhattan. It was hard to imagine the building without him.

3   Just before Walter came by, I had been unpacking groceries and reflecting on a conversation I had just had with Ali, the manager of my neighborhood grocery store. Ali is a devout[2] Muslim[3] from Bangladesh. He has a wife and three children and a PhD in geography. On visits to his native country, he often gives lectures on Islam.[4] He hopes to publish a book encouraging Bangladeshi people to see Jews as friends. It's a project he has been working on for some time, and to which he feels even more committed since September 11th. "This is what Allah[5] tells me I must do," he says. "I must love all people. I cannot hate people and love Allah."

---

1. **super:** superintendent, the person who serves as custodian in a building
2. **devout:** devoted to a religion
3. **Muslim:** a believer in Islam
4. **Islam:** a religion that worships one God
5. **Allah:** God

4   I have been shopping in this grocery store for years now, and Ali and I have always waved and said hello. But several months ago the hellos turned into conversation. When I told him that I am a rabbi,[1] we began discussing the connections between Judaism and Islam, the purpose of religion, the sorrow and anger we feel when people use religion as a justification for violence. Every time we talk I feel as if I have learned Torah[2]—the wisdom of my own faith tradition—from a man who quotes the Quran.[3]

5   I share these stories because they are a part of the puzzle of community. I am well aware that Walter and Ali do not fall into the simple categories of family member, coworker, or friend. We are from different backgrounds, different countries, and we occupy different socioeconomic[4] spheres. We don't go to each other's home for dinner or make plans to meet for coffee, and we probably won't. Our connections are site-specific and episodic.[5] And yet they make real claims on my heart and mind.

6   In the Book of Exodus, even as God continued to harden Pharaoh's heart, the Israelites began their journey out of Egypt. More than 600,000 packed up and headed out on foot, but they were not alone. An *erev rav*—a mixed multitude—went with them. The ancient rabbis' reviews are mixed when it comes to characterizing this anonymous crew. Some see them as a group of hangers-on ultimately responsible for the building of the golden calf. Others suggest that they were Egyptians who simply shared the basic human longing to be free. Either way, I imagine that by the time the travelers made it to shore and fanned out into the desert, called to different purposes and directions, they were bound to one another forever.

7   About a year ago, a guy came to replace the intercom system in my apartment. While he worked, he told me that he had been born in Ukraine, immigrated to Israel with his family and fought in the country's 1948 independence war. He explained that he was an atheist[6] and knew he could never believe in God. Nevertheless, as he was leaving he asked in Hebrew, "What blessing may I give you?" Before I could answer, he prayed that I would find my *bashert* (soulmate), kindly even suggesting one of his sons.

8   When he was gone I noticed that he had forgotten a bunch of different-colored wires. I saved them. I keep them in a tin with the quarters I use for doing laundry. They remind me that we are traveling not only with the people we have chosen but [also] with the ones who turn up along the way.

1. **rabbi:** a person ordained to lead a Jewish congregation
2. **Torah:** the Hebrew Bible
3. **Quran:** the sacred text of Islam
4. **socioeconomic:** involving both social and economic factors
5. **episodic:** temporary
6. **atheist:** one who denies the existence of God

The repairman, Walter, and Ali are part of my *erev rav,* and I am a part of theirs.

9   It's been months now since Walter and his family moved across the river to New Jersey. Soon Ali will take another trip to Bangladesh. I don't know what's next for me, but I know I won't be going alone.*

1. Which of the following sentences from the selection best expresses the main idea of the entire selection?
   a. "Not long ago my building super, Walter, stopped by my apartment." (paragraph 1)
   b. "It was hard to imagine the building without him." (paragraph 2)
   c. "In the Book of Exodus, even as God continued to harden Pharaoh's heart, the Israelites began their journey out of Egypt." (paragraph 6)
   d. "The repairman, Walter, and Ali are part of my *erev rav,* and I am a part of theirs." (paragraph 8)

2. Which of the following is the topic sentence of paragraph 6?
   a. "An *erev rav*—a mixed multitude—went with them."
   b. "The ancient rabbis' reviews are mixed when it comes to characterizing this anonymous crew."
   c. "Some see them as a group of hangers-on ultimately responsible for the building of the golden calf."
   d. "Others suggest that they were Egyptians who simply shared the basic human longing to be free."

3. Which of the following is a *major* supporting detail in paragraph 6?
   a. "More than 600,000 packed up and headed out on foot, but they were not alone."
   b. "An *erev rav*—a mixed multitude—went with them."
   c. "The ancient rabbis' reviews are mixed when it comes to characterizing this anonymous crew."
   d. "Some see them as a group of hangers-on ultimately responsible for the building of the golden calf."

4. What is the implied main idea of paragraph 3?
   a. Both Rabbi Krause and Ali are fascinated by geography.
   b. Ali's faith has made an impression on Rabbi Krause.
   c. Jews and Muslims have more in common than they realize.
   d. Rabbi Krause researches faiths other than her own.

* "The Ones Who Turn Up Along the Way" by Rabbi Jennifer Krause from *Newsweek,* November 26, 2001. Copyright © 2001 Newsweek. All rights reserved. Reprinted by permission.

5. Which of the following sentences does NOT begin with a transition?

   a. "But when I opened the door, he was holding the spare set of keys that he kept to my place." (paragraph 1)

   b. "Soon Ali will take another trip to Bangladesh." (paragraph 9)

   c. "In the Book of Exodus, even as God continued to harden Pharaoh's heart, the Israelites began their journey out of Egypt." (paragraph 6)

   d. "About a year ago, a guy came to replace the intercom system in my apartment." (paragraph 7)

6. Which pattern of organization arranges the details in paragraphs 7 through 9?

   a. cause/effect   c. series

   b. time order   d. definition

7. What can you infer about the author from paragraph 2?

   a. She is a Catholic.   c. She likes to read the Bible.

   b. She is not married.   d. She can't afford a house.

8. Which of the following sentences is a fact?

   a. "Not long ago my building super, Walter, stopped by my apartment." (paragraph 1)

   b. "It was hard to imagine the building without him." (paragraph 2)

   c. "And yet they make real claims on my heart and mind." (paragraph 5)

   d. "I don't know what's next for me, but I know I won't be going alone." (paragraph 9)

9. The author's tone in this selection is

   a. amused.   c. serious.

   b. sorrowful.   d. angry.

COMBINED SKILLS TEST 2

Read the article below and then respond to the questions that follow by circling the letter of each correct answer.

Lessons I Learned Staying Up All Night

1 Tiptoe through the stacks of any college library—especially around final exams—and you'll find them: college students so tired they've fallen asleep. "No matter what time of day," students are slumped over their textbooks, says Faye Backie, assistant director for public services at Michigan State

University. The library at the East Lansing, Michigan, school is open 24 hours every day but Saturday. "When I taught, I found them falling asleep in class too," adds Backie, a former professor.

2 Students, even the most prepared, sometimes have to cut back drastically on sleep to finish a term paper or cram for a final exam. "So many things are happening at once, in a really condensed[1] period of time, once or twice I'll have to stay up all night," explains Scott Kaplan, a senior political science major at the University of Pennsylvania.

3 Brian Babcock, a senior international relations and strategic history major at the U.S. Military Academy at West Point, NY, tries to avoid the full all-nighters, but he's still not getting his beauty sleep. "I usually call it quits around 4:30 or 5 [AM]." But being at a military academy means Babcock is at mandatory formation at 6:55 AM, and there is no wiggle room when it comes to sleeping or skipping classes. "When you feel tired, instead of falling asleep at your desk, you stand up for 10–15 minutes," he says; otherwise, you could end up in five-hour marching duty.

4 Dalia Alcazar, a sophomore at University of California at Berkeley, recalls staying up all night to write a paper for an 8 AM class. Around 6 AM she took a break to eat breakfast and decided to take some caffeine pills to boost her energy. It was a mistake, she says, leaving her nauseous and feeling sick.

5 Kelly Tanabe, founder of Supercollege.com, a website that helps students adjust to college life, says students will try anything to stay awake when it seems there just aren't enough hours in the day. Tanabe, a Harvard graduate who pulled her fair share of all-nighters, says a "coffee bomb" was very popular with her classmates. "Fill a cup halfway with (powdered) instant coffee. Fill the remainder with hot water. Drink. It's not pleasant, but the caffeine will power you through the night." Tanabe urges students to be realistic and accept that they're not going to learn everything they neglected the whole semester. Unfortunately, most don't grasp this until it's creeping toward 3 AM.

6 "Sometimes students who pull all-nighters sleep through the very exam they stayed up all night for," says Amy Wolfson, associate professor of psychology at College of the Holy Cross, in Worcester, Massachusetts. Wolfson says there are factors working against students that won't go away. "As we get further from where we last slept, we're likely to begin to feel more tired." According to Wolfson, it's generally recommended that college students get between 8.4 and 9.2 hours of sleep per night. "Every semester I have someone that falls asleep through a final exam," she adds. "Cramming has never been a recommended study habit. In fact, you're probably better off going to sleep, assuming you're someone who's attended class."

1. **condensed:** shortened

7   The author of *How to Ace Any Test* agrees. "It's absolutely, totally impossible to cram a whole semester's study in one night," says Ron Fry, who also wrote *How to Study* and *How to Improve Your Memory* (Career Press). Ideally, Fry says, students should be reviewing their notes on a weekly basis, but if that hasn't been the case and the semester is winding down, they should be choosy about what to study. "Selectivity is very important. Smart kids always figure this out; smart kids never study everything," he says. Fry suggests students go through their notes and see how much time a teacher dedicated to a particular subject. "If a teacher spent two weeks on one general topic and three days on another, chances are the two-week topic is going to be on [the exam]."

8   To recall facts, Fry notes there are several memorization techniques. If someone has a great musical memory, put a definition or fact to the rhythm of a song. Others have strong kinetic[1] memories and can easily associate some sort of body movement to it.

9   Another helpful shortcut at students' fingertips—one that previous generations didn't have—is online research. Many campus libraries offer free Internet access or a service such as Questia.com, which charges a small monthly fee and offers full-text reference materials in a user-friendly format. "When you cut and paste, we automatically create a footnote for you in the correct format. We even hyperlink it back to the right page on the service," says Troy Williams, founder and CEO.

10   But, adds Tanabe, hopefully one of the most important lessons learned while cramming for an exam is to space out assignments and study in the future. It will probably benefit students' grades as well as their sleeping habits. "What seems brilliant at 4 AM is oftentimes not truly brilliant."*

1. What is the topic of this selection?
   a. school
   b. bad planning
   c. cramming
   d. falling asleep

2. Which of the following is a *minor* supporting detail in paragraph 9?
   a. "Another helpful shortcut at students' fingertips—one that previous generations didn't have—is online research."
   b. "Many campus libraries offer free Internet access or a service such as Questia.com, which charges a small monthly fee and offers full-text reference materials in a user-friendly format."

1. **kinetic:** related to motion or movement

* From Maria Coder, "Lessons I Learned Staying Up All Night," Morganton, NC *News Herald*, December 2, 2001, 7C. Reprinted with permission of the Associated Press.

c. "'When you cut and paste, we automatically create a footnote for you in the correct format. We even hyperlink it back to the right page on the service,' says Troy Williams, founder and CEO."

3. What is the implied main idea of paragraph 1?
   a. College students do not get enough sleep.
   b. College students don't spend enough time in the library.
   c. College students don't read their textbooks thoroughly.
   d. The library is a boring place to be.

4. Which of the following sentences begins with a transition?
   a. "'So many things are happening at once, in a really condensed period of time, once or twice I'll have to stay up all night,' explains Scott Kaplan, a senior political science major at the University of Pennsylvania." (paragraph 2)
   b. "Ideally, Fry says, students should be reviewing their notes on a weekly basis, but if that hasn't been the case and the semester is winding down, they should be choosy about what to study." (paragraph 7)
   c. "But being at a military academy means Babcock is at mandatory formation at 6:55 AM, and there is no wiggle room when it comes to sleeping or skipping classes." (paragraph 3)
   d. "To recall facts, Fry notes there are several memorization techniques." (paragraph 8)

5. Which of the following patterns organizes many of the details in paragraph 5?
   a. comparison/contrast   c. process
   b. cause/effect   d. series

6. What can you infer about the U.S. Military Academy from paragraph 3?
   a. The Academy has strict rules that students must follow or face punishment.
   b. Only men attend that school.
   c. It is located in a beautiful section of New York State.
   d. The students march a lot.

7. Which of the following sentences is an opinion?
   a. "Students, even the most prepared, sometimes have to cut back drastically on sleep to finish a term paper or cram for a final exam." (paragraph 2)
   b. "Ideally, Fry says, students should be reviewing their notes on a weekly basis, but if that hasn't been the case and the semester is winding down, they should be choosy about what to study." (paragraph 7)

c. "The library at the East Lansing, Michigan, school is open 24 hours every day but Saturday." (paragraph 1)

d. "But being at a military academy means Babcock is at mandatory formation at 6:55 AM, and there is no wiggle room when it comes to sleeping or skipping class." (paragraph 3)

8. The author's tone in this selection is

a. outraged.   c. serious.

b. depressed.   d. silly.

COMBINED SKILLS TEST 3

Read the textbook passage below and then answer the questions that follow by circling the letter of each correct response.

Gangs

1   They may wear special colors, be involved in violent initiations, band together to violently protect their turf from other gangs, and terrorize neighborhoods. Gangs are a major source of violence both in and out of school. In 1999, 26,000 gangs with a membership of about 840,500 members existed.

2   The composition of gangs fluctuates[1] substantially over the years. In the early twentieth century, youth gangs were predominantly Irish, Jewish, and Italian, but today they are more likely to be African American and Latino. In one major study, 31 percent of adolescents claiming to be gang members were African American; 25 percent, Latino; 25 percent, Caucasian; 5 percent, Asian American; and 15 percent, "others". Most gang members are male.

3   Historically, gangs took root in urban areas, especially where poverty flourished.[2] Today, although urban youth gangs are still prominent,[3] gang activity has grown in rural counties, small cities and towns, and the suburbs. The average age of a youth gang member is about 17 to 18 years. The typical age range is from 12 to 24 years.

4   Youth gangs are responsible for a great deal of the crime and violence in the community. They commit violent offenses at a rate several times higher than do nongang adolescents. Years ago, gangs considered schools as neutral territory, but recently gang activity in schools has increased. Schools with gang activity report more violence, gun possession, and drug sales, and their

1. **fluctuates:** goes up and down   3. **prominent:** noticeable
2. **flourished:** thrived

students are much more likely to report fear of being a crime victim. Some gang violence is related to drug sales, but gangs also use violence to settle disputes,[1] define their turf and protect their honor. Of the nearly 1,000 homicides in Chicago between 1987 and 1994 committed by gangs, three-quarters were between gangs, 11 percent were within a gang, and 14 percent involved nongang victims. Gang members use violence to demonstrate their toughness and gain status. The willingness to use violence is a key characteristic distinguishing youth gangs from other adolescent peer groups. Many gang members have access to guns, which is why gang violence has turned deadly.

5   Adolescents offer many reasons for joining gangs. Some gangs provide a family-like relationship that appeals to adolescents who are isolated, drifting between a native and adopted culture, and feeling somewhat alienated[2] from both. Gang membership enhances prestige[3] and status, provides a social agenda and excitement, and offers a chance to make money through illegal activities. Social, economic, and cultural forces may push people to join gangs. Some individuals even join to gain protection from the violence perpetrated[4] by other gangs. These teens feel marginalized;[5] they feel they do not belong in school or in their communities, and they may have family problems. They find their sense of identity in gang membership.

6   Long-term studies find that the most important community risk factor for gang membership is growing up in neighborhoods with low social integration and attachment. Family characteristics include poverty, parental absence, low parental attachment to the adolescent, and little parental supervision. Three school-related characteristics are very significant: Low expectations for success in school by both parents and adolescents, low student commitment to school, and low attachment to teachers. Peers naturally have a substantial impact, and associating with delinquent[6] friends and unsupervised hanging around are a potent combination leading to gang membership. Individual risk factors include low self-esteem, numerous negative life events, depressive symptoms, easy access to drugs, and favorable views of drug use. The greater the number of risk factors operating, the greater the chances a person will join a gang.

7   A number of programs attempt to reduce gang violence. Some involve the use of outreach workers and other professionals to provide services and opportunities for community-based activities. Outreach workers encourage youth to attend schools, obtain job training, seek regular employment, and use social services.

1. **disputes:** disagreements
2. **alienated:** isolated
3. **prestige:** respect or high status
4. **perpetrated:** committed
5. **marginalized:** confined to a lower level of society
6. **delinquent:** failing to obey laws

8   Preventing adolescents from joining gangs is a cost-effective long-term strategy. The Gang Resistance Education and Training (GREAT) Program, which is directed at third and fourth graders and seventh and eighth graders, has obtained positive results. The middle school program consists of eight lessons promoting cultural sensitivity, improving conflict resolution, meeting basic needs without joining a gang, and establishing short- and long-term goals. In a summer program, the youth participate in numerous recreational and community projects, including food programs and painting over graffiti. Students completing the program report lower levels of gang affiliation[1] and delinquency, including drug use, minor offenses, and both property crimes and crimes against persons. Other effective programs, such as the Comprehensive Community Wide Gang Prevention, Intervention and Suppression program, mobilize[2] the community and outreach workers to provide social outlets, better monitoring of gang activities, and social interventions.

9   Progress has been made in identifying the major risk factors involved in joining gangs, although reducing these factors is not easy. Some successful programs combine social intervention, rehabilitation, and suppression, but few have been rigorously[3] evaluated. Combating gang violence and delinquency, which have a tremendous effect on everyone within the community, requires the cooperation of police, social workers, and members of the community.*

1. Which of the following sentence(s) from paragraph 3 begins with a time order transition?

   a. sentence 1   c. sentences 1 and 2
   b. sentence 2   d. sentences 3 and 4

2. What can you infer about many gang members from the information provided in paragraph 4?

   a. Many will end up in jail.
   b. Many try to get educations but can't do so.
   c. Many relocate to other parts of the country.
   d. Many gang members have big cars.

3. Would you say that this selection is made up mostly of facts or opinions?

   a. mostly facts   b. mostly opinions

4. What is the purpose of this selection?

   a. to entertain   c. to persuade
   b. to inform

1. **affiliation:** association; membership   3. **rigorously:** thoroughly or precisely
2. **mobilize:** assemble or coordinate

* From Paul S. Kaplan, *Adolescence* (Boston: Houghton Mifflin Co., 2004), 524–525. Copyright © 2004. Reprinted by permission of Houghton Mifflin Company.

5. What pattern organizes the details in paragraph 5?

   a. time order   c. series
   (b.) cause/effect   d. definition

6. What is the topic of paragraph 4?

   (a.) gang crime and violence in communities
   b. statistics on gang members in schools
   c. gangs and drugs
   d. gang-related homicides

7. What is the topic sentence of paragraph 5?

   (a.) the first sentence
   b. the second sentence
   c. the last sentence
   d. the first and last sentences

8. What is the implied main idea of paragraph 6?

   a. The neighborhood is the most important risk factor for gang membership.
   (b.) There are a number of risk factors for gang membership.
   c. Most gang members have not done well in school.
   d. Gangs are a big problem in certain urban communities.

COMBINED SKILLS TEST 4

Read the passage below and then answer the questions that follow by circling the letter of each correct response.

The Classroom

1 The sun beamed in through the dining room window, lighting up the hardwood floor. We had been talking there for nearly two hours. The phone rang yet again and Morrie asked his helper, Connie, to get it. She had been jotting the callers' names in Morrie's small black appointment book. Friends. Meditation teachers. A discussion group. Someone who wanted to photograph him for a magazine. It was clear I was not the only one interested in visiting my old professor—the *Nightline* appearance (on which Morrie discussed his illness and his philosophy on life and death) had made him something of a celebrity—but I was impressed with, perhaps even a bit envious of, all the friends that Morrie seemed to have. I thought about the "buddies" that circled my orbit back in college. Where had they gone?

2   "You know, Mitch, now that I'm dying, I've become much more interesting to people."

3   You were always interesting.

4   "Ho." Morrie smiled. "You're kind."

5   No, I'm not, I thought.

6   "Here's the thing," he said. "People see me as a bridge. I'm not as alive as I used to be, but I'm not yet dead. I'm sort of . . . in-between."

7   He coughed, then regained his smile. "I'm on the last great journey here—and people want me to tell them what to pack."

8   The phone rang again.

9   "Morrie, can you talk?" Connie asked.

10   "I'm visiting with my old pal now," he announced. "Let them call back."

11   I cannot tell you why he received me so warmly. I was hardly the promising student who had left him sixteen years earlier. Had it not been for *Nightline*, Morrie might have died without ever seeing me again. I had no good excuse for this, except the one that everyone these days seems to have. I had become too wrapped up in the siren song[1] of my own life. I was busy.

12   *What happened to me?* I asked myself. Morrie's high, smoky voice took me back to my university years, when I thought rich people were evil, a shirt and tie were prison clothes, and life without freedom to get up and go—motorcycle beneath you, breeze in your face, down the streets of Paris, into the mountains of Tibet—was not a good life at all. *What happened to me?*

13   The eighties happened. The nineties happened. Death and sickness and getting fat and going bald happened. I traded a lot of dreams for a bigger paycheck, and I never even realized I was doing it.*

1. What can you infer about Morrie's illness from paragraphs 6 and 7?

   (a.) His illness is incurable.
   b. He developed his illness while traveling.
   c. He is dying of tuberculosis.
   d. His lifestyle contributed to his illness.

---

1. siren song: a reference to the Sirens of Greek mythology, whose sweet songs were so entrancing that sailors couldn't do anything but listen and then ran their ships upon the rocks

---

* From *Tuesdays with Morrie* by Mitch Albom, copyright © 1997 by Mitch Albom. Used by permission of Doubleday, a division of Random House, Inc.

2. Which of the following statements best states the implied main idea in paragraph 12?

    a. The author regrets not graduating from college.

    (b.) The author is startled by how much he has changed since his college days.

    c. The author's ideas about good and evil were just beginning to form during college.

    d. The author now regrets the judgmental attitudes he had while in college.

3. Which of the following is the topic sentence of paragraph 13?

    a. "The eighties happened."

    b. "The nineties happened."

    c. "Death and sickness and getting fat and going bald happened."

    (d.) "I traded a lot of dreams for a bigger paycheck, and I never even realized I was doing it."

4. What can you infer about the relationship between the author and Morrie from paragraphs 10 and 11?

    a. They were best friends in college.

    (b.) Morrie was a college professor, and the author was one of his students.

    c. They parted ways after a terrible argument.

    d. Morrie is the author's father.

5. Which of the following sentences states a fact?

    (a.) "We had been talking there for nearly two hours." (paragraph 1)

    b. "'You know, Mitch, now that I'm dying, I've become much more interesting to people.'" (paragraph 2)

    c. "You were always interesting." (paragraph 3)

    d. "I was hardly the promising student who had left him sixteen years earlier." (paragraph 11)

6. What can you infer about the author's feelings from paragraphs 12 and 13?

    a. He is devastated by the possibility of losing Morrie.

    b. He is furious at himself for not contacting Morrie sooner.

    (c.) He regrets changing his values in order to make more money.

    d. He feels confused and alone.

COMBINED SKILLS TEST 5

Read the textbook passage on the next page and then answer the questions that follow by circling the letter of each correct response.

The "Fourth Law of Motion": The Automobile Air Bag

1   A major automobile safety feature is the air bag. Seat belts restrain you so you don't follow along with Newton's first law of motion ("An object will remain at rest or in uniform motion in a straight line unless acted on by an external, unbalanced force") when the car comes to a sudden stop. But where does the air bag come in, and what is its principle?

2   When a car has a head-on collision with another vehicle or hits an immovable object such as a tree, it stops almost instantaneously. Even with seat belts, the impact of a head-on collision could be such that seat belts might not restrain you completely, and injuries could occur.

3   Enter the air bag. This balloon-like bag inflates automatically on hard impact and cushions the driver. Passenger-side air bags are becoming more common, and back-seat air bags are available.

4   The air bag tends to "cushion" or increase the contact time in stopping a person, thereby reducing the impact force (as compared to hitting the dashboard or steering column). Also, the impact force is spread over a large general area and not applied to certain parts of the body as in the case of seat belts.

5   Being inquisitive,[1] you might wonder what causes an air bag to inflate and what inflates it. Keep in mind that this must occur in a fraction of a second to do any good. (How much time would there be between the initial collision contact and a driver hitting the steering wheel column?) The air bag's inflation is initiated by an electronic sensing unit. This unit contains sensors that detect rapid decelerations,[2] such as those in a high-impact collision. The sensors have threshold settings so that normal hard braking does not activate them, and they are equipped with their own electrical power source because, in a front-end collision, a car's battery and alternator are among the first things to go.

6   Sensing an impact, a control unit sends an electric current to an igniter in the air bag system that sets off a chemical explosion. The gases (mostly nitrogen) rapidly inflate the thin nylon bag. The total process of sensing to complete inflation takes about 25 thousandths of a second (0.025/s). Pretty fast, and a good thing, too!

7   However, a recent concern about air bags is the injuries and deaths resulting from their deployment.[3] An air bag is not a soft, fluffy pillow. When activated, it comes out of the dashboard at speeds of up to 200 miles per hour and could hit a person close by with enough force to cause severe injury and even death. Therefore, adults are advised to sit at least ten inches from the air

1. **inquisitive:** curious; asking questions
2. **decelerations:** decreases in motion
3. **deployment:** use or action

bag cover. This allows a margin of safety from the two- to three-inch "risk zone." Seats should be adjusted to allow for the proper safety distance.

8   Probably a more serious concern is associated with children. Children may get close to the dashboard if they are not buckled in or not buckled in securely so that they can see. Another bad situation is using a rear-facing child seat in the front passenger seat. An inflating air bag could have serious effects.

9   Sometimes it may be impossible to follow these safety rules. So air bag deactivation[1] may be authorized for one of four reasons. A rear-facing child restraint might need to be placed in the front seat because the car either has no back seat or has one that is too small. A child 12 years old or younger might need to ride in the front seat because of a medical condition that requires frequent monitoring. An individual who drives (or rides in the front seat) might have a medical condition that would make it safer to have the air bags turned off. A driver might need to sit within a few inches of the air bag (typically because of extremely short stature, 4 feet 6 inches or less).

10   Specific problems may exist, but air bags save many lives. All new passenger cars must have dual air bags, and manufacturers are beginning to install air bags that inflate with less force, so as to reduce the possibility of injuries. Even if your car is equipped with air bags, however, always remember to buckle up. (Maybe we should make that Newton's "fourth law of motion.")*

1. Which of the following sentences best states the thesis of the whole selection?

    a. "However, a recent concern about air bags is the injuries and deaths resulting from their deployment." (paragraph 7)

    (b.) "Specific problems may exist, but air bags save many lives." (paragraph 10)

    c. "A major automobile safety feature is the air bag." (paragraph 1)

    d. "So air bag deactivation may be authorized for one of four reasons." (paragraph 9)

2. What pattern organizes most of the supporting details in paragraphs 5 and 6?

    a. comparison/contrast   (c.) time order

    b. series   d. definition

1. **deactivation:** to make inactive or ineffective

---

* Adapted from James T. Shipman et al., *An Introduction to Physical Science,* 9th ed. (Boston: Houghton Mifflin Co., 2000), 54–55.

3. What pattern organizes the supporting details in paragraph 2?

   a. comparison/contrast   c. time order
   (b.) cause/effect   d. series

4. Which sentence expresses the main idea in paragraph 8?

   (a.) "Probably a more serious concern is associated with children."
   b. "Children may get close to the dashboard if they are not buckled in or not buckled in securely so that they can see."
   c. "Another bad situation is using a rear-facing child seat in the front passenger seat."
   d. "An inflating air bag could have serious effects."

5. Is the opinion stated in paragraph 8 informed or uninformed?

   a. informed   (b.) uninformed

6. What is the implied main idea of paragraph 4?

   a. Seat belts aren't as effective as air bags.
   b. People should drive more carefully.
   c. Automobile manufacturers could make cars safer from impacts.
   (d.) Air bags protect people from injuries.

7. Which of the following sentences is NOT a *major* supporting detail in paragraph 9?

   (a.) "So air bag deactivation may be authorized for one of four reasons."
   b. "A rear-facing child restraint might need to be placed in the front seat because the car either has no back seat or has one that is too small."
   c. "A child 12 years old or younger might need to ride in the front seat because of a medical condition that requires frequent monitoring."
   d. "An individual who drives (or rides in the front seat) might have a medical condition that would make it safer to have the air bags turned off."

8. Which of the following inferences can you make based on the information in paragraph 3?

   a. New cars have too many airbags.
   b. Air bags are not easy to pop.
   (c.) Air bags installed in the front seat have proven to be effective.
   d. Auto manufacturers think drivers are more important than passengers.

Index